Handbook of Antimicrobial Resistance

Matthias Gotte
Editor-in-Chief

Albert Berghuis • Greg Matlashewski
Mark A. Wainberg • Donald Sheppard
Editors

Handbook of Antimicrobial Resistance

With 48 Figures and 24 Tables

Springer

Editor-in-Chief
Matthias Gotte
Department of Microbiology
and Immunology
McGill University
Montreal, QC, Canada

Department of Medical Microbiology
and Immunology
University of Alberta
Edmonton, AB, Canada

Editors
Albert Berghuis
Department of Microbiology
and Immunology
McGill University
Montreal, QC, Canada

Greg Matlashewski
Department of Microbiology
and Immunology
McGill University
Montreal, QC, Canada

Mark A. Wainberg
Department of Microbiology
and Immunology
McGill University
Montreal, QC, Canada

Donald Sheppard
Department of Microbiology
and Immunology
McGill University
Montreal, QC, Canada

ISBN 978-1-4939-0693-2 ISBN 978-1-4939-0694-9 (eBook)
ISBN 978-1-4939-0695-6 (print and electronic bundle)
DOI 10.1007/978-1-4939-0694-9

Library of Congress Control Number: 2016955954

Printed on acid-free paper

This Springer imprint is published by Springer Nature
The registered company is Springer Science+Business Media LLC
The registered company address is: 233 Spring Street, New York, NY 10013, U.S.A

In Memoriam

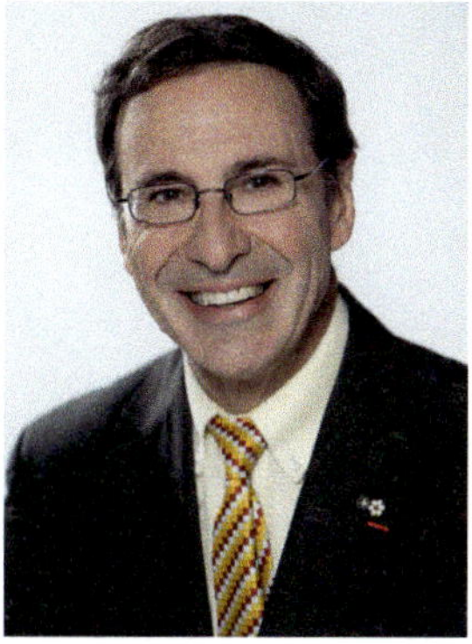

This *Handbook of Antimicrobial Resistance* was just finalized when we learned about the sudden and tragic passing of our dear friend and colleague Dr. Mark Wainberg. Mark was a professor at McGill University and the director of the McGill AIDS Centre at the Lady Davis Institute for Medical Research in Montreal.

His interests went beyond research and science, and he spoke loudly for those whose voices were too often not heard. He was well known for delivering talks and speeches with passion and conviction that were brilliant and injected with humor. Mark cared. He cared about people. He cared about significant problems and was always motivated to find solutions. It is therefore not surprising that he chose to work on HIV where he was among the true pioneers in the field. He was determined to help people living with HIV at so many levels. Mark was known for his contributions to the discovery of lamivudine, he was known for his tireless efforts to get life-saving antiretroviral drugs to those who were in desperate need, and he was known for his fight against stigmatization. Mark was a dedicated advocate and scientist in one person. His passion for the cause was unprecedented.

It is difficult to say whether Mark had a favorite research topic. The problem of resistance to antiviral drugs was certainly on top of the list. Mark and his team identified novel mutations that reduce drug susceptibility, he elucidated the underlying biochemical mechanisms, and he established resistance technologies, to name

The original version of this book was revised: 'In Memoriam' has been added to the book.

a few of his remarkable achievements. He immediately agreed to act as an editor and author of this handbook, and, as always, he delivered with passion. Mark will be missed by his loved ones, his friends, trainees, colleagues, and the many people whom he inspired.

Dr. Mark Wainberg died at the age of 71.

Matthias Gotte
Albert Berghuis
Greg Matlashewski
Donald Sheppard

Contents

Editorial Board

Contributors

Faiz Ahmad Khan Montreal Chest Institute, Montreal, QC, Canada

David Andes Department of Medicine, Department of Medical Microbiology and Immunology, University of Wisconsin, School of Medicine and Public Health, Madison, WI, USA

UW Medical Foundation Centennial Building, Madison, WI, USA

Nathan M. Beach Centro de Biología Molecular "Severo Ochoa" (CSIC-UAM), Consejo Superior de Investigaciones Científicas (CSIC), Madrid, Spain

Guy Boivin Research Center in Infectious Diseases, Laval University, Quebec City, QC, Canada

Paul S. Callaghan Department of Chemistry, Department of Biochemistry, Cellular and Molecular Biology, and Center for Infectious Disease, Georgetown University, Washington, DC, USA

Leah E. Cowen Department of Molecular Genetics, University of Toronto, Toronto, ON, Canada

Marsha Dillon-White Department of Microbiology, Icahn School of Medicine at Mount Sinai, New York, NY, USA

Esteban Domingo Centro de Biología Molecular "Severo Ochoa" (CSIC-UAM), Consejo Superior de Investigaciones Científicas (CSIC), Madrid, Spain

Centro de Investigación Biomédica en Red de Enfermedades Hepáticas y Digestivas (CIBERehd), Barcelona, Spain

Emilien Drouot Research Center in Infectious Diseases, Laval University, Quebec City, QC, Canada

Brooke D. Esquivel Division of Cell Biology and Biophysics, School of Biological Sciences, University of Missouri-Kansas City, Kansas City, MO, USA

Jed F. Fisher Department of Chemistry and Biochemistry, University of Notre Dame, Notre Dame, IN, USA

Greg Fox Woolcock Institute of Medical Research, The University of Sydney, Sydney, Australia

Lisa Frenkel Infectious Diseases/Departments of Pediatrics, Laboratory Medicine and Global Health, University of Washington and Seattle Children's Research Institute, Seattle, WA, USA

Axel Fun University of Cambridge, Cambridge, UK

Philippe Gallay Department of Immunology and Microbial Science, IMM-9, The Scripps Research Institute, La Jolla, CA, USA

Robert Grant Department of Medicine, University of California, San Francisco, CA, USA

Gladstone Institute of Virology and Immunology, San Francisco, CA, USA

San Francisco AIDS Foundation, San Francisco, CA, USA

Laura Marije Hofstra Department of Infection and Immunity, Luxembourg Institute of Health, Luxembourg, Luxembourg

Department of Medical Microbiology, University Medical Center Utrecht, Utrecht, The Netherlands

Jarrod W. Johnson Department of Chemistry and Biochemistry, University of Notre Dame, Notre Dame, IN, USA

Dustin T. King Department of Biochemistry and Molecular Biology and Center for Blood Research, University of British Columbia, Vancouver, BC, Canada

Victor G. Kramer Department of Experimental Medicine, McGill University, Montreal, QC, Canada

Danielle Légaré Centre de Recherche en Infectiologie du Centre de Recherche du CHU de Québec, Pavillon CHUL and Département de Microbiologie-Infectiologie et Immunologie, Faculté de Médecine, Université Laval, QC, Canada

Teri Liegler Department of Medicine, University of California, San Francisco, CA, USA

S. A. Locarnini Victorian Infectious Diseases Reference Laboratory, North Melbourne, VIC, Australia

Geoffrey McKay Department of Medicine, McGill University, Montreal, QC, Canada

Luis Menéndez-Arias Centro de Biología Molecular "Severo Ochoa" (CSIC-UAM), Consejo Superior de Investigaciones Científicas (CSIC), Madrid, Spain

Dick Menzies Respiratory Division, McGill University, Montreal, QC, Canada

Shahriar Mobashery Department of Chemistry and Biochemistry, University of Notre Dame, Notre Dame, IN, USA

Jeniel E. Nett Department of Medicine, Department of Medical Microbiology and Immunology, University of Wisconsin, School of Medicine and Public Health, Madison, WI, USA

Dao Nguyen Department of Medicine, McGill University, Montreal, QC, Canada

Research Institute of McGill University Health Centre, Montreal, QC, Canada

Monique Nijhuis Department of Medical Microbiology, Virology, University Medical Center Utrecht, Utrecht, The Netherlands

Scott Olson University of Washington, Seattle, WA, USA

Ana M. Ortega-Prieto Centro de Biología Molecular "Severo Ochoa" (CSIC-UAM), Consejo Superior de Investigaciones Científicas (CSIC), Madrid, Spain

Marc Ouellette Centre de Recherche en Infectiologie du Centre de Recherche du CHU de Québec, Pavillon CHUL and Département de Microbiologie-Infectiologie et Immunologie, Faculté de Médecine, Université Laval, QC, Canada

Ayşegül Özen Department of Biochemistry and Molecular Pharmacology, University of Massachusetts Medical School, Worcester, MA, USA

Celia Perales Centro de Biología Molecular "Severo Ochoa" (CSIC-UAM), Consejo Superior de Investigaciones Científicas (CSIC), Madrid, Spain

Centro de Investigación Biomédica en Red de Enfermedades Hepáticas y Digestivas (CIBERehd), Barcelona, Spain

David S. Perlin Department of Microbiology and Molecular Genetics, Public Health Research Institute, New Jersey Medical School, Rutgers, The State University of New Jersey, Newark, NJ, USA

Jocelyne Piret Research Center in Infectious Diseases, Laval University, Quebec City, QC, Canada

Paul D. Roepe Department of Chemistry, Department of Biochemistry, Cellular and Molecular Biology, and Center for Infectious Disease, Georgetown University, Washington, DC, USA

Christoph Sarrazin Medizinische Klinik 1, Universitätsklinikum, Frankfurt, Germany

Grant Schauer Department of Cell Biology, Rockefeller University, New York, NY, USA

Celia A. Schiffer Department of Biochemistry and Molecular Pharmacology, University of Massachusetts Medical School, Worcester, MA, USA

Jean-Claude Schmit Department of Infection and Immunity, Luxembourg Institute of Health, Luxembourg, Luxembourg

Seyedmojtaba Seyedmousavi Department of Medical Microbiology, Radboud University Medical Center, Nijmegen, The Netherlands

Department of Medical Microbiology and Infectious Diseases, Erasmus MC, Rotterdam, The Netherlands

Julie Sheldon Centro de Biología Molecular "Severo Ochoa" (CSIC-UAM), Consejo Superior de Investigaciones Científicas (CSIC), Madrid, Spain

Division of Experimental Virology, Twincore, Centre for Experimental and Clinical Infection Research, a joint venture between Medical School Hannover and Helmholtz Centre for Infection Research, Hannover, Germany

Viviana Simon Department of Microbiology, Icahn School of Medicine at Mount Sinai, New York, NY, USA

The Global Health and Emerging Pathogens Institute, Icahn School of Medicine at Mount Sinai, New York, NY, USA

Division of Infectious Diseases, Department of Medicine, Icahn School of Medicine at Mount Sinai, New York, NY, USA

Nicolas Sluis-Cremer Department of Medicine, Division of Infectious Diseases, University of Pittsburgh School of Medicine, Pittsburgh, PA, USA

Solmaz Sobhanifar Department of Biochemistry and Molecular Biology and Center for Blood Research, University of British Columbia, Vancouver, BC, Canada

Natalie C. J. Strynadka Department of Biochemistry and Molecular Biology and Center for Blood Research, University of British Columbia, Vancouver, BC, Canada

A. J. Thompson Department of Gastroenterology, St Vincent's Hospital Melbourne and The University of Melbourne, Fitzroy, VIC, Australia

Victorian Infectious Diseases Reference Laboratory, North Melbourne, VIC, Australia

Quy Ton University of Washington, Seattle, WA, USA

Johannes Vermehren Medizinische Klinik 1, Universitätsklinikum, Frankfurt, Germany

Paul E. Verweij Department of Medical Microbiology, Radboud University Medical Center, Nijmegen, The Netherlands

Mark A. Wainberg Department of Microbiology and Immunology, McGill University, Montreal, QC, Canada

Christoph Welsch Medizinische Klinik 1, Universitätsklinikum, Frankfurt, Germany

Annemarie M. J. Wensing Department of Medical Microbiology, University Medical Center Utrecht, Utrecht, The Netherlands

Theodore C. White Division of Cell Biology and Biophysics, School of Biological Sciences, University of Missouri-Kansas City, Kansas City, MO, USA

Martin Zavrel Institute of Organic Chemistry and Biochemistry, Prague 6, Czech Republic

Yanan Zhao Department of Microbiology and Molecular Genetics, Public Health Research Institute, New Jersey Medical School, Rutgers, The State University of New Jersey, Newark, NJ, USA

Part I

Virology

HBV Therapy and the Problem of Drug Resistance

A. J. Thompson and S. A. Locarnini

Contents

Abstract

The current goal of management for patients with chronic hepatitis B is to achieve sustained virological suppression. This has been shown to reduce the risk of liver disease progression, including cirrhosis, hepatic failure, and hepatocellular carcinoma. Nucleos(t)ide analogue monotherapy is commonly used as first-line therapy, and most patients will require long-term antiviral therapy. As for all

A.J. Thompson (✉)
Department of Gastroenterology, St Vincent's Hospital Melbourne and The University of Melbourne, Fitzroy, VIC, Australia

Victorian Infectious Diseases Reference Laboratory, North Melbourne, VIC, Australia
e-mail: alexander.thompson@svhm.org.au

S.A. Locarnini
Victorian Infectious Diseases Reference Laboratory, North Melbourne, VIC, Australia
e-mail: stephen.locarnini@mh.org.au

M. Gotte et al. (eds.), *Handbook of Antimicrobial Resistance*,
DOI 10.1007/978-1-4939-0694-9_4

direct-acting antiviral agents, the emergence of drug resistance is an important clinical concern. In this chapter, we discuss the principles of HBV antiviral resistance and clinical pathways for preventing the selection of drug-resistant variants, as well as appropriate management strategies for antiviral treatment failure.

Keywords
Hepatitis B • Tenofovir • Entecavir • Adefovir • Lamivudine • Telbivudine • Multidrug resistance • Hepatocellular cancer (HCC)

Introduction

More than 350 million individuals are chronically infected with hepatitis B virus (HBV). Chronic hepatitis B is associated with the long-term risk of progressive liver fibrosis and cirrhosis, liver failure, and hepatocellular carcinoma. CHB is a leading cause of human mortality, and more than 500,000 deaths are directly attributable to CHB annually (Lozano et al. 2012).

The risk of complications related to chronic HBV infection is linked to persistent high-level viral replication (Iloeje et al. 2006; Chen et al. 2006). Clinical guidelines therefore recommend antiviral therapy for patients with evidence of chronic hepatitis and HBV DNA levels >2,000 IU/mL (European Association for the Study of the Liver 2012; Lok and McMahon 2009; Liaw et al. 2012). The goal of therapy is to achieve sustained virological suppression (European Association for the Study of the Liver 2012; Lok and McMahon 2009; Liaw et al. 2012) which is associated with reduced risk of liver disease progression. Nucleos(t)ide analogue (NA) therapy is the treatment of choice for most patients, due to the limited efficacy and poor tolerability of peginterferon-α. Effective NA therapy for HBV is available, and five potent NAs have been approved for the treatment of CHB. Most patients will need long-term therapy to achieve sustained virological suppression, as the risk of virological relapse is high following cessation of NA. In this context, antiviral drug resistance is a critical determinant of long-term treatment success. Drug resistance is clinically important because virological breakthrough is associated with the loss of biochemical and eventually histological therapeutic gain. In the setting of advanced liver disease, virological breakthrough may lead to hepatitis flares, hepatic decompensation, and death (Liaw et al. 2004a, b).

Drug resistance can be prevented by selecting a potent NA with a high barrier to resistance as first-line therapy. The barrier to resistance is influenced by antiviral potency, genetic barrier, viral fitness, and treatment history (cross-resistance). The two first-line agents, tenofovir (TDF) and entecavir (ETV), are both high-barrier-to-resistance drugs. Second-line agents that continue to be used in resource-limited settings have lower barriers to resistance and include adefovir (ADV), telbivudine (LdT), and lamivudine (LMV). Once drug resistance occurs, it can be treated using salvage therapy with an agent that has a complementary cross-resistance profile, as will be discussed.

Understanding the basic principles of antiviral resistance is therefore important for planning appropriate selection of first-line and salvage NA therapies for CHB. In this chapter, we present an overview of the clinical aspects and molecular virology of HBV drug resistance, with a focus on prevention, early diagnosis, and rational management strategies.

Nucleos(t)ide Analogues Used to Treat HBV Infection

There are currently five drugs that belong to the class of nucleos(t)ide analogues (NAs) that have been approved for the treatment of CHB in most parts of the world (European Association for the Study of the Liver 2012). The NAs all directly inhibit the reverse transcriptase activity of the HBV polymerase (Pol). The approved NAs include lamivudine (LMV), a synthetic deoxycytidine analogue with an unnatural L-conformation, and the related L-nucleoside, telbivudine (LdT; β-L-thymidine). A second group, the acyclic phosphonates, includes adefovir dipivoxil (ADV), a prodrug for the acyclic 2′-deoxyadenosine monophosphate analog adefovir, and the structurally similar tenofovir (TFV). A third group of agents contains a D-cyclopentane sugar moiety linked to the base guanine and is the most potent anti-HBV drug discovered to date, entecavir (ETV) (Shaw and Locarnini 2004). This structural classification of the NA is useful clinically because it does help understand and classify the patterns and pathways of NA drug resistance (Table 1).

Antiviral Drug Resistance and HBV

Molecular Virology

The replication strategy of HBV involves two key steps. The major transcriptional template of the virus is the covalently closed circular (ccc)DNA minichromosome. This nuclear reservoir is inherently stable. The first step in the replication cycle is the transcription and nuclear export of pregenomic (pg)RNA to the cytoplasm. The pgRNA is the template for synthesis of the HBV polymerase (or reverse transcriptase, Pol) and the hepatitis B core proteins which form the nucleocapsid. Following its translation, the HBV Pol mediates reverse transcription of the same pgRNA transcript from which it was synthesized, a process which occurs inside the nascent nucleocapsid to form a replicating core complex (Harrison 2006). HBV replicates at an extremely high rate and the HBV Pol is inherently error-prone, resulting in a high nucleotide substitution rate and a population of viral variants or quasispecies capable of responding rapidly to endogenous (host immune response) or exogenous (antiviral therapy) selection pressures. This pool of quasispecies provides HBV with a survival advantage by generating a population of drug escape variants.

Antiviral drug-resistant variants are defined by a reduced susceptibility to the inhibitory effect of NA and emerge following the process of random mutation with adaptive selection under the pressure of antiviral therapy (Gish et al. 2012). Two types

Table 1 Patterns and pathways of antiviral drug resistance and cross-resistance in chronic hepatitis B

Pathway	HBV Pol / rt domains	LMV	LdT	ETV	ADV	TDV
Wildtype	A – B – C – D – E	S	S	S	S	S
L-nucleosides	M204V/I	R	R*	I	S	S
	A181T/V	R	R	S	R	I***
D-cyclopentanes	L180M, M204V/I; I169T, T184**, S202**, M250I/V	R	R	R	S	S
Acyclic phosphonates	N236T	S	S	S	R	I***
	A181T/V	R	R	S	R	I***
Multi-drug resistance^Φ	A181T/V, N236T, M250I/V	R	R	R	R	I***

* The main resistance substitution is the M204I
** T184 S/A/I/L/G/C/M, S202 C/G/I
*** Primary ADV resistance mutations have been associated with delayed kinetics of response to TDF in vivo [34]
Φ MDR has been associated with sequential monotherapy using drugs with overlapping resistance profiles

of mutations have been identified: primary resistance mutations, which are directly responsible for the associated drug resistance, and secondary or compensatory mutations. The latter occur in order to promote replication competence of resistance variants, because primary resistance mutations are typically associated with a reduction in replication fitness and competence. Compensatory mutations are important because they reduce the deleterious effects to the virus associated with acquisition of primary drug-resistant mutations (Domingo 2003) and allow the primary resistance mutations to be successfully archived in the intrahepatic cccDNA molecules.

Typically, the development of NA resistance depends on six factors: (1) magnitude and rate of virus replication, (2) fidelity of the viral polymerase, (3) selective pressure exerted by the NA (potency), (4) amount of available replication space in the liver (high ALT levels are associated with increased risk of resistance; high ALT levels are associated with hepatocyte proliferation creating replication space), (5) replication fitness of the emerging NA-resistant HBV, and (6) genetic barrier to resistance of the NA (Nafa et al. 2000; Yuen et al. 2001; Hadziyannis et al. 2006; Lai et al. 2007). Prior therapy with NAs also predicts for the development of drug resistance (Nafa et al. 2000; Yuen et al. 2001; Hadziyannis et al. 2006; Lai et al. 2007; Zoulim and Locarnini 2009).

Table 2 Definitions of antiviral resistance according to a recent expert consensus panel (REF)

Term	Definition
Primary nonresponse	Inability of nucleos(t)ide analogue (NA) treatment to reduce serum HBV DNA by ≥1 $\log_{10}$ IU/mL after the first 6 months of treatment
Partial response	Detectable HBV DNA using a real-time PCR assay during continuous therapy
	Note that the time point for the definition of partial response has not been well defined and will vary according to a drug's potency and genetic barrier to resistance (e.g., 24 weeks, LMV/LdT; 48 weeks, ADV; >48 weeks, ETV/TDF)
Virological breakthrough	Increase in serum HBV DNA by ≥1 $\log_{10}$ IU/mL above nadir on ≥2 occasions 1 month apart, in a treatment-compliant patient
Genotypic resistance	In the setting of antiviral therapy, the detection of viral populations bearing amino acid substitutions in the Pol/Rt region of the HBV genome that have been shown to confer resistance to antiviral drugs in phenotypic assays. These mutations are usually detected in patients with virological breakthrough, but they can also be present in patients with persistent viremia and no virological breakthrough
Phenotypic resistance	Decreased susceptibility of an HBV polymerase to an antiviral drug in vitro
Cross-resistance	Decreased susceptibility to more than one antiviral drug conferred by the same amino acid substitution or combination of amino acid substitutions

Clinical Definitions and Drug Resistance

Virological breakthrough is the consequence of the emergence of resistant variants and has defined as a >1 $\log_{10}$ (tenfold) increase in serum HBV DNA from nadir, in two consecutive samples taken 1 month apart, in a patient who had an initial virological response (Lok et al. 2007). Virological breakthrough is usually followed by biochemical breakthrough, with its associated risks of flare and decompensation. However, virological breakthrough may occur months and sometimes years before biochemical breakthrough; hence, early detection is possible prior to the development of clinical complications. This is particularly important in the setting of advanced liver disease. Standardized nomenclature for clinical, genotypic, and phenotypic resistance to NA therapy has been defined for CHB (Table 2).

NA and Treatment Failure

Lamivudine, LMV

Most of the literature describing the clinical consequences of resistance to NA in CHB has reported on the LMV experience. Lamivudine is a deoxycytidine analogue with an unnatural L-conformation (L-nucleoside). Lamivudine was the first NA approved and is regarded as a "first-generation" agent because of its low potency and low genetic barrier (Gish et al. 2012). The development of resistance begins with selection of mutations in the HBV Pol, followed by an increase in serum HBV DNA levels, and then, within weeks to months, a rise in serum alanine aminotransferase (ALT) levels and progression of liver disease (Nafa et al. 2000; Yuen et al. 2001; Lai et al. 2003). The risk of increased serum ALT in the setting of LMV resistance usually correlates with the duration of detectability of the resistant variant (Lok et al. 2003). These patients also have a significant risk of ALT flare and hepatic decompensation. The association between LMV resistance and progression of liver histology and then clinical deterioration was demonstrated by a placebo-controlled randomized clinical trial in patients with advanced fibrosis (Liaw et al. 2004a).

Lamivudine resistance is associated with amino acid substitutions in the tyrosine-methionine-aspartate-aspartate (YMDD) locus of the catalytic (C) domain of the HBV Pol (Table 1). Primary resistance mutations include the rtM204V/I. Although rtM204I can occur in isolation, rtM204V has been observed only in association with secondary compensatory mutations, most commonly the rtL180M (domain B). A second primary resistance mutation for LMV is the rtA181T/V. A number of other compensatory changes have been described in other domains of the HBV Pol, including the rtL80V/I (Ogata et al. 1999), trV173L (Delaney et al. 2003), and rtT184S (Bartholomeusz et al. 2005).

The frequency of LMV resistance increases progressively during treatment at rates of 14–32 % annually (Fig. 1), exceeding 70 % after 4 years of therapy

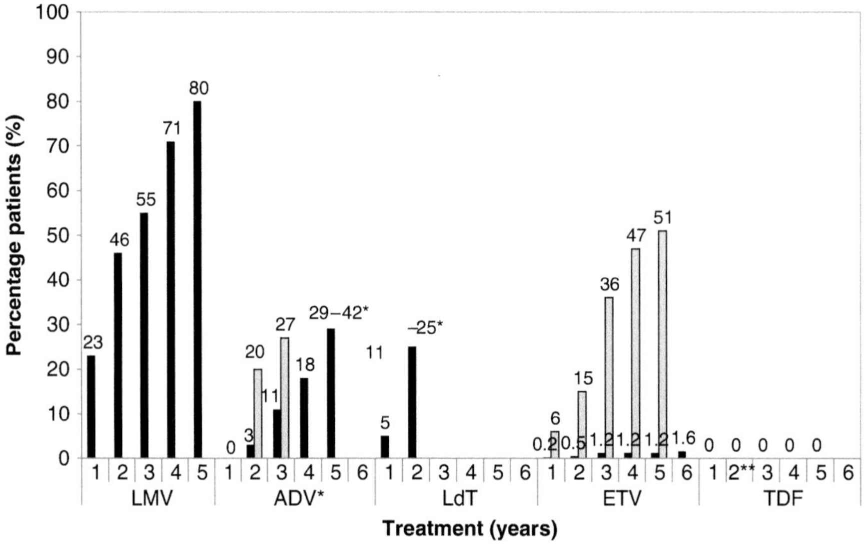

Fig. 1 Cumulative incidence of virological breakthrough due to the selection of resistant HBV variants. *Black columns* describe the prevalence of breakthrough in treatment-naïve patients. *Gray columns* describe the prevalence in lamivudine-experienced patients. *Rates in HBeAg-negative (*lower value*) and HBeAg-positive (*higher value*) patients, respectively. **For patients confirmed to be viremic at week 72+ in the registration studies, add-on emtricitabine was available at the clinician's discretion

(Lai et al. 2003). The rtM204V/I and rtA181T/V mutations both confer cross-resistance to the related L-nucleoside LdT and emtricitabine (FTC) (Table 1). The rtM204V/I does not confer cross-resistance to ADV or TDF, although the combination of M204V/I plus the L180M reduces susceptibility to ETV (Tenney et al. 2004). The rtA181T/V is also associated with resistance to ADV.

Adefovir, ADV

The kinetics of emergence of resistant variants to ADV are typically slower than was observed in the setting of LMV treatment (Fig. 1). In treatment-naïve patients, the prevalence of resistance is ~2 % at 2 years but rises progressively to 29 % after 5 years (Hadziyannis et al. 2006). Resistance to ADV emerges more rapidly in patients with prior LMV resistance (Fig. 1; Lee et al. 2006; Yeon et al. 2006; Fung et al. 2006). However, the same series of events occurs, with selection of genotypic resistant variants leading to sequential virological breakthrough, biochemical relapse/flare, and disease progression (Hadziyannis et al. 2006; Fung et al. 2005). Resistance to ADV has been associated with substitutions in the B domain (rtA181T/V) and/or the D (rtN236T) domain of HBV Pol (Angus et al. 2003; Villeneuve et al. 2003).

Only limited data are available on the clinical outcome of patients who are infected with ADV-, LdT-, ETV-, or TDF-resistant HBV, mainly because salvage treatment, usually based on in vitro cross-resistance data, has been initiated much earlier. The availability of antiviral drugs with complementary cross-resistance profiles (Table 1) has changed the management of patients with drug resistance, allowing physicians to prevent the worsening of clinical outcome resulting from the emergence of resistance.

Telbivudine, LdT

Telbivudine is cross-resistant with LMV, and the main resistance substitution is rtM204I (Table 1). Less common primary resistance mutations include the rtA181T/V and rtL229W/V. In the LdT registration studies, the prevalence of resistance to LdT increased from 4 % at 12 months to 30 % at 24 months of monotherapy (Fig. 1).

Entecavir, ETV

ETV has a high genetic barrier to resistance and requires the accumulation of multiple amino acid substitutions before drug sensitivity declines. Entecavir resistance requires the rtM204V/I plus L180M plus the selection of one of a number of signature ETV mutations: rtI169T, rtS184G, rtS202G/I, or rtM250V (Table 1). Primary resistance to ETV is uncommon in treatment-naïve individuals, being negligible in the first year and remaining low (approximately 1 %) even after 6 years of treatment (Fig. 1; Colonno et al. 2006; Tenney et al. 2009). Resistance was initially described in patients with a history of prior lamivudine resistance (Tenney et al. 2004), in whom it is far more common, reaching a prevalence of ~50 % after 4 years of treatment (Tenney et al. 2009). Entecavir is therefore not a suitable salvage therapy for patients with LMV resistance.

Tenofovir, TDF

Tenofovir disoproxil fumarate (TDF) is closely related to ADV and is also an acyclic phosphonate nucleotide analogue. Tenofovir is more potent than ADV and has a better toxicity profile, allowing higher standard dose (300 mg vs. 10 mg). To date, primary resistance mutations for TDF have not been identified. Tenofovir therefore also has a high genetic barrier to resistance. The primary resistance mutations for ADV, A181T/V and/or N236T, have been associated with small fold changes in sensitivity to TDF in vitro (<7-fold (Lok et al. 2007)). The clinical significance of this remains unclear. In three recent studies of TDF used for the treatment of patients failing ADV, continuous decline in HBV DNA was observed over time (Berg et al. 2010, 2014; Patterson et al. 2011). In one of the studies that recruited patients from the Asia-Pacific region, the presence of A181T/V and/or N236T substitutions at baseline was associated with delayed kinetics of viral decline. However, this was not seen in the European studies, where strong viral suppression was observed in the presence of preexisting LMV- or ADV-resistant mutations (Berg et al. 2010, 2014; van Bommel et al. 2010). No significant selection pressure on preexisting ADV- or LMV-resistant mutations was observed (Lavocat et al. 2013). There was no benefit of combination TDF plus FTC over TDF monotherapy following switch of therapy and no impact on long-term response (Berg et al. 2014). Further studies on whether ADV-associated substitutions reduce the antiviral response to TDF following switch of therapy are needed.

Pathways of Resistance

The primary resistance substitutions associated with drug failure for CHB are shown in Table 1. With the current five approved NAs, changes to eight codons in the HBV P ORF account for primary treatment failure. These eight substitutions can be understood based on NA chemistry and commit subsequent viral evolution to five different pathways:

- The L-nucleoside pathway (rtM204V/I). In this pathway, LMV and LdT treatment can select for rtM204V/I which predisposes to subsequent ETV resistance.
- The acyclic phosphonate pathway (rtN236T). ADV and TFV treatment can select for and/or consolidate rtN236T (van Bommel et al. 2010).
- Shared pathway (rtA181T/V). In this pathway, treatment with either L-nucleosides or acyclic phosphonates can select rtA181T/V, which occurs in about 40 % of cases of ADV failure but less than 5 % of cases of LMV failure. ADV and TFV treatment can consolidate rtA181T/V.
- The double pathway (rtA181T/V + rtN236T). In this pathway, treatment with TFV consolidates both of these variants, significantly blunting its antiviral efficacy (Patterson et al. 2011; van Bommel et al. 2010), resulting in persistent viremia (van Bommel et al. 2010).

- The D-cyclopentane-/ETV-naive resistance pathway (rtM204V/I ± rtL180M and one or more substitutions at rtI169, rtT184, rtS202, or rtM250). Three substitutions are required to be selected out on ETV, accounting for the very low resistance rates observed in NA-naïve patients (Fig. 1).
- Multidrug resistance (MDR) pathways. Monotherapy with low-potency and low-genetic-barrier NAs can promote selection for MDR strains of HBV. Multidrug-resistant HBV can also be selected out when patients are treated sequentially with drugs with overlapping resistance profiles, such as with LMV followed by ETV (Villet et al. 2007; Yim et al. 2006) or LMV followed by ADV (Liu et al. 2010; Villet et al. 2006; Brunelle et al. 2005) or ADV followed by TFV (Chang and Lai 2006; see Table 1).

Multidrug Resistance

Clonal analyses have shown that MDR usually occurs by the sequential acquisition of resistance mutations on the same viral genome; mutants that arise from this selection process may be fully resistant to multiple drugs. Studies have shown that MDR strains can arise if an "add-on" therapeutic strategy does not result in rapid viral suppression, particularly if there is sufficient replication space available for the mutants to spread (i.e., necro-inflammatory activity resulting in hepatocyte proliferation or liver graft not protected by HBIG because of the preexistence of escape mutants). These findings emphasize the need to achieve complete viral suppression during antiviral therapy: no replication (NR) = no resistance (NR). A specific single amino acid substitution may confer MDR (see Table 1). This was shown with the rtA181V/T substitutions, which are responsible not only for decreased susceptibility to the L-nucleosides LMV and LdT but also to the acyclic phosphonates ADV and TFV ((Warner and Locarnini 2008; Villet et al. 2008). This highlights the clinical usefulness of genotypic testing (drug resistance testing) in patients with treatment failure, as has been done for HIV therapy management (Clavel and Hance 2004), in order to determine the viral resistance mutation profile and thereby tailor therapy to the major viral circulating strain.

Management of Antiviral Resistance

Prevention

International guidelines recommend ETV and TDF as the best choice for first-line therapy (European Association for the Study of the Liver 2012; Lok and McMahon 2009; Liaw et al. 2012). These drugs are both potent and have a high genetic barrier to resistance. Lamivudine, LdT, and ADV should be considered as second-line choices. They will be continued to be used in resource-limited settings, however, as they are generally cheaper. It is important to emphasize the importance of compliance with patients. Patients should be tested for primary response, and we recommend testing for a reduction in HBV DNA >1 $\log_{10}$ IU/mL at 3 months (Table 2). It is then important to continue regular virological monitoring. We recommend repeating a serum HBV DNA level at 6 months in all patients. In patients taking ETV or TDF, we then monitor serum HBV DNA levels every 6 months.

In treatment-naïve patients for whom LMV, LdT, or ADV is used as first-line therapy, we recommend testing serum HBV DNA levels every 3 months, given the higher risk of virological resistance. This also allows treatment adjustment in the setting of suboptimal or partial response (Table 2). The hepatitis B "road map" concept has been proposed for resource-limited settings (Keeffe et al. 2007). The concept is based on data showing that patients with a profound and rapid virological response during treatment with LMV, LdT, or ADV have a lower risk of resistance than patients with a delayed virological response (Yuen et al. 2001; Zollner et al. 2001; Locarnini et al. 2005). Using this algorithm, patients who start treatment with a second-line agent are monitored for virological response at 3 and 6 months. In patients with a complete response at 6 months (undetectable serum HBV DNA), it is reasonable to continue therapy with virological monitoring every 3 months. In patients with an inadequate virological response (serum HBV DNA >2,000 IU/mL at 6 months), treatment should be intensified (e.g., L-nucleoside plus ADV) or switched to a first-line agent (ETV or TDF – TDF is most suitable for patients originally taking an L-nucleoside). In patients with a partial response (0 < serum HBV DNA <2,000 IU/mL), it is reasonable to maintain the original therapy until 48 weeks. If viremia persists at week 48, then add-on/switch treatment is appropriate because of the high risk of resistance with LMV, LdT, or ADV in the setting of persistent viremia.

In the setting of ETV or TDF therapy for treatment-naïve patients, the clinical significance of a partial virological response at week 24 or week 48 is less clear. Long-term follow-up studies have shown that resistance is very uncommon and that most patients will show continued virological decline. An emerging issue is persistent low-level viremia with HBV DNA levels $<10^{2-3}$ IU/mL. In per protocol analyses, up to 5 % of NA-naïve patients remain HBV DNA positive during long-term ETV or TDF therapy using sensitive real-time PCR assays (Snow-Lampart et al. 2011; Chang et al. 2010). HBV DNA sequencing is normally not possible given the low viral load, and virological rebound has not been reported to date in compliant patients. The long-term risk of selecting resistant variants is not known. In the setting of persistent viremia beyond week 96 of therapy with ETV or TDF, it seems reasonable to recommend treatment intensification with the add-on of another drug with no cross-resistance.

Combination therapy is required to prevent the selection of resistant variants in the setting of antiviral therapy for HIV or HCV. In the setting of HBV, combination of TDF plus ETV and TDF plus emtricitabine (FTC) has recently been shown to be associated with increased potency in patients with very high viral loads ($>10^8$ IU/mL) (Lok et al. 2012; Chan et al. 2013). However, combination therapy for HBV has not been proven to prevent resistance in treatment-naïve patients and cannot be recommended as a first-line strategy.

Table 3 Treatment strategies for antiviral drug resistance in chronic hepatitis B

Resistance	Management strategy	
LMV-R or LdT-R	Preferred option	Add-on or switch to TDF
	Alternate option (TDF not available)	Add-on ADV
ADV-R	Preferred option (NA naïve prior to ADV)	Switch to TDF plus LMV/FTC/LdT or switch to ETV
	Preferred option (prior LMV exposure)	Switch to TDF + LMV/FTC/LdT
	rtA181T/V identified	Switch to TDF + ETV
ETV-R	Preferred option	Add-on or switch to TDF
	Alternate option (TDF not available)	Add-on ADV
TDF-R[a]	Preferred option	Add-on ETV
	Alternate option (no history of LMV resistance)	Switch to ETV
Multidrug[b] **resistance**	Preferred option	ETV + TDF

[a]Note – primary resistance to TDF has not been confirmed to date and therefore there is no experience (genotypic analysis is recommended)
[b]A181T/V + N236T + M250I/V

Management of Treatment Failure

The most common cause of virological breakthrough remains poor compliance. Studies have shown that up to 40 % of patients taking long-term treatment for CHB may not be fully adherent (Pol and Sogni 2010). Therefore, assessment of treatment adherence is important in all patients who experience virological rebound. Patients must be educated about the importance of good compliance for maintaining maximal suppression of HBV DNA to reduce the risk of the selection of resistant variants.

Virological breakthrough in compliant patients occurs secondary to the emergence of resistant variants and necessitates salvage therapy. The choice of salvage therapy should be based on the knowledge of cross-resistance, so that the second agent has a resistance profile that differs from the failing drug (Table 1). This is particularly important as drug-resistant variants are thought to be archived in viral cccDNA reservoirs in the liver (Zhou et al. 1999). We recommend HBV Pol sequencing to define the resistance mutation associated with virological breakthrough and guide subsequent treatment. A guide to appropriate rescue therapies is presented in Table 3. There is a theoretical advantage to using add-on combination therapy, to raise the barrier of resistance and increase potency, making the subsequent development of drug resistance less likely.

Consequences of the Pol-HBsAg Overlap

The hepatitis B virus has a unique genome with overlapping reading frames. Two potentially important consequences emerge from the fact that almost every drug-resistant HBV has an associated change in its envelope (HBsAg), due to the overlapping nature of the HBV Pol and HBV S open reading frames.

Public Health Potential

The major public health issue related to the alteration in HBsAg antigenicity (Locarnini 1998) is the transmission of drug-resistant HBV (Kamili et al. 2009; Thibault et al. 2002) and therefore the possibility that these drug-resistant HBVs could represent a threat to the various immunization programs designed to control hepatitis B (Clements et al. 2010). These viruses have been termed antiviral drug-associated potential vaccine-escape mutants (ADAPVEMs) (Kamili et al. 2009).

The S protein of HBV, which is the main component of the envelope of the virion, carries the major target of the neutralizing antibody, the "a" determinant, and, on the genome, directly overlaps the catalytic domain of the Pol. Resistance mutations in the Pol usually result in non-synonymous changes in the S of HBsAg (Bartholomew et al. 1997; Ogura et al. 1999; Shields et al. 1999; Tipples et al. 1996), and the first study to demonstrate that these substitutions might affect HBsAg protein conformation, and more importantly its antigenicity, was carried out by Torresi et al. (2002a). These investigators showed that the common lamivudine (LMV)-resistant substitutions (rtM204V/sI195M, rtM204I/sW196S, rtM204I/sW196L, and rtV173L/sE164D plus rtL180M plus rtM204V/sI195M) resulted in reductions in the reactivity of the altered HBsAg with vaccine-induced antibody against HBsAg (anti-HBs). In addition, the converse has been shown in that changes in the S gene introduce changes in Pol that correspond with LMV-resistant compensatory-type mutations (Torresi et al. 2002b). These studies have now been independently confirmed using different in vitro models, including mammalian cell culture transfection and epitope "density" mapping (Sloan et al. 2008). The key findings are summarized in Fig. 2.

The true public health potential of these ADAPVEMs was realized when the common LMV-resistant mutation, rtV173L plus rtL180M plus rtM204V (Delaney et al. 2003), which displays the sE164D plus sI195M change in HBsAg, successfully infected hepatitis B-immunized chimpanzees that carried high titers of circulating anti-HBs pre-challenge (Kamili et al. 2009). This study also established the genetic stability of the drug-resistant ADAPVEM rtV173L plus rtL180M plus rtM204V variant in a non-immunized chimpanzee, in whom no revertants to wild type (WT) were detected over at least 6 months to a year compared with infection with the sG145R canonical vaccine-escape mutant, which quickly back-reverted to WT (Kamili et al. 2009). This latter observation reveals the important role of compensatory mutations such as rtV173L and rtL180M in "fixing the genetic archive," especially in the setting of transmission of NA resistance.

An important question is whether the emergence of ADAPVEMs poses a threat to the global hepatitis B immunization program. For a new viral species to pose a threat

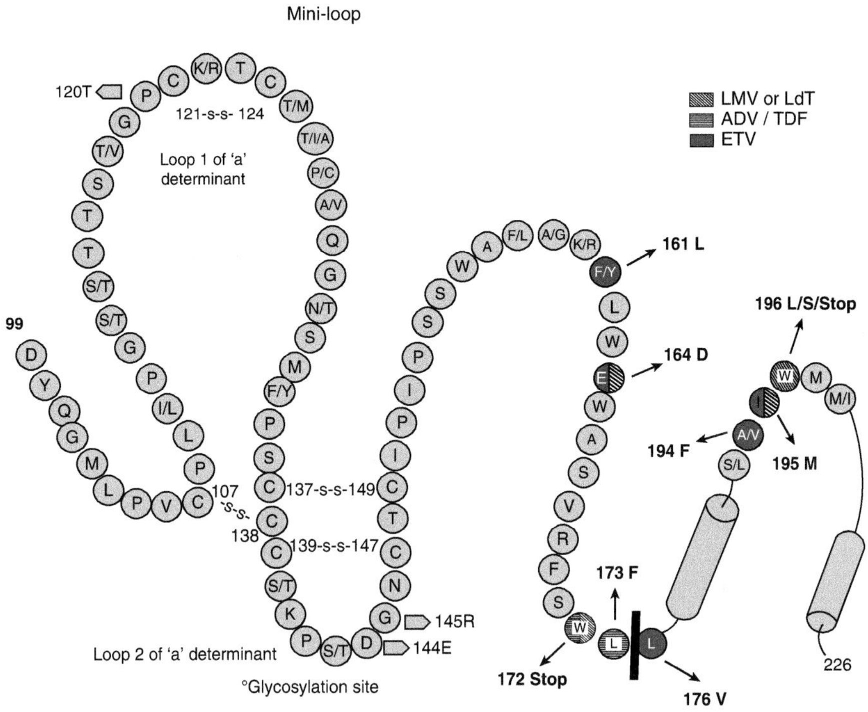

Fig. 2 The "a" determinant of HBsAg, highlighting the amino acid substitutions that have been associated with NA drug resistance due to the overlap between HBV Pol and S open reading frames

in this setting, Clements et al. have suggested that an ADAPVEM would need to possess at least four characteristics (Clements et al. 2010):

1. It needs to be a stable mutant.
2. It must have undergone sufficient changes in antigenicity such that anti-HBs generated by the current vaccine no longer neutralizes it.
3. It must be transmissible and cause infection in immunized individuals and so have the opportunity for ongoing spread.
4. It must cause disease (acute or chronic) in infected individuals.

From the studies reviewed to date, the first three have been achieved; it is not known if ADAPVEMs have the same propensity to cause disease as do current circulating strains of HBV (Clements et al. 2010), although one case of primary infection with a 3TC-resistant HBV was associated with acute hepatitis (Thibault et al. 2002). Clearly, further studies are needed to fully elucidate the clinical, pathological, and epidemiological significance of these emerging ADAPVEMs.

Molecular Pathogenesis and Oncogenic Potential

Several HBV proteins are involved in the development of HCC, transcribed from either integrated HBV DNA or the HBV genome. For example, truncated HBV surface proteins have been linked to the progression to HCC since they possess intrinsic transactivational activity, revealed by increased nuclear factor κB or activator protein 1 promoter activity (Schluter et al. 1994). It is known that NA therapy selects for point mutations in Pol that not only confer NA resistance but also result in truncated surface proteins and therefore could theoretically accelerate the progression to HCC (Lai et al. 2009; Lai and Yeh 2008; Warner and Locarnini 2008; Locarnini 1998). In particular, the point mutation that causes the rtA181T change in HBV Pol also encodes a stop codon (sW172*) in the overlapping surface proteins (Fig. 2), resulting in truncation of the last 55 amino acids of the C-terminal hydrophilic region of the HBsAg. The LMV-/LdT-resistant variant rtM204I/sW196* is another example. An extensive analysis of rtA181T/sW172* HBV in vitro has shown that it is defective in secretion of viral particles resulting in intracellular retention of surface proteins that have a dominant negative effect on WT virion secretion (Warner and Locarnini 2008). This can result in the observation of lower viral loads extracellularly and is what is often observed with the emergence of adefovir resistance (Warner and Locarnini 2008; Zoulim and Locarnini 2012). Two recent reports have now provided evidence for the involvement of HBV encoding the rtA181T/sW172* mutation in the pathogenesis of and progression to HCC (Lai et al. 2009; Lai and Yeh 2008). Analyses of HBV DNA from patients who developed HCC despite LMV therapy revealed stop codon mutations in the envelope gene in seven of eight patients compared with the control group, in which no patients developed HCC. Using expression constructs encoding the HBV surface proteins, these investigators demonstrated that surface proteins truncated at amino acids sL21, sW196, or sW172 (the last of which corresponds to the surface proteins expressed from rtA181T/sW172*) transactivated the c-myc and SV40 promoters. NIH-3T3 cells transfected with these constructs were also tumorigenic when injected into nude mice, whereas the WT full-length surface proteins were not (Warner and Locarnini 2008; Lai et al. 2009). Another common LMV/LdT resistance substitution is rtM204I/sW196* stop (Fig. 2), which is observed in up to 10 % of LMV-resistant patients and more commonly with LdT (Warner and Locarnini 2008; Yuen et al. 2007). To date, there has been no report available concerning its effects on viral replication or hepatocyte biology.

Although NA therapies significantly decrease viral load and improve patient survival in the short term (Liaw et al. 2004a) and have been shown to reduce the HCC risk by 50 % (REF), it appears that they might unexpectedly select for HBV variants that are potentially oncogenic, providing one possible mechanism for the observation that the incidence of HCC is increasing globally.

Conclusion

Current treatment for most patients with CHB involves long-term NA therapy. Antiviral drug resistance is a key factor determining the long-term outcomes. The likelihood of resistance is determined by a combination of genetic barrier, drug potency, patient adherence, treatment history, and cross-resistance. Drugs such as ETV and TDF are associated with very low rates of virological breakthrough and should be the choice for first-line therapy. Management of treatment failure requires close clinical and virological monitoring, as well as early treatment intervention with salvage antivirals according to cross-resistance profiles. Future challenges in the treatment of CHB include the development of treatment strategies that effectively inhibit HBV replication eliminating the risk of drug resistance, potentially through novel host-targeting mechanisms, as well as the development of antiviral therapies that do not select for potentially oncogenic drug-resistant HBV.

References

Angus P et al (2003) Resistance to adefovir dipivoxil therapy associated with the selection of a novel mutation in the HBV polymerase. Gastroenterology 125(2):292–297

Bartholomeusz A et al (2005) Mechanistic basis for HBV resistance to acyclic nucleoside phosphonate analogues, adefovir and tenofovir. Hepatology 42:594A

Bartholomew MM et al (1997) Hepatitis-B-virus resistance to lamivudine given for recurrent infection after orthotopic liver transplantation. Lancet 349(9044):20–22

Berg T et al (2010) Tenofovir is effective alone or with emtricitabine in adefovir-treated patients with chronic-hepatitis B virus infection. Gastroenterology 139(4):1207–1217

Berg T et al. (2014) Long-term efficacy and safety of emtricitabine plus tenofovir DF vs. tenofovir DF monotherapy in adefovir-experienced chronic hepatitis B patients. J Hepatol. 60(4):715–22

Brunelle MN et al (2005) Susceptibility to antivirals of a human HBV strain with mutations conferring resistance to both lamivudine and adefovir. Hepatology 41(6):1391–1398

Chan HL et al (2013) Tenofovir df (tdf) compared to emtricitabine (ftc)/tdf in hbeag-positive, chronic hepatitis b (chb) virusinfected patients in the immune tolerant (it) phase. J Hepatol Vol 52 (Suppl 1): S45 (A101)

Chang TT, Lai CL (2006) Hepatitis B virus with primary resistance to adefovir. N Engl J Med 355:322–323; author reply 323

Chang TT et al (2010) Long-term entecavir therapy results in the reversal of fibrosis/cirrhosis and continued histological improvement in patients with chronic hepatitis B. Hepatology 52(3):886–893

Chen CJ et al (2006) Risk of hepatocellular carcinoma across a biological gradient of serum hepatitis B virus DNA level. JAMA 295(1):65–73

Clavel F, Hance AJ (2004) HIV drug resistance. N Engl J Med 350(10):1023–1035

Clements CJ et al (2010) Global control of hepatitis B virus: does treatment-induced antigenic change affect immunization? Bull World Health Organ 88(1):66–73

Colonno RJ et al (2006) Entecavir resistance is rare in nucleoside naive patients with hepatitis B. Hepatology 44(6):1656–1665

Delaney WE et al (2003) The hepatitis B virus polymerase mutation rtV173L is selected during lamivudine therapy and enhances viral replication in vitro. J Virol 77(21):11833–11841

Domingo E (2003) Quasispecies and the development of new antiviral strategies. Prog Drug Res 60:133–158
European Association for the Study of the Liver (2012) EASL clinical practice guidelines: management of chronic hepatitis B virus infection. J Hepatol 57(1):167–185
Fung SK et al (2005) Adefovir-resistant hepatitis B can be associated with viral rebound and hepatic decompensation. J Hepatol 43(6):937–943
Fung SK et al (2006) Virologic response and resistance to adefovir in patients with chronic hepatitis B. J Hepatol 44(2):283–290
Gish R et al (2012) Selection of chronic hepatitis B therapy with high barrier to resistance. Lancet Infect Dis 12(4):341–353
Hadziyannis SJ et al (2006) Long-term therapy with adefovir dipivoxil for HBeAg-negative chronic hepatitis B for up to 5 years. Gastroenterology 131(6):1743–1751
Harrison TJ (2006) Hepatitis B virus: molecular virology and common mutants. Semin Liver Dis 26(2):87–96
Iloeje UH et al (2006) Predicting cirrhosis risk based on the level of circulating hepatitis B viral load. Gastroenterology 130(3):678–686
Kamili S et al (2009) Efficacy of hepatitis B vaccine against antiviral drug-resistant hepatitis B virus mutants in the chimpanzee model. Hepatology 49(5):1483–1491
Keeffe EB et al (2007) Report of an international workshop: roadmap for management of patients receiving oral therapy for chronic hepatitis B. Clin Gastroenterol Hepatol 5(8):890–897
Lai MW, Yeh CT (2008) The oncogenic potential of hepatitis B virus rtA181T/ surface truncation mutant. Antivir Ther 13(7):875–879
Lai CL et al (2003) Prevalence and clinical correlates of YMDD variants during lamivudine therapy for patients with chronic hepatitis B. Clin Infect Dis 36(6):687–696
Lai CL et al (2007) Telbivudine versus lamivudine in patients with chronic hepatitis B. N Engl J Med 357(25):2576–2588
Lai MW et al (2009) Identification of nonsense mutations in hepatitis B virus S gene in patients with hepatocellular carcinoma developed after lamivudine therapy. Antivir Ther 14(2):249–261
Lavocat F et al (2013) Similar evolution of hepatitis B virus quasispecies in patients with incomplete adefovir response receiving tenofovir/emtricitabine combination or tenofovir monotherapy. J Hepatol 59(4):684–695
Lee YS et al (2006) Increased risk of adefovir resistance in patients with lamivudine-resistant chronic hepatitis B after 48 weeks of adefovir dipivoxil monotherapy. Hepatology 43 (6):1385–1391
Liaw YF et al (2004a) Lamivudine for patients with chronic hepatitis B and advanced liver disease. N Engl J Med 351(15):1521–1531
Liaw YF, Chien RN, Yeh CT (2004b) No benefit to continue lamivudine therapy after emergence of YMDD mutations. Antivir Ther 9(2):257–262
Liaw Y-F et al (2012) Asian-Pacific consensus statement on the management of chronic hepatitis B: a 2012 update. Hepatol Int 6:531–561
Liu Y et al (2010) Evolution and suppression of HBV strains with multidrug resistance to lamivudine, adefovir dipivoxil and entecavir in a patient with chronic hepatitis B. Antivir Ther 15(8):1185–1190
Locarnini SA (1998) Hepatitis B virus surface antigen and polymerase gene variants: potential virological and clinical significance. Hepatology 27(1):294–297
Locarnini S, Qi X, Arterturn S (2005) Incidence and predictors of emergence of adefovir resistant HBV during 4 years of adefovir dipivoxil therapy for patients with chronic hepatitis B. J Hepatol 42(Suppl 1):754A
Lok AS, McMahon BJ (2009) Chronic hepatitis B: update 2009. Hepatology 50(3):661–662
Lok AS et al (2003) Long-term safety of lamivudine treatment in patients with chronic hepatitis B. Gastroenterology 125(6):1714–1722
Lok AS et al (2007) Antiviral drug-resistant HBV: standardization of nomenclature and assays and recommendations for management. Hepatology 46(1):254–265

Lok AS et al (2012) Efficacy of entecavir with or without tenofovir disoproxil fumarate for nucleos (t)ide-naive patients with chronic hepatitis B. Gastroenterology 143(3):619–628.e1

Lozano R et al (2012) Global and regional mortality from 235 causes of death for 20 age groups in 1990 and 2010: a systematic analysis for the Global Burden of Disease Study 2010. Lancet 380(9859):2095–2128

Nafa S et al (2000) Early detection of viral resistance by determination of hepatitis B virus polymerase mutations in patients treated by lamivudine for chronic hepatitis B. Hepatology 32(5):1078–1088

Ogata N et al (1999) Novel patterns of amino acid mutations in the hepatitis B virus polymerase in association with resistance to lamivudine therapy in Japanese patients with chronic hepatitis B. J Med Virol 59(3):270–276

Ogura Y et al (1999) Prevalence and significance of naturally occurring mutations in the surface and polymerase genes of hepatitis B virus. J Infect Dis 180(5):1444–1451

Patterson SJ et al (2011) Tenofovir disoproxil fumarate rescue therapy following failure of both lamivudine and adefovir dipivoxil in chronic hepatitis B. Gut 60(2):247–254

Pol S, Sogni P (2010) Treatment of chronic hepatitis B: adherence and safety. Gastroenterol Clin Biol 34(Suppl 2):S142–S148

Schluter V et al (1994) Integrated hepatitis B virus X and 3′ truncated preS/S sequences derived from human hepatomas encode functionally active transactivators. Oncogene 9(11):3335–3344

Shaw T, Locarnini S (2004) Entecavir for the treatment of chronic hepatitis B. Expert Rev Anti Infect Ther 2(6):853–871

Shields PL et al (1999) Selection of hepatitis B surface "escape" mutants during passive immune prophylaxis following liver transplantation: potential impact of genetic changes on polymerase protein function. Gut 45(2):306–309

Sloan RD et al (2008) Antiviral resistance mutations potentiate hepatitis B virus immune evasion through disruption of its surface antigen a determinant. Antivir Ther 13(3):439–447

Snow-Lampart A et al (2011) No resistance to tenofovir disoproxil fumarate detected after up to 144 weeks of therapy in patients monoinfected with chronic hepatitis B virus. Hepatology 53(3):763–773

Tenney DJ et al (2004) Clinical emergence of entecavir-resistant hepatitis B virus requires additional substitutions in virus already resistant to Lamivudine. Antimicrob Agents Chemother 48(9):3498–3507

Tenney DJ et al (2009) Long-term monitoring shows hepatitis B virus resistance to entecavir in nucleoside-naive patients is rare through 5 years of therapy. Hepatology 49(5):1503–1514

Thibault V et al (2002) Primary infection with a lamivudine-resistant hepatitis B virus. AIDS 16(1):131–133

Tipples GA et al (1996) Mutation in HBV RNA-dependent DNA polymerase confers resistance to lamivudine in vivo. Hepatology 24(3):714–717

Torresi J et al (2002a) Reduced antigenicity of the hepatitis B virus HBsAg protein arising as a consequence of sequence changes in the overlapping polymerase gene that are selected by lamivudine therapy. Virology 293(2):305–313

Torresi J et al (2002b) Restoration of replication phenotype of lamivudine-resistant hepatitis B virus mutants by compensatory changes in the "fingers" subdomain of the viral polymerase selected as a consequence of mutations in the overlapping S gene. Virology 299(1):88–99

van Bommel F et al (2010) Long-term efficacy of tenofovir monotherapy for hepatitis B virus-monoinfected patients after failure of nucleoside/nucleotide analogues. Hepatology 51(1):73–80

Villeneuve JP et al (2003) Selection of a hepatitis B virus strain resistant to adefovir in a liver transplantation patient. J Hepatol 39(6):1085–1089

Villet S et al (2006) Selection of a multiple drug-resistant hepatitis B virus strain in a liver-transplanted patient. Gastroenterology 131(4):1253–1261

Villet S et al (2007) Stepwise process for the development of entecavir resistance in a chronic hepatitis B virus infected patient. J Hepatol 46(3):531–538

Villet S et al (2008) Impact of hepatitis B virus rtA181V/T mutants on hepatitis B treatment failure. J Hepatol 48(5):747–755
Warner N, Locarnini S (2008) The antiviral drug selected hepatitis B virus rtA181T/sW172* mutant has a dominant negative secretion defect and alters the typical profile of viral rebound. Hepatology 48(1):88–98
Yeon JE et al (2006) Resistance to adefovir dipivoxil in lamivudine resistant chronic hepatitis B patients treated with adefovir dipivoxil. Gut 55(10):1488–1495
Yim HJ et al (2006) Evolution of multi-drug resistant hepatitis B virus during sequential therapy. Hepatology 44(3):703–712
Yuen MF et al (2001) Factors associated with hepatitis B virus DNA breakthrough in patients receiving prolonged lamivudine therapy. Hepatology 34(4 Pt 1):785–791
Yuen LK et al (2007) SeqHepB: a sequence analysis program and relational database system for chronic hepatitis B. Antiviral Res 75(1):64–74
Zhou T et al (1999) Emergence of drug-resistant populations of woodchuck hepatitis virus in woodchucks treated with the antiviral nucleoside lamivudine. Antimicrob Agents Chemother 43(8):1947–1954
Zollner B et al (2001) Correlation of hepatitis B virus load with loss of e antigen and emerging drug-resistant variants during lamivudine therapy. J Med Virol 65(4):659–663
Zoulim F, Locarnini S (2009) Hepatitis B virus resistance to nucleos(t)ide analogues. Gastroenterology 137(5):1593–1608.e1-2
Zoulim F, Locarnini S (2012) Management of treatment failure in chronic hepatitis B. J Hepatol 56 (Suppl 1):S112–S122

Protease Inhibitor Resistance

Johannes Vermehren, Christoph Welsch, and Christoph Sarrazin

Contents

Abstract

The recent development of hepatitis C virus (HCV)–specific direct-acting antivirals (DAAs) has marked a major milestone in the treatment of chronic HCV infection, allowing for viral elimination in the majority of treated patients. The first two drugs to be approved for the treatment of HCV genotype 1 infection were the HCV NS3/4A protease inhibitors telaprevir and boceprevir. However, their administration in combination with pegylated interferon alfa and ribavirin was associated with poor tolerability despite showing improved overall efficacy. In

J. Vermehren (✉) • C. Welsch • C. Sarrazin
Medizinische Klinik 1, Universitätsklinikum, Frankfurt, Germany
e-mail: johannes.vermehren@kgu.de; christoph.welsch@kgu.de; sarrazin@em.uni-frankfurt.de

M. Gotte et al. (eds.), *Handbook of Antimicrobial Resistance*,
DOI 10.1007/978-1-4939-0694-9_6

addition, as in DAAs targeting other viruses, concerns were raised with regard to the selection of drug-resistant viral variants. Selection of resistance-associated variants (RAVs) allows the virus to escape from drug pressure with subsequent treatment failure. The emergence of RAVs depends on a number of drug-, host-, and virus-related factors that are reviewed here. In addition, detailed resistance profiles of approved protease inhibitors and those that are still in clinical development are also discussed.

Keywords
Hepatitis C virus • Protease inhibitor • Ribavirin • Pegylated interferon alfa • Resistance • Resistance associated variant • NS3-4A • Telaprevir • Boceprevir • Simeprevir • Paritaprevir

Introduction

For the past decade, treatment of chronic hepatitis C infection was confined to pegylated interferon alfa (PEG-IFN) and ribavirin (RBV), both of which do not directly target viral proteins. Overall, rates of viral eradication have been poor, ranging from 20 % to 80 %, depending on the disease stage, viral genotype, and polymorphisms within the host interleukin 28B gene locus (Fried et al. 2002; Lange and Zeuzem 2011; Manns et al. 2001). Achievement of a sustained virologic response (SVR) defined as HCV-RNA negativity 12 or 24 weeks after treatment cessation has been particularly difficult in patients with HCV genotype 1 which constitutes the most prevalent genotype in Europe and North America, with SVR rates in the range of 40–50 % only (Fried et al. 2002; Manns et al. 2001).

Improved knowledge of the viral life cycle that followed the development of several different cell-based culture systems as well as experimental structure models of viral proteins led to the development of small molecules that directly target the viral replication machinery (Lohmann et al. 1999). The proof of principle for these direct-acting antivirals (DAAs) was established in 2003 with the development of ciluprevir, a small molecule inhibitor of the NS3-4A serine protease that led to a significant reduction of HCV-RNA (Lamarre et al. 2003). The further development of ciluprevir, however, was halted due to animal toxicity issues (Hinrichsen et al. 2004). Therefore, it was another 8 years until regulatory approval of the first two HCV NS3-4A protease inhibitors telaprevir and boceprevir for the treatment of chronic HCV genotype 1 infection in 2011. Each of these protease inhibitors (PI) are administered in combination with pegylated interferon alfa (PEG-IFN) and ribavirin (RBV), and the respective pivotal trials have demonstrated increased cure rates by 20–30 % when compared to PEG-IFN-based dual combination therapies as well as shortened treatment duration for the majority of patients that were treatment-naïve or previous relapsers (Bacon et al. 2011; Jacobson et al. 2011; Poordad et al. 2011; Sherman et al. 2011a; Zeuzem et al. 2011). However, in the wake of the first experiments with PIs administered as monotherapy, concerns were raised regarding the development of drug resistance–associated amino acid variants (RAVs).

These concerns were based on the knowledge of the high replication rate of HCV along with the lack of proofreading activity that leads to a genetically diverse population of viral variants within an infected patient, the so-called quasispecies. The quasispecies population contains both wildtype (WT) viruses and and viral variants with every possible single- and double-nucleotide variant and subsequently every RAV generated several times each day, according to mathematical modeling (Rong et al. 2010). RAVs within the NS3-4A protease domain are often less fit in terms of replication capacity and/or virus production (Shimakami et al. 2011; Welsch et al. 2012a) and are therefore usually present in much smaller numbers within the quasispecies population compared to WT variants. However, in the presence of selective drug pressure, outgrowth of RAVs can lead to treatment failure. Rapid selection of RAVs was observed in vitro and in vivo following the administration of telaprevir and boceprevir monotherapy. Hence, viral eradication with these drugs was not achievable by monotherapy but only in triple therapy combination with PEG-IFN and RBV (Kieffer et al. 2007; Sarrazin et al. 2007a, b). A detailed knowledge of the key parameters of PI resistance development and their clinical implications for combination therapies with PEG-IFN or drugs that target other viral structures is crucial for successful HCV eradication.

Molecular Basis of HCV NS3-4A as a Drug Target

The molecular and structural properties of the NS3-4A protease as a drug target have been reviewed in detail by Welsch (Welsch 2014) and Bartenschlager (Bartenschlager et al. 2013). The nonstructural protein 3 (NS3) is a 70 kDa cleavage product (631 amino acids in length) of the HCV polyprotein that is bound to the membrane of the host cell endoplasmatic reticulum. NS3 is bifunctional, possessing a protease and a helicase domain. The carboxy-terminal two-thirds of NS3 constitute a superfamily 2 DExH/D-box RNA helicase that also shows NTPase activity. Both activities are essential for HCV replication. Development of DAAs that target the helicase has proven difficult, mainly due to structural similarities with cellular RNA helicases (Bartenschlager et al. 2013). The N-terminal ~180 amino acids of NS3, together with the cofactor NS4A, constitute a serine-type protease domain of chymotrypsin fold, NS3-4A (Morikawa et al. 2011), which is required for processing of the viral polyprotein downstream of the NS2-3 junction. NS3-4A is also considered a key contributor to viral persistence as it is involved in blocking innate immune signaling cascades by cleavage of cellular substrates such as MAVS, mitochondrial antiviral signaling protein (also known as Cardif, IPS-1, and VISA), and TRIF (toll-IL-1 receptor domain-containing adaptor inducing IFN-ß), two key adaptor molecules in the RIG-I and TLR3 viral RNA-sensing pathways and as such involved in induction of type I interferons (Li et al. 2005; Meylan et al. 2005). Direct inhibition of the NS3-4A protease does not only interfere with viral replication but may also support viral clearance by restoring the innate immune response as shown previously (Johnson et al. 2007). Besides MAVS and TRIF, NS3-4A has been found also to target several other cellular proteins.

Given its implications for the host innate immunity, the elimination threshold of an NS3-4A RAV depends not only on its drug resistance level but also its interference with such signaling cascades and consecutively the host cell IFN responsiveness. Such mechanisms are thought to play a key role in the second slope decay and late phase of viral eradication under DAA pressure by (i) complete suppression of viral replication and/or (ii) eradication of residual virus and virus-infected cells (Welsch 2014). Variants that escape such immune mechanisms likely relate to some relapses observed in recent clinical trials with PIs (Poordad et al. 2014). It is shown that a poorly fit virus can replicate for weeks within the liver of a persistently infected chimpanzee in the absence of detectable viremia even with the very sensitive TMA assay and that when the virus does mutate to a more fit phenotype, the mutations that had made it unfit are eventually no longer detectable. As a consequence, caution must be taken in inferring the absence of virologic resistance from the absence of detectable RAVs following the reappearance of virus in relapsing patients (Yi et al. 2014).

The relatively shallow active site of the NS3-4A protease has been a major challenge for the development of NS3-4A inhibitors. However, based on the observation of N-terminal product inhibition of the enzyme, potent peptidomimetic inhibitors were later developed (Summa et al. 2012).

DAAs that directly target the NS3-4A protease can be divided into three chemical classes: linear peptidomimetics that derive their potency from covalent but reversible linkage with the active site residue serine 139 of the protease, linear peptidomimetics that do not form covalent adducts with the active site, and macrocyclic inhibitors that are chemically distinct as they utilize structural constraints instead of covalent linkage. Overall, HCV PIs have a low-to-medium genetic barrier to resistance, and selection of RAVs has been observed in vitro and in vivo. Moreover, a significant overlap of resistance profiles has been observed as shown in Table 1. In addition, the structure of the NS3-4A serine protease with bound inhibitor and RAV sites is depicted in Fig. 1.

The first class of PIs comprises the two NS3-4A inhibitors telaprevir and boceprevir. Monotherapy studies of both compounds had led to a rapid and profound reduction of HCV-RNA (Sarrazin et al. 2007b; Reesink et al. 2006). However, viral rebound was observed in all patients upon treatment cessation, and viral breakthrough due to the selection of RAVs was frequently documented (Sarrazin et al. 2007a; Susser et al. 2009). Thus for the first time, the concept of antiviral drug resistance, which had not been relevant in patients receiving PEG-IFN and RBV only, had become a major issue in the context of anti-HCV therapy. Subsequent studies of telaprevir or boceprevir given in combination with PEG-IFN and RBV showed an even more pronounced decline in HCV RNA and reduced frequency of resistance-associated viral breakthrough (Sarrazin et al. 2007b; Forestier et al. 2007).

More recently, second-generation PIs including simeprevir, faldaprevir, asunaprevir, paritaprevir, and grazoprevir have been developed for therapy in combination with PEG-IFN and RBV but also as part of interferon-free all-oral direct antiviral combination therapy regimens (Pawlotsky 2014).

Table 1 Cross resistance table of mutations at amino acid positions within the HCV NS3-4A protease associated with PI resistance. Blue boxes represent first generation linear PIs, green boxes represent first-generation macrocyclic PIs and the purple boxes represent second-generation PIs

	36	54	55	80	155	156A	156B	168	170
Telaprevir (linear)									
Boceprevir (linear)									
Faldaprevir (linear)									
Simeprevir (macrocyclic)									
Asunaprevir (macrocyclic)									
Paritaprevir (macrocyclic)									
Grazoprevir (macrocyclic)									
Sovaprevir (linear)								a	

36: V36A/M; 54: T54S/A; 55: V55A; 80: Q80R/K; 155: R155K/T/Q; 156A: A156S; 156B: A156T/V; 168: D168A/V/T/H; 170: A/T. [a]mutations associated with in vitro resistance only

Parameters of Resistance Development

Virus-Related Parameters

Naturally Occurring RAVs

Direct sequencing analyses revealed a number of RAVs (e.g., substitutions at positions V36, T54, V55, Q80, R155, D168, and V170) to preexist at varying frequencies in patients who had been naïve to direct antiviral treatment (Bartels et al. 2008; Kuntzen et al. 2008). The more recent utilization of next-generation sequencing (NGS) methods provided evidence that RAVs preexist within the quasispecies cloud in virtually all patients but mostly at very low frequencies (Chevaliez et al. 2011).

The clinical consequences of preexisting RAVs were further elucidated by analyzing data of patients who had not responded to PEG-IFN-based treatment regimens (prior null response or 1 log HCV RNA decline during 4 weeks of PEG-IFN/RBV). In these patients who were a priori insensitive to the PEG-IFN backbone, addition of a PI as de facto monotherapy in the setting of preexisting RAVs led to treatment failure in all cases (De Meyer et al. 2012a; Howe et al. 2013a). However, as primary PEG-IFN nonresponsiveness is rare and the probability to detect a preexisting RAV as a major variant is low (3–8 %), there was no significant impact of baseline RAVs on treatment outcome in patients who received telaprevir- or boceprevir-based triple therapies (Howe et al. 2013a; Barnard et al. 2013; Bartels et al. 2013; Hezode et al. 2014; Poordad et al. 2012; McHutchison et al. 2010).

For the second-generation protease inhibitor simeprevir, a previously unknown RAV within the NS3-4A protease domain was described that conferred

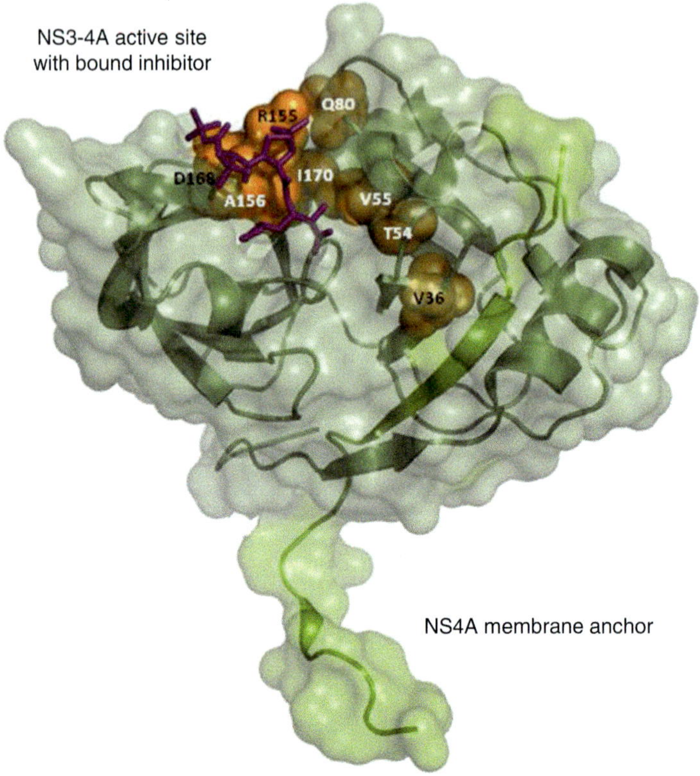

Fig. 1 Structure of the NS3-4A serine protease with bound inhibitor and resistance-associated amino acid sites. NS3-4A protease structure from Protein Databank entry 2OC8, showing the NS3 protease domain and NS4A as *dark green* and *light green* ribbon models respectively with transparent surface representation. A bound NS3-4A protease inhibitor is given as *purple* stick model. Resistance-associated sites (according to Table 1) are given as orange spheres (CPK models)

low-to-medium-level resistance in vitro (Q80K). Importantly, Q80K was confirmed to be a commonly observed RAV in untreated patients, specifically for genotype 1a, as it can be found in 19 % and 48 % of untreated HCV genotype 1a patients in Europe and the United States, respectively (Lenz et al. 2011), while it is rarely seen in genotype 1b (0.5 %). Although the resistance level for Q80K against PIs was determined to be rather low (only approximately tenfold change), its clinical consequences are all the more striking: In large phase 2 and phase 3 clinical trials, Q80K was highly associated with treatment failure in subtype 1a patients leading to response rates that were statistically not superior to the PEG-IFN/RBV control groups (Jacobson et al. 2014; Lenz et al. 2012; Manns et al. 2014c). However, the underlying molecular mechanisms remain yet to be determined.

Currently, IFN-free treatment regimens that also include NS3-4A PIs are being evaluated in phase 2–3 clinical trials. For example, simeprevir in combination with the nucleoside NS5B polymerase inhibitor sofosbuvir and a multidrug regimen including the ritonavir-boosted PI paritraprevir in combination with the NS5A inhibitor ombitasvir and the non-nucleoside NS5B polymerase inhibitor dasabuvir are all evaluated in patients with HCV genotype 1 infection. While the clinical impact of baseline RAVs has yet to be determined for these multidrug regimens (Poordad et al. 2014; Feld et al. 2014; Zeuzem et al. 2014), some data are available for the combination of simeprevir and sofosbuvir. In a relatively small study of this drug regimen, virologic failure was observed in subtype 1a patients only. However, despite an association of Q80K with treatment failure (Q80K was noted as a baseline RAV in four out of six patients with treatment failure), the majority of patients with preexisting Q80K (>90 %) still achieved sustained virologic response (SVR) (Lawitz et al. 2014). Ongoing larger phase 3 studies will have to determine the potential impact of baseline RAVs on treatment response in patients with all-oral PI-containing DAA treatment regimens.

Genetic Barrier

The likelihood of breakthrough is not entirely dependent on the mere presence or the number of preexisting RAVs but also relates to the genetic barrier to resistance, which is defined as the number of nucleotide changes for a resistance mutation to occur (Gish et al. 2012). NS3-4A PIs have a relatively low genetic barrier to resistance with significant differences between HCV subtypes due to the nucleotide sequence pattern at respective resistance-associated amino acid residues (Kieffer et al. 2007; Sarrazin et al. 2007a). For example, HCV subtype 1b possesses a higher genetic barrier to resistance compared to subtype 1a, which is in part related to the number of mutations required for resistance development that is higher in 1b than 1a (Sarrazin et al. 2007a). For example, a resistance-associated nucleotide change at codon 155 for generation of the R155K mutation requires two nucleotide changes in subtype 1b but only one change in subtype 1a (Welsch 2014). As a consequence, RAVs develop more frequently in patients with subtype 1a who fail to achieve SVR following a PI-based treatment regimen (Bacon et al. 2011; Poordad et al. 2011). The quality of the nucleotide change may also contribute to the genetic barrier to resistance. It is shown that a mutational bias in favor of nucleotide transitions over transversions may directly affect the emergence of RAVs (Grammatikos et al. 2014; Powdrill et al. 2011).

Variant Fitness

Another important aspect is the fitness phenotype of a RAV, which has been defined as the ability to replicate in the setting of natural selection (Domingo et al. 1997). RAVs are usually less fit compared to wild-type virus. However, under selective drug pressure, the virus wild type can be rapidly suppressed whereas RAVs continue to replicate and may eventually become the dominant viral strain in a given host environment.

Compensatory Mutations

Upon discontinuation of antiviral therapy, variants that harbor resistance mutations are usually replaced by wild-type virus due to inferior variant fitness. However,

RAVs may eventually become fixed in the viral quasispecies population due to compensatory second-site mutations. The selection of such compensatory mutations may also allow for efficient replication in the presence of drug pressure. Few data exist on the underlying mechanisms and potential clinical implications of such compensatory mutations. However, complex patterns of mutations were recently described from patients treated with boceprevir or telaprevir that showed an increasing complexity of linked variant combinations in patients with viral breakthrough during therapy (Susser et al. 2012), whereas other data suggest that compensatory substitutions are not observed in patients with telaprevir treatment failure (Sullivan et al. 2011). Such second-site mutations may also explain why some RAVs persist upon treatment cessation and why RAVs that negatively impact the virus replication capacity in a cell culture model of HCV infection can dominate in untreated patients (Welsch et al. 2012b).

Drug-Related Parameters

The probability of RAVs to be selected in the presence of PI therapy depends on a number of factors related to the specific compound. One such factor is the potency of the drug, which is a function of viral susceptibility and drug exposure, where susceptibility depends on the molecular structure of the drug target site whereas the drug exposure depends on its ADME properties, absorption, distribution, metabolism, and excretion. The close interplay between drug exposure and barrier to resistance has been demonstrated for telaprevir, where trough plasma concentration levels of the drug did correlate with the emergence of RAVs and hence viral breakthrough (Sarrazin et al. 2007a). However, the specific accumulation of active drug metabolites in the liver renders plasma drug levels with only limited predictive power for antiviral efficacy of NS3-4A PIs.

Host-Related Parameters

Patient adherence is crucial for the avoidance of RAV development and associated viral breakthrough. So far, failure of DAA-based therapies was mostly restricted to post-treatment relapse whereas breakthrough during antiviral therapy was more rarely observed in clinical trials of PIs. Here, breakthrough was mostly related to poor treatment adherence. Similarly, subtherapeutic plasma trough levels of antiretroviral drugs in patients infected with the human immunodeficiency virus (HIV) were found in association with treatment failure (Gardner et al. 2009). Despite this, exposure–response analyses did not show a significant association between higher PI exposure and increased SVR rates (FDA 2011).

Another important issue is potential drug–drug interactions (DDIs) that can pose an additional threat to successful HCV eradication. As all NS3-4A PIs are metabolized to some extent by cytochrome P450 3A4 (CAP3A4), their effect on other CYP3A4 substrates that are commonly used therapeutics (e.g., antiretrovirals, antibiotics, antimycotics, antidepressants, and immunosupressants) needs to be taken into account when starting antiviral therapy and preferably avoided during the course of antiviral treatment or the dosing of either the PI or the concomitant medication need to be adjusted.

Host factors that are relevant for immune responses and/or delivery of drugs to the target cells in the liver can be important cofounders for treatment success, i.e., host genetics such as polymorphisms within the interleukin (IL) 28B gene locus on chromosome 19. The disease stage seems to have a particular impact on treatment outcome. Patients with cirrhosis tend to achieve lower SVR rates even when treated with the most advanced PI-based all-oral drug combinations. Whether this is due to cirrhosis-related alterations in the patient's endogenous immune response and/or alterations in the pharmacokinetics/pharmacodynamics in the setting of portal hypertension requires further elucidation (Afdhal et al. 2014).

Resistance Profiles of Protease Inhibitors During Antiviral Therapy

Telaprevir

Telaprevir (VX-950; Vertex Pharmaceuticals, Cambridge, MA, USA) is a linear peptidomimetic ketoamide NS3-4A PI that forms a covalent, reversible enzyme–inhibitor complex. Telaprevir led to a median reduction of 4.4 $\log_{10}$ IU/ml and 5.49 $\log_{10}$ IU/ml HCV RNA when given as monotherapy (750 mg every 8 h) and in combination with PEG-IFN/RBV, respectively, in patients with HCV genotype 1 infection (Reesink et al. 2006; Forestier et al. 2007). Additional phase 1 and 2 studies showed that telaprevir has good antiviral activity in HCV genotype 2 but only minimal activity in patients with genotype 3 and 4 (Benhamou et al. 2013; Foster et al. 2011). Telaprevir has been approved only for the treatment of HCV genotype 1 infection.

RAVs against telaprevir were first identified at position A156 of the NS3/4A protease catalytic domain using HCV replicon cell lines (Lin et al. 2004). In vivo analysis of phase 1 trials confirmed residue 156 as a key site for telaprevir resistance (Kieffer et al. 2007; Sarrazin et al. 2007a). However, additional RAVs were also detected either as single or double mutations, such as the low-level resistance mutations V36A/M, T54A, R155K/T, and A156S that show higher fitness in terms of viral replication compared to variants with high-level resistance, such as A156V/T and V36A/M + A156V/T (Sarrazin et al. 2007a).

A comprehensive analysis of the telaprevir phase 3 trials revealed that 77 % of patients not responding to telaprevir-based triple therapy had detectable RAVs at the time of treatment failure. In patients with HCV genotype 1a infection, the most frequently detected variants were V36M and R155K or the combination of both whereas in genotype 1b patients, V36A, T54A/S, and A156S/T were mainly observed (Sullivan et al. 2013). The occurrence of RAVs was more frequently observed in HCV genotype 1a patients compared to genotype 1b but did not appear to depend on the prior treatment status. Despite this, virologic failure occurred in 52 % of prior null responders and was associated with higher-level resistance whereas the failure rate in prior relapsers was only 1 %. In treatment-naïve patients, who represent a mixture of patients with different sensitivities to PEG-IFN/RBV, the virologic failure rate was 7 % (De Meyer et al. 2012b). Taken together, these findings suggest that the likelihood of failure to telaprevir-based triple therapy mainly depends on the responsiveness to the PEG-IFN/RBV backbone.

Follow-up investigation of telaprevir-treated patients who did not achieve SVR revealed a median time to loss of RAVs of 10.6 and 0.9 months for genotype 1a and 1b, respectively (Sullivan et al. 2013).

Long-term follow-up (median duration, 29 months) of patients ($n = 126$) treated in phase 2/3 trials with telaprevir demonstrates a loss of RAVs in 85 % of patients by using population sequencing (Fig. 2) (Sherman et al. 2011b). However, more sensitive techniques such as clonal sequencing and deep sequencing did reveal additional low-level resistant variants even at much later time points (Dierynck et al. 2013). Despite this, at baseline of retreatment with telaprevir-based triple therapy, no RAVs were detectable using deep sequencing up to 5.7 years after short-term exposure to telaprevir in phase 1 trials (Fig. 3) (Sarrazin et al. 2013). Finally, in a small study, patients exposed to telaprevir during phase 1 trials were retreated with a full course of telaprevir-based triple therapy. Here, in four patients

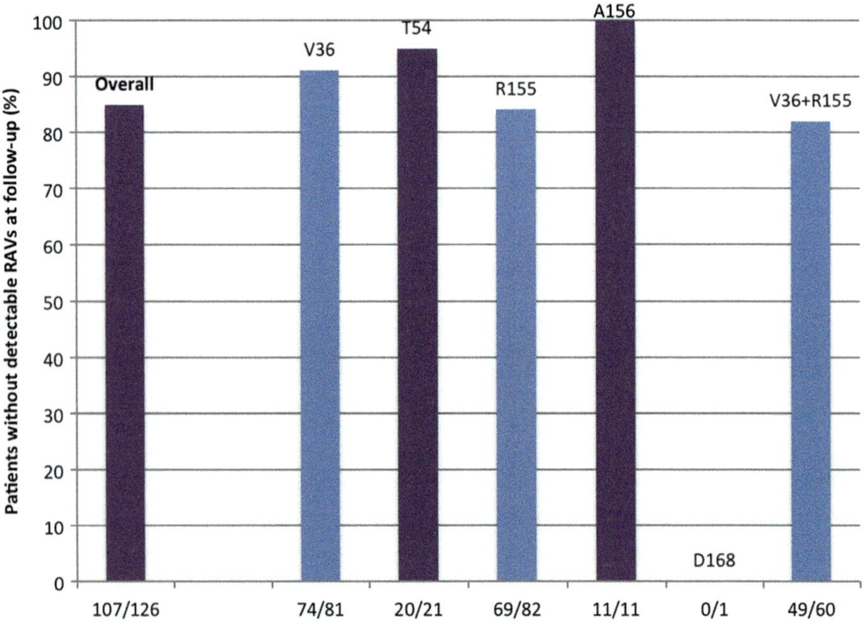

Fig. 2 Long-term follow-up of of telaprevir RAVs. The proportion of patients without detectable RAVs at a median follow-up of 29 months upon treatment failure is shown. Variant positions within the NS3-4A protease domain are shown above each column (Adapted from Sherman et al. (2011b))

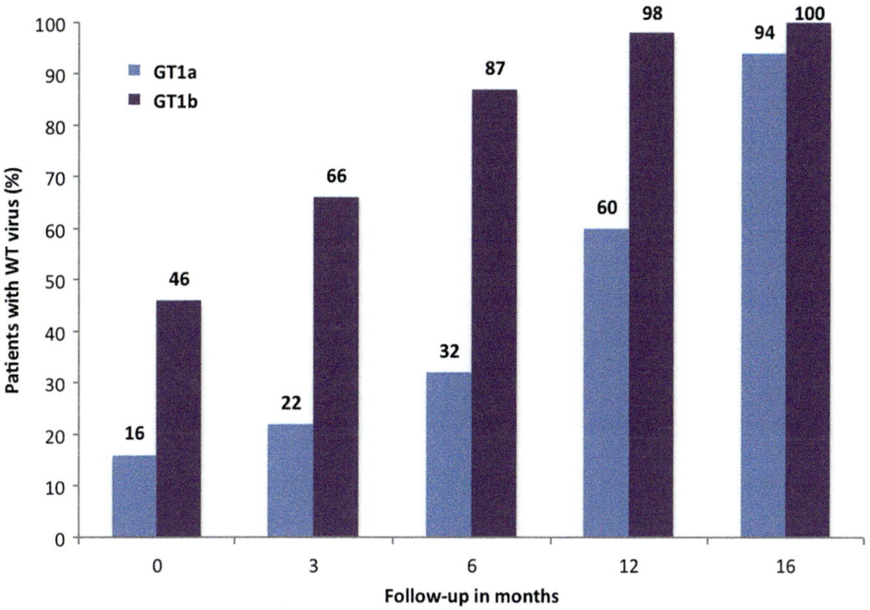

Fig. 3 RAV reversal to wild-type. Time to reversal to wild-type in months after telaprevir-based treatment in patients with HCV genotype 1a versus 1b infection (Adapted from Sullivan et al. (2013))

with treatment failure, viral variants were analyzed by means of sequential deep sequencing during the first and second telaprevir exposure. Interestingly, a heterogeneous evolution of viral isolates was observed, and no general rule for (re) selection of resistant variants after a second exposure to telaprevir could be established (Susser et al. 2015).

Boceprevir

Boceprevir (SCH 503034; Merck and Co., Whitehouse Station, NJ, USA) is a linear ketoamide PI that has led to a mean maximum reduction in HCV RNA of 1.61 and 2.88 $\log_{10}$ IU/ml after 1–2 weeks of monotherapy (400 mg three times daily) and in combination with PEG-IFN, respectively, in patients with HCV genotype 1 (Sarrazin et al. 2007b). Boceprevir has limited antiviral activity in HCV genotypes 2 and 3 (Silva et al. 2013) and was only approved for the treatment of genotype 1 infection.

Boceprevir has a largely overlapping resistance profile with telaprevir (Table 1). RAVs have been detected at positions V36, T54, R155, A156, and V170 in vitro (Tong et al. 2006) whereas additional mutations at positions Q41, F43, V55, and V158 were detected in phase 1 clinical trials (Susser et al. 2009; Vermehren et al. 2012). The mutations V36G, T54S, and R155L confer low-level resistance whereas medium-level resistance is observed for T54A, V55A, R155K, A156S, and V170A. Of note, variant V170A has been observed more frequently during boceprevir treatment and showed higher resistance levels compared to telaprevir (Sarrazin and Zeuzem 2010). Finally, A156T is known to confer the highest resistance level to boceprevir (Susser et al. 2009).

Population sequencing analyses from patients in the phase 3 trials SPRINT-2 (Poordad et al. 2011) and RESPOND-2 (Bacon et al. 2011) with boceprevir in triple combination with PEG-IFN and RBV showed that V36M, T54S, and R155K were found more frequently with HCV genotype 1a infection whereas variants T54A, V55A, A156S, and V170A were found more frequently in genotype 1b patients. As with telaprevir, the overall frequency of RAVs was higher in genotype 1a patients. Overall, postbaseline RAVs were detectable in 53 % of non-SVR patients, showing a decline to 22.8 % within 6–14 months upon treatment discontinuation (Barnard et al. 2013). The median time for all RAVs to disappear was 1.11 (1.05–1.2) years, which is not significantly different between subtypes 1a and 1b (Howe et al. 2013b). However, when applying the more sensitive clonal sequencing approach, boceprevir-resistant variants were detectable up to 4 years following short-term boceprevir exposure in phase 1 studies (Susser et al. 2011).

As for telaprevir, a second short-term low-dose exposure to boceprevir in phase 1 studies showed a heterogeneous evolution of RAVs with reoccurrence of variants selected during a previous course of boceprevir therapy in only a minority of patients (Vermehren et al. 2012).

Simeprevir

Simeprevir (TMC435; Janssen Pharmaceutica, Beerse, Belgium) was the first macrocyclic NS3-4A PI to be approved for the treatment of HCV genotype 1 infection. Simeprevir monotherapy (200 mg once daily) led to a median maximal reduction of 3.9 $\log_{10}$ IU/ml HCV RNA after 5 days in patients with HCV genotype 1 infection. Antiviral activity was comparably high in genotypes 4 and 6, followed by genotypes 2 and 5 (2.2–2.7 $\log_{10}$ decline), whereas no antiviral activity was evident for genotype 3 (Moreno et al. 2012), and these findings correlated with preexisting RAVs that are known to reduce or abolish the binding efficiency of simeprevir to the NS3-4A protease (Lenz et al. 2013).

The main resistance loci identified in clinical trials were Q80, R155, and D168, whereas RAVs at positions F43 and A156 have been detected only in experimental studies (Lenz et al. 2010; Reesink et al. 2010). Levels of resistance range from <10-fold for Q80K to about 2,000-fold for D168V and D168I. At residue 156, the fold change ranges from 16–44 for A156G/T to 177 for A156V, depending on the specific amino acid change (Lenz et al. 2010).

Due to significantly reduced SVR rates in patients with HCV genotype 1a infection treated with simeprevir in combination with PEG-IFN/RBV in the presence of Q80K-baseline RAVs, the FDA recommended for the first time a routine resistance testing prior to antiviral treatment. Interestingly, the majority of genotype 1a patients with preexisting Q80K RAVs seem to exhibit R155K at the time of treatment failure. Therefore, it has been concluded that a facilitated selection of additional RAVs in the presence of Q80K as opposed to Q80K alone may be responsible for treatment failure in these patients (Lenz et al. 2013, 2015). Small phase 2 studies of simeprevir as part of all-oral drug combinations consistently showed high SVR rates in patients with and without Q80K-baseline RAVs in genotype 1a patients (Lawitz et al. 2014), whereas larger phase 3 studies that elaborate the importance of Q80K for treatment failure are to be awaited. Median time until loss of Q80K was 36 and 24 months for genotype 1a and 1b, respectively. Loss of R155K in the presence of Q80K took 32 months whereas R155K alone disappeared after 64 months only (Lenz et al. 2015).

Faldaprevir

RAV selection during treatment with the linear tripeptide faldaprevir (BI201335; Boehringer Ingelheim, Ingelheim, Germany) is mainly restricted to mutations at residues 155 and 168. However, mutations at positions R155, A156, and D168 were all associated with resistance development in preclinical studies (Lagace et al. 2012). Clinically important RAVs that confer moderate (130-fold change) to high-level (up to 1,800-fold change) resistance include R155K and D168V, respectively (Berger et al. 2013). Chances of virologic failure are significantly higher in genotype 1a patients where R155K is predominantly selected (Sulkowski et al. 2013a, b). The more common Q80K variant was not associated with reduced SVR rates, and S61L was observed as a second-site mutation with D168V (Berger et al. 2014). No clinical data are available for antiviral activity of faldaprevir in genotypes 2–6. The company that developed faldaprevir recently decided not to move forward with the approval process due to the growing market of potentially more successful competitor drugs.

Asunaprevir

Asunaprevir is a linear tripeptide (BMS-650032; Bristol-Myers Squibb; New York, NY, USA) that has been approved as part of a PEG-IFN-free all-oral drug regimen that also includes the HCV NS5A replication complex inhibitor daclatasvir for the treatment of HCV genotype 1 infection in Japan. Preclinical studies identified R155K, D168G, and I170T to confer low- to moderate-level resistance against asunaprevir in genotype 1a (5- to 21-fold), whereas in genotype 1b, the main site for RAVs to occur is at position D168 with high-level asunaprevir resistance of 16- to 280-fold (McPhee et al. 2012). In clinical studies, the predominant baseline RAV was once again Q80K, which had an impact on virologic response rates in a single-ascending-dose study, but less so after administration of multiple doses of asunaprevir (McPhee et al. 2012).

In an all-oral combination therapy comprising asunaprevir and daclatasvir, 643 genotype 1b–infected patients showed preexisting RAVs in the NS3-4A protease domain in 11 % of cases. While overall SVR rates in the different study arms were high (82–90 %), only 38 % of patients with naturally occurring RAVs achieved SVR (Kao et al. 2014; Manns et al. 2014a). Thus, RAVs had an obvious influence on virologic response in this DAA regimen with a low barrier to resistance.

Paritaprevir

Preclinical resistance data on the linear PI inhibitor paritaprevir (ABT-450; AbbVie; North Chicago, IL, USA) have not yet been disclosed, and clinical data have only been published in abstract form. The R155K and D168V RAVs were detected by population sequencing after only 3 days of dosing in most patients treated with low doses of ritonavir-boosted paritaprevir (paritaprevir/r) whereas higher doses of paritaprevir/r appeared to suppress early resistance emergence (Pilot-Matias et al. 2011). A multidrug DAA regimen comprising paritaprevir/r, the NS5A inhibitor ombitasvir, and the non-nucleoside NS5B polymerase inhibitor dasabuvir was shown to be highly effective in genotype 1a and 1b–infected patients with SVR rates of 91–99 %. The rare occurrence of treatment failure in these patients was primarily observed in subtype 1a and was typically associated with the selection of RAVs against more than one DAA. The impact of rarely observed baseline RAVs on treatment outcomes has not yet been addressed (Poordad et al. 2014; Feld et al. 2014; Zeuzem et al. 2014). As of now, the question whether multidrug combinations have the potential to reduce the impact of naturally occurring RAVs on single DAA agents remains to be determined and certainly requires further attention. No clinical (resistance) data are available for HCV genotypes 2–6.

NS3-4A Protease Inhibitor Pipeline

The structural constraints of first-generation macrocyclic inhibitors allow for high drug potency but limit their efficacy in genotypes other than HCV genotype 1 (danoprevir, vaniprevir, GS-9256, GS-9451, IDX-320) (Sarrazin et al. 2012). Thus, recent developments include compounds that are highly potent and broadly active against different HCV genotypes as well as active against variants known to confer resistance against first-generation PIs. The macrocyclic PI grazoprevir (Merck & Co, Whithouse Station, NJ, USA) is the first compound with antiviral activity against HCV strains harboring the R155K mutation (Summa et al. 2012). While clinical data suggest that R155K can be still selected during grazoprevir therapy in HCV genotype 1, the resistance level seems to be too low for virologic breakthrough to occur (Strizki et al. 2012). Due to liver toxicity at higher doses that were associated with high antiviral activity in HCV genotype 3, the further development was restricted to lower doses and genotype 1 only (Summa et al. 2012; Manns et al. 2014b).

Sovaprevir (ACH-1625; Achillion, New Haven, CT, USA) is a linear peptidomimetic PI that noncovalently binds to the active site thereby showing high potency and broad genotypic coverage in early clinical trials. While Q80K was detected in both phase 1 and phase 2 studies, virologic response was not affected in the respective patients suggesting that drug exposure was sufficient to inhibit this variant to be selected (Fabrycki et al. 2012). Additional therapeutic trials are ongoing.

Conclusion

NS3/4A PIs represent the first class of DAAs that were approved for the treatment of chronic HCV infection. While adding a PI to the PEG-IFN-based treatment backbone has substantially increased cure rates, the selection of drug-resistant viral variants has evolved as an important limiting factor.

RAVs may be present in the viral quasispecies cloud already before treatment is started. However, while a clear association between some baseline RAVs (e.g., Q80K in simeprevir-treated patients) and treatment failure has been observed for PEG-IFN-based combination therapies, their clinical impact on the outcome of IFN-free DAA regimens is unclear to date. Parameters that determine RAV selection during antiviral therapy include genetic barriers and variant fitness phenotypes. The genetic barrier of HCV PIs is comparatively low, and combination regimes with DAAs that possess a higher genetic barrier (e.g., nucleotide polymerase inhibitors) have been more effective. However, it is the variant fitness that impacts RAV persistence most and the ability to compete with wild-type virus upon treatment cessation. Whether drug resistance will have any clinically meaningful impact on current and future DAA combination therapies remains to be determined. This will, however, require in-depth knowledge of the exact molecular escape mechanisms of each antiviral class available.

References

Afdhal NH, Everson G, Calleja JL, McCaughan G, Symonds WT, Denning J et al (2014) Sofosbuvir and ribavirin for the treatment of chronic HCV with cirrhosis and portal hypertension with and without decompensation: early virologic response and safety. J Hepatol 60:S28

Bacon BR, Gordon SC, Lawitz E, Marcellin P, Vierling JM, Zeuzem S et al (2011) Boceprevir for previously treated chronic HCV genotype 1 infection. N Engl J Med 364(13):1207–1217

Barnard RJ, Howe JA, Ogert RA, Zeuzem S, Poordad F, Gordon SC et al (2013) Analysis of boceprevir resistance associated amino acid variants (RAVs) in two phase 3 boceprevir clinical studies. Virology 444(1–2):329–336

Bartels DJ, Zhou Y, Zhang EZ, Marcial M, Byrn RA, Pfeiffer T et al (2008) Natural prevalence of hepatitis C virus variants with decreased sensitivity to NS3.4A protease inhibitors in treatment-naive subjects. J Infect Dis 198(6):800–807

Bartels DJ, Sullivan JC, Zhang EZ, Tigges AM, Dorrian JL, De Meyer S et al (2013) Hepatitis C virus variants with decreased sensitivity to direct-acting antivirals (DAAs) were rarely observed in DAA-naive patients prior to treatment. J Virol 87(3):1544–1553

Bartenschlager R, Lohmann V, Penin F (2013) The molecular and structural basis of advanced antiviral therapy for hepatitis C virus infection. Nat Rev Microbiol 11(7):482–496

Benhamou Y, Moussalli J, Ratziu V, Lebray P, De Backer K, De Meyer S et al (2013) Telaprevir activity in treatment-naive patients infected hepatitis C virus genotype 4: a randomized trial. J Infect Dis 208(6):1000–1007
Berger KL, Lagace L, Triki I, Cartier M, Marquis M, Lawetz C et al (2013) Viral resistance in hepatitis C virus genotype 1-infected patients receiving the NS3 protease inhibitor Faldaprevir (BI 201335) in a phase 1b multiple-rising-dose study. Antimicrob Agents Chemother 57(10):4928–4936
Berger K, Sarrazin C, Ferenci P, Jensen DM, Jacobson IM, Stern JO et al (2014) NS3 Q80K did not impact efficacy or treatment-emergent resistance patterns in HCV genotype 1-infected patients receiving faldaprevir + peginterferon/ribavirin in three phase III trials. J Hepatol 60:S497
Chevaliez S, Rodriguez C, Soulier A, Ahmed-Belkacem A, Hezode C, Pawlotsky JM (2011) Molecular characterization of HCV resistance to telaprevir by means of ultra-deep pyrosequencing: preexisting resistant variants and dynamics of resistant populations. J Hepatol 54:S30
De Meyer S, Thys K, Dierynck I, Ghys A, Aerssens J, Picchio G (2012a) Deep sequencing screening for telaprevir-resistant viral variants in previous null responders fails to identify those patients at risk of failing telaprevir plus peginterferon/ribavirin therapy. J Hepatol 56:S465
De Meyer S, Dierynck I, Ghys A, Beumont M, Daems B, Van Baelen B et al (2012b) Characterization of telaprevir treatment outcomes and resistance in patients with prior treatment failure: results from the REALIZE trial. Hepatology 56(6):2106–2115
Dierynck I, Thys K, Bartels DJ, Ghys A, Van Rossem E, Zhang E et al (2013) Post-treatment viral evolution assessment using ultra-deep pyrosequencing in samples from patients with hepatitis C virus infection: the EXTEND study. Hepatology 58:939A
Domingo E, Menendez-Arias L, Holland JJ (1997) RNA virus fitness. Rev Med Virol 7(2):87–96
Fabrycki J, Patel D, Yang G, Zhao Y, Podos S, Robison H et al (2012) Characterization of HCV NS3 protease variants from patients enrolled in a 28-day phase 2a trial of ACH-1625 daily dosing plus PegIFN-alpha 2a/RBV. J Hepatol 56:S468
FDA (2011) Advisory Committee Briefing Document for NDA 201-917 Telaprevir 375 mg tablets. http://www.fda.gov/downloads/AdvisoryCommittees/CommitteesMeetingMaterials/Drugs/AntiviralDrugsAdvisoryCommittee/UCM252561.pdf
Feld JJ, Kowdley KV, Coakley E, Sigal S, Nelson DR, Crawford D et al (2014) Treatment of HCV with ABT-450/r-ombitasvir and dasabuvir with ribavirin. N Engl J Med 370(17):1594–1603
Forestier N, Reesink HW, Weegink CJ, McNair L, Kieffer TL, Chu HM et al (2007) Antiviral activity of telaprevir (VX-950) and peginterferon alfa-2a in patients with hepatitis C. Hepatology 46(3):640–648
Foster GR, Hezode C, Bronowicki JP, Carosi G, Weiland O, Verlinden L et al (2011) Telaprevir alone or with peginterferon and ribavirin reduces HCV RNA in patients with chronic genotype 2 but not genotype 3 infections. Gastroenterology 141(3):881–889
Fried MW, Shiffman ML, Reddy KR, Smith C, Marinos G, Goncales FL Jr et al (2002) Peginterferon alfa-2a plus ribavirin for chronic hepatitis C virus infection. N Engl J Med 347(13):975–982
Gardner EM, Burman WJ, Steiner JF, Anderson PL, Bangsberg DR (2009) Antiretroviral medication adherence and the development of class-specific antiretroviral resistance. AIDS 23(9):1035–1046
Gish R, Jia JD, Locarnini S, Zoulim F (2012) Selection of chronic hepatitis B therapy with high barrier to resistance. Lancet Infect Dis 12(4):341–353
Grammatikos G, Jabara CB, Ahmad MQ, Herrmann E, Zeuzem S, Welsch C (2014) Genetic background for development of resistance mutations within the HCV NS3 protease-helicase in patients naive to direct antivirals. Antivir Ther 19(5):455–461
Hezode C, Fontaine H, Dorival C, Zoulim F, Larrey D, Canva V et al (2014) Effectiveness of telaprevir or boceprevir in treatment-experienced patients with HCV genotype 1 infection and cirrhosis. Gastroenterology 147(1):132–142

Hinrichsen H, Benhamou Y, Wedemeyer H, Reiser M, Sentjens RE, Calleja JL et al (2004) Short-term antiviral efficacy of BILN 2061, a hepatitis C virus serine protease inhibitor, in hepatitis C genotype 1 patients. Gastroenterology 127(5):1347–1355

Howe JA, Long JM, Black S, Chase R, McMonagle P, Curry S et al (2013a) Pooled clinical trial analyses of detectable basline HCV NS3/4A resistance associated variants on the efficacy of boceprevir plus pegylated interferon/ribavirin. Hepatology 58:1097A

Howe AY, Long JM, Thompson S, Barnard RJ, Alves K, Howe JA et al (2013b) Analysis of the durability of response and persistance of resistance associated variants during long term follow Up after boceprevir plus pegylated interferon/ribavirin therapy – 3 year analysis. Hepatology 58:1095A

Jacobson IM, McHutchison JG, Dusheiko G, Di Bisceglie AM, Reddy KR, Bzowej NH et al (2011) Telaprevir for previously untreated chronic hepatitis C virus infection. N Engl J Med 364(25):2405–2416

Jacobson IM, Dore GJ, Foster GR, Fried MW, Radu M, Rafalsky VV et al. (2014) Simeprevir with pegylated interferon alfa 2a plus ribavirin in treatment-naive patients with chronic hepatitis C virus genotype 1 infection (QUEST-1): a phase 3, randomised, double-blind, placebo-controlled trial. Lancet 384(9941):403–13

Johnson CL, Owen DM, Gale M Jr (2007) Functional and therapeutic analysis of hepatitis C virus NS3.4A protease control of antiviral immune defense. J Biol Chem 282(14):10792–10803

Kao J-H, Heo J, Yoffe B, Sievert W, Jacobson IM, Bessone F et al (2014) Efficacy and safety of daclatasvir in combination with asunaprevir (DCV+ASV) in cirrhotic and Non-cirrhotic patients with HCV genotype 1B: results of the hallmark dual study. J Hepatol 60:S527

Kieffer TL, Sarrazin C, Miller JS, Welker MW, Forestier N, Reesink HW et al (2007) Telaprevir and pegylated interferon-alpha-2a inhibit wild-type and resistant genotype 1 hepatitis C virus replication in patients. Hepatology 46(3):631–639

Kuntzen T, Timm J, Berical A, Lennon N, Berlin AM, Young SK et al (2008) Naturally occurring dominant resistance mutations to hepatitis C virus protease and polymerase inhibitors in treatment-naive patients. Hepatology 48(6):1769–1778

Lagace L, White PW, Bousquet C, Dansereau N, Do F, Llinas-Brunet M et al (2012) In vitro resistance profile of the hepatitis C virus NS3 protease inhibitor BI 201335. Antimicrob Agents Chemother 56(1):569–572

Lamarre D, Anderson PC, Bailey M, Beaulieu P, Bolger G, Bonneau P et al (2003) An NS3 protease inhibitor with antiviral effects in humans infected with hepatitis C virus. Nature 426(6963):186–189

Lange CM, Zeuzem S (2011) IL28B single nucleotide polymorphisms in the treatment of hepatitis C. J Hepatol 55(3):692–701

Lawitz E, Sulkowski MS, Ghalib R, Rodriguez-Torres M, Younossi ZM, Corregidor A et al (2014) Simeprevir plus sofosbuvir, with or without ribavirin, to treat chronic infection with hepatitis C virus genotype 1 in non-responders to pegylated interferon and ribavirin and treatment-naive patients: the COSMOS randomised study. Lancet 384(9956):1756–1765

Lenz O, Verbinnen T, Lin TI, Vijgen L, Cummings MD, Lindberg J et al (2010) In vitro resistance profile of the hepatitis C virus NS3/4A protease inhibitor TMC435. Antimicrob Agents Chemother 54(5):1878–1887

Lenz O, Fevery B, Vijgen L, Verbeeck J, Peeters M, Beumont M et al (2011) TMC435 in combination with peginterferon alpha-2a/ribavirin in treatment-naive patients infected with HCV genotype 1: virology analysis of the pillar study. Hepatology 54:985A

Lenz O, de Bruijne J, Vijgen L, Verbinnen T, Weegink C, Van Marck H et al (2012) Efficacy of re-treatment with TMC435 as combination therapy in hepatitis C virus-infected patients following TMC435 monotherapy. Gastroenterology 143(5):1176–1178.e1171-1176

Lenz O, Vijgen L, Berke JM, Cummings MD, Fevery B, Peeters M et al (2013) Virologic response and characterisation of HCV genotype 2–6 in patients receiving TMC435 monotherapy (study TMC435-C202). J Hepatol 58(3):445–451

Lenz O, Fevery B, Verbinnen T, Tambuyzer L, Vijgen L, Peeters M et al (2015) Resistance analyses of HCV isolates from patients treated with simeprevir in phase 2b/3 studies. Hepatology 62(5):1008–14

Li XD, Sun L, Seth RB, Pineda G, Chen ZJ (2005) Hepatitis C virus protease NS3/4A cleaves mitochondrial antiviral signaling protein off the mitochondria to evade innate immunity. Proc Natl Acad Sci U S A 102(49):17717–17722

Lin C, Lin K, Luong YP, Rao BG, Wei YY, Brennan DL et al (2004) In vitro resistance studies of hepatitis C virus serine protease inhibitors, VX-950 and BILN 2061: structural analysis indicates different resistance mechanisms. J Biol Chem 279(17):17508–17514

Lohmann V, Korner F, Koch J, Herian U, Theilmann L, Bartenschlager R (1999) Replication of subgenomic hepatitis C virus RNAs in a hepatoma cell line. Science 285(5424):110–113

Manns MP, McHutchison JG, Gordon SC, Rustgi VK, Shiffman M, Reindollar R et al (2001) Peginterferon alfa-2b plus ribavirin compared with interferon alfa-2b plus ribavirin for initial treatment of chronic hepatitis C: a randomised trial. Lancet 358(9286):958–965

Manns MP, Pol S, Jacobson IM, Marcellin P, Gordon SC, Peng C-Y et al (2014a) All-oral daclatasvir plus asunaprevir for hepatitis C virus genotype 1b: a multinational, phase 3, multicohort study. Lancet 384(9954):1597–1605

Manns MP, Vierling JM, Bacon BR, Bruno S, Shibolet O, Baruch Y et al (2014b) The combination of MK-5172, peginterferon, and ribavirin is effective in treatment-naive patients with hepatitis C virus genotype 1 infection without cirrhosis. Gastroenterology 147(2):366–376

Manns M, Marcellin P, Poordad F, de Araujo ES, Buti M, Horsmans Y et al. (2014c) Simeprevir with pegylated interferon alfa 2a or 2b plus ribavirin in treatment-naive patients with chronic hepatitis C virus genotype 1 infection (QUEST-2): a randomised, double-blind, placebo-controlled phase 3 trial. Lancet 384(9941):414–26

McHutchison JG, Manns MP, Muir AJ, Terrault NA, Jacobson IM, Afdhal NH et al (2010) Telaprevir for previously treated chronic HCV infection. N Engl J Med 362(14):1292–1303

McPhee F, Friborg J, Levine S, Chen C, Falk P, Yu F et al (2012) Resistance analysis of the hepatitis C virus NS3 protease inhibitor asunaprevir. Antimicrob Agents Chemother 56(7):3670–3681

Meylan E, Curran J, Hofmann K, Moradpour D, Binder M, Bartenschlager R et al (2005) Cardif is an adaptor protein in the RIG-I antiviral pathway and is targeted by hepatitis C virus. Nature 437(7062):1167–1172

Moreno C, Berg T, Tanwandee T, Thongsawat S, Van Vlierberghe H, Zeuzem S et al (2012) Antiviral activity of TMC435 monotherapy in patients infected with HCV genotypes 2–6: TMC435-C202, a phase IIa, open-label study. J Hepatol 56(6):1247–1253

Morikawa K, Lange CM, Gouttenoire J, Meylan E, Brass V, Penin F et al (2011) Nonstructural protein 3-4A: the Swiss army knife of hepatitis C virus. J Viral Hepat 18(5):305–315

Pawlotsky JM (2014) New hepatitis C virus (HCV) drugs and the hope for a cure: concepts in anti-HCV drug development. Semin Liver Dis 34(1):22–29

Pilot-Matias T, Tripathi R, Dekhtyar T, Menon R, Gaultier IA, Cohen D et al (2011) Genotypic and phenotypic characterization of NS3 variants selected in HCV-infected patients treated with ABT-450. J Hepatol 54:S485

Poordad F, McCone J Jr, Bacon BR, Bruno S, Manns MP, Sulkowski MS et al (2011) Boceprevir for untreated chronic HCV genotype 1 infection. N Engl J Med 364(13):1195–1206

Poordad F, Bronowicki JP, Gordon SC, Zeuzem S, Jacobson IM, Sulkowski MS et al (2012) Factors that predict response of patients with HCV infection to boceprevir. Gastroenterology 143(3):608–618

Poordad F, Hezode C, Trinh R, Kowdley KV, Zeuzem S, Agarwal K et al (2014) ABT-450/r-ombitasvir and dasabuvir with ribavirin for hepatitis C with cirrhosis. N Engl J Med 370(21):1973–1982

Powdrill MH, Tchesnokov EP, Kozak RA, Russell RS, Martin R, Svarovskaia ES et al (2011) Contribution of a mutational bias in hepatitis C virus replication to the genetic barrier in the development of drug resistance. Proc Natl Acad Sci U S A 108(51):20509–20513

Reesink HW, Zeuzem S, Weegink CJ, Forestier N, van Vliet A, van de Wetering de Rooij J et al (2006) Rapid decline of viral RNA in hepatitis C patients treated with VX-950: a phase Ib, placebo-controlled, randomized study. Gastroenterology 131(4):997–1002

Reesink HW, Fanning GC, Farha KA, Weegink C, Van Vliet A, Van 't Klooster G et al (2010) Rapid HCV-RNA decline with once daily TMC435: a phase I study in healthy volunteers and hepatitis C patients. Gastroenterology 138(3):913–921

Rong L, Dahari H, Ribeiro RM, Perelson AS (2010) Rapid emergence of protease inhibitor resistance in hepatitis C virus. Sci Transl Med 2(30):30ra32

Sarrazin C, Zeuzem S (2010) Resistance to direct antiviral agents in patients with hepatitis C virus infection. Gastroenterology 138(2):447–462

Sarrazin C, Kieffer TL, Bartels D, Hanzelka B, Muh U, Welker M et al (2007a) Dynamic hepatitis C virus genotypic and phenotypic changes in patients treated with the protease inhibitor telaprevir. Gastroenterology 132(5):1767–1777

Sarrazin C, Rouzier R, Wagner F, Forestier N, Larrey D, Gupta SK et al (2007b) SCH 503034, a novel hepatitis C virus protease inhibitor, plus pegylated interferon alpha-2b for genotype 1 nonresponders. Gastroenterology 132(4):1270–1278

Sarrazin C, Hezode C, Zeuzem S, Pawlotsky JM (2012) Antiviral strategies in hepatitis C virus infection. J Hepatol 56(Suppl 1):S88–S100

Sarrazin C, Reesink HW, Zeuzem S, Dierynck I, Luo D, Witek J et al (2013) Treatment with telaprevir/PEG-IFN/RBV after 14-day telaprevir exposure in phase I studies: results from the phase IIIB C219 rollover study. J Hepatol 58:S369

Sherman KE, Flamm SL, Afdhal NH, Nelson DR, Sulkowski MS, Everson GT et al (2011a) Response-guided telaprevir combination treatment for hepatitis C virus infection. N Engl J Med 365(11):1014–1024

Sherman KE, Sulkowski MS, Zoulim F, Alberti A, Wei LJ, Sullivan J et al (2011b) Follow-up of SVR durability and viral resistance in patients with chronic hepatitis C treated with telaprevir-based regimens: interim analysis of the extend study. Hepatology 54:485A

Shimakami T, Welsch C, Yamane D, McGivern DR, Yi M, Zeuzem S et al (2011) Protease inhibitor-resistant hepatitis C virus mutants with reduced fitness from impaired production of infectious virus. Gastroenterology 140(2):667–675

Silva MO, Treitel M, Graham DJ, Curry S, Frontera MJ, McMonagle P et al (2013) Antiviral activity of boceprevir monotherapy in treatment-naive subjects with chronic hepatitis C genotype 2/3. J Hepatol 59(1):31–37

Strizki JM, Barnard RJO, Cheney C, McHale C, Graham D, Himmelberger A et al (2012) Evaluation of NS3 amino acid variants in a phase 1b study of genotype 1 (Gt1) and Gt3 infected patients with the Hcv protease inhibitor, MK-5172. J Hepatol 56:S479

Sulkowski MS, Asselah T, Lalezari J, Ferenci P, Fainboim H, Leggett B et al (2013a) Faldaprevir combined with pegylated interferon alfa-2a and ribavirin in treatment-naive patients with chronic genotype 1 HCV: SILEN-C1 trial. Hepatology 57(6):2143–2154

Sulkowski MS, Bourliere M, Bronowicki JP, Asselah T, Pawlotsky JM, Shafran SD et al (2013b) Faldaprevir combined with peginterferon alfa-2a and ribavirin in chronic hepatitis C virus genotype-1 patients with prior nonresponse: SILEN-C2 trial. Hepatology 57(6):2155–2163

Sullivan JC, De Meyer S, Bartels DJ, Dierynck I, Zhang E, Spanks J et al (2011) Evolution of treatment-emergent resistant variants in telaprevir phase 3 clinical trials. J Hepatol 54:S4

Sullivan JC, De Meyer S, Bartels DJ, Dierynck I, Zhang EZ, Spanks J et al (2013) Evolution of treatment-emergent resistant variants in telaprevir phase 3 clinical trials. Clin Infect Dis 57(2):221–229

Summa V, Ludmerer SW, McCauley JA, Fandozzi C, Burlein C, Claudio G et al (2012) MK-5172, a selective inhibitor of Hepatitis C Virus NS3/4a protease with broad activity across genotypes and resistant variants. Antimicrob Agents Chemother 56(8):4161–4167

Susser S, Welsch C, Wang Y, Zettler M, Domingues FS, Karey U et al (2009) Characterization of resistance to the protease inhibitor boceprevir in hepatitis C virus-infected patients. Hepatology 50(6):1709–1718

Susser S, Vermehren J, Forestier N, Welker MW, Grigorian N, Fuller C et al (2011) Analysis of long-term persistence of resistance mutations within the hepatitis C virus NS3 protease after treatment with telaprevir or boceprevir. J Clin Virol 52(4):321–327

Susser S, Schelhorn SE, Lange CM, Welsch C, Vermehren J, Perner D et al (2012) 454 deep sequencing analysis of hepatitis C virus NS3 protease resistance mutations A87T, R117H, and S174F in patients treated with telaprevir or boceprevir. Hepatology 56:714A

Susser S, Flinders M, Reesink HW, Zeuzem S, Lawyer A, Ghys A et al (2015) Re-treatment with telaprevir-based triple therapy after telaprevir exposure in phase 1 studies: deep sequence analysis for persistence of resistant variants. Antimicrob Agents Chemother 59(5):2746–55

Tong X, Chase R, Skelton A, Chen T, Wright-Minogue J, Malcolm BA (2006) Identification and analysis of fitness of resistance mutations against the HCV protease inhibitor SCH 503034. Antivir Res 70(2):28–38

Vermehren J, Susser S, Lange CM, Forestier N, Karey U, Hughes E et al (2012) Mutations selected in the hepatitis C virus NS3 protease domain during sequential treatment with boceprevir with and without pegylated interferon alfa-2b. J Viral Hepat 19(2):120–127

Welsch C (2014) Genetic barrier and variant fitness in hepatitis C as critical parameters for drug resistance development. Drug Discov Today Technol 11:19–25

Welsch C, Schweizer S, Shimakami T, Domingues FS, Kim S, Lemon SM et al (2012a) Ketoamide resistance and hepatitis C virus fitness in val55 variants of the NS3 serine protease. Antimicrob Agents Chemother 56(4):1907–1915

Welsch C, Shimakami T, Hartmann C, Yang Y, Domingues FS, Lengauer T et al (2012b) Peptidomimetic escape mechanisms arise via genetic diversity in the ligand-binding site of the hepatitis C virus NS3/4A serine protease. Gastroenterology 142(3):654–663

Yi M, Hu F, Joyce M, Saxena V, Welsch C, Chavez D et al (2014) Evolution of a cell culture-derived genotype 1a hepatitis C virus (H77S.2) during persistent infection with chronic hepatitis in a chimpanzee. J Virol 88(7):3678–3694

Zeuzem S, Andreone P, Pol S, Lawitz E, Diago M, Roberts S et al (2011) Telaprevir for retreatment of HCV infection. N Engl J Med 364(25):2417–2428

Zeuzem S, Jacobson IM, Baykal T, Marinho RT, Poordad F, Bourliere M et al (2014) Retreatment of HCV with ABT-450/r-ombitasvir and dasabuvir with ribavirin. N Engl J Med 370(17):1604–1614

Contribution of APOBEC3-Driven Mutagenesis to HIV Evolution and HIV Drug Resistance

Marsha Dillon-White and Viviana Simon

Contents

Selection of the Bibliography: An extensive review of the current literature was performed using the keywords "APOBEC3, APOBEC3G, Vif, and/or HIV drug resistance." Due to space constraints, we sometimes had to refer to reviews summarizing a given topic rather than citing original articles.

M. Dillon-White
Department of Microbiology, Icahn School of Medicine at Mount Sinai, New York, NY, USA
e-mail: marsha.dillon-white@mssm.edu

V. Simon (✉)
Department of Microbiology, Icahn School of Medicine at Mount Sinai, New York, NY, USA

The Global Health and Emerging Pathogens Institute, Icahn School of Medicine at Mount Sinai, New York, NY, USA

Division of Infectious Diseases, Department of Medicine, Icahn School of Medicine at Mount Sinai, New York, NY, USA
e-mail: viviana.simon@mssm.edu

M. Gotte et al. (eds.), *Handbook of Antimicrobial Resistance*,
DOI 10.1007/978-1-4939-0694-9_8

Abstract
Sequence variation is central to the ability of HIV-1 to evade immune responses and antiretroviral therapeutics. APOBEC3 editing enzymes are potent mutagens of retroviral genomes. In humans, the APOBEC3 family comprises seven different proteins (APOBEC3A [A3A] to A3H), whose cytidine deaminase activity – if left unchecked – results in extensive mutagenesis of the HIV-1 genome. There is emerging evidence that cytidine deaminases other than A3G play an important role in restricting the spread and replication of HIV-1. APOBEC3 molecules, indeed, differ not only in catalytic activity and expression but also in susceptibility to HIV-1 Vif-mediated degradation. The interplay between these intracellular host defenses and HIV counterstrategies is discussed in this chapter with a special emphasis on viral evolution and drug resistance.

Keywords
A3G • A3H • Acquired immunodeficiency syndrome (AIDS) • Drug resistance • Hypermutations • Mutagenesis • Restriction factor • Reverse transcriptase (RT) • Viral evolution • Viral-host interaction

Introduction

The APOBEC3 family comprises seven members (A3A, A3B, A3C, A3DE, A3F, A3G, and A3H) whose genes are located in tandem on human chromosome 22 (Fig. 1, Jarmuz 2002; Wedekind et al. 2003). They constitute the most recent addition to the superfamily of cytidine deaminases (Jarmuz 2002) of which APOBEC1 and AID (activation-induced deaminase) were the first described representatives (Wedekind et al. 2003). This group of mammalian proteins with DNA-editing activity can introduce genetic modifications in retroviral genomes through cytosine deamination (Jarmuz 2002). Recent studies have shown that A3G, A3F, A3DE, and certain A3H haplotypes not only display a range of antiretroviral activities but also differ in their susceptibility to degradation by the different circulating HIV Vif variants (Albin et al. 2013; Malim 2009). Importantly, the

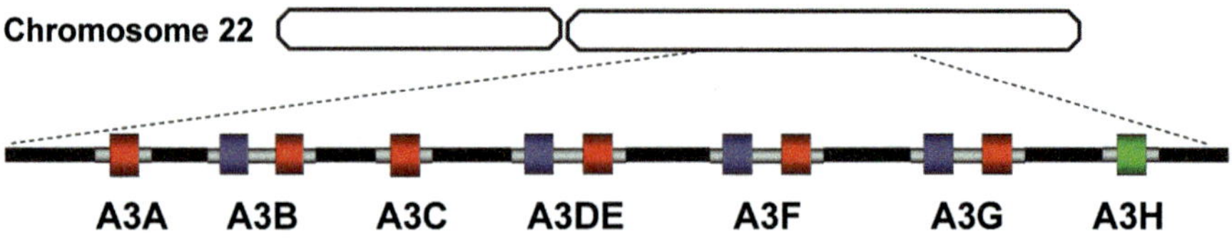

Fig. 1 Schematic representation of the human APOBEC3 locus. These proteins are composed of either one or two deaminase domains (*red*, *blue*, or *green*). A3H is identified in a different color to illustrate the fact that it has different haplotypes that differ in antiviral activity

APOBEC3 proteins are co-expressed in cell populations susceptible to HIV infection (e.g., primary human T lymphocytes and macrophages (Albin et al. 2013; Harris et al. 2003; Mangeat 2003; Koning et al. 2009)).

Cellular Cytidine Deaminases with Antiretroviral Activity

The identification of the human gene APOBEC3G (initially referred to as CEM15, abbreviated here throughout the text as A3G) as the target of the HIV Vif in 2002 (Sheehy et al. 2002) spurred a series of studies aimed at elucidating this novel host defense mechanism (see Albin and Harris 2010; Bieniasz 2004; Neuberger 2003; Refsland and Harris 2013 for reviews). Indeed, the presence of the accessory lentiviral protein Vif in "nonpermissive" (=APOBEC3 expressing) producer cells is essential for the generation of HIV particles that can productively infect other cells (e.g., T lymphocytes). Conversely, viral particles generated in the presence of A3G but in the absence of Vif yield proviruses with reduced viral infectivity due to the high frequency of G-to-A mutations (Lecossier 2003; Mariani et al. 2003).

Our current understanding of the APOBEC3 mode of action is as follows. APOBEC3 are incorporated into newly generated viral particles in the absence of Vif. Upon infection of a new cell, APOBEC3 enzymes deaminate deoxycytidine to deoxyuracil in the retroviral minus-strand cDNA generated during the reverse transcription step, which, in turn, results in guanosine-to-adenosine (G-to-A) mutations in the plus-strand cDNA (Harris et al. 2003; Mangeat 2003). Depending on the frequency and the position of these G-to-A mutations, the resulting provirus may be defective or display an attenuated phenotype (Fig. 2). In addition to this editing-dependent restriction mechanism, APOBEC3 can block HIV replication by non-editing means (Gillick et al. 2013).

All lentiviruses with the exception of equine infectious anemia virus express Vif ("viral infectivity factor"). In doing so, they have developed an efficient way to protect their genome from the deleterious effects associated with cellular cytidine deaminases. Vif reduces the level of APOBEC3 in the producer cell by targeting it for proteasomal degradation (Sheehy et al. 2002; Stopak et al. 2003; Marin 2003; Conticello et al. 2003a; Liu et al. 2004; Zennou et al. 2004). HIV Vif interacts with a complex of four cellular proteins (Cullin 5, Elongin B and C, and Rbx1 as well as APOBEC3) which leads to ubiquitination/proteasomal degradation of the deaminase (Yu et al. 2003, 2004; Yu 2004). Recently, it has been revealed that a transcription factor, CBF-beta, is essential for stabilizing HIV Vif (Zhang et al. 2012; Jager et al. 2012; Kim et al. 2013) (Fig. 3). The first crystal structure of HIV Vif was solved in 2014 in complex with the E3 ligase Cullin 5 and the transcription factor CBF-beta (Guo et al. 2014).

It was initially thought that A3G was the most potent antiretroviral deaminase, but in the past couple of years, a more nuanced picture has emerged. It is now well accepted that A3B, A3DE, A3F, and A3H, in addition to A3G, display activity against HIV variants lacking active Vif alleles (Albin et al. 2013; Sato et al. 2014; Chaipan et al. 2013; Hultquist et al. 2011).

For example, the role of A3F on HIV-1 restriction in human primary blood mononuclear cells (PBMCs) was investigated using a full-length HIV-1 NL4-3 Vif

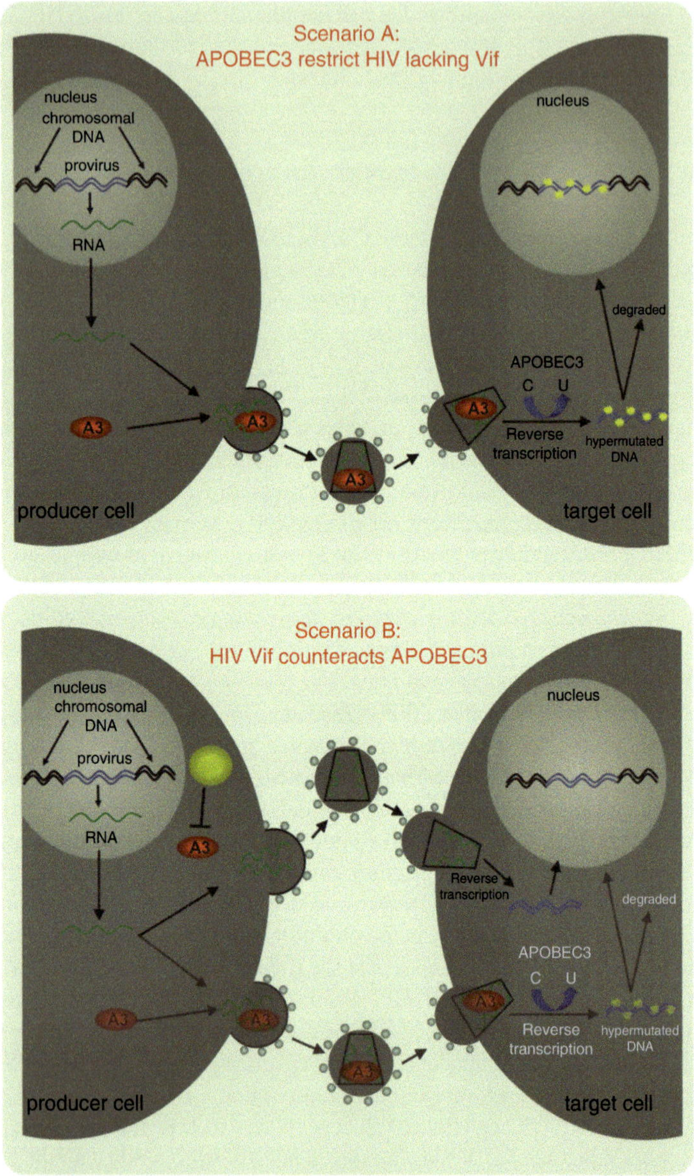

Fig. 2 The mode of action of APOBEC3 restriction is depicted. In the absence of HIV Vif, APOBEC3 proteins are incorporated into the egressing virions and deaminate the minus-strand cDNA in the next round of infection (scenario A). However, circulating HIV strains express the accessory protein Vif which excludes APOBEC3 from the virions resulting in fully infectious viral particles (scenario B)

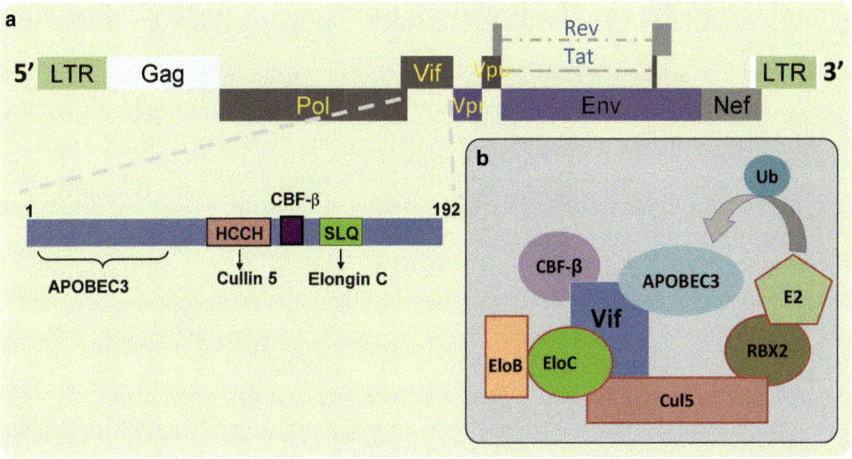

Fig. 3 The accessory protein Vif counteracts APOBEC3 by inducing their proteasomal degradation. Regions in Vif which are important for interacting with the host cell machinery as well as with the APOBEC3 protein are highlighted: (**a**) Vif binds CBF-beta and APOBEC3 and assembles a E3 ligase complex which results in the degradation of the deaminase. Abbreviations: *Ub*, Ubiquitin; *EloC*, Elongin C; *EloB*, Elongin B; *Cul5*, Cullin 5. Note that the identity of the E2 remains unknown to date

mutant (HIV W11R) that normally degrades A3G but does not target A3F (Mulder et al. 2010). This Vif mutant virus replicated as efficiently as the wild-type NL4-3 in human PBMCs suggesting a marginal contribution for A3F to HIV-1 restriction. This notion was further corroborated by the low A3F expression levels in PBMCs when compared to A3G (Mulder et al. 2010). The same mutant HIV W11R is restricted in the frequently used nonpermissive MT2 T-cell line, which expresses comparable levels of A3G and A3F. Recently, the modest activity of A3F has also been reported by others using stable cell lines (Miyagi et al. 2010).

Emerging evidence points to the importance of A3H in restricting HIV replication. A series of publications established that multiple A3H protein variants with distinct properties exist in human populations. Indeed, a cluster of single nucleotide polymorphisms (SNPs) determines protein stability, lentiviral restriction, as well as susceptibility to Vif-mediated degradation (Tan et al. 2009; OhAinle et al. 2008a, b; Harari et al. 2009; Dang et al. 2008). The Emerman laboratory reported that these destabilizing SNPs occurred twice independently during human evolution. The stable A3H variants (e.g., haplotype II) are found at high frequencies in populations of African descent (e.g., Yoruba), while they are less prevalent in European or Asian populations (OhAinle et al. 2008b). A3H is not only polymorphic in sequence but also subjected to alternative splicing (Harari et al. 2009). Evidence for HIV Vif adaptation to specific A3H haplotypes can be found in HIV-infected patients suggesting that A3H is a bona fide restriction factor (Ooms et al. 2013).

Deamination Target Site Preference of Human APOBEC3 Proteins

All APOBEC3 proteins are expressed to a varying degree in different human cell populations. Deamination by any of the APOBEC3 proteins is not specifically aimed at retroviral sequences but rather targets any single-stranded DNA. Indeed, APOBEC3-driven mutagenesis is not only apparent in retroviral genomes but also in human cancer genomes (Harris 2013; Kuong and Loeb 2013; Razzak 2013).

In contrast to this broad activity, APOBEC3 proteins display distinct target site discrimination (Albin and Harris 2010). For example, A3G favors a 5′-dCdC dinucleotide context ("GG" in the provirus), while the other deaminases with anti-HIV activity (A3DE, A3F, and A3H) favor a 5′-dTdC dinucleotide context ("GA" in the provirus). A3B has been shown to introduce mutations in both dinucleotide contexts (Albin and Harris 2010). Patient-derived proviral sequences display G-to-A mutations in both GG and GA dinucleotide contexts (Albin and Harris 2010; Fourati et al. 2014).

Vif Sequence Motifs Required for Anti-APOBEC3 Function

The HIV Vif protein promotes the ubiquitin/proteasome-dependent degradation of A3C, A3G, A3F, A3D, and A3H hapII (Albin and Harris 2010; Mehle et al. 2004). Of note, all functional domains of Vif have been mapped using Vif from subtype B molecular clones such as NL4-3, LAI or HXB2, and APOBEC3 reference proteins. Based on these analyses, the N-terminal region of Vif is important for Vif binding to A3G, A3F, and possibly other APOBEC3 proteins (Mariani et al. 2003; Mehle et al. 2004; Russell and Pathak 2007; Conticello et al. 2003b; Kao et al. 2003; Simon et al. 2005; Mehle et al. 2007; Schrofelbauer et al. 2006; Tian et al. 2006; Wichroski et al. 2005). Site-directed mutagenesis studies revealed that a number of residues located throughout the protein are essential for infectivity and viral replication in nonpermissive cells (Simon et al. 1999; Fujita et al. 2003). Mutations of the two cysteine residues (positions 114 and 133; Ma et al. 1994) as well as alanine substitutions in the conserved SLQ sequence motif (residues 144–147) abolish Vif activity. The C-terminal region of Vif contains the SLQYLAXXXX SOCS-box (residues 145–154) which is important for Vif binding to Elongin C in the E3 ubiquitin ligase complex (Yu et al. 2004; Stanley et al. 2008). Mutations of this domain abrogate Vif activity against A3G and A3F due to loss of interaction between Vif and Elongin C (Liu et al. 2004; Simon et al. 1999). This region also contains the zinc-binding HCCH motif consisting of residues H108, C114, C133, and H139, which is necessary for Vif binding to Cullin 5. By binding to Cullin 5 and Elongin C, Vif mediates polyubiquitination of APOBEC3 proteins and subsequent degradation via the 26S proteasome (Albin and Harris 2010; Paul et al. 2006; Luo et al. 2005; Mehle et al. 2006; Xiao et al. 2007a, b). In summary, the N-terminal region of Vif allows APOBEC3-specific interactions, while the C-terminal region connects to the host cell machinery.

The ability of HIV-1 Vif to "neutralize" APOBEC3-mediated HIV-1 mutagenesis varies in circulating strains. Our group found that about 20 % of naturally occurring Vif proteins are defective with some Vif proteins being selectively able to neutralize particular APOBEC3 enzymes and not others (Simon et al. 2005). Most Vif alleles from different subtypes neutralize A3G but display differences with respect to recognizing A3F and A3H haplotype (hap) II. Importantly, some subtype C and F Vif variants efficiently counteracted A3H hapII (Binka et al. 2012).

The Importance of the Vif-APOBEC3 Axis for Viral Diversity and the Shaping of the HIV Pandemic

The accessory HIV protein Vif counteracts the antiretroviral activity of some but not all APOBEC3 proteins (A3G/A3F, highly Vif sensitive; A3B/A3H, only partially Vif sensitive). HIV strains with Vif alleles unable to neutralize A3G have been identified in vivo, suggesting that complete neutralization of A3G is not necessary for the survival of HIV as a population (Mulder et al. 2008; Piantadosi et al. 2009). Indeed, the partial neutralization of APOBEC3 by Vif may be beneficial for HIV's diversity and spread. However, it remains controversial to what extent APOBEC3-driven mutagenesis contributes to viral evolution and disease control in vivo: some studies find a correlation between frequency of G-to-A mutations and viral loads (Pace et al. 2006), whereas others fail to find such association (Piantadosi et al. 2009; Gandhi et al. 2008). Work from several groups suggests that differences in Vif activity shape the phenotype of circulating viruses and facilitate emergence of drug resistance (Mulder et al. 2008; Fourati et al. 2010). For example, HIV can exploit APOBEC3 to escape from the antiretroviral drug 3TC (Mulder et al. 2008). HIV mutant viruses carrying single nucleotide Vif-inactivating mutations displayed attenuated growth in human PBMCs. In the absence of any drug selection, these infections, however, resulted in a diverse proviral population with high frequency of 3TC drug resistance-associated mutations. Moreover, wild-type HIV produced in the presence of hypermutated proviruses rapidly acquired drug resistance, likely by recombination, and thrived at 3TC concentrations that were lethal for the wild-type virus (Mulder et al. 2008). These results suggest that hypermutated, defective proviruses can shape the phenotype of circulating viruses. This observation represents a novel concept since hypermutated proviruses are generally regarded as evolutionary dead ends. The clinical and immunological relevance of deaminated long-lived proviral reservoirs will need to be reevaluated in the light of these findings. Of note, these initial observations have been reproduced and extended by other laboratories (Sadler et al. 2010; Kim et al. 2010).

Further evidence that APOBEC3 modulation drives viral evolution was provided by the examination of protease (PR), reverse transcriptase (RT), and Vif sequences of viruses derived from plasma of HIV-1-infected individuals failing antiretroviral treatment and compared them to HIV-1 from antiretroviral-naive patients (Fourati et al. 2010). In this patient cohort, a specific substitution in Vif (Vif K22H) was positively associated with treatment failure. Indeed, RT and PR sequences derived from patients harboring Vif K22H showed a significantly higher number of G-to-A (GA and GG dinucleotide contexts) drug resistance-associated mutations. Upon infection of the nonpermissive MT2 cells, most of the K22H proviral clones encoded increased numbers of G-to-A mutations. Among these mutations, the 3TC drug resistance-associated mutation M184I in RT was detected in 25 % of the clones in the absence of any 3TC exposure. These data provide evidence that patients experiencing antiretroviral treatment failure may harbor defective Vif alleles (i.e., K22H). Such Vif variants, which may occur more frequently in certain HIV subtypes, impact virological responses to antiretroviral therapy as they lose their ability to counteract APOBEC3 proteins leading to an increased number of G-to-A mutations that facilitate the emergence of antiretroviral resistance mutations (Fourati et al. 2010; Yebra and Holguin 2011).

The Challenges Arising from HIV-1 Viral Diversity

Extensive viral diversity on both an individual and a population level is the hallmark of RNA virus infection (Moya et al. 2004). High viral replication rate, low fidelity of reverse transcription, and the ability to recombine are the viral determinants that lead to the assortment of heterogeneous HIV-1 species found in chronically infected individuals. Variations in sequence may determine changes in viral phenotype and/or fitness and allow for rapid adaptation in the face of inhibitors. Thus, the continuously evolving HIV-1 diversity poses an immense challenge to any therapeutic interventions.

Viral Diversity from a Molecular Epidemiological Perspective

From an evolutionary point of view, HIV-1 diversification takes place at two different levels: within the infected individual (intra-host) and within the entire host population (inter-host). Different forces influence these processes, and there is evidence for positive selection only within intra-host evolution.

The propensity of HIV to rapidly mutate facilitated the spread of this virus through susceptible populations. Based on phylogenetic analyses, the HIV pandemic is estimated to have originated in the first decades of the twentieth century (Korber et al. 2000). The HIV subtype 1 genome resembles most closely lentiviral sequences derived from chimpanzees in western and central Africa (Gao et al. 1999). Approximately a century after the initial cross-species transmission events, HIV has diversified into numerous clades (e.g., subtypes A-H, "main group") as well as a number of circulating recombinant forms (CRF) that differ to some extent in their biological characteristics (e.g., co-receptor usage, anti-APOBEC3 activity of Vif alleles). Nonetheless, all HIV strains elicit a gradual depletion of CD4+ T lymphocytes leading to the clinical picture of acquired immunodeficiency syndrome (AIDS).

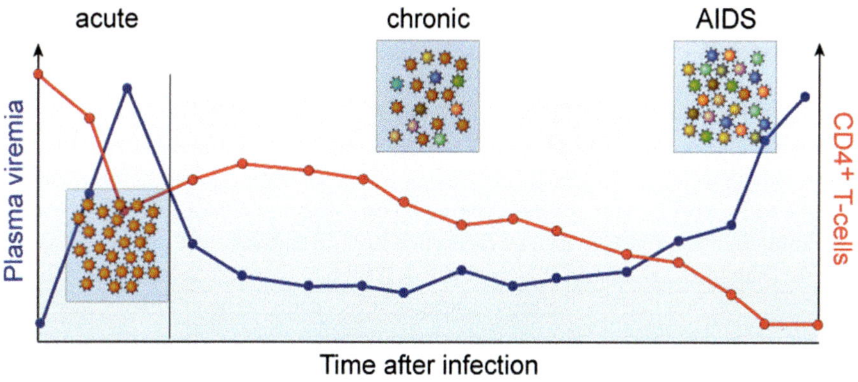

Fig. 4 Viral diversification throughout the infection is depicted. The transmitted founder virus diversifies rapidly in the new host in order to achieve optimal fitness. The interplay between APOBEC3 repertoire and HIV Vif phenotype of the transmitted HIV strain may impact AIDS disease outcome

Thus, HIV variation likely contributed to necessary viral adaptation to the human species.

HIV replication is very dynamic in nature, with the half-life of a virion being so short that half of the entire plasma virus population is replaced in less than 6 h (Simon and Ho 2003). Consequently, the total number of virions produced and released in an untreated HIV-infected person can reach on the order of $>10^{10}$ particles per day (see review by Simon and Ho 2003). The HIV virion contains two RNA copies of its genome which may differ if the producer cell was infected by more than one provirus. Since viral reverse transcription has no proofreading function, approximately 0.2–1 errors are introduced per genome in each replication cycle (Coffin 1995; Martinez et al. 1994). Consequently every single mutation at every possible position of the 9,500 nucleotide-long HIV-1 genome will arise daily (Coffin 1995). Moreover, APOBEC3-driven mutagenesis can introduce additional mutations (Simon et al. 2005). Additionally, crossover events between two genomes during the process of reverse transcription can result in the generation of recombinant forms. Recent evidence suggests that recombination takes place at a significantly higher rate than initially predicted (Levy et al. 2004). Thus, mutations – introduced by RT or APOBEC3 – and recombination fueled by a high turnover rate of virus production are the main features underlying intra-host HIV-1 variation (Fig. 4).

Viral Diversity from a Molecular Biology Perspective

HIV-1 is a complex retrovirus that encodes regulatory genes (e.g., vif, rev, nef) in addition to the gag, pol, and env genes found in all other retrovirus species (Freed and Martin 2001). Although the codon usage of retroviruses generally displays a nucleotide composition that is skewed toward adenosine in their nucleotide composition, the HIV-1 genome reflects a remarkable preference for adenosine (A, 36 %; G, 24 %; T, 22 %; C, 18 %; Berkhout et al. 2002). Possible explanations that have been proposed to explain the bias include RT-associated preferential incorporation rate in the viral plus-strand and unbalanced intracellular nucleotide pools (Martinez et al. 1994). It has also been speculated that selection pressures could be exerted on the retroviral genome by host-specific constraints such as host restriction factors (van Hemert and Berkhout 1995; Rambaut et al. 2004).

The situation is further complicated by the phenomenon of "G-to-A hypermutation," defined as the monotonous and extensive substitution of guanosine by adenosine. Hypermutated viral genes have first been described as arising during in vitro culture of certain HIV-1 isolates (Vartanian et al. 1991). Independently of in vitro propagation, hypermutations have been described throughout the entire genome of certain viral isolates (e.g., HIV-1 group O strain Vau; Vartanian et al. 2002), resulting in a level of mutations that renders these genomes replication defective. Hypermutated HIV-1 sequences have also been amplified from PBMC of long-term nonprogressors (LTNP; Wei et al. 2004) as well as chronically infected patients (Huang et al. 1998; Janini 2001; Koulinska et al. 2003). HIV undergoes a rapid evolution as the result of the action of error-prone reverse transcriptase, fast replication turnover, and recombination (Ho et al. 1995; Jirillo et al. 1994; Wei et al. 1995). It is attractive to speculate that APOBEC3-driven mutagenesis is another mechanism for HIV-1 diversification. Viruses derived from early infections frequently encode G-to-A mutations in CTL epitopes (Wood et al. 2009) in agreement with the fact that APOBEC3s are part of the early innate immune defense system (Koning et al. 2009; Neil and Bieniasz 2009). Mutagenesis of proviral sequences has been used as a surrogate marker for past APOBEC3 activity in vivo. Endogenous expression levels of APOBEC3 and phenotypic Vif function are important elements that modify the outcome of APOBEC3 restriction. APOBEC3 expression is very variable in HIV target cells in vivo given that these proteins are constitutively expressed but are also inducible by interferons (Chen et al. 2006; Peng et al. 2006). APOBEC3 transcripts are detectable in peripheral blood mononuclear cells as well as many other human tissues (Koning et al. 2009; Cullen 2006; Refsland et al. 2010). Moreover, expression levels are cell type-dependent (Albin and Harris 2010; Refsland et al. 2010; Peng et al. 2007) and could change during cell differentiation. For example, Th1 CD4+ T cells were reported to express more A3G compared to Th2 CD4+ T-cells subsets (Vetter and D'Aquila 2009).

Taken together, hypermutations can be produced artificially in vitro by modulating the dNTP balance (Vartanian et al. 1994, 1997), but the identification of cDNA deamination by the APOBEC3 proteins suggests that intrinsic host defenses provide an additional source of in vivo mutagenesis. Both the adenosine bias of the HIV-1 genome and the occasionally observed extensive G-to-A mutations could, indeed, be interpreted as footprints of more or less successful Vif-mediated protection from intracellular deamination (Hache et al. 2006).

HIV-1 Adaptation to Antiretroviral Selection Pressure

An increasing body of evidence demonstrates that cytotoxic T-cell (CTL) escape variants as well as drug-resistant HIV are transmissible. The evolution of drug-resistant viral variants can be divided into two phases. Initially, drug-resistant viruses are selected solely based on their ability to replicate in the presence of a given pharmacological inhibitor, but typically display an impaired replication capacity in a drug-free environment. Ongoing viral evolution in the presence of suboptimal inhibitor concentrations leads, however, to the selection of variants with additional mutations that compensate for the impaired fitness of drug-resistant variants selected during the first phase. It has also been shown that an alteration of the endogenous dNTP pool can influence the emergence of drug-resistant mutants.

Is HIV Drug Resistance Mediated by G→A Mutations?

The HIV-1 genome is adenosine rich, suggesting that the protection from cytidine deamination mediated by Vif may not be complete in vivo. Moreover, the frequency of G→A mutations resulting from the antiviral activity of APOBEC3G exceeds the rate of mutations randomly generated by HIV-1 RT by almost an order of magnitude (Mariani 2003). Twenty-one percent of all drug resistance-conferring mutations in PR, RT, and envelope are due to G-to-A substitutions (Berkhout and De Ronde 2004; Jern et al. 2009). More specifically, in 6/20 (30 %) codons in protease (PR – D30N, V32I, M36I, M46I, A71T, V77I), 8/22 (33 %) codons in reverse transcriptase (RT – D67N, V75I, V106M/I, V108I, V118I, M184I, E138K, G190E), and 2/10 (20 %) codons in the heptad repeat 1 (HR1) of gp41 (G36S/D, V38M), G-to-A substitutions result in drug resistance-associated mutations. One can speculate that some Vif alleles in vivo will likely be less efficient at mediating DNA deaminase degradation, and the generation of drug resistance mutations involving G-to-A transitions may be favored in this scenario.

Not every G-to-A mutation, however, should be considered a cytidine deaminase-induced hypermutation. The latter has been shown to occur in a nucleotide context-dependent manner (GA or GG), and hypermutated HIV sequences may display a range of nucleotide transitions with up to 60 % of all guanosine being replaced by adenosine (OhAinle et al. 2008b). As mentioned previously, the intrinsic sequence preference of A3G, A3F, A3DE, or A3H leads to cytidine deamination in a dinucleotide context-dependent manner with GG, respectively, GA being the favorite target (Malim 2009). These observations may be relevant to the mutational process leading to the selection of drug-resistant mutants. It seems possible that the generation of a subset of drug resistance-associated mutations involving G-to-A mutations in a GG or GA context (e.g., the primary mutations D30N in HIV protease and M184I, E138K in HIV RT) may be favored in cytidine deaminase expressing cell populations (e.g., T lymphocytes). This would be especially true in the genetic context of a partially active Vif allele.

Resistance to the nucleoside analogue lamivudine (3TC) emerges within weeks of treatment since only a single nucleotide mutation is required to change the methionine (M) codon to valine (V) or isoleucine (I) at position 184 of RT. Residue 184 is located in the conserved YMDD motif at the polymerase active site. M184I/V mutations have been reported to alter RT processivity and reduce the viral replication rate over multiple rounds of infection although single cycle replication rates are only modestly reduced compared to that of wild-type viruses. Both M184I and M184V lead to a more than 500-fold reduced susceptibility to 3TC. Interestingly, it has been reported that mutant M184I emerges first and disappears when viral variants encoding M184V appear. These divergent kinetics have been attributed in the past to differences in replication capacity and RT polymerase function. Of note, M184I mutation results from a single G-to-A substitution, whereas a single A-to-G mutation leads to M184V. Cell culture experiments suggest that A3G-mediated mutagenesis editing facilitates emergence of M184I variants in the presence of the antiretroviral drug lamivudine (Kim et al. 2010). Moreover, HIV can exploit APOBEC3 to escape from 3TC by allowing hypermutated, defective proviruses to shape the phenotype of circulating viruses via recombination (Mulder et al. 2008).

Conclusions

All pandemic HIV strains are (multi)-APOBEC3 resistant through the expression of the accessory protein Vif. The genetic variation within HIV-1 Vif itself has the potential to determine the spread of HIV subtypes on a global level as well as HIV/AIDS disease progression on an individual level. Taken together, a better understanding of the underlying viral-host interactions will have direct implications for the prevention and treatment of HIV/AIDS disease. Additional studies aimed at dissecting the forces driving HIV drug resistance and viral evolution in the presence of APOBEC3 expression are urgently needed. This is especially relevant since future inhibitors targeting the HIV-APOBEC3 interaction will likely be administered as part of combination antiretroviral treatments.

Acknowledgments We thank the members of the Simon laboratory for helpful discussions, critical review of the chapter, and assistance with the figures.

References

Albin JS, Harris RS (2010) Interactions of host APOBEC3 restriction factors with HIV-1 in vivo: implications for therapeutics. Expert Rev Mol Med 12:e4

Albin JS, Anderson JS, Johnson JR, Harjes E, Matsuo H, Krogan NJ, Harris RS (2013) Dispersed sites of HIV Vif-dependent polyubiquitination in the DNA deaminase APOBEC3F. J Mol Biol 425:1172–1182

Berkhout B, De Ronde A (2004) APOBEC3G versus reverse transcriptase in the generation of HIV-1 drug-resistance mutations. AIDS 18:1861–1863

Berkhout B, Grigoriev A, Bakker M, Lukashov VV (2002) Codon and amino acid usage in retroviral genomes is consistent with virus-specific nucleotide pressure. AIDS Res Hum Retroviruses 18:133–141
Bieniasz PD (2004) Intrinsic immunity: a front-line defense against viral attack. Nat Immunol 5:1109–1115
Binka M, Ooms M, Steward M, Simon V (2012) The activity spectrum of Vif from multiple HIV-1 subtypes against APOBEC3G, APOBEC3F, and APOBEC3H. J Virol 86:49–59
Chaipan C, Smith JL, Hu WS, Pathak VK (2013) APOBEC3G restricts HIV-1 to a greater extent than APOBEC3F and APOBEC3DE in human primary CD4+ T cells and macrophages. J Virol 87:444–453
Chen K, Huang J, Zhang C, Huang S, Nunnari G, Wang FX, Tong X, Gao L, Nikisher K, Zhang H (2006) Alpha interferon potently enhances the anti-human immunodeficiency virus type 1 activity of APOBEC3G in resting primary CD4 T cells. J Virol 80:7645–7657
Coffin JM (1995) HIV population dynamics in vivo: implications for genetic variation, pathogenesis, and therapy. Science 267:483–489
Conticello S, Harris R, Neuberger M (2003a) The Vif protein of HIV triggers degradation of the human antiretroviral DNA deaminase APOBEC3G. Curr Biol 13:2009–2013
Conticello SG, Harris RS, Neuberger MS (2003b) The Vif protein of HIV triggers degradation of the human antiretroviral DNA deaminase APOBEC3G. Curr Biol 13:2009–2013
Cullen BR (2006) Role and mechanism of action of the APOBEC3 family of antiretroviral resistance factors. J Virol 80:1067–1076
Dang Y, Siew LM, Wang X, Han Y, Lampen R, Zheng YH (2008) Human cytidine deaminase APOBEC3H restricts HIV-1 replication. J Biol Chem 283:11606–11614
Fourati S, Malet I, Binka M, Boukobza S, Wirden M, Sayon S, Simon A, Katlama C, Simon V, Calvez V, Marcelin AG (2010) Partially active HIV-1 Vif alleles facilitate viral escape from specific antiretrovirals. AIDS 24:2313–2321
Fourati S, Lambert-Niclot S, Soulie C, Wirden M, Malet I, Valantin MA, Tubiana R, Simon A, Katlama C, Carcelain G, Calvez V, Marcelin AG (2014) Differential impact of APOBEC3-driven mutagenesis on HIV evolution in diverse anatomical compartments. AIDS 28:487–491
Freed EO, Martin MA (2001) Chapter 59: HIVs and their replication. In: Knipe DM, Howley PM (eds) Fields virology, 4th edn. Lippincott Williams & Wilkins, Philadelphia, pp 1971–2042
Fujita M, Sakurai A, Yoshida A, Miyaura M, Koyama AH, Sakai K, Adachi A (2003) Amino acid residues 88 and 89 in the central hydrophilic region of human immunodeficiency virus type 1 Vif are critical for viral infectivity by enhancing the steady-state expression of Vif. J Virol 77:1626–1632
Gandhi SK, Siliciano JD, Bailey JR, Siliciano RF, Blankson JN (2008) Role of APOBEC3G/F-mediated hypermutation in the control of human immunodeficiency virus type 1 in elite suppressors. J Virol 82:3125–3130
Gao F, Bailes E, Robertson DL, Chen Y, Rodenburg CM, Michael SF, Cummins LB, Arthur LO, Peeters M, Shaw GM, Sharp PM, Hahn BH (1999) Origin of HIV-1 in the chimpanzee Pan troglodytes troglodytes. Nature 397:436–441
Gillick K, Pollpeter D, Phalora P, Kim EY, Wolinsky SM, Malim MH (2013) Suppression of HIV-1 infection by APOBEC3 proteins in primary human CD4(+) T cells is associated with inhibition of processive reverse transcription as well as excessive cytidine deamination. J Virol 87:1508–1517
Guo Y, Dong L, Qiu X, Wang Y, Zhang B, Liu H, Yu Y, Zang Y, Yang M, Huang Z (2014) Structural basis for hijacking CBF-beta and CUL5 E3 ligase complex by HIV-1 Vif. Nature 505:229–233
Hache G, Mansky LM, Harris RS (2006) Human APOBEC3 proteins, retrovirus restriction, and HIV drug resistance. AIDS Rev 8:148–157
Harari A, Ooms M, Mulder LC, Simon V (2009) Polymorphisms and splice variants influence the antiretroviral activity of human APOBEC3H. J Virol 83:295–303
Harris RS (2013) Cancer mutation signatures, DNA damage mechanisms, and potential clinical implications. Genome Med 5:87

Harris RS, Bishop KN, Sheehy AM, Craig HM, Petersen-Mahrt SK, Watt IN, Neuberger MS, Malim MH (2003) DNA deamination mediates innate immunity to retroviral infection. Cell 113:803–809

Ho DD, Neumann AU, Perelson AS, Chen W, Leonard JM, Markowitz M (1995) Rapid turnover of plasma virions and CD4 lymphocytes in HIV-1 infection. Nature 373:123–126

Huang Y, Zhang L, Ho DD (1998) Characterization of gag and pol sequences from long-term survivors of human immunodeficiency virus type 1 infection. Virology 240:36–49

Hultquist JF, Lengyel JA, Refsland EW, Larue RS, Lackey L, Brown WL, Harris RS (2011) Human and rhesus APOBEC3D, APOBEC3F, APOBEC3G, and APOBEC3H demonstrate a conserved capacity to restrict Vif-deficient HIV-1. J Virol 8:11220–11234

Jager S, Kim DY, Hultquist JF, Shindo K, LaRue RS, Kwon E, Li M, Anderson BD, Yen L, Stanley D, Mahon C, Kane J, Franks-Skiba K, Cimermancic P, Burlingame A, Sali A, Craik CS, Harris RS, Gross JD, Krogan NJ (2012) Vif hijacks CBF-beta to degrade APOBEC3G and promote HIV-1 infection. Nature 481:371–375

Janini M (2001) Human immunodeficiency virus type 1 DNA sequences genetically damaged by hypermutation are often abundant in patient peripheral blood mononuclear cells and may be generated during near-simultaneous infection and activation of CD4+ T cells. J Virol 75:7973–7986

Jarmuz A (2002) An anthropoid-specific locus of orphan C to U RNA-editing enzymes on chromosome 22. Genomics 79:285–296

Jern P, Russell RA, Pathak VK, Coffin JM (2009) Likely role of APOBEC3G-mediated G-to-A mutations in HIV-1 evolution and drug resistance. PLoS Pathog 5:e1000367

Jirillo E, Covelli V, Maffione AB, Greco B, Pece S, Fumarola D, Antonaci S, De Simone C (1994) Endotoxins, cytokines, and neuroimmune networks with special reference to HIV infection. Ann N Y Acad Sci 741:174–184

Kao S, Khan MA, Miyagi E, Plishka R, Buckler-White A, Strebel K (2003) The human immunodeficiency virus type 1 Vif protein reduces intracellular expression and inhibits packaging of APOBEC3G (CEM15), a cellular inhibitor of virus infectivity. J Virol 77:11398–11407

Kim EY, Bhattacharya T, Kunstman K, Swantek P, Koning FA, Malim MH, Wolinsky SM (2010) Human APOBEC3G-mediated editing can promote HIV-1 sequence diversification and accelerate adaptation to selective pressure. J Virol 84:10402–10405

Kim DY, Kwon E, Hartley PD, Crosby DC, Mann S, Krogan NJ, Gross JD (2013) CBFbeta stabilizes HIV Vif to counteract APOBEC3 at the expense of RUNX1 target gene expression. Mol Cell 49:632–644

Koning FA, Newman EN, Kim EY, Kunstman KJ, Wolinsky SM, Malim MH (2009) Defining APOBEC3 expression patterns in human tissues and hematopoietic cell subsets. J Virol 83:9474–9485

Korber B, Muldoon M, Theiler J, Gao F, Gupta R, Lapedes A, Hahn BH, Wolinsky S, Bhattacharya T (2000) Timing the ancestor of the HIV-1 pandemic strains. Science 288:1789–1796

Koulinska IN, Chaplin B, Mwakagile D, Essex M, Renjifo B (2003) Hypermutation of HIV type 1 genomes isolated from infants soon after vertical infection. AIDS Res Hum Retroviruses 19:1115–1123

Kuong KJ, Loeb LA (2013) APOBEC3B mutagenesis in cancer. Nat Genet 45:964–965

Lecossier D (2003) Hypermutation of HIV-1 DNA in the absence of the Vif protein. Science 300:1112

Levy DN, Aldrovandi GM, Kutsch O, Shaw GM (2004) Dynamics of HIV-1 recombination in its natural target cells. Proc Natl Acad Sci U S A 101:4204–4209, Epub 2004 Mar 4209

Liu B, Yu X, Luo K, Yu Y, Yu XF (2004) Influence of primate lentiviral Vif and proteasome inhibitors on human immunodeficiency virus type 1 virion packaging of APOBEC3G. J Virol 78:2072–2081

Luo K, Xiao Z, Ehrlich E, Yu Y, Liu B, Zheng S, Yu XF (2005) Primate lentiviral virion infectivity factors are substrate receptors that assemble with cullin 5-E3 ligase through a HCCH motif to suppress APOBEC3G. Proc Natl Acad Sci U S A 102:11444–11449

Ma XY, Sova P, Chao W, Volsky DJ (1994) Cysteine residues in the Vif protein of human immunodeficiency virus type 1 are essential for viral infectivity. J Virol 68:1714–1720

Malim MH (2009) APOBEC proteins and intrinsic resistance to HIV-1 infection. Philos Trans R Soc Lond B Biol Sci 364:675–687

Mangeat B (2003) Broad antiretroviral defence by human APOBEC3G through lethal editing of nascent reverse transcripts. Nature 424:99–103

Mariani R (2003) Species-specific exclusion of APOBEC3G from HIV-1 virions by Vif. Cell 114:21–31

Mariani R, Chen D, Schrofelbauer B, Navarro F, Konig R, Bollman B, Munk C, Nymark-McMahon H, Landau NR (2003) Species-specific exclusion of APOBEC3G from HIV-1 virions by Vif. Cell 114:21–31

Marin M (2003) HIV-1 Vif protein binds the editing enzyme APOBEC3G and induces its degradation. Nat Med 9:1398–1403

Martinez MA, Vartanian JP, Wain-Hobson S (1994) Hypermutagenesis of RNA using human immunodeficiency virus type 1 reverse transcriptase and biased dNTP concentrations. Proc Natl Acad Sci U S A 91:11787–11791

Mehle A, Strack B, Ancuta P, Zhang C, McPike M, Gabuzda D (2004) Vif overcomes the innate antiviral activity of APOBEC3G by promoting its degradation in the ubiquitin-proteasome pathway. J Biol Chem 279:7792–7798, Epub 2003 Dec 7713

Mehle A, Thomas ER, Rajendran KS, Gabuzda D (2006) A zinc-binding region in Vif binds Cul5 and determines cullin selection. J Biol Chem 281:17259–17265

Mehle A, Wilson H, Zhang C, Brazier AJ, McPike M, Pery E, Gabuzda D (2007) Identification of an APOBEC3G binding site in human immunodeficiency virus type 1 Vif and inhibitors of Vif-APOBEC3G binding. J Virol 81:13235–13241

Miyagi E, Brown CR, Opi S, Khan M, Goila-Gaur R, Kao S, Walker RC Jr, Hirsch V, Strebel K (2010) Stably expressed APOBEC3F has negligible antiviral activity. J Virol 84: 11067–11075

Moya A, Holmes EC, Gonzalez-Candelas F (2004) The population genetics and evolutionary epidemiology of RNA viruses. Nat Rev Microbiol 2:279–288

Mulder LC, Harari A, Simon V (2008) Cytidine deamination induced HIV-1 drug resistance. Proc Natl Acad Sci U S A 105:5501–5506

Mulder LC, Ooms M, Majdak S, Smedresman J, Linscheid C, Harari A, Kunz A, Simon V (2010) Moderate influence of human APOBEC3F on HIV-1 replication in primary lymphocytes. J Virol 84:9613–9617

Neil S, Bieniasz P (2009) Human immunodeficiency virus, restriction factors, and interferon. J Interferon Cytokine Res 29:569–580

Neuberger MS (2003) Immunity through DNA deamination. Trends Biochem Sci 28:305–312

OhAinle M, Kerns JA, Li MMH, Malik HS, Emerman M (2008a) Antiretroelement activity of APOBEC3H was lost twice in recent human evolution. Cell Host Microbe 4:249–259

OhAinle M, Kerns JA, Li MM, Malik HS, Emerman M (2008b) Antiretroelement activity of APOBEC3H was lost twice in recent human evolution. Cell Host Microbe 4:249–259

Ooms M, Brayton B, Letko M, Maio SM, Pilcher CD, Hecht FM, Barbour JD, Simon V (2013) HIV-1 Vif adaptation to human APOBEC3H haplotypes. Cell Host Microbe 14:411–421

Pace C, Keller J, Nolan D, James I, Gaudieri S, Moore C, Mallal S (2006) Population level analysis of human immunodeficiency virus type 1 hypermutation and its relationship with APOBEC3G and vif genetic variation. J Virol 80:9259–9269

Paul I, Cui J, Maynard EL (2006) Zinc binding to the HCCH motif of HIV-1 virion infectivity factor induces a conformational change that mediates protein-protein interactions. Proc Natl Acad Sci U S A 103:18475–18480

Peng G, Lei KJ, Jin W, Greenwell-Wild T, Wahl SM (2006) Induction of APOBEC3 family proteins, a defensive maneuver underlying interferon-induced anti-HIV-1 activity. J Exp Med 203:41–46, Epub 2006 Jan 2017

Peng G, Greenwell-Wild T, Nares S, Jin W, Lei KJ, Rangel ZG, Munson PJ, Wahl SM (2007) Myeloid differentiation and susceptibility to HIV-1 are linked to APOBEC3 expression. Blood 110:393–400

Piantadosi A, Humes D, Chohan B, McClelland RS, Overbaugh J (2009) Analysis of the percentage of human immunodeficiency virus type 1 sequences that are hypermutated and markers of disease progression in a longitudinal cohort, including one individual with a partially defective Vif. J Virol 83:7805–7814

Rambaut A, Posada D, Crandall KA, Holmes EC (2004) The causes and consequences of HIV evolution. Nat Rev Genet 5:52–61

Razzak M (2013) Genetics: APOBEC-a double-edged sword. Nat Rev Clin Oncol 10:488

Refsland EW, Harris RS (2013) The APOBEC3 family of retroelement restriction factors. Curr Top Microbiol Immunol 371:1–27

Refsland EW, Stenglein MD, Shindo K, Albin JS, Brown WL, Harris RS (2010) Quantitative profiling of the full APOBEC3 mRNA repertoire in lymphocytes and tissues: implications for HIV-1 restriction. Nucleic Acids Res 38:4274–4284

Russell RA, Pathak VK (2007) Identification of two distinct HIV-1 Vif determinants critical for interactions with human APOBEC3G and APOBEC3F. J Virol 83:1992–2003

Sadler HA, Stenglein MD, Harris RS, Mansky LM (2010) APOBEC3G contributes to HIV-1 variation through sublethal mutagenesis. J Virol 84:7396–7404

Sato K, Takeuchi JS, Misawa N, Izumi T, Kobayashi T, Kimura Y, Iwami S, Takaori-Kondo A, Hu WS, Aihara K, Ito M, An DS, Pathak VK, Koyanagi Y (2014) APOBEC3D and APOBEC3F potently promote HIV-1 diversification and evolution in humanized mouse model. PLoS Pathog 10:e1004453

Schrofelbauer B, Senger T, Manning G, Landau NR (2006) Mutational alteration of human immunodeficiency virus type 1 Vif allows for functional interaction with nonhuman primate APOBEC3G. J Virol 80:5984–5991

Sheehy A, Gaddis N, Choi J, Malim M (2002) Isolation of a human gene that inhibits HIV-1 infection and is suppressed by the viral Vif protein. Nature 418:646–650

Simon V, Ho DD (2003) HIV-1 dynamics in vivo: implications for therapy. Nat Rev Microbiol 1:181–190

Simon JH, Sheehy AM, Carpenter EA, Fouchier RA, Malim MH (1999) Mutational analysis of the human immunodeficiency virus type 1 Vif protein. J Virol 73:2675–2681

Simon V, Zennou V, Murray D, Huang Y, Ho DD, Bieniasz PD (2005) Natural variation in Vif: differential impact on APOBEC3G/3F and a potential role in HIV-1 diversification. PLoS Pathog 1:e6

Stanley BJ, Ehrlich ES, Short L, Yu Y, Xiao Z, Yu XF, Xiong Y (2008) Structural insight into the human immunodeficiency virus Vif SOCS box and its role in human E3 ubiquitin ligase assembly. J Virol 82:8656–8663

Stopak K, de Noronha C, Yonemoto W, Greene WC (2003) HIV-1 Vif blocks the antiviral activity of APOBEC3G by impairing both its translation and intracellular stability. Mol Cell 12:591–601

Tan L, Sarkis PT, Wang T, Tian C, Yu XF (2009) Sole copy of Z2-type human cytidine deaminase APOBEC3H has inhibitory activity against retrotransposons and HIV-1. FASEB J 23:279–287

Tian C, Yu X, Zhang W, Wang T, Xu R, Yu XF (2006) Differential requirement for conserved tryptophans in human immunodeficiency virus type 1 Vif for the selective suppression of APOBEC3G and APOBEC3F. J Virol 80:3112–3115

van Hemert FJ, Berkhout B (1995) The tendency of lentiviral open reading frames to become A-rich: constraints imposed by viral genome organization and cellular tRNA availability. J Mol Evol 41:132–140

Vartanian JP, Meyerhans A, Asjo B, Wain-Hobson S (1991) Selection, recombination, and G→A hypermutation of human immunodeficiency virus type 1 genomes. J Virol 65:1779–1788

Vartanian JP, Meyerhans A, Sala M, Wain-Hobson S (1994) G→A hypermutation of the human immunodeficiency virus type 1 genome: evidence for dCTP pool imbalance during reverse transcription. Proc Natl Acad Sci U S A 91:3092–3096

Vartanian JP, Plikat U, Henry M, Mahieux R, Guillemot L, Meyerhans A, Wain-Hobson S (1997) HIV genetic variation is directed and restricted by DNA precursor availability. J Mol Biol 270:139–151

Vartanian JP, Henry M, Wain-Hobson S (2002) Sustained G→A hypermutation during reverse transcription of an entire human immunodeficiency virus type 1 strain Vau group O genome. J Gen Virol 83:801–805

Vetter ML, D'Aquila RT (2009) Cytoplasmic APOBEC3G restricts incoming Vif-positive human immunodeficiency virus type 1 and increases two-long terminal repeat circle formation in activated T-helper-subtype cells. J Virol 83:8646–8654

Wedekind JE, Dance GS, Sowden MP, Smith HC (2003) Messenger RNA editing in mammals: new members of the APOBEC family seeking roles in the family business. Trends Genet 19:207–216

Wei X, Ghosh SK, Taylor ME, Johnson VA, Emini EA, Deutsch P, Lifson JD, Bonhoeffer S, Nowak MA, Hahn BH et al (1995) Viral dynamics in human immunodeficiency virus type 1 infection. Nature 373:117–122

Wei M, Xing H, Hong K, Huang H, Tang H, Qin G, Shao Y (2004) Biased G-to-A hypermutation in HIV-1 proviral DNA from a long-term non-progressor. AIDS 18:1863–1865

Wichroski MJ, Ichiyama K, Rana TM (2005) Analysis of HIV-1 viral infectivity factor-mediated proteasome-dependent depletion of APOBEC3G: correlating function and subcellular localization. J Biol Chem 280:8387–8396

Wood N, Bhattacharya T, Keele BF, Giorgi E, Liu M, Gaschen B, Daniels M, Ferrari G, Haynes BF, McMichael A, Shaw GM, Hahn BH, Korber B, Seoighe C (2009) HIV evolution in early infection: selection pressures, patterns of insertion and deletion, and the impact of APOBEC. PLoS Pathog 5:e1000414

Xiao Z, Ehrlich E, Luo K, Xiong Y, Yu XF (2007a) Zinc chelation inhibits HIV Vif activity and liberates antiviral function of the cytidine deaminase APOBEC3G. FASEB J 21:217–222

Xiao Z, Xiong Y, Zhang W, Tan L, Ehrlich E, Guo D, Yu XF (2007b) Characterization of a novel Cullin5 binding domain in HIV-1 Vif. J Mol Biol 373:541–550

Yebra G, Holguin A (2011) Mutation Vif-22H, which allows HIV-1 to use the APOBEC3G hypermutation to develop resistance, could appear more quickly in certain non-B variants. J Antimicrob Chemother 66:941–942

Yu Q (2004) Single-strand specificity of APOBEC3G accounts for minus-strand deamination of the HIV genome. Nat Struct Mol Biol 11:435–442

Yu X, Yu Y, Liu B, Luo K, Kong W, Mao P, Yu XF (2003) Induction of APOBEC3G ubiquitination and degradation by an HIV-1 Vif-Cul5-SCF complex. Science 302:1056–1060, Epub 2003 Oct 1016

Yu Y, Xiao Z, Ehrlich ES, Yu X, Yu XF (2004) Selective assembly of HIV-1 Vif-Cul5-ElonginB-ElonginC E3 ubiquitin ligase complex through a novel SOCS box and upstream cysteines. Genes Dev 18:2867–2872

Zennou V, Perez-Caballero D, Gottlinger H, Bieniasz PD (2004) APOBEC3G incorporation into human immunodeficiency virus type 1 particles. J Virol 78:12058–12061

Zhang W, Du J, Evans SL, Yu Y, Yu XF (2012) T-cell differentiation factor CBF-beta regulates HIV-1 Vif-mediated evasion of host restriction. Nature 481:376–379

Resistance to Cyclophilin Inhibitors

Philippe Gallay

Contents

Abstract

The best approach to avoid hepatitis C virus (HCV) resistance to a specific therapy is rapid and massive suppression of viral replication. This is best accomplished by combining several drugs with potent antiviral activity across multiple genotypes, with each possessing a high barrier to resistance, different mechanisms of action, and no cross-resistance. A novel class of anti-HCV agents that have shown great promise in HCV patients – the cyclophilin inhibitors (CypI) – possess such properties. CypI are host-targeting antivirals (HTAs) with a mechanism of action that differs from those of all existing direct-acting antivirals (DAAs). CypI are pan-genotypic due to their distinct mechanism of action that targets the host protein cyclophilin A (CypA), which is required for HCV replication. HCV has to develop a lengthy mutational strategy to efficiently replicate in vitro independently of the host factor CypA leading to a high genetic barrier that the virus has to cross to develop resistance to CypI. CypI mediate rapid and profound viral load suppression in patients. Very low viral breakthrough rates are associated with the CypI treatment, which result mostly from suboptimal drug exposure rather than viral resistance. The high genetic barrier and the lack of cross-resistance to DAAs make CypI attractive drug candidates to

P. Gallay (✉)
Department of Immunology and Microbial Science, IMM-9, The Scripps Research Institute, La Jolla, CA, USA
e-mail: gallay@scripps.edu

M. Gotte et al. (eds.), *Handbook of Antimicrobial Resistance*,
DOI 10.1007/978-1-4939-0694-9_3

be part of a regimen with one or two DAAs that may constitute the backbone of a new, safe, and effective IFN-free therapy. The characteristic resistance profile of CypI offers an exceptional opportunity to cure HCV.

Keywords
Hepatitic • cyclophilin • cyclophilia inhibitas • NSSA • resistance

Abbreviations

BID	Taken twice a day
cEVR	Complete early virological response = no virus detected after 12 weeks
eRVR	Extended rapid virological response = no virus detected at week 4 and week 12
EVR	Early virological response = 2 log drop of HCV RNA after 12 weeks
QD	Taken once a day
RVR	Rapid virological response = no virus detected at week 4
SVR12	Sustained virological response = no virus detected at 12 weeks after completion of treatment
SVR24	No virus detected at 24 weeks after completion of treatment

Introduction

HCV is the major causative agent of acute and chronic liver diseases. Chronic infection is associated with higher risks of hepatocellular carcinoma and liver cirrhosis (Dienstag and McHutchison 2006). Nearly 200 million people worldwide (3 % of the population), including four to five million in the USA, are chronically infected with HCV, and four million new infections occur every year (Alter 2007; Soriano et al. 2008a; Global surveillance and control of HCV 1999; World Health Organization 2012). In the developed world, HCV accounts for 2/3 of all cases of liver cancer and transplants, and in the USA, ~12,000 people are estimated to die from HCV each year (Shepard et al. 2005; Armstrong et al. 2006). The weekly injection of pegylated IFNα together with the daily administration of the nucleoside analog ribavirin greatly enhanced the percentage of chronically HCV-infected patients able to reach a sustained antiviral response (SVR) – defined as a clearance of blood HCV RNA 24 weeks after treatment termination (Sy and Jamal 2006; Tong et al. 1997; Fried et al. 2002). However, the combination of pegylated IFNα and ribavirin has a success rate of merely ~50 % in patients with genotypes 1 and 4, often causing severe side effects as well (Cross et al. 2008; Simmonds et al. 2005; Manns et al. 2006). Not only is genotype 1 the most prevalent HCV genotype in Europe, North and South America, China, and Japan, it is also the most difficult to treat (Global Surveillance and Control of Hepatitis C 1999). There is thus an urgent need for the development of new potent pan-genotypic anti-HCV agents in order to improve, shorten, simplify, and lower the cost of HCV management.

Direct-Acting Agents. HCV treatment has been revolutionized by the development and recent FDA approval of direct-acting agents (DAAs). In contrast to the nonspecific antiviral activities of IFNα and ribavirin, DAAs target viral proteins. The binding of the DAA to its viral target neutralizes a function of the viral protein that is vital for the HCV replication cycle. The complexity of the viral cycle afforded the identification of several viral targets with DAAs such as the NS3/4A serine protease, the NS5B RNA-dependent RNA polymerase, and the NS5A protein. The NS3/4A protease inhibitors telaprevir and boceprevir were the first two DAAs to be approved by the FDA in 2011. The combination of boceprevir or telaprevir with pegylated IFNα and ribavirin significantly improved treatment efficacy to 75 % SVR in genotype 1 patients. This represented a major milestone in HCV therapy.

The persistence of the side effects associated with IFNα has lead to a novel therapeutic strategy. This approach entails an IFN-free treatment that would offer high efficacy, with manageable side effects. Three classes of DAAs could currently be part of this IFN-free regimen including second-generation NS3/4A protease inhibitors, NS5B polymerase inhibitors, and NS5A inhibitors. Recent phase II studies provided the proof of concept that combination therapy with DAAs can provide high efficacy in the absence of pegylated IFNα. Specifically, the combination of a nucleoside NS5B polymerase inhibitor and an NS5A inhibitor, with or without ribavirin, showed high SVR in treatment-naïve HCV-infected patients (Sulkowski et al. 2012; Gane et al. 2012). Moreover, the combination of an NS5A inhibitor, a protease inhibitor, and a non-nucleoside NS5B polymerase inhibitor also delivered high SVR in treatment-naïve genotype 1a-infected patients (Kowdley et al. 2012; Everson et al. 2012). These phase II studies provide the proof of concept that chronic infection can be cured using novel combinations of orally available DAAs in the absence of IFN. These regimens represent the future of HCV therapy. It is anticipated that in the coming years, the combination of existing or new DAAs without IFNα will reduce chronic infection to an easily treatable disease with the goal of cure being achieved in the vast majority of patients using simplified dosing regimens with minimal toxicity.

Host-Targeting Agents. Another promising therapeutic strategy consists of targeting host factors that are absolutely required for HCV replication, rather than viral factors (Pawlotsky 2012). Emerging host-targeting agent (HTA) candidates include inhibitors of viral entry, internal ribosome entry site-mediated viral translation, and viral RNA replication, along with viral assembly and release. Figure 1 shows the list of HTAs, which are in preclinical or clinical development. Importantly, one class of HTAs has showed great promise in HCV patients – cyclophilin inhibitors (CypI).

To date, three CypI – alisporivir (previously called DEB025), NIM-811, and SCY-635 – have demonstrated safety and efficacy in HCV-infected patients in phase I and II studies (Flisiak et al. 2007; Gallay 2009; Fischer et al. 2010; Pockros 2010; Liu 2010; von Hahn et al. 2011; Vermehren and Sarrazin 2011; Hopkins and Gallay 2012; Pawlotsky et al. 2012a). All three CypI are synthetic derivates of the immunosuppressive drug cyclosporine A (CsA) (Fig. 2). Slight chain modifications of the parental cyclic undecapeptide CsA enhance the binding affinity of alisporivir,

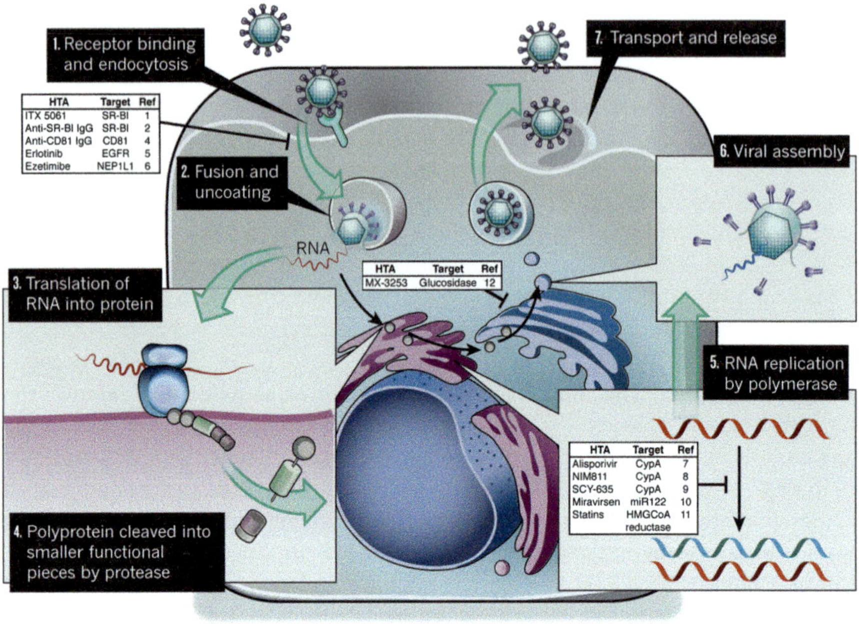

Fig. 1 Existing HTAs that interfere at various steps of the HCV replication cycle (Modified from Schlütter, *Nature*, 474 (2010))

Cyp Inhibitor:	Cyclosporin A	NIM811	Alisporivir	SCY-635
Structure:	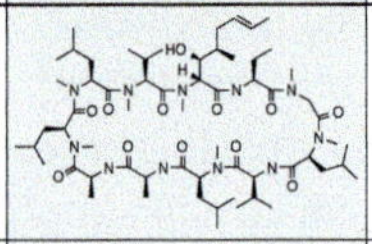	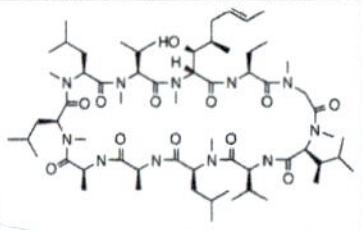	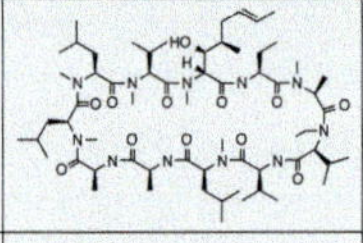	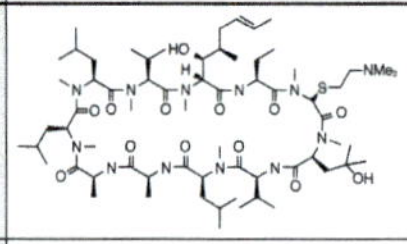
Anti-HCV Activity (EC_{50}):	0.3 μM	0.06 μM	0.04 μM	0.1 μM
Cyp PPIase Inhibition (KI):	9.79 nM	2.11 nM	0.34 nM	1.8 nM
Immunosuppression Activity (IL-2 Inhibition):	0.006 μg/mL	>10 μg/mL	21.5 μg/mL	13 μg/mL

Fig. 2 Antiviral, anti-PPIase, and anti-immunosuppressive activities of CypI

NIM-811, and SCY-635 to their host ligands – the cyclophilins – and abolish their binding to calcineurin, resulting in the elimination of their immunosuppressive activity (Fig. 2).

Cyclosporine A and Cyclophilins. The isolation of CsA from the fungus *Tolypocladium inflatum* in 1971 launched a new era in immunopharmacology (Borel 2002). It was the first immunosuppressive drug, which mediates specific down-immunoregulation of T cell expansion without excessive toxicity. CsA was approved in 1983 for its use to prevent graft rejection during organ transplantation

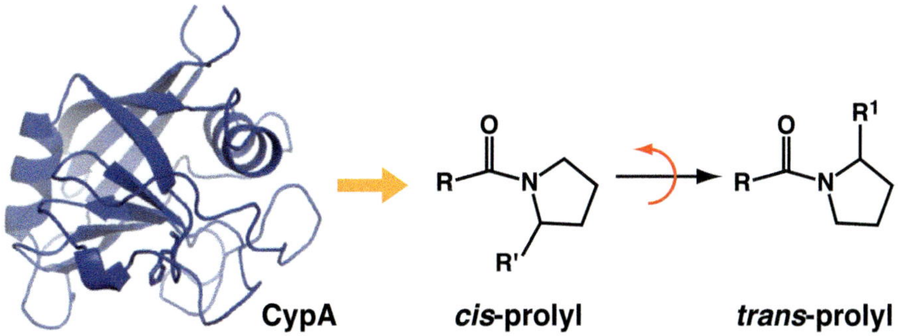

Year	Findings	References
1971	Discovery of cyclosporine A	Borel *et al.*, 2002
1983	Approval of the use cyclosporine A for organ transplantation	Flechner *et al.*, 1983
1984	Discovery of cyclophilin A as ligand for cyclosporine A	Handschumacher *et al.*, 1984
1984	Discovery of enzymes that accelerate the isomerization of peptidyl-prolyl bonds	Fischer *et al.*, 1984
1987	Classification of the peptidyl-prolyl *cis-trans* isomerases (PPIases)	Lang *et al.*, 1987
1989	Cyclophilin A is a peptidyl-prolyl *cis-trans* isomerase	Fischer *et al.*, 1989
1991	Cyclosporine A is a potent inhibitor of the peptidyl-prolyl *cis-trans* isomerase activity of cyclophilin A	Kofron *et al.*, 1991

Fig. 3 Discovery of the PPIase CypA

(Flechner 1983). The following year, cyclophilin A (CypA) was identified as the primary host cytosolic ligand of CsA (Handschumacher et al. 1984) as well as the main in vivo target for CsA in preventing tissue rejection by inhibition of the activation of T lymphocyte subsets (Borel 2002). Remarkably, the same year, a new type of enzymes, which accelerates the isomerization of peptidyl-prolyl bonds, was discovered (Fischer et al. 1984) (Fig. 3). These enzymes were classified as peptidyl-prolyl cis-trans isomerases (PPIases) (Lang et al. 1987). The isomerization to the *cis* form is required for de novo protein folding and refolding processes following membrane trafficking. Five years later, CypA was identified as the PPIase, which is responsible for the isomerization of peptidyl-prolyl bonds (Fischer et al. 1989). By binding to the hydrophobic pocket of CypA, CsA neutralizes its isomerase activity (Kofron et al. 1991).

Cyclophilin Inhibitors and HCV Replication. The connection between HCV and cyclophilins was made by several independent labs, which demonstrated that CypI including CsA, NIM811, SCY-635, and alisporivir block HCV replication in vitro (Watashi et al. 2003; Nakagawa et al. 2004; Goto et al. 2006; Ishii et al. 2006; Ma et al. 2006; Paeshuyse et al. 2006; Houck et al. 2006). Using stable knockdown approaches, CypA was found to be the major cyclophilin member vital for HCV replication (Yang et al. 2008; Chatterji et al. 2009; Kaul et al. 2009). The isomerase activity of CypA was found to be critical to support HCV replication (Chatterji et al. 2009; Liu et al. 2009; Kaul et al. 2009). Together these findings suggested that CypI exert their antiviral effect by targeting host CypA. The existence of knockout mice (Colgan et al. 2005) and knockout human cell lines (Braaten and Luban 2001), suggest that CypA is not only optional for cell growth and survival, but that it also represents a viable target for CypI in HCV therapy.

Mechanisms of Action of Cyclophilin Inhibitors. It has been postulated that CypI block HCV replication, by binding to the hydrophobic pocket of CypA, thereby neutralizing the isomerase activity of CypA. However, the precise mechanism of antiviral action of CypI remains to be fully elucidated. Several observations suggest that the HCV NS5A protein is the main viral ligand for CypA (Hanoulle et al. 2009; Waller et al. 2010; Fernandes et al. 2010; Chatterji et al. 2010; Yang et al. 2010; Coelmont et al. 2010; Foster et al. 2011; Verdegem et al. 2011). First, under CypI pressure, HCV develops resistance mutations mostly in the NS5A gene (Fernandes et al. 2007; Hopkins et al. 2010; Kaul et al. 2009; Chatterji et al. 2010; Yang et al. 2010; Coelmont et al. 2010). Second, CypA was found to interact directly with NS5A (Hanoulle et al. 2009; Chatterji et al. 2010; Yang et al. 2010; Coelmont et al. 2010; Fernandes et al. 2010). Third, CypI including CsA, alisporivir, SCY-635, and even the non-CsA derivate sanglifehrins prevent CypA-NS5A interactions (Hanoulle et al. 2009; Chatterji et al. 2010; Yang et al. 2010; Coelmont et al. 2010; Fernandes et al. 2010; Gregory et al. 2011; Hopkins et al. 2012). Fourth, NS5A proteins derived from all genotypes tested so far (1a, 1b, 2a, 2b, and 3) bind CypA directly, suggesting that CypA-NS5A interactions are conserved among HCV genotypes (Chatterji et al. 2010), which correlates well with the fact that CypI possess a pan-genotypic anti-HCV activity in HCV-infected patients (Flisiak et al. 2007; Gallay 2012; Fischer et al. 2010; Pockros 2010; von Hahn et al. 2011; Vermehren and Sarrazin 2011; Hopkins and Gallay 2012; Pawlotsky et al. 2012). Fifth, nuclear magnetic resonance (NMR) studies showed that CypA, via its enzymatic pocket, interacts with proline residues located within domains II and III of NS5A (Hanoulle et al. 2009; Coelmont et al. 2010; Verdegem et al. 2011; Rosnoblet et al. 2012). This is in accordance with the fact that CypA possesses the ability to catalyze the *cis* to *trans* isomerization of proline-containing peptides (Fischer et al. 1984). Altogether these data indicate that NS5A is the main viral ligand for CypA and that the abrogation of CypA-NS5A contacts by CypI is lethal to the virus.

Further work is required to determine how CypA interacting with NS5A assists HCV replication. Several findings obtained by independent labs suggest different functions for CypA in viral replication. The first finding was that CypA stimulates the RNA binding of NS5A and that the addition of CypI or the introduction of mutations in the isomerase pocket of CypA attenuates the CypA-mediated stimulation of the NS5A RNA binding (Foster et al. 2011). Thus, one can envision that the CypA-mediated enhancement of NS5A binding to the viral RNA is a critical event in HCV RNA replication. Previous work showed that NS5A, as a dimer, represents the RNA-binding-competent form of the protein (Hwang et al. 2010). NS5A, by binding to G/U-rich regions of the HCV genome, may play a key role in both HCV regulation and cellular gene expression (Huang et al. 2005; Hwang et al. 2010). The second finding was that the NS5B polymerase binds NS5A (Shirota et al. 2002) and that CypA and NS5B share a binding region in the domain II of NS5A (Rosnoblet et al. 2012). One thus can envision that CypA modulates an NS5A and/or NS5B function. For example, NS5A, by binding to NS5B, could inhibit its polymerase activity. In this scenario, CypA, by binding to NS5A, prevents its binding to NS5B, enabling the polymerase to replicate the viral genome. In this model, CypI, by blocking CypA-NS5A contacts, allows NS5A to bind to NS5B leading to inefficient RNA replication. In another example, CypA-NS5A complexes could promote either the viral RNA binding of NS5B and/or its enzymatic activity. In this scenario, the elimination of CypA-NS5A contacts by CypI blocks the NS5A-mediated activation of the NS5B polymerase activity, resulting in defective RNA replication. The action of CypA upon NS5B should be indirect since CypA does not bind to NS5B (Rosnoblet et al. 2012). Further work is required to determine which, if any, of these interesting findings represent the biologically relevant functionality of NS5A-CypA interactions.

A recent study suggested that the daily administration of a CypI (SCY-635) to HCV-infected patients causes fast increases in plasma concentrations of IFNα, $\lambda 1$, $\lambda 3$, 2′5′OAS-1, and neopterin (Hopkins et al. 2012). No changes were observed in either placebo-treated HCV patients or SCY-635-treated non-HCV-infected volunteers (Hopkins et al. 2012). These data suggest that in HCV-infected patients, the CypI administration and subsequent CypA neutralization reduce the plasma amounts of viruses and transiently increase the concentration of components in the IFN response. NS5A was shown to possess the ability to counter the rising IFN response that a cell develops during HCV invasion (He et al. 2006). Therefore, CypI, by preventing and disrupting CypA-NS5A interactions, may cause both a block in HCV replication and a rescue of the IFN response. It is likely that the rapid and transient increase of plasma concentration of components of the IFN response observed in SCY-635-treated HCV-infected patients originates from the block of HCV replication by the CypI and the prompt stoppage of the expression of viral proteins, which normally counter the IFN response (i.e., NS3, NS5A, core, and E2) (He et al. 2006). The SCY-635 in vivo findings remain to be confirmed for other CypI members. Indeed, it remains to be determined whether other or even all CypI also cause this rapid and transient raise of the plasma concentrations of components of the IFN response. A recent study obtained apparent conflicting results. Specifically, a comparison analysis of the expression of IFN-stimulated genes (ISGs) between baseline and week 4 of treatment demonstrated a downregulation rather than an upregulation of the expression of ISGs upon the administration of the CypI alisporivir (Pawlotsky et al. 2012). An elevated upregulation of the expression of ISG was observed in IFN-treated patients (Pawlotsky et al. 2012), demonstrating the accuracy of the ISG analysis.

To fully elucidate the mechanisms of antiviral action of CypI, several questions remain to be answered: (a) whether the binding activity or the isomerase activity of CypA is vital for HCV replication, (b) what is the precise activity of CypA on NS5A (i.e., folding, trafficking, protein-protein interactions, etc.), (c) how does the CypA activity promote HCV replication (i.e., enhancing NS5A and/or NS5B activities), and (d) whether CypA binds viral or host proteins other than NS5A and whether these interactions are critical for HCV replication. If these questions can be addressed, our understanding of both the role of CypA in HCV replication and the mechanisms of action of CypI will be greatly improved.

Clinical Safety and Efficacy of Cyclophilin Inhibitors. Clinical trials with the CypI NIM811 and SCY-635 were restricted to exploratory phase I and II trials with small and well-defined patient populations. In contrast, the safety and efficacy profiles of alisporivir were examined using a large patient population (~1,800). Alisporivir is currently being tested for safety and efficacy in phase III studies.

NIM811: The CypI NIM811 was administered orally at total daily doses ranging from 25 to 1,600 mg in treatment-experienced and treatment-naïve genotype 1 patients ($n = 72$) (Lawitz et al. 2011). NIM811 was well tolerated in all groups; however, suppression of plasma viremia was not observed at any dose level tested as monotherapy including the maximum daily dose of 1,200 mg. One cohort of patients was added at the completion of the monotherapy to assess the antiviral activity of NIM811 when administered in combination with pegylated IFNα. Patients received placebo or NIM811 at a dose of 600 mg given twice daily. At day 14, significant reductions from baseline in viral load were reported for patients who received combination therapy (2.85 ± 1.02 $\log^{10}$ IU/mL) when compared to patients who received pegylated IFNα only (0.65 ± 0.77 $\log^{10}$ IU/mL). The development of NIM811 was discontinued due to its weaker antiviral effect compared to that of alisporivir.

SCY-635: Ascending oral doses of SCY-635 (300, 600, or 900 mg/day) were administered for 15 days in genotype 1 patients (Hopkins et al. 2012). No evidence of clinical or laboratory toxicity was identified. SCY-635 at total daily doses of 300 or 600 mg was associated with insignificant changes in viral load, whereas patients who received 900 mg/day exhibited declines in viral load (1.90 $\log^{10}$ IU/mL below baseline), demonstrating the clinical efficacy of SCY-635.

Alisporivir: Alisporivir is the most advanced CypI in clinical development. The safety and efficacy results of sequential phase I and II studies, in which alisporivir was used as part of the anti-HCV treatment are described below. A phase III study was initiated in 2012; however, no public data is currently available.

The DEB-025-103 Study: Clinical proof of concept was provided in a 15-day phase I study in HIV-1 and HCV coinfected patients, who received alisporivir (1,200 mg bid) or placebo (Flisiak et al. 2008). The maximal HCV RNA reduction from baseline for patients who received alisporivir was 3.63 $\log^{10}$ IU/mL compared to 0.73 for placebo-treated patients. The antiviral activity of alisporivir was observed irrespective of viral genotype. Several cases of reversible hyperbilirubinemia were also observed in alisporivir-treated patients.

The DEB-025-HCV-203 Study: Lower doses of alisporivir were tested in combination with pegylated IFNα in a 29-day phase II study in treatment-naive patients ($n = 90$) (Flisiak et al. 2009). In the first four arms, patients received placebo or increasing doses of alisporivir (200, 600, or 1,000 mg) in combination with pegylated IFNα. In the last arm, patients received 1,000 mg alisporivir alone. Patients received alisporivir twice daily during the first week and once daily during weeks 2 through 4. The viral load reductions for patients who received 1,000 mg alisporivir monotherapy, pegylated IFNα alone, 200 mg alisporivir plus pegylated IFNα, 600 mg alisporivir plus pegylated IFNα, and 1,000 mg alisporivir plus pegylated IFNα were 2.87, 3.56, 3.30, 5.07, and 5.09 $\log^{10}$ IU/mL, respectively.

Alisporivir was also tested in combination with pegylated IFNα and ribavirin in a 29-day phase II study in genotype 1 null responders (Nelson et al. 2009). In arm 1, patients received pegylated IFNα plus ribavirin with 400 mg alisporivir; in arm 2, patients received 400 mg alisporivir; in arm 3, patients received pegylated IFNα with 400 mg alisporivir; in arm 4, patients received pegylated IFNα and ribavirin with 800 mg alisporivir; and in arm 5, patients received pegylated IFNα and ribavirin with 400 mg alisporivir twice daily for one week and once daily until the end of the study. No decline of viral replication was observed in patients who received alisporivir alone. The antiviral activity of alisporivir combined with IFNα was similar in patients who received 800 mg qd (2.38 $\log^{10}$ IU/mL) or 400 mg bid alisporivir (1.96 $\log^{10}$ IU/mL), demonstrating that the combination of the CypI alisporivir, pegylated IFNα, and ribavirin is an attractive treatment strategy for patients who previously failed to respond to an IFN-based therapy.

The DEB-025-HCV-205 Study: *ESSENTIAL* – Larger alisporivir phase II studies were conducted. In the ESSENTIAL study (Flisiak et al. 2011), all treatment-naïve genotype 1 patients ($n = 288$) received pegylated IFNα and ribavirin. In arm 1, patients received placebo once daily for 48 weeks. In arms 2, 3, and 4, patients received 600 mg alisporivir twice daily during the first week and once daily until the end of the study. In arm 2, patients received alisporivir in combination with pegylated IFNα and ribavirin for 48 weeks. In arm 3, response-guided therapy (RGT) was used to determine the duration of treatment with alisporivir in combination with pegylated IFNα and ribavirin. In arm 3, patients who demonstrated a rapid virological response (RVR) were eligible to receive 24 weeks of treatment. Patients, who did not demonstrate an RVR, continued the treatment for 48 weeks. In arm 4, patients received alisporivir in combination with pegylated IFNα and ribavirin for 24 weeks. Alisporivir was well tolerated in all arms. The frequency of reversible hyperbilirubinemia was 1.4, 32.9, 25.4, and 41.7 % in arms 1, 2, 3, and 4, respectively.

The primary endpoint of the study was to determine the proportion of patients in each arm who achieved SVR at week 24 (SVR_{24}) using 10 IU/mL as limit detection for HCV plasma RNA. SVR_{24} were 55, 76, 69, and 53 % in arms 1 (control), 2 (48 weeks of alisporivir), 3 (24 or 48 weeks of alisporivir RGT), and 4 (24 weeks of alisporivir), respectively. Only arm 2 reached statistical significance ($p = 0.008$). End-of-treatment responses were elevated in CC IL28B patients (100 % of patients exhibited undetectable HCV plasma RNA) and were preserved at the 24-week follow-up (100 % SVR_{24}) for patients who received the originally scheduled treatment duration of 48 weeks or 24 weeks of RGT with alisporivir. End-of-treatment responses were diminished at the 24-week evaluation for CC IL28B patients who received control treatment or a planned 24-week treatment with alisporivir. The benefit of adding alisporivir to pegylated IFNα and ribavirin was evident in TT IL28B patients. SVR_{24} were 17, 33, 62, and 73 % for TT IL28B patients in arm 1, 2, 3, and 4, respectively. RVR was enhanced in all arms that contain alisporivir (arms 2–4) compared to the control arm (arm 1). The frequency of viral breakthrough was low (2.8 %) in patients who received the CypI alisporivir. In conclusion, the addition of 48 weeks of 600 mg alisporivir to pegylated IFNα and ribavirin improves SVR_{24} in treatment-naïve genotype 1 patients.

The CDEB025A2211 Study: *VITAL-1* – The goals of the phase II VITAL-1 study were to test the safety and efficacy of alisporivir administered alone, with ribavirin or with ribavirin and pegylated IFNα for 24 weeks. The addition of pegylated IFNα and ribavirin was delayed in treatment-naïve genotype 2 or 3 patients (Pawlotsky et al. 2012a). In arm 1, patients received 1,000 mg alisporivir ($n = 83$); in arm 2, patients received 600 mg alisporivir with ribavirin ($n = 84$); in arm 3, patients received 800 mg alisporivir with ribavirin ($n = 94$); in arm 4, patients received 600 mg alisporivir with pegylated IFNα ($n = 84$); and in arm 5, patients received pegylated IFNα and ribavirin ($n = 40$). All patients received 600 mg alisporivir twice daily for a week, after which patients started their randomized dose of alisporivir. Follow-up evaluations were scheduled at week 36 and 48 to measure SVR_{12} and SVR_{24}, respectively. Viral load was measured at week 4 for RVR rates and for the decision to modify the original randomized treatment. If a patient demonstrated RVR (viral load <25 IU/mL), the patient continued his original treatment. If a patient exhibited viral load >25 IU/mL, he would switch at week 6 to a treatment combining 600 mg alisporivir, pegylated IFNα, and ribavirin until the end of treatment at week 24.

Alisporivir was well tolerated in all arms. SVR_{12} rates were superior in all arms that contained alisporivir compared to the control arm (pegylated IFNα and ribavirin). SVR_{12} rates were 81 %, 83 %, 81 %, 77 %, and 58 % for arms 1, 2, 3, 4, and 5, respectively. RVR rates were 29 %, 37 %, and 42 % for arms 1, 2, and 3, respectively. Patients with RVR rates of 82 %, 93 %, and 91 % in arms 1, 2, and 3 achieved SVR_{12}, demonstrating that alisporivir as monotherapy or in combination with ribavirin is an attractive treatment strategy for treatment-naïve genotype 2 or 3 patients who demonstrated RVR at week 4. Yet, the majority of patients in all arms did not reach RVR and switched at week 6 to 600 mg alisporivir combined with pegylated IFNα and ribavirin. For these patients, SVR_{12} rates were 94 %, 92 %, and

96 % for arms 1, 2, and 3, respectively, demonstrating that the addition of pegylated IFNα and ribavirin to alisporivir by week 6 promotes viral clearance in genotype 2 or 3 patients who did not achieve RVR.

A subsequent analysis demonstrated that alisporivir improved SVR_{24} rates in all arms compared to pegylated IFNα and ribavirin (Pawlotsky et al. 2012b). SVR_{24} rates were 80 %, 85 %, 81 %, 80 %, and 58 % in arms 1, 2, 3, 4, and 5, respectively. Alisporivir treatments (arms 1–4) decreased the relapse rates compared to the control pegylated IFNα and ribavirin (arm 5): 11 %, 8 %, 6 %, 10 %, and 25 % in arms 1, 2, 3, 4, and 5, respectively. These latest results demonstrate that the combination of alisporivir and ribavirin yields high SVR_{24} rates as either IFN-free regimen or as IFN-add-on regimen in treatment-naive genotype 2 or 3 patients with rapid viral clearance, low viral breakthrough, and low relapse rates.

The CDEB025A2210 Study: FUNDAMENTAL – The goals of the 48-week phase II FUNDAMENTAL study were to test the safety and efficacy of alisporivir in combination with pegylated IFNα and ribavirin in genotype 1 patients with a documented history of relapse or nonresponse to prior treatment with pegylated IFNα and ribavirin (Alberti et al. 2012). In arm 1, patients received 600 mg alisporivir once daily ($n = 121$); in arm 2, patients received 800 mg alisporivir once daily ($n = 117$); in arm 3, patients received 400 mg alisporivir twice daily ($n = 109$); and in arm 4, patients received placebo once or twice daily ($n = 114$). All patients received pegylated IFNα and ribavirin. In arms 1 and 2, patients received 600 mg alisporivir twice daily for a week after which patients started their randomized dose of alisporivir. Scheduled follow-up evaluations were conducted at week 60 and 72 to measure SVR_{12} and SVR_{24}, respectively. The primary endpoint of the study was to determine at week 12 the percentage of patients who achieved complete early virologic response (cEVR) (HCV RNA <25 IU/mL). Viral load was assessed at week 4 for the determination of RVR rates.

Alisporivir was well tolerated. Alisporivir enhanced the percentage of patients who achieved cEVR with values of46.4 %, 61.1 %, 71.3 %, and 32.7 % in arms 1, 2, 3, and 4, respectively. The 400 mg bid alisporivir administration (arm 3) yielded a superior percentage of cEVR than that of the 800 mg qd administration (arm 2). Among relapsers, alisporivir produced a higher percentage of patients who achieved cEVR, with values of 62.5, 77.6, 72.9, and 51.9 for arms 1, 2, 3, and 4, respectively. The same trend was observed for nonresponders in arms 2 (47.5 % cEVR) and 3 (70 % cEVR). The 400 mg bid alisporivir treatment was highly potent in null nonresponders (69.7 % cEVR) and partial nonresponders (68.0 % cEVR). A low viral breakthrough was observed – 3.6, 3.7, 1.8, and 2.7 % – in arms 1, 2, 3, and 4, respectively. In conclusion, the addition of the CypI alisporivir to pegylated IFNα and ribavirin is a novel and attractive choice for difficult-to-treat patients, particularly for genotype 1 patients who did not respond previously to IFN-based regimens.

A subsequent analysis was executed at week 24 and further demonstrated that the addition of alisporivir greatly improves the efficacy of the treatments (Davis et al. 2012). Specifically, alisporivir enhanced the percentage of patients who achieved cEVR with values of 48.2 %, 61.1 %, 72.5 %, and 35.5 % in arms 1, 2, 3, and 4, respectively. RVR values were 20.9 %, 25.0 %, 40.4 %, and 7.3 %, and

VR_{24} values were 64.5 %, 70.4 %, 73.4 %, and 31.8 % in arms 1, 2, 3, and 4, respectively. Alisporivir enhanced VR_{24} (70.8–79.2 %) in relapsers compared to pegylated IFNα and ribavirin (55.6 %). The 400 mg bid alisporivir treatment (arm 3) yielded not only higher VR_{24} (75.4 %) in nonresponders compared to the pegylated IFNα and ribavirin treatment (8.9 %) but also in the most difficult-to-treat null responders (70.6 %) compared to pegylated IFNα and ribavirin (5.6 %). The viral breakthrough rates were 11.8 %, 7.3 %, 1.8 %, and 4.5 % in arms 1, 2, 3, and 4, respectively. In some patients, hyperbilirubinemia was transient and reversible and not associated with liver toxicity.

HCV Resistance to Direct-Antiviral Agents. HCV replication comprises a rapid turnover rate and a lack of proofreading by the NS5B polymerase, resulting in high genetic diversity among HCV virions. These extremely variable viral quasi-species contain a mixture of viruses with numerable mutational variants. It is important to emphasize that the mutated variants are present in patients prior to the administration of antiviral therapy and may become the dominant viral population under selective drug pressure. As anticipated, quick selection of resistant variants was observed in HCV-infected patients upon administration of various DAAs including the protease and NS5A inhibitors when given as monotherapy (Wyles 2013). Thus, the development of resistance to DAAs targeting HCV can compromise successful therapy.

The mechanisms that determine prevalence and frequency of resistance-conferring mutations remain elusive. Several parameters control resistance to DAAs. Among them are viral, host, and pharmacokinetic factors.

Viral Parameters: As mentioned above, estimates of HCV replication in chronically infected patients suggest that viral production may be as high as 10^{10}–10^{12} virions per day. Accordingly, the clearance of free virions in plasma is exceedingly rapid yielding values of 2–3 h for the half-life of viral particles (Neumann et al. 1998). The lack of proofreading by the RNA-dependent RNA polymerase NS5B results in the accumulation of genetically distinct viral variants called quasi-species (Martell et al. 1992). Since de novo mutant variants are continuously produced, it has been proposed that in any untreated HCV-infected patient, any possible mutant variant exists (Rong et al. 2010). A recent study showed that the NS5B polymerase does not incorporate incorrect nucleotides at identical rates (Powdrill et al. 2011). Specifically, enzyme kinetic measurements revealed surprisingly elevated error rates for G:U/U:G mismatches. The observation that G:U/U:G mismatches occur at a greater frequency than all other misincorporation events correlates well with a mutational predisposition for transitions over transversions. Therefore, the probability of viral breakthrough throughout DAA therapy is contingent upon the nucleotide exchange (transition versus transversion) necessary to create a resistance-associated mutation. Thus, the nature of the nucleotide change can contribute to the genetic barrier in the development of resistance to DAAs (Powdrill et al. 2011).

In HCV-infected patients, the fitness of a mutant variant is characterized by its capacity to replicate. It is common for mutant variants that are resistant to DAAs to exhibit diminished fitness compared to wild-type virus. Wild-type viruses are the dominant viruses within the quasi-species (Sarrazin and Zeuzem 2010; Soriano et al. 2008b), but under DAA pressure they are promptly eliminated. However, the mutant variants that contain adequate mutations to escape the effects of the drug will replicate and then represent the predominant viral population. Prolonged drug treatment then leads to the emergence of additional or secondary mutational changes, which contribute to both the fitness of the mutant virus and the resistance of the virus to the drug.

The genotype of the virus represents an additional critical parameter for DAA resistance. Since the first-generation protease inhibitors were originally designed to neutralize the protease activity of genotype 1, these DAAs exert poor antiviral activity against other genotypes (Gottwein et al. 2011). Importantly, the second-generation protease inhibitors, which are already tested for safety and efficacy in phase II and III studies, exhibit broader antiviral activities against other genotypes. Unlike the first-generation protease inhibitors, non-nucleoside polymerase inhibitors exhibit antiviral activity broadly against multiple diverse genotypes and subtypes. Nucleos(t)ide polymerase inhibitors target the highly conserved active site of the NS5B polymerase; they are potent against all genotypes (Sarrazin and Zeuzem 2010). This broad antiviral activity among genotypes is referred to as pan-genotypic antiviral activity. First-generation NS5A inhibitors also exhibited varying degrees of potency between genotypes (Fridell et al. 2010; Gao et al. 2010) likely due to the relatively high heterogeneity of the NS5A gene among genotypes, however, second-generation NS5A inhibitors (i.e., PPI-668, ACH-3102) afford pan-genotypic antiviral activity.

The subtype of the virus also contributes to the genetic barrier to resistance of DAAs. Specifically, the R155K mutation, which mediates resistance to the protease inhibitors boceprevir and telaprevir, requires only one nucleotide change in subtype 1a patients but requires two mutations in 1b patients. Since the single nucleotide exchange for the R155K mutation in 1a is created by a simple transition, whereas one of the two nucleotide exchanges for the R155K mutation in 1b is created by a transversion (Powdrill et al. 2011; Sullivan et al. 2011), R155K mutations are more often found in 1a patients treated with boceprevir or telaprevir. This is consistent with the observation that virologic failures, which are associated with HCV resistance to the DAAs boceprevir or telaprevir, are more frequently found in 1a patients than in 1b patients (Jacobson et al. 2011a; Poordad et al. 2011). It is important to emphasize that analogous transition/transversion nucleotide exchanges were also observed in HCV variants exhibiting resistance to NS5B polymerase and NS5A inhibitors (Sarrazin and Zeuzem 2010).

Because monotherapies with protease (i.e., boceprevir or telaprevir) or NS5A (i.e., BMS-790052) inhibitors resulted in the rapid (15 days) selection of resistant variants (viral breakthrough) (Sarrazin et al. 2007a, b; Fridell et al. 2011), clinicians and researchers postulated that DAA-resistant variants exist within the quasi-species prior to the beginning of the treatment. Supporting this hypothesis, resistant variants carrying NS3 mutations at specific positions (i.e., V36, T54, V55, Q80, R155, D168, and V170) that confer resistance to protease inhibitors were found at varying frequencies in untreated patients (Bartels et al. 2008; Kuntzen et al. 2008; Lenz et al. 2011; Vicenti et al. 2012). Similarly, resistant variants carrying NS5A (M28V,

Q30R/H, Q54H, Y93H) or NS5B mutations (S282T/R, C316Y/F/S, M423T/I, and V499A) that confer resistance to NS5A and non-nucleoside polymerase inhibitors, respectively, were also found to exist in untreated patients (Bartels et al. 2008; Kuntzen et al. 2008; Lenz et al. 2011; Vicenti et al. 2012). Variants, which are resistant to nucleos(t)ide polymerase inhibitors, have rarely been identified in patients (Fridell et al. 2011; Margeridon et al. 2011; Gaudieri et al. 2009; Sun et al. 2011). Novel DNA sequencing techniques, referred to as "next-generation" sequencing (NGS), provide high-speed throughput that can produce an enormous volume of sequences. The most important advantage provided by these platforms is the identification of sequence data from single DNA fragments within a library, eliminating the use of amplification techniques that can introduce spurious mutations prior to sequence acquisition. Deep sequencing by NGS techniques is being increasingly used in clinical practice to detect low abundance drug-resistant HCV variants. Although these new sequencing methodologies resulted in the detection of DAA-resistant variants with NS3, NS5A, and NS5B mutations in a majority of untreated patients (Chevaliez et al. 2011), the role of these preexisting resistant variants within quasi-species remains to be determined. Further sequencing studies will also determine whether or not these DAA-resistant variants present in quasi-species turn out to be critical in previous pegylated IFNα and ribavirin nonresponders or unfavorable CT or TT IL28 genotype patients.

Pharmacokinetic Parameters: Both the potency of the DAA and the genetic barrier to resistance define the likelihood of the emergence of a viral variant under drug selection pressure. Drug potency is characterized by the drug concentration required to inhibit 50 % or 90 % of the viral growth (IC_{50} and IC_{90}). Drug concentrations above the IC_{50} and IC_{90} are needed to inhibit drug-resistant variants. There is a direct correlation between the emergence of DAA-resistant variants (viral breakthrough) and drug exposure. The genetic barrier to resistance is characterized by an optimal transition/transversion nucleotide exchange and the number of mutations needed to develop resistance. Resistance to DAAs with a low genetic barrier to resistance necessitates only one or two amino acid substitutions and/or transitions, whereas resistance to DAAs with a high genetic barrier to resistance necessitates three or more nucleotide changes and/or transversions (Powdrill et al. 2011). DAAs with a high genetic barrier to resistance, but with a low potency, represent a therapeutic concern.

Host Parameters: Resistance emergence is highly contingent upon patient adherence. It has been clearly shown that adherence to highly active antiretroviral therapies (HAART) is correlated with suppression of detectable HIV-1 replication, reduced rates of resistance, increased survival, and improved quality of life (Kitahata et al. 1996; Kitahata et al. 2000). One thus can anticipate that a correlation between drug resistance and treatment adherence will also be observed in HCV-infected patients. Specifically, if compliance is low, plasma drug levels will drop below IC_{50} and IC_{90} levels, resulting in the emergence of resistant HCV variants. This may be particularly true for the two DAAs boceprevir and telaprevir, which exhibit fairly short half-lives. Thus, adherence to treatment as prescribed is a critical parameter to avoid drug resistance. Other host parameters important for the emergence of drug resistance are genetic predispositions and fibrosis stage at the time of drug treatment. For example, a low fibrosis stage and the CC genotype of a single nucleotide polymorphism (rs12979860) in the IL28B gene are positive prognostic factors for high virologic response rates to DAA combination therapies (Zeuzem et al. 2012; Poordad et al. 2012; Jacobson et al. 2011b).

In Vitro HCV Resistance to Cyclophilin Inhibitors. The development of HTAs is mainly a consequence of our increasing understanding of the molecular biology of the HCV replication cycle and the interplay between the virus and the host. Targeting host factors rather than viral factors must combine a specific antiviral effect with a higher barrier to resistance and a broader genotypic activity. In contrast to viral factors, host factors are encoded by host chromosomes and therefore are not subject to the high genetic variability of the viral genome. Targeting a host factor rather than a viral factor may increase the potential for side effects such as cellular toxicity. While far less common to viral genomes, sequence variations in host genes (i.e., single nucleotide polymorphisms (SNPs)) occur and occasionally affect the development of a disease or the response to a therapy (Balagopal et al. 2010). Supporting this hypothesis, a recent study investigated the effects of non-synonymous SNPs in the CypA gene on HCV replication (von Hahn et al. 2012). Interestingly, they identified three SNPs in the CypA gene that protect cells from HCV replication. The single amino acid changes appeared to provoke rapid degradation of CypA. However, it is important to reemphasize that the existence of knockout mice (Colgan et al. 2005) and human cell lines (Braaten and Luban 2001) without evident deleterious phenotypes further suggests that CypA is a valuable target for CypI in HCV therapy. Together these findings strongly suggest that CypA is a relevant therapeutic target.

Numerous studies demonstrated that HCV variants resistant to CypI including CsA, NIM811, alisporivir, and SCY-635 can emerge under drug selection pressure in hepatoma cell in vitro systems (Fernandes et al. 2007, 2010; Robida et al. 2007; Kaul et al. 2009; Yang et al. 2010; Coelmont et al. 2010; Hopkins et al. 2012; Garcia-Rivera et al. 2012a). Importantly, the time required for CypI resistance selection is particularly lengthy (3–6 months) compared to that required for DAA resistance (2–3 weeks) including protease, NS5B polymerase, and NS5A inhibitors (Coelmont et al. 2010). The slow development of resistance to CypI represents a major benefit of using them as part of a future anti-HCV regimen.

The level of HCV resistance to CypI is relatively low compared to other DAAs such as protease, NS5B polymerase, and NS5A inhibitors (Ma et al. 2006; Coelmont et al. 2010). Specifically, the inhibition of CypI-resistant variants in vitro requires relatively low concentrations of CypI compared to that of wild-type virus (5- to 10-fold higher concentrations). In contrast, inhibition of DAA-resistant variants in vitro requires high concentrations of DAA compared to that of wild-type virus (>100-fold higher concentrations). Attempts to further increase CypI (i.e., alisporivir) concentration were unsuccessful. Prolonged exposure of HCV replicon cells resulted in viral clearance rather than the selection of increasingly resistant replicon cells (Coelmont et al. 2009).

A large number of in vitro studies investigated the resistance of HCV to various CypI (Fernandes et al. 2007; Robida et al. 2007; Kaul et al. 2009; Fernandes et al. 2010; Yang et al. 2010; Coelmont et al. 2010; Hopkins et al. 2012; Garcia-Rivera et al. 2012a). The sequencing of CypI-resistant subgenomic and genomic HCV clones showed that mutations emerged in several genes including NS3, NS5A, and NS5B (Fig. 4). Importantly, the reintroduction of the mutations into the wild-type viral genome and the subsequent examination of the sensitivity of resulting HCV mutants to CypI determined the true significance of the mutations for CypI resistance. Although early work suggested that mutations, which arose in NS5B (i.e., P540A and I432V), are important for CypI resistance (Robida et al. 2007), more recent studies indicate that only mutations in NS5A are critical for HCV resistance to CypI including CsA, alisporivir, SCY-635, sanglifehrin A, or a combination of CypI (sanglifehrin A plus NIM811 or CsA plus NIM811) (Fig. 4). This is in accordance with the fact that NS5A serves as a binding locus for CypA (Hanoulle et al. 2009; Chatterji et al. 2010; Yang et al. 2010; Coelmont et al. 2010; Fernandes et al. 2010). Note that the relevant resistance mutations occur only in the viral NS5A protein and not in the host CypA protein. Individual and combinational analyses of NS5A mutations, which emerged during CypI resistance selection, revealed that the D320E NS5A mutation frequently arose in CypI-resistant variants (Fig. 4). Specifically, the D320E mutation was identified in genotype 1b (Con1) HCV variants resistant to CsA (Goto et al. 2009), alisporivir (Coelmont et al. 2010; Garcia-Rivera et al. 2012a), sanglifehrin A (Puyang et al. 2010), sanglifehrin A plus NIM811 (Puyang et al. 2010), CsA plus NIM811 (Puyang et al. 2010), and SCY-635 (Hopkins et al. 2012). Moreover, the D320E mutation (position D316 in JFH-1) was also found in genotype 2a HCV variants which, in contrast to wild-type virus, replicate in CypA-knockdown cells (Yang et al. 2010) (Fig. 4). Importantly, the reintroduction of the D320E mutation into the wild-type genome renders the resulting subgenomic and genomic mutants either partially resistant to CypI or independent of CypA (Goto et al. 2009; Coelmont et al. 2010; Puyang et al. 2010; Yang et al. 2010; Hopkins et al. 2012; Garcia-Rivera et al. 2012a). Altogether these data strongly suggest not only that the D320E mutation is key to provide partial HCV resistance to CypI, but they also suggest that the D320E NS5A mutation partially bypasses the need for CypA.

As mentioned above, the level of HCV resistance to CypI is relatively low compared to other DAAs. Supporting this notion, the D320E NS5A mutation only reduced the HCV susceptibility to CypI by ~2- to 5-fold (Goto et al. 2009; Coelmont et al. 2010; Puyang et al. 2010; Hopkins et al. 2012; Garcia-Rivera et al. 2012a). The D320E mutation does not influence the fitness of the resistant replicons. Additional in vitro studies suggest that by itself the single D320E mutation in the domain II of NS5A does not confer high-level resistance to CypI. A combination of multiple simultaneously occurring mutations is required to render HCV more resistant to CypI (Coelmont et al. 2010; Puyang et al. 2010; Garcia-Rivera et al. 2012a). Indeed, two independent studies showed that a mutation adjacent to the D320E NS5A mutation, the Y321N mutation, is also important for CypI resistance (Fig. 4). One study showed that HCV (JFH-1) develops D320E and Y321N NS5A mutations

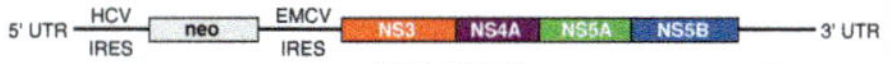

Cyclophilin Inhibitor	Genotype	Resistance Mutations	References
CsA	1b	E260G, F288S, V284A, L307Q, R360G, V448A } NS5A; P538T, S556G } NS5B	Fernandes *et al.*, 2007
CsA	1b	I432V, P540A, I432V + P540A } NS5B	Robida *et al.*, 2007
CsA	1b	Q86R, I252T } NS3; ***D320E*** } NS5A	Goto *et al.*, 2009
Alisporivir	2a	Y391F } NS3; D253G, L290F, V464A/L } NS5A	Kaul *et al.*, 2009
CsA + NIM811	1b	Q42H, S341I } NS3; L183P, D333N, R356Q, T360P, P426R } NS5A; C575G } NS5B	Puyang *et al.*, 2010
Sanglifehrin A	1b	I71V, Q80R, G262S } NS3; V9I, M51V } NS4; L27I, C446S } NS5A; W571R } NS5B	Puyang *et al.*, 2010
Sanglifehrin A + NIM811	1b	I71V, Q80R, G262S } NS3; V9I, M51V } NS4; V278A, P353S, W433R, C446S } NS5A; N142S, W571R } NS5B	Puyang *et al.*, 2010
Alisporivir	1b	A241P } NS3; R262Q, R328W, ***D320E*** } NS5A	Coelmont *et al.*, 2010
shCypA	2a	***D320E***, ***Y321N*** } NS5A	Yang *et al.*, 2010
SCY-635	1b	***D320E***, ***Y321N*** } NS5A	Hopkins *et al.*, 2012
Alisporivir	1b	***D320E***, ***Y321N*** } NS5A	Garcia-Rivera *et al.*, 2012

```
GT-1a        ARALPVWARPDYNPPLVETWKKPDYEPPVVHG
GT-1b        PRAMPIWARPDYNPPLLESWKDPDYVPPVVHG
GT-2a[J6]    PPALPAWARPDYNPPLVESWKRPDYQPATVAG
GT-2a[JFH]   PRALPAWARPDYNPPLVESWRRPDYQPPTVAG
GT-2b        PPALPPWARPEYNPPVIETWKRPDYEPPTVLG
GT-3         PPALPIWARPDYNPPLLDRWKAPDYVPPTVHG
GT-4         PPALPIWARPDYNPPLTETWKQQDYQAPTVHG
GT-5         PPALPVWARPGYDPPLLETWKRPDYDPPQVWG
GT-6         PPALPIWARPDYNPPLLQKWQMPGYEPPVVSG
             PPALP.WARPDYNPPL.E.WK.PDY PPTV G
```

■ = DY motif (*D320E* and *Y321N*)

Fig. 4 In vitro development of CypI resistance mutations

(D316E and Y317N in JFH1) when cultured in CypA-knockdown cells (Yang et al. 2010). Another study showed that HCV develops a combination of D320E and Y321N NS5A mutations when cultured under the CypI alisporivir selection (Garcia-Rivera et al. 2012a). The D320 residue is conserved among HCV genotypes (GT1a, GT1b, GT2a, GT3, GT4, and GT6) except for GT2b (D320E) and GT5 (D320G), whereas the Y321 residue is highly conserved among all genotypes (Fig. 4). The D320E or Y321N mutation alone confers only partial replication in CypA-knockdown cells (Yang et al. 2010) and only a slight resistance to alisporivir (Garcia-Rivera et al. 2012a). However, the combination of the two mutations renders HCV more resistant to alisporivir in vitro and is able to robustly replicate in CypA-knockdown cells (Yang et al. 2010; Garcia-Rivera et al. 2012a). The combination of D320E and Y321N mutations renders HCV universally resistant to CypI in vitro including CsA, alisporivir, SCY-635, sanglifehrins, and sanglifehrin derivates (Garcia-Rivera et al. 2012b). Together these data not only suggest that the mutations found in the NS5A gene of CypI-resistant variants are truly responsible for the observed drug resistance, they also suggest that not a single NS5A mutation but rather the development of multiple mutations is necessary for robust CypI resistance as well as CypA independence, at least in vitro. This further suggests that CypI impose a high genetic barrier for the development of viral resistance.

The D320E and Y321 mutations that emerged for CypI resistance in vitro do not influence NS5A binding to CypA or the sensitivity of CypA-NS5A interactions to CypI (Chatterji et al. 2010; Yang et al. 2010; Fernandes et al. 2010; Garcia-Rivera et al. 2012a). This suggests that these mutations do not render CypA-NS5A interactions impervious to CypI-mediated dissociation. The D320E and Y321 mutations do not alter NS5A dimerization, NS5A binding to NS5B, or NS5A binding to RNA (). CypA enhances the binding of the domain II of NS5A to RNA, and the addition of CypI blocks the CypA effect (Foster et al. 2011). Importantly, the RNA binding of the domain II of NS5A that contains the D320E mutation was unaffected by CypA (Foster et al. 2011), suggesting that the CypI resistance mutation bypasses the need for CypA in the in vitro binding of NS5A to RNA.

Comparative NMR studies with NS5A peptides that contain either the D320 or the E320 residue revealed a shift in population between major and minor *cis-trans* conformers (Hanoulle et al. 2009). Specifically, residues preceding Pro319 in wild-type D320 peptide exist on average for 24.1 % in a minor conformation attributed to the Pro319 *cis* form. This minor conformer in D320 peptide becomes the dominant conformer in the E320 peptide, with a relative population of 70.4 % (Hanoulle et al. 2009). The CypI resistance NS5A mutations apparently relieve the CypA dependence by acquiring a conformational inversion mediated by the D320E mutation that normally is mediated by CypA. The prolyl *cis-trans* isomerization activity of CypA would thereby not be strictly required anymore, explaining the HCV resistance to CypI. The CypI resistance mutations may generate a particular conformation of NS5A that is directly or indirectly necessary for optimal HCV replication. Further work is required to unravel the precise structural origin of this conformational inversion.

The fact that HCV has to develop a lengthy mutational strategy to efficiently replicate in vitro independently of a host factor explains the high genetic barrier that the virus has to cross to develop resistance to CypI. The characteristic resistance profile of CypI offers an exceptional opportunity to cure HCV as part of a combination therapy with other antivirals such as DAAs in treatment-naive patients or as part as a rescue therapy for patients harboring resistance mutations to other classes of anti-HCV agents such as DAAs.

In Vivo HCV Resistance to Cyclophilin Inhibitors. Very low viral breakthroughs arose in CypI-treated patients such as alisporivir-treated patients (Tiongyip et al. 2011). Viral breakthrough was only observed in TT or CT IL28B allele patients in the alisporivir ESSENTIAL study (Flisiak et al. 2011). Population sequencing of HCV genomes did not identify any genotypic change consistently associated with viral breakthrough, assessed by clonal sequencing of NS5A, the putative in vivo viral target of CypA. Interestingly, the D320E mutation was seen at the time of initial viral breakthrough in one patient (Li et al. 2011). However, phenotypic assays demonstrated only a slight (~3-fold) decrease in susceptibility to alisporivir with GT1b replicons bearing D320E alone or the entire NS5A gene of the patient isolate. These data suggest that the emergence of D320E or viral resistance is not the primary cause of the viral breakthrough. Importantly, a number of mutations that confer resistance to DAAs including NS5A inhibitors were seen at baseline for patients who achieved RVR and subsequently SVR_{24} with alisporivir (Li et al. 2011), supporting the in vitro data of lack of cross-resistance between alisporivir and DAAs. Altogether these data strongly suggest a low potential for development of resistance to CypI in treated patients.

Viral breakthrough was associated with decrease in dose or stoppage of pegylated IFNα and ribavirin or with low drug exposure. Specifically, while on full dose of the CypI alisporivir, 6/215 patients experienced viral breakthrough compared to 4/73 patients in the control arm (placebo with pegylated IFNα and ribavirin) (Li et al. 2011). No viral breakthrough occurred until week 12. In three of the six alisporivir-treated patients, viral breakthrough occurred after dose adjustment or stoppage of pegylated IFNα and ribavirin dose. Pharmacokinetic analyses demonstrated suboptimal plasma concentrations of alisporivir in two of the other three patients who exhibited viral breakthroughs.

In the alisporivir VITAL-1 study, several residue changes were recognized in the NS5A gene in patients, who underwent viral breakthrough. When certain of these mutations were introduced together in the wild-type viral genome, the resulting mutants exhibited a mild to moderate resistance to alisporivir in vitro ($<$17-fold increase in EC_{50}) (Li et al. 2011). These findings further suggest that, in contrast to DAAs, multiple mutations are necessary to provide substantial resistance to CypI, at least to alisporivir. Importantly, the alisporivir-resistant variants isolated from treated patients continued to be susceptible to DAAs (Li et al. 2011). Altogether these observations convincingly demonstrate that CypI offer a high barrier to the development of HCV resistance in treated patients.

The Future of Cyclophilin Inhibitors

A novel therapeutic approach is currently being tested for safety and efficacy in various clinical trials. This approach entails an IFN-free treatment that offers both high efficiency and low frequency of adverse events. This IFN-free treatment may consist of a combination of two or three DAAs, two or three HTAs including a CypI, or a combination of DAAs and HTAs. Remarkably, data generated from a rapidly growing number of phase II and III studies strongly suggests that IFN-free DAAs combination therapies represent the future for therapy for curing chronic HCV infection.

Here we briefly describe a few IFN-free regimens, which exhibited apparent successful therapeutic results. The AVIATOR study from Abbot tested a combination of the protease inhibitor ABT-450, the NS5A inhibitor ABT-267, and the NS5B polymerase inhibitor ABT-333, without pegylated IFNα and ribavirin. High SVR_{12} were observed in treatment-naive genotype 1a (83 %) and 1b (96 %) patients. The addition of ribavirin to the combination of the three DAAs yielded high SVR_{12} in null responders (89 % and 100 % for genotype 1a and 1b patients, respectively) (Kowdley et al. 2012). Based on these promising results, Abbot recently announced the design of phase III studies, which will evaluate the safety and efficacy of a 12-week regimen of the three DAAs with and without ribavirin, for the treatment of

HCV in genotype 1 non-cirrhotic, treatment-naïve and treatment-experienced patients. An additional phase III study will be conducted with ribavirin in patients with cirrhosis for 12 or 24 weeks. Another phase II study from Bristol-Myers Squibb that combined the NS5A inhibitor daclatasvir (BMS-790062), the protease inhibitor asunaprevir (BMS-650032), and the NS5B polymerase inhibitor BMS-791325, without ribavirin, yielded high SVR_{12} (94 %) in treatment-naïve genotype 1a patients without major adverse events (Everson et al. 2012). Phase III studies are anticipated to begin in 2014. The ELECTRON study from Gilead, which combined the NS5B polymerase inhibitor sofosbuvir (GS-7977), the NS5A inhibitor GS-5885, and ribavirin, yielded high SVR_{12} in treatment-naïve genotype 1 patients (Gane et al. 2012). Gilead just announced preliminary results from their FISSION study, which evaluated a 12-week course of the once-daily sofosbuvir with ribavirin in treatment-naïve genotype 2 or 3 patients. The study met its primary efficacy endpoint of non-inferiority of the sofosbuvir plus ribavirin treatment compared to control pegylated-IFNα plus ribavirin treatment, with 67 % SVR_{12} for both treatments. No major adverse events occurred. Altogether these studies provide the proof of concept that IFN-free regimens represent the future for an HCV therapy or cure.

The combination of the CypI alisporivir with ribavirin exhibited high efficiency in treatment-naïve genotype 2 and 3 patients. However, one or even two DAAs will certainly have to be added to alisporivir to yield high SVR in treatment-naïve patients infected with all genotypes, relapsers, and nonresponders (Pawlotsky et al. 2012; Alberti et al. 2012). For example, the combination of alisporivir (or another CypI) with a second-generation protease inhibitor, a NS5B polymerase inhibitor, and/or an NS5A inhibitor represents attractive IFN-free regimens. Indeed, targeting both viral and host factors critical for HCV replication should greatly improve the efficacy of the regimen, especially in difficult-to-treat patients. Combination studies of a CypI with one or two DAAs should be evaluated initially in vitro and subsequently in vivo to pinpoint the best CypI/DAA combination, which would combine synergistic and pan-genotypic properties. An appealing combination would be a CypI with an NS5A inhibitor given that CypI prevent the binding of CypA to the domain II of NS5A and that NS5A inhibitors target the domain I of NS5A (Gao et al. 2010; Lemm et al. 2010). The combination of CypI and NS5A inhibitors may be particularly effective because this combination strategy may present an unusually high genetic barrier to resistance by requiring the virus to develop several mutations simultaneously in two distinct domains of NS5A in order to escape the selection pressure of the two classes of inhibitors. Nevertheless, the in vivo efficacy of the combination of CypI and NS5A inhibitors remains to be established.

Conclusion

CypI represent a novel class of anti-HCV agents with a mechanism of action that differs from those of all existing DAAs. Because of their distinct mechanisms of action that target the host protein cyclophilin A, CypI are pan-genotypic. A very low viral breakthrough rate was associated with CypI treatments, and no consistent genotypic change was associated with viral breakthrough. The high genetic barrier and the lack of cross-resistance to DAAs make CypI excellent drug candidates for a rescue regimen for patients who did not respond to DAAs combined with pegylated IFNα and ribavirin. More importantly, CypI, as part of a regimen with one or two DAAs (i.e., NS5A or NS5B inhibitors), may constitute the backbone of a new, safe, and effective IFN-free therapy.

Acknowledgments We thank Drs Baugh, Chatterji, Garcia-Rivera, Lin, Hopkins, and Borroto-Esoda for the careful reading of the manuscript. We also thank J. Kuhns for the administrative assistance. We acknowledge financial support from the US Public Health Service grant no. AI087746 (P.A.G.). This is publication no. 23007 from the Department of Immunology and Microbial Science, The Scripps Research Institute, La Jolla, CA.

References

Alberti M, Chuang WL, Flisiak R et al (2012) Alisporivir (ALV) plus peg-interferon/ribavirin (PR) in HCV G1 treatment-experienced patients achieves primary endpoint with superior efficacy at treatment week 12 compared to retreatment with PR. J Hepatol 56:S553–S554. Abstract 1406

Alter MJ (2007) Epidemiology of hepatitis C virus infection. World J Gastroenterol 13:2436–2441

Armstrong GL, Wasley A, Simard EP, McQuillan GM, Kuhnert WL, Alter MJ (2006) The prevalence of hepatitis C virus infection in the United States, 1999 through 2002. Ann Intern Med 144:705–714

Balagopal A, Thomas DL, Thio CL (2010) IL28B and the control of hepatitis C virus infection. Gastroenterology 139(6):1865–1876. doi:10.1053/j.gastro.2010.10.004. Epub 2010 Oct 13. Review

Bartels DJ, Zhou Y, Zhang EZ, Marcial M, Byrn RA, Pfeiffer T et al (2008) Natural prevalence of hepatitis C virus variants with decreased sensitivity to NS3/4A protease inhibitors in treatment-naive subjects. J Infect Dis 198(6):800–807

Borel JF (2002) History of the discovery of cyclosporin and of its early pharmacological development. Wien Klin Wochenschr 114(12):433–437

Braaten D, Luban J (2001) Cyclophilin A regulates HIV-1 infectivity, as demonstrated by gene targeting in human T cells. EMBO J 20:1300–1309

Chatterji U, Bobardt M, Selvarajah S, Yang F, Tang H, Sakamoto N, Vuagniaux G, Parkinson T, Gallay P (2009) The isomerase active site of cyclophilin A is critical for hepatitis C virus replication. J Biol Chem 284:16998–17005

Chatterji U, Lim P, Bobardt MD, Wieland S, Cordek DG, Vuagniaux G, Chisari F, Cameron CE, Targett-Adams P, Parkinson T, Gallay PA (2010) HCV resistance to cyclosporin A does not correlate with a resistance of the NS5A-cyclophilin A interaction to cyclophilin inhibitors. J Hepatol 53:50–56

Chevaliez S, Rodriguez C, Soulier A, Ahmed-Belkacem A, Hezode C, Pawlotsky JM (2011) Molecular characterization of HCV resistance to telaprevir by means of ultra-deep pyrosequencing: preexisting resistant variants and dynamics of resistant populations. J Hepatol 54:S30

Coelmont L, Kaptein S, Paeshuyse J et al (2009) Debio 025, a cyclophilin binding molecule, is highly efficient in clearing hepatitis C virus (HCV) replicon-containing cells when used alone or in combination with specifically targeted antiviral therapy for HCV (STAT-C) inhibitors. Antimicrob Agents Chemother 53(3):967–976. doi:10.1128/AAC.00939-08

Coelmont L, Hanoulle X, Chatterji U, Berger C, Snoeck J, Bobardt M, Lim P, Vliegen I, Paeshuyse J, Vuagniaux G, Vandamme AM, Bartenschlager R, Gallay P, Lippens G (2010)

Neyts. DEB025 (Alisporivir) inhibits hepatitis C virus replication by preventing a cyclophilin A induced *cis*-trans isomerisation in domain II of NS5A. J PLoS One 5:e13687
Colgan J, Asmal M, Yu B, Luban J (2005) Cyclophilin A-deficient mice are resistant to immunosuppression by cyclosporine. J Immunol 174:6030–6038
Cross TJ, Antoniades CG, Harrison PM (2008) Current and future management of chronic hepatitis C infection. Postgrad Med J 84:172–176
Davis G, Kao J, Alberti A et al (2012) Alisporivir (ALV) plus Peg-interferon/Ribavirin (P/R) achieves high on-treatment undetectable HCV RNA levels among the most difficult to treat HCV G1 patients. Results of a planned treatment week 24 interim analysis of a randomized, double blind, placebo controlled trial (FUNDAMENTAL study). In: 63rd annual meeting of the American Association for the Study of Liver Diseases, Boston, 9–12 Nov 2012
Dienstag JL, McHutchison JG (2006) American Gastroenterological Association technical review on the management of hepatitis C. Gastroenterology 130:231–264
Everson GT, Sims KD, Rodriguez-Torres M et al (2012) An interferon-free, ribavirin-free 12-week regimen of daclatasvir (DCV), asunaprevir (ASV), and BMS-791325 yielded SVR4 of 94 % in treatment-naive patients with genotype (GT) 1 chronic hepatitis C virus (HCV) infection. In: 63rd annual meeting of the American Association for the Study of Liver Diseases (AASLD 2012), Boston, 9–13 Nov 2012. Abstract LB-3
Fernandes F, Poole DS, Hoover S, Middleton R, Andrei AC, Gerstner J, Striker R (2007) Sensitivity of hepatitis C virus to cyclosporine A depends on nonstructural proteins NS5A and NS5B. Hepatology 46(4):1026–33
Fernandes F, Ansari IU, Striker R (2010) Cyclosporine inhibits a direct interaction between cyclophilins and hepatitis C NS5A. PLoS One 5:e9815
Fischer G, Bang H, Berger E, Schellenberger A (1984) Conformational specificity of chymotrypsin toward proline-containing substrates. Biochim Biophys Acta 791(1):87–97
Fischer G, Wittmann-Liebold B, Lang K et al (1989) Cyclophilin and peptidyl-prolyl *cis-trans* isomerase are probably identical proteins. Nature 337(6206):476–478
Fischer G, Gallay P, Hopkins S (2010) Cyclophilin inhibitors for the treatment of HCV infection. Curr Opin Investig Drugs 11(8):911–918
Flechner SM (1983) Cyclosporine: a new and promising immunosuppressive agent. Urol Clin N Am 10(2):263–275
Flisiak R, Dumont JM, Crabbé R (2007) Cyclophilin inhibitors in hepatitis C viral infection. Expert Opin Investig Drugs 16:1345–1354
Flisiak R, Horban A, Gallay P, Bobardt M, Selvarajah S, Wiercinska-Drapalo A, Siwak E, Cielniak I, Higersberger J, Kierkus J, Aeschlimann C, Grosgurin P, Nicolas-M'etral V, Dumont JM, Porchet H, Crabb'e R, Scalfaro P (2008) The cyclophilin inhibitor Debio-025 shows potent anti–hepatitis C effect in patients coinfected with hepatitis C and human immunodeficiency virus. Hepatology 47:817–826
Flisiak R, Feinman SV, Jablkowski M, Horban A, Kryczka W, Pawlowska M, Heathcote JE, Mazella G, Vandelli C, Nicolas-M'etral V, Grosgurin P (2009) The cyclophilin inhibitor Debio 025 combined with Peg-Ifna2a significantly reduces viral load in treatment naïve hepatitis C patients. Hepatology 49:1460–1468
Flisiak R, Pawlotsky JM, Crabbe R, Calistru P, Kryczka W, Haussinger D, Mazella G, Romero M, Purcea D, Vuagniaux G, Bao W, Avila C, Zeuzem S (2011) Once daily alisporivir (DEB025) plus Peg-IFN-alfa-2A/ribavirin results in superior sustained virologic response (SVR24) in chronic hepatitis C genotype 1 treatment-naïve patients – the ESSENTIAL study. J Hepatol 55(Suppl 1): S2. Abstract 190
Foster TL, Gallay P, Stonehouse NJ, Harris M (2011) Cyclophilin A interacts with domain II of hepatitis C virus NS5A and stimulates RNA binding in an isomerase-dependent manner. J Virol. 85(14):7460–4. doi: 10.1128/JVI. 00393-11
Fridell RA, Qiu DK, Wang CF, Valera L, Gao M (2010) Resistance analysis of the hepatitis C virus NS5A inhibitor BMS-790052 in an in vitro replicon system. Antimicrob Agents Chemother 54 (9):3641–3650

Fridell RA, Wang CF, Sun JH, O'Boyle DR, Nower P, Valera L et al (2011) Genotypic and phenotypic analysis of variants resistant to hepatitis C virus nonstructural protein 5A replication complex inhibitor BMS-790052 in humans: in vitro and in vivo correlations. Hepatology 54 (6):1924–1935

Fried MW, Shiffman ML, Reddy KR, Smith C, Marinos G, Goncales FL Jr et al (2002) Peginterferon alfa-2a plus ribavirin for chronic hepatitis C virus infection. N Engl J Med 347 (13):975–982

Gallay PA (2009) Cyclophilin inhibitors. Clin Liver Dis 13:403–417

Gallay PA (2012) Cyclophilin inhibitors: a novel class of promising host-targeting anti-HCV agents. Immunol Res. 52(3):200–10. doi:10.1007/s12026-011-8263-5

Gane EJ, Stedman CA, Hyland RH et al (2012) Once daily sofosbuvir (GS-7977) plus ribavirin in patients with HCV genotypes 1, 2, and 3: the ELECTRON trial. In: 63rd annual meeting of the American Association for the Study of Liver Diseases (AASLD 2012), Boston, 9–13 Nov 2012. Abstract 229

Gao M, Nettles RE, Belema M, Snyder LB, Nguyen VN, Fridell RA et al (2010) Chemical genetics strategy identifies an HCV NS5A inhibitor with a potent clinical effect. Nature 465 (7294):96–100. doi:10.1038/nature08960

Garcia-Rivera JA, Bobardt MD, Chatterji U, Hopkins S, Gregory MA, Wilkinson B, Lin K, Gallay PA (2012a) Multiple mutations in HCV NS5A domain II are required to confer a significant level of resistance to alisporivir. Antimicrob Agents Chemother 56:5113–5121. doi:10.1128/AAC.00919-12. Epub 2012 Jul 16. PMCID: PMC3457393 (Available on 2013/4/1)

Garcia-Rivera JA, Lin K, Hopkins S, Gregory MA, Wilkinson B, Gallay PA (2012b) Development of a flow cytometry live cell assay for the screening of inhibitors of hepatitis C virus (HCV) replication. Open Virol J 6:97–102. doi:10.2174/1874357901206010097. Epub 2012 Nov 26. Pub Med Central PMCID: PMC3514710

Gaudieri S, Rauch A, Pfafferott K, Barnes E, Cheng W, McCaughan G et al (2009) Hepatitis C virus drug resistance and immune driven adaptations: relevance to new antiviral therapy. Hepatology 49(4):1069–1082

Global Surveillance and Control of Hepatitis C (1999) Report of a WHO Consultation organized in collaboration with the Viral Hepatitis Prevention Board, Antwerp, Belgium. J Viral Hepat 6:35–47

Goto K, Watashi K, Murata T et al (2006) Evaluation of the anti-hepatitis C virus effects of cyclophilin inhibitors, cyclosporin A, and NIM811. Biochem Biophys Res Commun 343:879–884

Goto K, Watashi K, Inoue D, Hijikata M, Shimotohno K (2009) Identification of cellular and viral factors related to anti-hepatitis C virus activity of cyclophilin inhibitor. Cancer Sci 100 (10):1943–1950. doi:10.1111/j.1349-7006.2009.01263.x. Epub 2009 Jun 26

Gottwein JM, Scheel TKH, Jensen TB, Ghanem L, Bukh J (2011) Differential efficacy of protease inhibitors against HCV genotypes 2a, 3a, 5a, and 6a NS3/4A protease recombinant viruses. Gastroenterology 141(3):1067–1079

Gregory MA, Moss SJ, Coates N, Foster T, Bobardt M, Chatterji U, Gallay PA, Leyssen P, Neyts J, Nur-E-Alam M, Piraee M, Suthar D, Warneck T, Zhang M-Q, Wilkinson B (2011) Preclinical characterization of naturally occurring polyketide cyclophilin inhibitors from the sanglifehrin family. Antimicrob Agents Chemother 55:1975–1981

Handschumacher RE, Harding MW, Rice J et al (1984) Cyclophilin: a specific cytosolic binding protein for cyclosporin A. Science 226(4674):544–547

He Y, Staschke KA, Tan SL (2006) HCV NS5A: a multifunctional regulator of cellular pathways and virus replication, Chapter 9. In: Tan SL (ed) Hepatitis C viruses: genomes and molecular biology. Horizon Bioscience, Norfolk

Hopkins S, Scorneaux B, Huang Z, Murray MG, Wring S, Smitley C, Harris R, Erdmann F, Fischer G, Ribeill Y (2010) SCY-635, a novel nonimmunosuppressive analog of cyclosporine that exhibits potent inhibition of hepatitis C virus RNA replication in vitro. Antimicrob Agents Chemother. 54(2):660–72. doi:10.1128/AAC. 00660-09

Hopkins S, Gallay P (2012) Cyclophilin inhibitors: an emerging class of therapeutics for the treatment of chronic hepatitis C infection. Viruses 4(11):2558–2577. doi:10.3390/v4112558

Hopkins S, Bobardt M, Chatterji U, Garcia-Rivera JA, Lim P, Gallay PA (2012a) The cyclophilin inhibitor SCY-635 disrupts hepatitis C virus NS5A-cyclophilin A complexes. Antimicrob Agents Chemother 56:3888–3897. doi:10.1128/AAC.00693-12. Epub 2012 May 14. PMCID: PMC3393457

Hopkins S, DiMassimo B, Rusnak P, Heuman D, Lalezari J, Sluder A, Scorneaux B, Mosier S, Kowalczyk P, Ribeill Y, Baugh J, Gallay PA (2012b) The cyclophilin inhibitor SCY-635 suppresses viral replication and induces endogenous interferons in patients with chronic HCV genotype 1 infection. J Hepatol 57:47–54. doi:10.1016/j.jhep.2012.02.024. Epub 2012 Mar 13

Houck DR, Hopkins S (2006) Preclinical evaluation of SCY-635, a cyclophilin inhibitor with potent anti-HCV activity. Hepatology 44(Suppl 1):S534–S535. Abstract 934

Huang L, Hwang J, Sharma SD, Hargittai MR, Chen Y, Arnold JJ, Raney KD, Cameron CE (2005) Hepatitis C virus nonstructural protein 5A (NS5A) is an RNA-binding protein. J Biol Chem 280 (43):36417–36428. Epub 2005 Aug 25

Hwang J, Huang L, Cordek DG, Vaughan R, Reynolds SL, Kihara G, Raney KD, Kao CC, Cameron CE (2010) Hepatitis C virus nonstructural protein 5A: biochemical characterization of a novel structural class of RNA-binding proteins. J Virol 84(24):12480–12491. doi:10.1128/JVI.01319-10. Epub 2010 Oct 6

Ishii N, Watashi K, Hishiki T et al (2006) Diverse effects of cyclosporine on hepatitis C virus strain replication. J Virol 80:4510–4520

Jacobson IM, Catlett I, Marcellin P, Bzowej NH, Muir AJ, Adda N et al (2011a) Telaprevir substantially improved SVR rates across all IL28B genotypes in the advance trial. J Hepatol 54:S542–S543

Jacobson IM, McHutchison JG, Dusheiko G, Di Bisceglie AM, Reddy KR, Bzowej NH et al (2011b) Telaprevir for previously untreated chronic hepatitis C virus infection. N Engl J Med 364(25):2405–2416

Kaul A, Stauffer S, Berger C, Pertel T, Schmitt J, Kallis S, Zayas M, Lohmann V, Luban J, Bartenschlager R (2009) Essential role of cyclophilin A for hepatitis C virus replication and virus production and possible link to polyprotein cleavage kinetics. PLoS Pathog 5:e1000546

Kitahata MM, Koepsell TD, Deyo RA et al (1996) Physicians' experience with the acquired immunodeficiency syndrome as a factor in patients' survival. N Engl J Med 334(11):701–706

Kitahata MM, Van Rompaey SE, Shields AW (2000) Physician experience in the care of HIV-infected persons is associated with earlier adoption of new antiretroviral therapy. J Acquir Immune Defic Syndr 24(2):106–114

Kofron JL, KuzmiE P, Kishore V, Colon-Bonilla E, Rich DH (1991) Determination of kinetic constants for peptidyl-prolyl *cis-trans* isomerases by an improved spectrophotometric assay. Biochemistry 30:6127–6134

Kowdley KV, Lawitz E, Poordad F et al (2012) A 12-week interferon-free treatment regimen with ABT-450/r, ABT-267, ABT-333 and ribavirin achieves SVR rates (observed data) of 99 % in treatment-naive patients and 93 % in prior null responders with HCV genotype 1 infection. In: 63rd annual meeting of the American Association for the Study of Liver Diseases (AASLD 2012), Boston, 9–13 Nov 2012. Abstract LB-1

Kuntzen T, Timm J, Berical A, Lennon N, Berlin AM, Young SK et al (2008) Naturally occurring dominant resistance mutations to hepatitis C virus protease and polymerase inhibitors in treatment-naive patients. Hepatology 48(6):1769–1778

Lang K, Schmid FX, Fischer G (1987) Catalysis of protein folding by prolyl isomerase. Nature 329 (6136):268–270

Lawitz E, Godofsky E, Rouzier R, Marbury T, Nguyen T, Ke J, Huang M, Praestgaard J, Serra D, Evans TG (2011) Safety, pharmacokinetics, and antiviral activity of the cyclophilin inhibitor NIM811 alone or in combination with pegylated interferon in HCV-infected patients receiving 14 days of therapy. Antivir Res 89:238–245

Lemm JA, O'Boyle D 2nd, Liu M et al (2010) J Virol 84(1):482–491. doi:10.1128/JVI.01360-09

Lenz O, Fevery B, Vijgen L, Verbeeck J, Peeters M, Beumont M et al (2011) TMC435 in combination with peginterferon alpha-2a/ribavirin in treatment-naive patients infected with HCV genotype 1: virology analysis of the pillar study. Hepatology 54:985A

Li B, Snoeck J, Tang Y, Jones CT, Tiongyip C, Bao W, Yu J, Vandamme A, Vuagniaux G, Crabbe R, Avila C, Naoumov NV, Lin K (2011) Alisporivir – a host-targeting antiviral, provides low viral breakthrough rate and high barrier to resistance in HCV genotype 1 treatment-naïve patients in the phase IIb ESSENTIAL study. American Association for Study of the Liver Congress, San Francisco

Lin K (2010) Development of novel antiviral therapies for hepatitis C virus. Virol Sin 25:246–266

Liu Z, Yang F, Robotham JM, Tang H (2009) Critical role of cyclophilin A and its prolyl-peptidyl isomerase activity in the structure and function of the hepatitis C virus replication complex. J Virol 83:6554–6565

Ma S, Boerner JE, TiongYip C et al (2006) NIM811, a cyclophilin inhibitor, exhibits potent in vitro activity against hepatitis C virus alone or in combination with alpha interferon. Antimicrob Agents Chemother 50:2976–2982

Manns MP, Wedemeyer H, Cornberg M (2006) Treating viral hepatitis C: efficacy, side effects, and complications. Gut 55:1350–1359

Margeridon S, Le Pogam S, Liu TF, Hanczaruk B, Simen BB, Shulman N et al (2011) No detection of variants bearing NS5B S282T mericitabine (MCB) resistance mutation in DAA treatment-naive HCV genotype 1 (G1)-infected patients using ultra-deep pyrosequencing (UDPS). Hepatology 54:532A

Martell M, Esteban JI, Quer J, Genesca J, Weiner A, Esteban R et al (1992) Hepatitis C virus (HCV) circulates as a population of different but closely related genomes: quasispecies nature of HCV genome distribution. J Virol 66(5):3225–3229

Nakagawa M, Sakamoto N, Enomoto N et al (2004) Specific inhibition of hepatitis C virus replication by cyclosporin A. Biochem Biophys Res Commun 313:42–47

Nelson DR, Ghalib RH, Sulkowski M, Schiff E, Rustgi V, Pockros PJ, Wang C, Kerhuel GD, Grosgurin P, Porchet H, Crabb'e R (2009) Efficacy and safety of the cyclophilin inhibitor Debio 025 in combination with pegylated interferon alpha-2A and ribavirin in previously null responder genotype 1 HCV patients. J Hepatol 50:S1. Abstract 95

Neumann AU, Lam NP, Dahari H, Gretch DR, Wiley TE, Layden TJ et al (1998) Hepatitis C viral dynamics in vivo and the antiviral efficacy of interferon-alpha therapy. Science 282 (5386):103–107

Paeshuyse J, Kaul A, De Clercq E et al (2006) The non-immunosuppressive cyclosporin DEBIO 025 is a potent inhibitor of hepatitis C virus replication in vitro. Hepatology 43:761–770

Pawlotsky JM (2012) The science of direct-acting antiviral and host-targeted agent therapy. Antivir Ther 17(6 Pt B):1109–1117. doi:10.3851/IMP2423. Epub 2012 Oct 5

Pawlotsky JM, Sarin SK, Foster GR, Peng CY, Rasenack J, Flisiak R, Piratvisuth T, Wedemeyer H, Chuang WL, Zhang WM, Naoumov NV (2012a) Alisporivir plus ribavirin is highly effective as interferon-free or interferon-add-on regimen in previously untreated HCV-G2 or G3 patients: SVR12 results from VITAL-1 phase 2b study. J Hepatol 56(Suppl 2):S553. Abstract 1405

Pawlotsky JM, Sarin SK, Foster GR et al (2012b) Alisporivir plus Ribavirin achieves high rates of sustained HCV clearance (SVR24) as interferon (IFN)-free or IFN-add-on regimen in treatment-naive patients with HCV GT2 or GT3: final results from VITAL-1 study. In: 63rd annual meeting of the American Association for the Study of Liver Diseases, Boston, 9–12 Nov 2012. Abstract 233

Pockros PJ (2010) New direct-acting antivirals in the development for hepatitis C virus infection. Therap Adv Gastroenterol 3:191–202

Poordad F, McCone J Jr, Bacon BR, Bruno S, Manns MP, Sulkowski MS et al (2011) Boceprevir for untreated chronic HCV genotype 1 infection. N Engl J Med 364(13):1195–1206

Poordad F, Bronowicki JP, Gordon SC, Zeuzem S, Jacobson IM, Sulkowski MS et al (2012) Factors that predict response of patients with HCV infection to boceprevir. Gastroenterology. Epub ahead of print

Powdrill MH, Tchesnokov EP, Kozak RA, Russell RS, Martin R, Svarovskaia ES et al (2011) Contribution of a mutational bias in hepatitis C virus replication to the genetic barrier in the development of drug resistance. Proc Natl Acad Sci U S A 108(51):20509–20513

Puyang X, Poulin DL, Mathy JE, Anderson LJ, Ma S, Fang Z, Zhu S, Lin K, Fujimoto R, Compton T, Wiedmann B (2010) Mechanism of resistance of hepatitis C virus replicons to structurally distinct cyclophilin inhibitors. Antimicrob Agents Chemother 54(5):1981–1987. doi:10.1128/AAC.01236-09. Epub 2010 Feb 22

Robida JM, Nelson HB, Liu Z, Tang H (2007) Characterization of hepatitis C virus subgenomic replicon resistance to cyclosporine in vitro. J Virol 81(11):5829–40

Rong L, Dahari H, Ribeiro RM, Perelson AS (2010) Rapid emergence of protease inhibitor resistance in hepatitis C virus. Sci Transl Med 2(30):30ra2

Rosnoblet C, Fritzinger B, Legrand D, Launay H, Wieruszeski JM, Lippens G, Hanoulle X (2012) Hepatitis C virus NS5B and host cyclophilin A share a common binding site on NS5A. J Biol Chem 287(53):44249–44260. doi:10.1074/jbc.M112.392209. Epub 2012 Nov 14

Sarrazin C, Zeuzem S (2010) Resistance to direct antiviral agents in patients with hepatitis C virus infection. Gastroenterology 138(2):447–462

Sarrazin C, Kieffer TL, Bartels D, Hanzelka B, Muh U, Welker M et al (2007a) Dynamic hepatitis C virus genotypic and phenotypic changes in patients treated with the protease inhibitor telaprevir. Gastroenterology 132(5):1767–1777

Sarrazin C, Rouzier R, Wagner F, Forestier N, Larrey D, Gupta SK et al (2007b) SCH 503034, a novel hepatitis C virus protease inhibitor, plus pegylated interferon alpha-2b for genotype 1 nonresponders. Gastroenterology 132:1270–1278

Shepard CW, Finelli L, Alter MJ (2005) Global epidemiology of hepatitis C virus infection. Lancet Infect Dis 5:558–567

Shirota Y, Luo H, Qin W, Kaneko S, Yamashita T, Kobayashi K, Murakami S (2002) Hepatitis C virus (HCV) NS5A binds RNA-dependent RNA polymerase (RdRP) NS5B and modulates RNA-dependent RNA polymerase activity. J Biol Chem 277:11149–11155

Simmonds P, Bukh J, Combet C et al (2005) Consensus proposals for a unified system of nomenclature of hepatitis C virus genotypes. Hepatology 42:962–973

Soriano V, Madejon A, Vispo E et al (2008a) Emerging drugs for hepatitis C. Expert Opin Emerg Drugs 13:1–19

Soriano V, Perelson AS, Zoulim F (2008b) Why are there different dynamics in the selection of drug resistance in HIV and hepatitis B and C viruses? J Antimicrob Chemother 62(1):1–4

Sulkowski MS, Gardiner DF, Rodriguez-Torres M et al (2012) High rate of sustained virologic response with the all-oral combination of daclatasvir (NS5A inhibitor) plus sofosbuvir (nucleotide NS5B inhibitor), with or without ribavirin, in treatment-naive patients chronically infected with HCV genotype 1, 2, or 3. In: 63rd annual meeting of the American Association for the Study of Liver Diseases (AASLD 2012), Boston, 9–13 Nov 2012. Abstract LB-2

Sullivan JC, De Meyer S, Bartels DJ, Dierynck I, Zhang E, Spanks J et al (2011) Evolution of treatment-emergent resistant variants in telaprevir phase 3 clinical trials. J Hepatol 54:S4

Sun SCC, Bae A, Qi X, Harris J, Wong KA, Miller MD et al (2011) Natural variation in drug susceptibility to HCV polymerase inhibitors in treatment-naive HCV patient isolates. J Viral Hepat 18(12):861–870

Sy T, Jamal MM (2006) Epidemiology of hepatitis C virus (HCV) infection. Int J Med Sci 3:41–46

Tiongyip X, Badillo A, Wieruszeski JM, Verdegem D, Landrieu I, Bartenschlager R, Penin F, Lippens G (2009) Hepatitis C virus NS5A protein is a substrate for the peptidyl-prolyl cis/trans isomerase activity of cyclophilins A and B. J Biol Chem 284:13589–13601

Tiongyip C, Jones CT, Tang Y et al (2011) Host targeting cyclophilin inhibitor alisporivir presents a high barrier to resistance with no cross-resistance to direct acting antivirals. In: 6th international workshop on hepatitis C, resistance and new compounds, Cambridge, MA, 24 June 2011

Tong MJ, Reddy KR, Lee WM et al (1997) Treatment of chronic hepatitis C with consensus interferon: a multicenter, randomized, controlled trial. Consens Interferon Study Group Hepatol 26:747–754

Verdegem D, Badillo A, Wieruszeski JM, Landrieu I, Leroy A, Bartenschlager R, Penin F, Lippens G, Hanoulle X (2011) Domain 3 of NS5A protein from the hepatitis C virus has intrinsic alpha-helical propensity and is a substrate of cyclophilin A. J Biol Chem 286:20441–20454

Vermehren J, Sarrazin C (2011) New hepatitis C therapies in clinical development. Eur J Med Res 16:303–314

Vicenti I, Rosi A, Saladini F, Meini G, Pippi F, Rossetti B et al (2012) Naturally occurring hepatitis C virus (HCV) NS3/4A protease inhibitor resistance-related mutations in HCV genotype 1-infected subjects in Italy. J Antimicrob Chemother 67(4):984–987

von Hahn T, Ciesek S, Manns MP (2011) Arrest all accessories – inhibition of hepatitis C virus by compounds that target host factors. Discov Med 12:237–244

von Hahn T, Schiene-Fischer C, Van ND, Pfaender S, Karavul B, Steinmann E, Potthoff A, Strassburg C, Hamdi N, Abdelaziz AI, Sarrazin C, Müller T, Berg T, Trépo E, Wedemeyer H, Manns MP, Pietschmann T, Ciesek S (2012) Hepatocytes that express variants of cyclophilin A are resistant to HCV infection and replication. Gastroenterology 143(2):439.e1–447.e1. doi:10.1053/j.gastro.2012.04.053. Epub 2012 May 8

Waller H, Chatterji U, Gallay P, Parkinson T, Targett-Adams P (2010) The use of AlphaLISA technology to detect interaction between hepatitis C virus-encoded NS5A and cyclophilin A. J Virol Methods 165:202–210

Watashi K, Hijikata M, Hosaka M et al (2003) Cyclosporin A suppresses replication of hepatitis C virus genome in cultured hepatocytes. Hepatology 38:1282–1288

World Health Organization (2012) Hepatitis C factsheet no. 164. http://www.whoint/mediacentre/factsheets/fs164/en/index. Accessed online on 28 June 2012

Wyles DL (2013) Antiviral resistance and the future landscape of hepatitis C virus infection therapy. J Infect Dis 207(Suppl 1):S33–S39. doi:10.1093/infdis/jis761

Yang F, Robotham JM, Nelson HB, Irsigler A, Kenworthy R, Tang H (2008) Cyclophilin A is an essential cofactor for hepatitis C virus infection and the principal mediator of cyclosporine resistance in vitro. J Virol 82:5269–5278

Yang F, Robotham JM, Grise H, Frausto S, Madan V, Zayas M, Bartenschlager R, Robinson M, Greenstein AE, Nag A, Logan TM, Bienkiewicz E, Tang H (2010) A major determinant of cyclophilin dependence and cyclosporine susceptibility of hepatitis C virus identified by a genetic approach. PLoS Pathog 6:e1001118

Zeuzem S, Soriano V, Asselah T, Bronowicki JP, Lohse A, Mullhaupt B et al (2012) SVR4 and SVR12 with an interferon-free regimen of BI 201335 and BI 207127, +/− ribavirin, in treatment-naive patients with chronic genotype-1 HCV infection: interim results of sound-C2. J Hepatol 56:S45

Antiviral Drug Resistance in Herpesviruses

Jocelyne Piret, Emilien Drouot, and Guy Boivin

Contents

Abstract

The discovery of acyclovir (ACV), a nucleoside analogue, more than 30 years ago, represents a milestone in the management of herpes simplex virus (HSV) and varicella-zoster virus (VZV) infections. The modest activity of ACV against human cytomegalovirus (HCMV) has prompted the development of another nucleoside analogue, ganciclovir (GCV), for the management of systemic and organ-specific HCMV diseases. Second-line agents such as the pyrophosphate analogue foscarnet (FOS) and the nucleotide analogue cidofovir (CDV) have

J. Piret • E. Drouot • G. Boivin (✉)
Research Center in Infectious Diseases, Laval University, Quebec City, QC, Canada
e-mail: jocelyne.piret@crchudequebec.ulaval.ca; emilien.drouot@crchudequebec.ulaval.ca; Guy.Boivin@crchudequebec.ulaval.ca

M. Gotte et al. (eds.), *Handbook of Antimicrobial Resistance*,
DOI 10.1007/978-1-4939-0694-9_7

been approved subsequently. In contrast to ACV and GCV, the latter drugs do not require an initial phosphorylation step by viral protein kinases to be converted into their active forms. Since the introduction of these antivirals, the emergence of drug-resistant mutants has been constantly reported particularly in severely immunocompromised patients such as bone marrow and solid organ transplant recipients as well as human immunodeficiency virus (HIV)-infected individuals. In this chapter, we review the characteristics of the antiviral agents currently approved for the management of HSV, VZV, and HCMV diseases, the laboratory methods for assessing drug susceptibilities, and the clinical significance of drug-resistant infections and their management.

Keywords

Herpesvirus • Herpes simplex virus • Varicella-zoster virus • Human cytomegalovirus • Antiviral drug • Resistance • Mutations • Phenotypic testing • Genotypic testing • Clinical significance • Management • Immunocompromised patient

Introduction

Herpesviridae is a large family of DNA viruses including nine different human viruses which belong to the *α-herpesvirinae* [herpes simplex virus types 1 and 2 (HSV-1 and HSV-2) and varicella-zoster virus (VZV)], the *β-herpesvirinae* [human cytomegalovirus (HCMV) and human herpesviruses 6 and 7 (HHV-6 A/B and HHV-7)], and the *γ-herpesvirinae* [Epstein-Barr virus (EBV) and (HHV-8)] subfamilies. These ubiquitous viruses cause different types of pathologies which vary considerably according to the immune status of the infected individuals. They all have the ability to establish latency and to reactivate under certain circumstances. Among members of the Herpesviridae family, four of them (HSV-1, HSV-2, VZV, and HCMV) will be discussed in this chapter since they are the targets of antiviral strategies. HSV-1 and HSV-2 cause orolabial and genital infections as well as keratitis, encephalitis, and neonatal infections. VZV is the causative agent of varicella and herpes zoster. HCMV is responsible for mononucleosis-like syndromes as well as systemic and organ-specific diseases in immunocompromised patients.

Antiviral Agents for Herpesvirus Infections

All antiviral agents currently approved for the treatment of HSV, VZV, and HCMV infections ultimately target the viral DNA polymerase (Andrei et al. 2009). First-line antiviral agents for the treatment of HSV and VZV infections include acyclovir (ACV, Zovirax®, GlaxoSmithKline) and penciclovir (PCV) and their respective ester prodrugs valacyclovir (VACV, Valtrex®, GlaxoSmithKline) and famciclovir (FCV, Famvir®, Novartis). Acyclovir and PCV are deoxyguanosine analogues that must be phosphorylated by HSV- or VZV-encoded thymidine kinase (TK) and then by

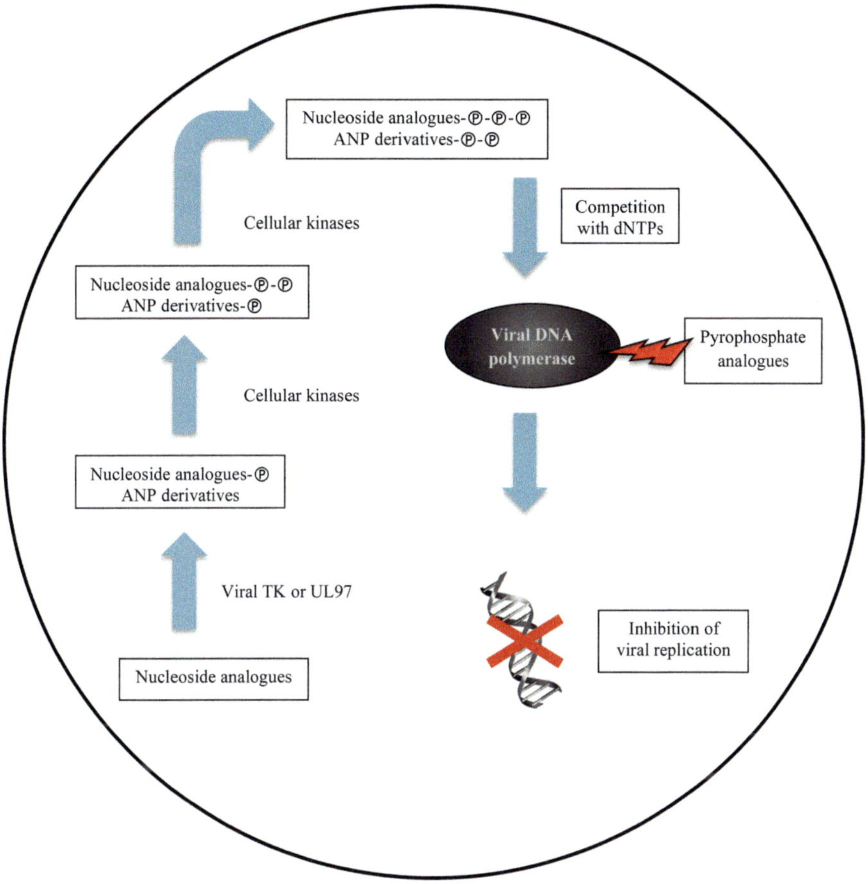

Fig. 1 Mechanisms of action of the different classes of antiviral agents. The nucleoside analogues such as acyclovir, penciclovir, and ganciclovir must be first phosphorylated by the viral thymidine kinase or UL97 protein kinase and then by cellular kinases to be converted into their active forms. The acyclic nucleoside phosphonate (*ANP*) derivatives such as cidofovir must be phosphorylated by cellular kinases only to be active. The nucleoside analogue triphosphate and the ANP derivative diphosphate compete with deoxynucleotide triphosphates (dNTPs) to inhibit the viral replication. The pyrophosphate analogues such as foscarnet directly inhibit the activity of the DNA polymerase. Key: Ⓟ represents the phosphate groups

cellular kinases to exert their antiviral activity. The triphosphate forms are competitive inhibitors of the viral DNA polymerase (Fig. 1) (Reardon and Spector 1989). Moreover, ACV triphosphate is incorporated into the replicating DNA and acts as a chain terminator of the DNA polymerase. Oral ACV, VACV, and FCV are used for short-term therapy of primary and recurrent HSV infections (particularly genital herpes), long-term suppressive therapy of recurrent genital herpes, as well as treatment of herpes zoster. The intravenous (IV) formulation of ACV is indicated for the management of severe HSV (including encephalitis and neonatal herpes) and VZV infections. Topical formulations of ACV and PCV (Denavir®, Novartis) are used for the treatment of herpes labialis and keratitis.

Ganciclovir (GCV, Cytovene®, Roche) is the first-line antiviral drug for the prevention and treatment of HCMV diseases. Ganciclovir is a deoxyguanosine analogue that requires a first phosphorylation by the protein kinase encoded by the *UL97* gene and two subsequent phosphorylations by cellular kinases to exert its antiviral activity. Ganciclovir triphosphate acts as a potent inhibitor of the DNA polymerase encoded by the *UL54* gene by competing with deoxyguanosine triphosphate for incorporation into replicating DNA where it slows down DNA polymerization and eventually stops chain elongation (Fig. 1) (Biron et al. 1985). Ganciclovir can be given orally, intravenously, or as an intravitreal implant (Vitrasert, Chiron) for the treatment of HCMV retinitis. The poor bioavailability of GCV (~6 %) following oral administration prompted the development of its L-valyl ester prodrug, valganciclovir (VGCV, Valcyte®, Roche), which exhibits approximately 10-fold increase in oral bioavailability (Pescovitz et al. 2000). Oral VGCV and IV GCV are indicated in the treatment of established HCMV diseases in immunocompromised patients and in the prevention of symptomatic episodes, especially in transplant recipients. Two preventive strategies may be used depending on the risk for patients to develop severe HCMV diseases. The "universal prophylaxis" strategy consists of administering the antiviral to all patients after transplantation for a 3- to 6-month period, whereas the "preemptive" approach requires laboratory monitoring evidence of HCMV replication in the blood (typically monitored once weekly) based on the detection of pp65 antigen or viral DNA by real-time PCR (Boeckh et al. 2004; Piiparinen et al. 2004; Gimeno et al. 2008) before initiation of antiviral treatment.

Second-line antiviral drugs for the treatment of HCMV diseases include foscarnet (FOS, Foscavir®, AstraZeneca) and cidofovir (CDV, Vistide®, Gilead). Due to their toxicity profiles and the absence of oral formulations, they are usually reserved for patients failing or not tolerating therapy with nucleoside analogues. Foscarnet is a pyrophosphate analogue which does not require phosphorylation by viral or cellular kinases. It directly inhibits the viral DNA polymerase by binding to the pyrophosphate binding site and preventing pyrophosphate cleavage from incoming deoxynucleotide triphosphates (dNTPs), which then results in cessation of chain elongation (Fig. 1) (Oberg 1989). The IV formulation of FOS is indicated for the treatment of HCMV retinitis in individuals with the acquired immunodeficiency syndrome (AIDS) and for GCV-resistant HCMV infections in immunocompromised patients. Foscarnet may also be used in the treatment of infections caused by nucleoside analogue-resistant HSV and VZV mutants. Cidofovir is an acyclic deoxycytidine monophosphate which requires only two phosphorylations by cellular enzymes to be converted into its active form, which acts as a DNA chain terminator (Fig. 1) (Xiong et al. 1997). The IV formulation of CDV is indicated in the treatment of HCMV retinitis in AIDS patients and is occasionally also used in transplant recipients. Topical and IV formulations of CDV may be used "off label" in the treatment of ACV- and/or FOS-resistant HSV infections (Andrei et al. 2009).

Herpes Simplex Virus and Varicella-Zoster Virus Antiviral Drug Resistance

Phenotypic and Genotypic Testing for Detection of HSV and VZV Drug Resistance

Suspected HSV or VZV drug-resistant infections can be confirmed by testing the susceptibility of clinical isolates against antiviral agents in cell culture (phenotypic assays) or by the identification of specific mutations conferring drug resistance directly in clinical samples (genotypic assays).

The plaque reduction assay (PRA) is the gold standard phenotypic method to determine the susceptibility of HSV isolates to antiviral drugs and is approved as a standard protocol by the Clinical and Laboratory Standard Institute (Swierkosz et al. 2004). In this assay, cells are infected with a constant viral inoculum. The virus is then allowed to grow in the presence of serial drug dilutions for 2–3 days before fixing and staining the cells. The cytopathic effects (CPE) or viral plaques are then counted under an inverted microscope. The drug concentration that reduces the CPE by 50 % compared to controls (without antiviral) is defined as the 50 % effective concentration (EC_{50}). Breakpoint values that are widely accepted to define HSV resistance to ACV and FOS are EC_{50} equal to or greater than 9 and 330 μM, respectively (Swierkosz et al. 2004). No consensus value has been proposed for PCV. Drug resistance can also be defined by an increase in the EC_{50} value greater than three to five times that of the baseline isolate from the same patient.

The low rate of VZV isolation from vesicle samples (from 20 % to 43 %) and its slow growth in cell culture (5–6 days) limit the use of the PRA in that context (Sauerbrei et al. 1999). An increase in the EC_{50} value equal to or greater than four times that of a sensitive reference strain (e.g., the Oka strain) is generally accepted to define VZV resistance to ACV (Saint-Leger et al. 2001).

It is worth mentioning that the difficulty in obtaining an appropriate clinical specimen for cell culture, the length of time required for the propagation of the viral isolate in cultured cell lines, the subjectivity of counting plaques, and the possible selection bias introduced during the growth of heterogeneous viral populations in cell culture can all potentially limit the clinical utility of the PRA. The objectivity of the readout was improved in several phenotypic methods based on the detection of specific antigens (by ELISA, flow cytometry, or immunoperoxidase staining) or the detection of DNA (by hybridization or real-time PCR).

Genotypic testing is based on the amplification of HSV or VZV genes involved in drug resistance by PCR and the identification of specific mutations by DNA sequencing. Standard dideoxy sequencing can detect an emerging resistance mutation when it exceeds approximately 20 % of the total population. It is thus estimated that a viral load of at least 1,000 copies/ml of clinical sample is required to obtain reliable genotypic profiles (Schuurman et al. 1999). Mutations conferring resistance to nucleoside analogues occur in *UL23* (HSV) or *ORF36* (VZV) genes encoding the TKs and/or in *UL30* (HSV) or *ORF28* (VZV) genes encoding the DNA polymerases. As some degrees of inter-strain variability exist in these genes, mutations conferring drug resistance must be discriminated from natural polymorphisms. In this respect, results of genotypic testing must be interpreted by comparison with mutations already assigned to natural polymorphism or confirmed drug resistance in the literature. Mutations with unknown significance in drug resistance must be confirmed by recombinant phenotyping which consists in the introduction of an individual mutation into the genome of a control-sensitive laboratory strain followed by the determination of the resulting drug-susceptibility phenotype (Bestman-Smith and Boivin 2003; Sergerie and Boivin 2006).

An ACV-resistant HSV or VZV mutant may exhibit a TK-deficient (lack of enzyme activity), a TK low-producer (reduced level of enzymatic activity), a TK-altered (substrate-specific enzyme which phosphorylates thymidine but not ACV and/or PCV), or a DNA polymerase-altered (altered enzyme activity) phenotype. Approximately, 95 % of HSV or VZV clinical isolates resistant to ACV possess TK-negative or TK low-producer phenotypes, whereas a minority consists of TK-altered and DNA polymerase-altered mutants (Roberts et al. 1991; Pottage and Kessler 1995; Gaudreau et al. 1998; Gilbert et al. 2002; Burrel et al. 2012; Malartre et al. 2012; Sauerbrei et al. 2012, 2013).

Both TK and DNA polymerase mutants resistant to ACV exhibit a decrease in so-called in vivo "fitness" and neurovirulence. The HSV TK is not essential for viral growth in cell culture, but this enzyme plays an important role in the pathogenesis as demonstrated in animal models (Coen et al. 1989; Efstathiou et al. 1989; Chen et al. 2004). It has been suggested that mutations arising in the TK may eliminate or markedly reduce the enzyme activity that could not fulfill the greater requirement of thymidine phosphorylation for virus replication in neurons compared to other cells (Chen et al. 1998). Indeed, TK low-producer mutants show some reduction in pathogenicity compared with wild-type strains but are generally able to reactivate (Coen 1994; Bernstein et al. 2000). In contrast, TK-deficient mutants have impaired pathogenicity, established latency in sensory ganglia with a lower efficiency than wild-type strains, and reactivate poorly. However, some TK-deficient HSV clinical isolates express ultra-low levels of enzyme activity that could be sufficient to allow reactivation (Coen 1994; Besecker et al. 2007). Moreover, phylogenetically related HSV-1 strains sensitive and resistant to ACV were shown to coexist in latently-infected trigeminal ganglia of immunocompetent individuals (van Velzen et al. 2012). Therefore, immunocompromised patients are at risk of reactivating ACV-resistant mutants that can cause infections refractory to nucleoside analogue therapy. Mutants with altered DNA polymerase activity have been less studied, but they seem to exhibit different degrees of attenuation of neurovirulence in mice (Field and Coen 1986; Pelosi et al. 1998; Andrei et al. 2007; Dambrosi et al. 2010). As the HSV DNA polymerase is essential for viral replication, mutations emerging in this enzyme must be functionally conservative. It is proposed that DNA polymerase mutants could have a lower affinity for dNTPs leading to an altered viral replication in neurons which only contain small amounts of nucleic acid precursors (Field and Coen 1986).

Role of *UL23/ORF36* and *UL30/ORF28* Gene Mutations in Conferring HSV/VZV Drug Resistance

In clinical HSV isolates, resistance to ACV is mediated in 95 % of the cases by mutations in the *UL23* gene and, in the remaining cases, by mutations in the *UL30* gene (Gaudreau et al. 1998; Gilbert et al. 2002; Morfin and Thouvenot 2003; Frobert et al. 2007; Piret and Boivin 2011, 2014). Six highly conserved domains have been identified among Herpesviridae TKs (Balasubramaniam et al. 1990). The most important regions involved in the enzyme activity are the ATP-binding site, the nucleoside-binding site, and the cysteine at codon 336 which maintains the three-dimensional structure of the active site (Evans et al. 1998). Resistance hot spots in the *UL23* gene correspond to homopolymer stretches of guanines or cytosines (Fig. 2a) (Sasadeusz et al. 1997; Gaudreau et al. 1998; Morfin et al. 2000). Approximately half (up to 80 % in a study (Burrel et al. 2013a)) of the clinical cases of ACV resistance consist in addition or deletion of nucleotides in these regions. The resulting frameshift reading introduces premature termination codons and the expression of a truncated TK polypeptide. The remaining cases of ACV resistance result from single amino acid substitutions that are usually located in the six conserved domains (especially the ATP-binding and nucleoside-binding sites) as well as at amino acid 336 of the TK (Gaudreau et al. 1998; Morfin et al. 2000; Chibo et al. 2004; Stranska et al. 2004b; Duan et al. 2009; Burrel et al. 2010; Sauerbrei et al. 2010, 2011a). Some mutations located outside these highly conserved regions may also confer resistance to ACV (Gaudreau et al. 1998; Morfin et al. 2000; Stranska et al. 2004b; Duan et al. 2009). Resistance to PCV generally maps to mutations within the *UL23* gene (Sarisky et al. 2002, 2003) and consists of 4 % single-nucleotide substitutions distributed throughout the gene and 96 % frameshift mutations (Suzutani et al. 2003).

Mutations conferring resistance to ACV, FOS, and CDV in HSV clinical isolates have been identified in the catalytic or conserved domains of the DNA polymerase (Fig. 2b) (Gilbert et al. 2002; Morfin and Thouvenot 2003; Frobert et al. 2007; Piret and Boivin 2011, 2014). The Herpesviridae DNA polymerases belong to the family of α-like DNA polymerases (Wong et al. 1988) which share regions of homology numbered I to VII. These regions correspond to the degree of conservation among these enzymes, with region I being the most conserved. Moreover, Herpesviridae DNA polymerases also contain a δ-region C, which is shared by enzymes related to eukaryotic DNA polymerases δ (Zhang et al. 1991). The HSV DNA polymerase is formed by six conserved structural domains, namely, pre-NH_2 and NH_2 domains, polymerase palm, fingers, and thumb domains, and a 3′–5′ exonuclease domain (Liu and Homa 2009). The polymerase palm domain contains regions I, II, and VII, and the thumb domain contains region V. These four regions appear to flank the catalytic site in the palm domain and contain the catalytic triad of aspartic acid residues (at positions 717, 886, and 888) that are essential for polymerase activity. Regions III and VI belong to the finger domain and may play a role in positioning the template

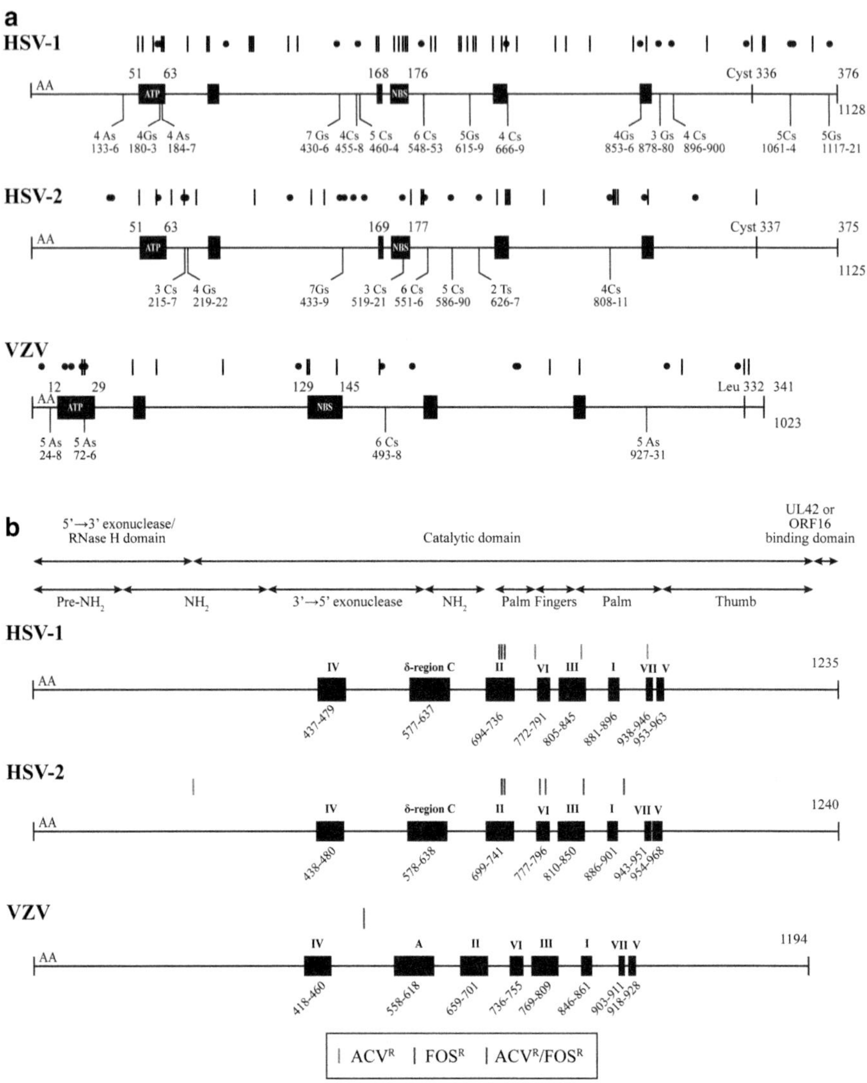

Fig. 2 Confirmed drug-resistance mutations identified in clinical HSV-1, HSV-2, and VZV isolates (laboratory-derived strains are not shown for clarity). Panel a shows mutations in the *UL23* gene of HSV-1 and HSV-2 and in the *ORF36* gene of VZV conferring resistance to acyclovir. Conserved regions among the thymidine kinase of Herpesviridae including the ATP-binding site (*ATP*) and the nucleoside-binding site (*NBS*) are represented by the black boxes. Bars (|) indicate amino acid (*AA*) substitutions, whereas dots (•) represent nucleotide additions and/or deletions. The homopolymer runs, as well as the nucleotides involved, are indicated below vertical bars. Panel b shows mutations in the *UL30* gene of HSV-1 and HSV-2 and in the *ORF28* gene of VZV conferring resistance to acyclovir (ACV^R) and/or foscarnet (FOS^R). Conserved regions among the Herpesviridae DNA polymerase are represented by the black boxes. The roman numbers (I–VII) and δ-region C corresponding to each of these regions are indicated above the boxes. Bars (|) indicate amino acid substitutions

and primer strands. The 3′–5′ exonuclease domain contains three highly conserved sequence motifs Exo I, Exo II (region IV), and Exo III (δ-region C). Single amino acid substitutions associated with ACV resistance are mostly located in regions II, III, VI, and VII of the enzyme; the greatest clusters of mutations being found in regions II and III (Schmit and Boivin 1999; Sauerbrei et al. 2011a). Only a few mutations have been described within the other conserved domains or outside such regions (Schmit and Boivin 1999). Most FOS-resistant clinical isolates contain single amino acid substitutions in conserved regions II, III, or VI and in a non-conserved region (between regions I and VII) of the DNA polymerase (Schmit and Boivin 1999; Bestman-Smith and Boivin 2002). Some of these isolates retain susceptibility or, at least, borderline levels of susceptibility to ACV and CDV (Schmit and Boivin 1999; Bestman-Smith and Boivin 2002). However, mutations within conserved regions II and VI are frequently associated with resistance to both ACV and FOS. The mutations S724N (region II) and L778M (region VI) in HSV-1, which confer cross-resistance to ACV and FOS, also cause reduced susceptibility to CDV (Bestman-Smith and Boivin 2003). Genotypic analyses of drug-sensitive HSV isolates reveal a high degree of polymorphism in the *UL23* and *UL30* genes (Frobert et al. 2008; Burrel et al. 2010; Bohn et al. 2011).

In VZV clinical isolates, resistance to ACV is mostly associated with mutations in the viral TK and, less frequently, with mutations in the viral DNA polymerase (Gilbert et al. 2002; Piret and Boivin 2014). The genome of VZV has a lower GC content (46 %) than those of HSVs (68 %) and only a few homopolymer stretches are present in the *ORF36* gene (Andrei et al. 2012). The string of six cytosines located at codon positions 493–498 within this gene emerged as a hot spot for the insertion or deletion of nucleotides involved in ACV resistance (Fig. 2a) (Boivin et al. 1994; Morfin et al. 1999; Andrei et al. 2012; van der Beek et al. 2013). In addition, non-synonymous nucleotide substitutions conferring resistance to ACV are widely dispersed in the *ORF36* gene (Sawyer et al. 1988; Talarico et al. 1993; Boivin et al. 1994; Fillet et al. 1998; Morfin et al. 1999; Saint-Leger et al. 2001; Sauerbrei et al. 2011b). However, these amino acid changes occur more frequently in the ATP-binding and nucleoside-binding sites and at amino acid 231 of the TK (Morfin et al. 1999).

A few reports have described ACV- and/or FOS-resistant clinical VZV isolates with mutations in the *ORF28* gene (Fig. 2b) (Visse et al. 1998; Kamiyama et al. 2001; Sauerbrei et al. 2011b). These amino acid substitutions are mainly found in the catalytic site and in the conserved regions of the DNA polymerase and may confer cross-resistance to ACV and FOS. The TK and DNA polymerase of VZV are highly conserved compared to those of HSVs and only very few natural polymorphisms have been identified in the *ORF36* and *ORF28* genes (Sauerbrei et al. 2011b).

Clinical Significance, Prevalence, and Risk Factors for Drug-Resistant HSV and VZV Infections

Cases of HSV infections unresponsive to treatment in immunocompetent patients are usually associated with diagnoses of recurrent genital herpes, keratitis, and encephalitis. In general, most unresponsive cases in immunocompetent patients are not due to antiviral drug resistance. Furthermore, the rare instances of resistance in that setting are not associated with prolonged active lesions due to a functional immune system. In immunocompromised patients, infections caused by ACV-resistant isolates are associated with significant morbidity, including persistent and/or disseminated diseases refractory to antiviral therapy. Patients with AIDS can develop extensive mucocutaneous lesions usually not associated with visceral or central nervous system infections (Levin et al. 2004). A few cases of lethal disseminated visceral HSV infections due to ACV-resistant mutants have been reported in bone marrow transplant (BMT) recipients (Ljungman et al. 1990), and a case of meningoencephalitis was described in an AIDS patient (Gateley et al. 1990).

The prevalence of nucleoside analogue-resistant HSV isolates differs greatly for immunocompetent and immunocompromised patients. A low prevalence of 0.3–0.7 % was reported for HSV resistance to ACV in immunocompetent patients during extensive surveys between 1980 and 1992 (Collins and Ellis 1993). The prevalence of ACV resistance has remained constant since then ranging from 0.1 % to 0.7 % (Christophers et al. 1998; Boon et al. 2000; Bacon et al. 2002, 2003; Danve-Szatanek et al. 2004; Stranska et al. 2005). A more recent report has documented a relatively high prevalence (6.4 %) of ACV-resistant HSV-1 isolates in immunocompetent patients with herpetic keratitis (Duan et al. 2008), and some of these cases were clinically refractory to ACV therapy (Burrel et al. 2013b; James and Prichard 2013; van Velzen et al. 2013; Pan et al. 2014). The higher incidence of ACV resistance in this setting may be related to the fact that the cornea can be considered as an immune-privileged site where low immune surveillance favors the rapid selection of resistant viruses (Andrei and Snoeck 2013). Similarly, a low prevalence of 0.19–0.22 % was reported for PCV resistance in immunocompetent patients (Sarisky et al. 2003). A prevalence of less than 0.3 % was also observed in persons who used the topical formulation of PCV to treat recurrent herpes labialis (Shin et al. 2003).

Prolonged treatment with ACV, VACV, or FCV is required to prevent or to manage HSV infections in the immunocompromised host, which may result in the selection of viral isolates with reduced drug susceptibility. The prevalence of HSV infections caused by ACV-resistant isolates in these populations varies from 3.5 % to 11 % (Englund et al. 1990; Nugier et al. 1992; Christophers et al. 1998; Bacon et al. 2003; Stranska et al. 2005). The prevalence for ACV resistance ranged from 3.5 % to 7 % in human immunodeficiency virus (HIV)-positive patients (Englund et al. 1990; Reyes et al. 2003; Danve-Szatanek et al. 2004; Levin et al. 2004; Ziyaeyan et al. 2007; Lolis et al. 2008), from 2.5 % to 10 % in solid organ transplant (SOT) recipients (Christophers et al. 1998; Danve-Szatanek et al. 2004), and from 4.1 % to 10.9 % in hematopoietic stem cell transplant (HSCT) recipients (Wade et al. 1983; Chakrabarti et al. 2000; Chen et al. 2000; Morfin et al. 2000; Danve-Szatanek et al. 2004; Erard et al. 2007; Frangoul et al. 2007). An even higher frequency (36 %) of ACV resistance was also reported in the latter population (Langston et al. 2002). In one study, patients receiving either autologous or allogeneic BMT developed HSV infections at a similar rate (9.2 %), but resistance occurred only in allogeneic transplants reaching a prevalence of 27 % (Morfin et al. 2004). The emergence of PCV-resistant HSV isolates among immunocompromised patients has been less studied but found to be 2.1 % and not associated with treatment failure in one report summarizing different clinical trials (Sarisky et al. 2003). Few reports have described the emergence of FOS-resistant HSV isolates mainly in AIDS patients failing therapy (Hwang et al. 1992; Safrin et al. 1994a, b; Chakrabarti et al. 2000; Bestman-Smith and Boivin 2002; Langston et al. 2002; Saijo et al. 2002; Danve-Szatanek et al. 2004; Stranska et al. 2004a). For instance, nine HSV strains resistant to FOS have been isolated in HIV-infected individuals for whom ACV and FOS therapy sequentially failed, but mutations conferring FOS resistance identified in the viral DNA polymerase were not associated with reduced ACV or CDV susceptibility (Schmit and Boivin 1999; Bestman-Smith and Boivin 2003).

The severity of immunosuppression and the dose and duration of ACV prophylaxis/treatment are likely important risk factors in the development of drug resistance. In the setting of T cell-depleted haploidentical transplantation, all HSV patients who received short courses of low-doses ACV for prophylaxis experienced clinical reactivation at a median $CD4^+$ T cell count of 3.5/μl (Langston et al. 2002). Lesion healing was correlated with immune recovery, but one patient had recurrent ACV-resistant HSV lesions due to a drop in the $CD4^+$ T cell count. The treatment regimen used was inadequate in this setting and drug resistance occurred less frequently when a prophylaxis with higher doses was given for longer periods. It was also reported that HSV-1 visceral infection (9.8 % versus 2.2 %) and ACV resistance (5.8 % versus 1.8 %) were more common in type-discordant [seronegative donor (D^-)/seropositive recipient (R^+)] than in type-concordant (D^+/R^+) HSCT patients, respectively (Nichols et al. 2003). However, drug-resistant HSV mutants have been isolated in some patients in the absence of known history of ACV exposure (Malvy et al. 2005; Schulte et al. 2010) and likely represent the natural rates of TK mutations.

The emergence of VZV isolates resistant to ACV has not been reported in immunocompetent individuals with primary VZV infections or herpes zoster. Cases of resistance to ACV have been described in AIDS patients, SOT and HSCT recipients, as well as hemato-oncological patients with VZV reactivations unresponsive to therapy (Talarico et al. 1993; Boivin et al. 1994; Fillet et al. 1998; Visse et al. 1998; Morfin et al. 1999). In these patients, VZV infections unresponsive to ACV therapy persist in the form of chronic skin lesions and are associated with significant morbidity and mortality due to visceral dissemination. A chronic verrucous form of VZV infections caused by ACV-resistant mutants has also been described in some of these patients (Crassard et al. 2000; Bryan et al. 2008). Two cases of immunocompromised children presenting herpes zoster due to the Oka vaccine strain and who developed chronic disseminated drug-resistant VZV infections following ACV therapy have been reported (Levin et al. 2003; Bryan et al. 2008). However, the prevalence of ACV-resistant cases in these different populations is unknown because only case reports have been published so far. In a recent study, it was reported that 27 % of hemato-oncological patients, including

HSCT recipients, with persistent VZV infections had mutations possibly associated with resistance to ACV (van der Beek et al. 2013). The isolation of PCV-resistant VZV mutants in the clinic has not been described so far possibly because this drug is not used as often as VACV. Few reports have described the emergence of VZV strains resistant to FOS in immunocompromised patients (Fillet et al. 1995; Visse et al. 1998, 1999).

Management of Infections Caused by Drug-Resistant HSV and VZV Mutants

An algorithm for the management of infections caused by drug-resistant HSV mutants is proposed in Fig. 3. The persistence of active lesions due to HSV for 7–10 days after initiation of high-dose oral ACV, VACV, or FCV therapy without appreciable decrease in size, an atypical appearance, or the emergence of satellite lesions is suggestive of treatment failure. When drug resistance is suspected, a change of therapy should be considered depending on the clinical severity of the disease. Most ACV-resistant HSV isolates harbor a mutation in the TK enzyme. Therefore, a patient failing to respond to ACV or VACV will usually not respond to FCV as there will be probably cross-resistance between the two nucleoside analogues. An initial step in case of treatment failure with oral drugs is to initiate high doses of IV ACV (10 mg/kg of body weight every 8 h adjusted for renal function). If there is no improvement after 7 days, a switch to IV FOS should be considered. Indeed, a few reports have described some efficacy of FOS therapy against ACV-resistant infections in AIDS patients (Chatis et al. 1989; Erlich et al. 1989; Safrin et al. 1990; Alvarez-McLeod et al. 1999) and BMT recipients (Verdonck et al. 1993; Reusser et al. 1996). The recommended dosage for the treatment of ACV-resistant HSV infections is 40 mg/kg every 8 h (with reduction in dose for renal dysfunction). In parallel, isolates from the lesions should be submitted for phenotypic susceptibility testing (starting with ACV and FOS and then CDV, if required) and/or genotypic assays if the patient is failing therapy. Continuous infusion of high-dose ACV (e.g., 1.5–2.0 mg/kg per hour) could also be administered as it is a well-tolerated alternative for severe ACV- or multidrug-resistant HSV infections (Engel et al. 1990; Kim et al. 2011). A switch to IV CDV (5 mg/kg once a week for 3–4 weeks) could also be considered. Cidofovir has a long intracellular half-life which makes infrequent dosing possible. Because of its nephrotoxicity, CDV is routinely administered with probenecid and requires IV hydration. Intravenous CDV has shown some efficacy in the treatment of progressive ACV- and/or FOS-resistant mucocutaneous HSV infections in immunocompromised patients (Snoeck et al. 1994; LoPresti et al. 1998; Kopp et al. 2002; Castelo-Soccio et al. 2010) but is not approved for this indication.

Topical formulations of FOS, including a 1 % cream (Javaly et al. 1999) and a 2.4 % solution (Pechere et al. 1998), were effective in the treatment of mucocutaneous HSV infections unresponsive to ACV. Topical formulations of CDV have been also used successfully for the treatment of drug-resistant mucocutaneous HSV infections

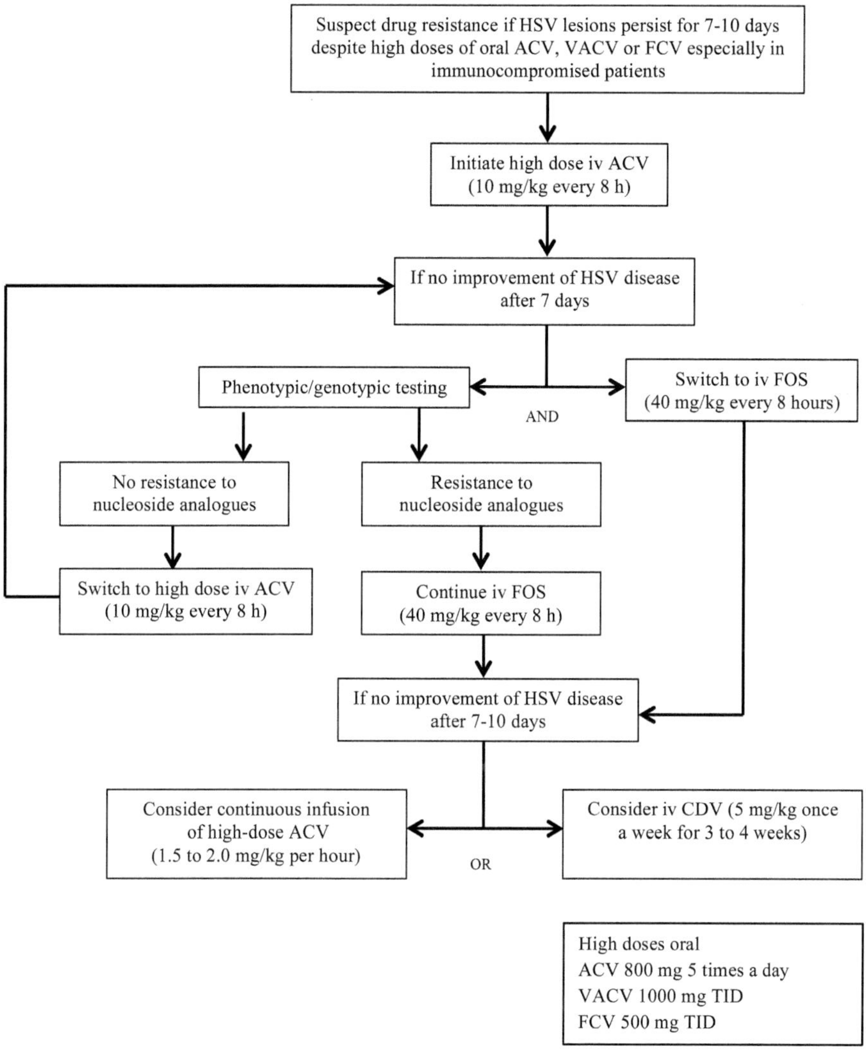

Fig. 3 Suggested algorithm for the management of suspected nucleoside analogue-resistant HSV infections. Key: *ACV* acyclovir, *VACV* valaciclovir, *FCV* famciclovir, *FOS* foscarnet, *CDV* cidofovir, *IV* intravenous

(Lalezari et al. 1997; Sacks et al. 1998; Sims et al. 2007; Evans et al. 2011). Although the use of these topical formulations could avoid the adverse effects associated with IV administration of FOS and CDV, they are not commercially available. A topical formulation containing 5 % imiquimod, an immunomodulatory drug, was effective in the treatment of recurrent and severe mucocutaneous lesions due to ACV- and FOS-resistant HSV-2 isolates in HIV-infected individuals (Lascaux et al. 2012). A 1 % topical solution of trifluorothymidine (TFT), a fluorinated pyrimidine nucleoside analogue that inhibits thymidylate synthase, is usually administered in cases of ophthalmic herpetic infections that do not respond to ACV (Chilukuri and Rosen 2003).

The persistence of clinical signs of VZV infections for more than 10–14 days after initiation of high-dose oral ACV is suggestive of treatment failure, and it should lead to alternate therapy depending on the clinical severity of the disease (Ahmed et al. 2007). Genotypic testing of the *ORF36* gene coding for the TK protein could be performed in biopsy of mucocutaneous lesions or other body compartments when necessary (Brink et al. 2011). Foscarnet is generally used for the management of VZV infections due to suspected or confirmed ACV-resistant mutants, as described mainly in HIV-infected individuals (Safrin et al. 1991; Breton et al. 1998) and some oncology patients (Crassard et al. 2000; Levin et al. 2003; Bryan et al. 2008). The recommended IV dosage is 60 mg/kg every 8 h adjusted for renal function for at least 10 days or until complete lesion healing is observed (Ahmed et al. 2007). Clinical experience with the use of CDV in the treatment of drug-resistant VZV diseases is very limited (Schliefer et al. 1999).

Human Cytomegalovirus Antiviral Drug Resistance

Phenotypic and Genotypic Testing for Detection of HCMV Drug Resistance

The method of choice to determine HCMV drug susceptibility is the PRA, which has been standardized in a consensus protocol to decrease high inter-assay and interlaboratory variabilities (Landry et al. 2000). This assay is time-consuming (6–8 weeks) and subjective. Proposed cutoff values defining resistance to GCV, CDV, and FOS are 6, 2, and 400 μM, respectively (Drew et al. 1993; Chou 2008). An increase in the EC_{50} value greater than two- to three-fold over that of a sensitive reference strain or a baseline isolate is also a widely accepted breakpoint value (Chou 2010).

In line with their mechanisms of action, drug-resistance mutations are detected primarily in the *UL97* gene encoding the protein kinase (GCV) and/or in the *UL54* gene encoding the viral DNA polymerase (GCV, CDV, and FOS). Genotypic testing can be performed directly on clinical specimens either by restriction fragment length polymorphism (RFLP) of PCR products amplified from the *UL97* gene, melting point PCR analysis using hybridization probes specific for each mutation site in the *UL97* gene, or DNA sequencing of PCR products amplified from the *UL97* (typically codons 400–670) and/or *UL54* (typically codons 300–1,000) genes (Lurain and Chou 2010). Genotypic testing is fast (1–3 days) and objective. However, mutations conferring drug resistance must be discriminated from those associated with natural polymorphisms. Drug-resistance mutations identified in the *UL97* and *UL54* genes can be linked to resistance phenotypes by using a web-based search tool (http://www.informatik.uni-ulm.de/ni/staff/HKestler/hcmv) (Chevillotte et al. 2010).

If their significance in drug resistance is unknown, these mutations must be subjected to recombinant phenotyping (Lurain and Chou 2010; Drouot et al. 2013).

Role of *UL97* and *UL54* Gene Mutations in Conferring HCMV Drug Resistance

The great majority (>90 %) of drug-resistant HCMV clinical isolates selected from initial treatment with GCV contain one or more mutations in the UL97 kinase, whereas mutations in the UL54 DNA polymerase are less frequently encountered (Erice 1999). The catalytic domain of protein kinases consists of eleven major conserved regions numbered I to XI, with region I corresponding to the highest level of homology (Hanks et al. 1988). The ATP-binding site, the phosphate transfer domain, and the substrate-recognition site correspond to codon ranges located at positions 337–345 (region I), 453–462 (region VIB), and 574–579 (region IX), respectively. Laboratory-engineered UL97-negative HCMV mutant demonstrated a severe replicative deficiency compared to the wild-type parental strain highlighting the essential role of this enzyme in the viral replicative cycle (Prichard et al. 1999). Therefore, only a small number of mutations clustered in a relatively short genomic region of the *UL97* gene have been reported to confer resistance to GCV (Fig. 4a) (Gilbert et al. 2002; Gilbert and Boivin 2005; Lurain and Chou 2010; James and Prichard 2011; Komatsu et al. 2014). Ganciclovir-resistance mutations in the *UL97* gene consist in single-nucleotide substitutions or in-frame deletions (Gilbert et al. 2002; Gilbert and Boivin 2005). More than 80 % of GCV-resistant clinical isolates typically contain one of the seven canonical mutations (M460V/I, H520Q, C592G, A594V, L595S, and C603W) in the *UL97* gene (Lurain et al. 1994; Chou et al. 1995a, b; Wolf et al. 1995a, b). These non-synonymous mutations impair GCV phosphorylation without altering the normal kinase functions and result in EC_{50} value increases of five- to ten-fold, except for C592G which confers a three-fold increase (Gilbert and Boivin 2005; Lurain and Chou 2010). Other less frequently encountered mutations can emerge at codon 460 and between codons 590 and 607. Such mutations confer various degrees of resistance to GCV with EC_{50} increases of up to 15-fold (Chou et al. 2002). Mutation V466G, located outside typical codon ranges, confers low-grade GCV resistance (3.5-fold) and is associated with a significant replicative defect (Martin et al. 2010a). The replicative capacity of UL97 mutants has not been extensively studied. It was demonstrated that substitutions or small deletions in the *UL97* gene had no major impact on the viral replicative capacity (Emery et al. 1999; Chou and Meichsner 2000; Chou et al. 2002; Gill et al. 2009). In contrast, a virus with a deletion accounting for 70 % of the *UL97* gene (Prichard et al. 1999) and a recombinant virus with a truncated protein kinase domain (Chou et al. 2007b) had severely impaired replicative capacity. Amino acid changes associated with natural polymorphisms in the *UL97* gene are mainly clustered in two distinct regions (codons 1–249 and 427–674) (Boutolleau et al. 2011).

Ganciclovir-resistant HCMV clinical isolates with an altered DNA polymerase activity result from numerous mutations widely distributed among the different

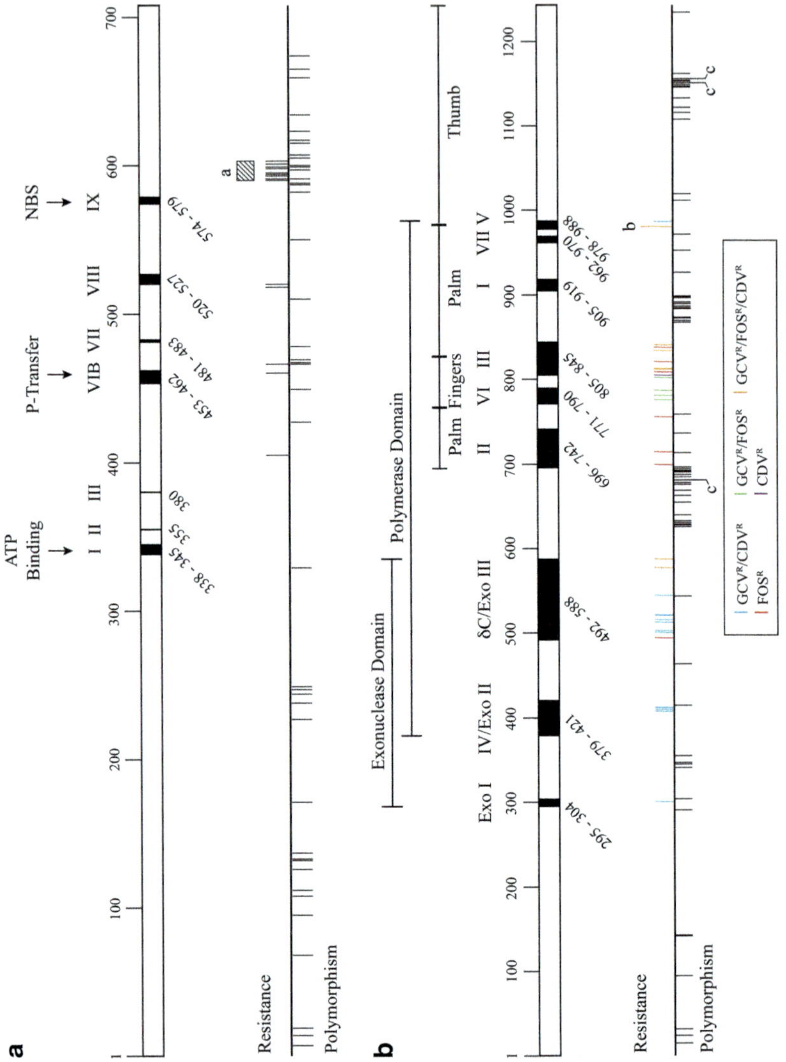

Fig. 4 (continued)

conserved domains of the enzyme, but mostly occur at codons 395–545 and 809–987 (Fig. 4b) (Gilbert et al. 2002; Gilbert and Boivin 2005; Lurain and Chou 2010; James and Prichard 2011; Komatsu et al. 2014). The catalytic domain of the UL54 DNA polymerase consists of eight conserved domains (i.e., I to VII and δ-region C) at its carboxyl-terminal portion. Moreover, a 3′–5′ exonuclease domain (containing Exo I, Exo II, and Exo III conserved motifs) maps to the N-terminal region of the polypeptide. The mechanisms of drug resistance occurring in the DNA polymerase involve either a prevention of the active drug binding to the enzyme or an alteration of the balance between exonuclease and polymerase activities which favor the removal of the incorporated drug (Hall et al. 1995; Cihlar et al. 1998b). In general, mutations in the *UL54* gene emerge after prolonged GCV exposure and increase the level of resistance conferred by mutations already present in the *UL97* gene (Lurain and Chou 2010). However, occasional reports have described mutations restricted to the *UL54* gene only after initial therapy with GCV (Boivin et al. 2005a; Hantz et al. 2010). DNA polymerase mutations that emerge under GCV therapy can confer cross-resistance to CDV and, less frequently, to FOS. Cross-resistance to GCV and CDV is associated with mutations located in the exonuclease domains (codons 301, 408–413, 501–545) and in region V (codons 981–987) of the enzyme (Sullivan et al. 1993; Chou et al. 1997, 2003, 2008; Cihlar et al. 1998a; Marfori et al. 2007; Scott et al. 2007). Resistance mutations to FOS are widely dispersed in the conserved domains of the *UL54* gene. However, clusters of mutations are mainly found in regions II, VI, and III and are associated with resistance to FOS alone, to both FOS and GCV, and to all three available antiviral agents, respectively (Baldanti et al. 1996; Chou et al. 1997, 2003, 2007a; Cihlar et al. 1998a; Weinberg et al. 2003; Scott et al. 2007). Mutations D588N (Exo III), A834P, and G841A (region III) as well as the deletion of codons 981–982 (region V) cause cross-resistance to GCV, CDV, and FOS (Chou et al. 2000; Scott et al. 2007). Regions I and VII have not been associated with drug resistance so far (Lurain and Chou 2010) probably because of their essential role in the enzyme activity. In

Fig. 4 Confirmed drug-resistance mutations identified in clinical HCMV isolates. *Panel a* shows mutations in the *UL97* gene conferring resistance to ganciclovir or associated with natural polymorphism. The ATP-binding site, the phosphate transfer (P-transfer) domain, the nucleoside-binding site (*NBS*), and some regions conserved among the protein kinase family (i.e., I, II, III, VIB, VII, VIII, and IX) are represented by the black boxes. Bars (|) indicate amino acid substitutions associated with resistance (*upper bars*) or with polymorphism (*lower bars*). [a], shaded area corresponds to the codon 590–603 region where different amino acid deletions were identified (i.e., deletions 590–593, 591–594, 591–603, 595–603, 598–601, 599–603, 600, and 601–603). *Panel b* shows mutations in the *UL54* gene conferring resistance to ganciclovir (GCV^R), foscarnet (FOS^R), and/or cidofovir (CDV^R) or associated with natural polymorphism. Conserved regions among the Herpesviridae DNA polymerase are represented by the black boxes. The roman numbers (I–VII) and δ-region C corresponding to each of these regions are indicated above the boxes. Conserved motifs (Exo I, Exo II, and Exo III) in the exonuclease domain are also indicated above the boxes. Bars (|) indicate amino acid substitutions associated with resistance (*upper bars*) or with polymorphism (*lower bars*). [b], represents amino acid deletion 981–982 that confers resistance to all three antivirals; [c], indicates amino acid deletions associated with polymorphism (i.e., deletions 681–688, 1151, and 1156) contrast to the situation with UL97 mutants, isolates with DNA polymerase mutations conferring drug resistance usually exhibit an attenuated or slow-growth phenotype in cell culture compared to wild-type strains (Baldanti et al. 1996; Cihlar et al. 1998b). It has been suggested that these mutations could affect substrate recognition which might decrease the affinity of the viral DNA polymerase for dNTPs. Finally, the natural polymorphism is more common in the *UL54* gene than in the *UL97* gene and occurs most often at non-conserved residues (between codons 614 and 697) where little homology exists among herpesvirus DNA polymerases (Chou et al. 1999; Fillet et al. 2004). This high degree of inter-strain variability in the *UL54* gene complicates the interpretation of genotypic testing.

Clinical Significance, Prevalence, and Risk Factors for Drug-Resistant HCMV Infections

Drug-resistant HCMV isolates are associated with different clinical presentations from asymptomatic to severe organ invasive or fatal disseminated diseases. In SOT recipients, infections caused by HCMV drug-resistant isolates can manifest as asymptomatic and symptomatic viremic episodes, an earlier onset of HCMV disease, graft loss, and an increased risk of mortality (Bhorade et al. 2002).

Shortly after the introduction of GCV, the emergence of drug-resistant HCMV strains was reported particularly in untreated or poorly treated AIDS patients who developed HCMV retinitis at a high frequency (ranging from 20 % to 45 %) (Jabs 1995). Several studies in AIDS patients who had received prolonged antiviral treatment for HCMV retinitis demonstrated that the emergence of drug-resistant isolates was directly related to the duration of therapy. Indeed, no drug-resistant isolate could be recovered in AIDS patients who had received GCV therapy for less than 3 months, whereas the incidence of resistance reached 8 % after a treatment period exceeding 3 months (Drew et al. 1991). The rates of emergence of drug-resistant mutants in AIDS patients with HCMV retinitis who had received GCV for 9 months and VGCV for 12 months were found to be 27 % and 13 %, respectively (Jabs et al. 1998a; Boivin et al. 2001). The lower incidence of GCV resistance in the latter study could be due to improved AIDS therapy. Indeed, the introduction of highly active antiretroviral therapy (HAART) substantially reduced the incidence of HCMV retinitis in AIDS patients, and this was associated with a concomitant decrease in the rate of emergence of drug resistance. Another study reported a reduction in the incidence of GCV resistance from 28 % to 9 % in the pre-HAART and HAART eras, respectively (Martin et al. 2007). Patients with AIDS, especially those with $CD4^+$ T cell counts below 50 cells/µl, remain at risk of developing HCMV retinitis and eventually GCV-resistant infections even nowadays (Sugar et al. 2012).

Thereafter, the more widespread use of oral GCV (with a low bioavailability of 6 %) and the intensification of immunosuppressive regimen resulted in an increased prevalence of HCMV drug resistance in SOT recipients. The prevalence of drug resistance in transplant recipients who have received GCV therapy for more than

2 months is approximately 10 % in general and up to 30 % in high-risk patients (D^+/R^- lung transplant recipients) (Limaye et al. 2002; Lurain et al. 2002; Hantz et al. 2010). The emergence of drug resistance in R^+ patients is rarely observed except in lung transplant recipients (Lurain et al. 2002). A retrospective study that evaluated 240 SOT patients reported an incidence of GCV resistance of 2.1 % in the overall population and of 7 % in D^+/R^- patients (Limaye 2002). More specifically, drug resistance was more frequently observed among recipients of kidney-pancreas or pancreas alone (21 %) than among patients transplanted with kidney (5 %) or liver (0 %). In two US centers, phenotypic evaluation of HCMV drug resistance demonstrated incidence rates varying from less than 0.5 % to 5.6 % and from 2.2 % to 15.2 % in non-lung and lung transplant recipients, respectively (Lurain et al. 2002). It is noteworthy to mention that HCMV infections caused by GCV-resistant isolates represented 20 % of all HCMV disease that developed during the first year after transplantation in one US study (Limaye et al. 2000).

In contrast to oral GCV, VGCV is highly absorbed leading to an improved systemic exposure (about 60 %) that could limit the emergence of drug-resistant HCMV mutants. The clinical efficacy and safety profile of a daily dose of VGCV were shown to be similar to thrice-daily doses of oral GCV for the prevention of HCMV diseases in high-risk SOT recipients (Paya et al. 2004). Several studies compared the emergence of drug resistance in SOT recipients who had received one of these two prophylactic regimens. A first study investigated the emergence of drug resistance in 364 high-risk D^+/R^- patients (including liver, kidney, heart, kidney-pancreas, and liver-kidney recipients) who had received oral GCV or VGCV prophylaxis for 100 days based on *UL97* (Boivin et al. 2004) and *UL54* (Boivin et al. 2005a, b) genotypic testing. The resistance rates at the end of the prophylactic period were 0 % and 3 % in the VGCV and GCV arms, respectively. The incidence of drug resistance in lung transplant recipients who had received IV GCV (D^+/R^- patients), oral GCV (R^+ patients), or oral VGCV prophylaxis was also found to be low (Boivin et al. 2005b; Humar et al. 2005). Finally, a low incidence of drug resistance was reported in adult D^+/R^- transplant patients and pediatric liver and heart transplant recipients who had received VGCV prophylaxis (Eid et al. 2008; Martin et al. 2010b). The low frequency of drug resistance in SOT recipients receiving VGCV (compared to oral GCV) could be related to an improved GCV exposure and to a better compliance of the patients to the once daily dosing.

High-risk patients who receive VGCV prophylaxis for 100 days post transplant might still be at risk of developing late-onset HCMV disease. However, extending the prophylactic regimen may increase the risk of emergence of drug resistance. Therefore, the impact of extending VGCV prophylaxis from 100 to 200 days on the incidence of resistance was investigated in 318 D^+/R^- kidney transplant recipients based on genotypic testing (Boivin et al. 2012). The rates of drug resistance were similar (1.8 % versus 1.9 %) in patients who had received VGCV prophylaxis for 100 and 200 days suggesting that extending the prophylactic period up to 200 days did not significantly affect the incidence of GCV resistance. Of note, almost all cases of resistance occurred during VGCV prophylaxis and rarely thereafter. Prophylaxis with VGCV for 200 days after transplantation could thus be an interesting option in high-risk kidney transplant recipients.

It is still under debate whether a prophylactic or a preemptive approach is more effective in preventing HCMV disease in high-risk transplant patients. In D^+/R^- kidney transplant recipients, both prophylaxis and preemptive therapy seem to have similar efficacy. Several studies also evaluated the effect of these treatment regimens on the emergence of drug resistance. In a first study, GCV-resistance mutations were detected in 2.2 % of the overall renal transplant recipients and, more specifically, in 12.5 % of D^+/R^- patients who had received once daily VGCV preemptive therapy (Myhre et al. 2011). Another study compared the emergence of resistance in D^+/R^- renal transplant recipients who had received VGCV prophylaxis for 3 months or VGCV preemptive therapy (Couzi et al. 2012). HCMV drug resistance was more frequent in the preemptive compared to the prophylactic group (16 % versus 3 %). The author suggested that, during preemptive therapy, patients may be exposed to suboptimal drug levels which favor an active viral replication state, thus increasing the risk of emergence of GCV resistance. Therefore, it is proposed that the use of prophylaxis may be more appropriate than the preemptive therapy in high-risk transplant recipients, although other studies are still needed to confirm this point.

Valganciclovir was shown to be noninferior to IV GCV for the treatment of established HCMV disease in SOT recipients (Asberg et al. 2007, 2009). A secondary endpoint of this trial was the evaluation of the emergence of drug resistance in 275 SOT patients (including heart, kidney, liver, and lung recipients) treated for HCMV disease with a 21-day induction dose of IV GCV or VGCV followed by VGCV maintenance dose for 49 days in both arms (Boivin et al. 2009). Probable or confirmed drug-resistance mutations were low and found to be similar for VGCV (3.6 %) and IV GCV (2.3 %) treatments. Overall, incidences of GCV drug resistance were low in kidneys (3.7 %), intermediate in livers and hearts (4.3–5.0 %), and highest in lungs (17.6 %).

Valganciclovir is also widely used for the management of HCMV disease in HSCT recipients. The incidence of drug resistance among HSCT recipients who had received preemptive therapy with GCV or VGCV was low in several studies (Gilbert et al. 2001; Nichols et al. 2001; Allice et al. 2009; Hantz et al. 2010; van der Beek et al. 2012) and cannot explain the high rate of treatment failure observed in this setting that is probably more related to the profound immunosuppression. In a recent study, a high rate of drug resistance (14.5 %) was exclusively identified in haploidentical-HSCT recipients receiving preemptive therapy with GCV (Shmueli et al. 2014).

Overall, proposed risk factors for the emergence of GCV resistance in transplant recipients include the lack of HCMV-specific immunity (typically the D^+/R^- group), lung or kidney-pancreas transplantation, high HCMV loads due to potent immunosuppressive therapy and/or suboptimal GCV levels, extended duration of therapy, and the type of antiviral regimen (i.e., treatment, prophylaxis, or preemptive therapy) (Gilbert and Boivin 2005).

As FOS and CDV constitute second-line antivirals for the treatment of HCMV diseases, only a few reports have described the emergence of resistance to these drugs in the clinic. In one study, baseline frequencies of resistance were reported to be less than 3 % for FOS and less than 7 % for CDV in AIDS patients with HCMV retinitis (Jabs et al. 1998b). These rates reached 37 % in patients treated with FOS for 9 months and 29 % in patients treated with CDV for 3 months. Globally, resistance to FOS and CDV occurs at similar rates as those typically reported for GCV.

Management of Infections Caused by Drug-Resistant HCMV Mutants

Guidelines for the management of GCV-resistant HCMV disease have been developed following a consensus meeting organized by the Transplantation Society International CMV Consensus Group (Kotton et al. 2013) with a suggested algorithm shown in Fig. 5. Antiviral drug resistance should be suspected in case of cumulative GCV exposure for more than 6 weeks and sustained or rising viral loads (especially DNAemia levels) despite more than 2 weeks of full dose of IV GCV (5 mg/kg twice daily, adjusted for renal function). However, a rise in pp65 antigenemia or DNAemia levels during the first 2 weeks of antiviral therapy in HSCT recipients has been associated mostly with host and other transplant-related factors rather than with the emergence of drug-resistance mutations (Nichols et al. 2001). The first change to be considered could be a reduction in the immunosuppressive therapy although this may lead to organ rejection (which would require intensifying immunosuppression). As the modulation of immunosuppression is rarely sufficient to control HCMV, the use of adjunctive immunoglobulins containing HCMV antibodies could be considered, but these agents are expensive and their supply is limited. At this initial step, a clinical decision about antiviral modification is empirical but should be based on the evaluation of host risk factors (e.g., D^+/R^- recipients, lung transplant recipients) and disease severity (sight- or life-threatening disease). Full or higher doses of IV GCV (5 or 10 mg/kg twice daily, respectively, adjusted for renal function) can be administered to low-risk patients with mild disease, whereas FOS alone or combined with GCV can be initiated for high-risk patients with severe disease. Of note, clear evidence of the superiority of GCV and FOS combination over FOS alone has not yet been demonstrated (Drew 2006). As resistance mutations to GCV typically emerge in the protein kinase, *UL97* gene sequencing is first recommended. Genotypic assays are performed typically on whole-blood or plasma specimens (Lisboa et al. 2011). However, some studies have demonstrated a compartmentalization of drug-resistant HCMV strains which suggests that resistance assessment based solely on blood samples may be suboptimal in some instances (Hamprecht et al. 2003; Jeong et al. 2012). Therefore, genotypic testing of cerebrospinal fluid, bronchoalveolar lavages, or biopsy specimens could be occasionally performed in high-risk patients.

If no mutation is identified in the *UL97* gene, full dose of IV GCV (5 mg/kg twice daily, adjusted for renal function) should be continued together with an optimization of host factors. If a major UL97 mutation (more than 5-fold increase in GCV EC_{50} value) is identified, a switch to IV FOS is recommended. If a minor UL97 mutation (less than 5-fold increase in GCV EC_{50} value) is detected, IV GCV can be increased

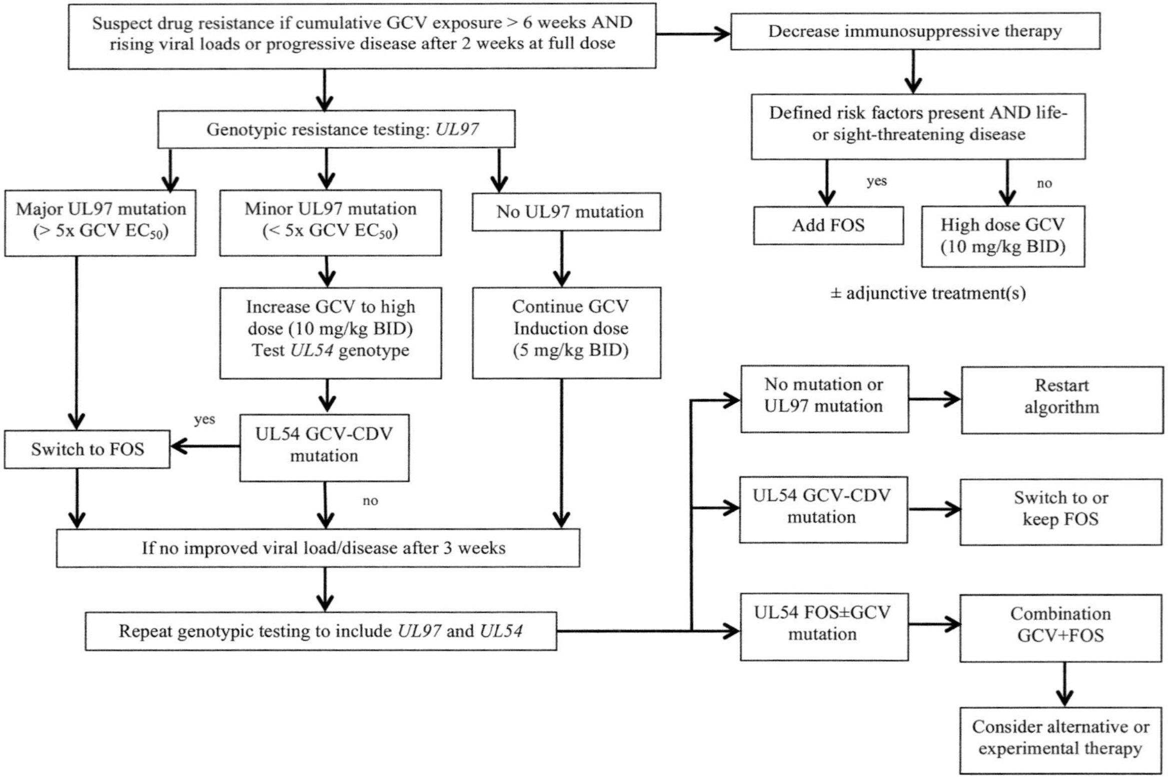

Fig. 5 Suggested algorithm for management of suspected HCMV drug resistance. Key: *GCV* ganciclovir, *FOS* foscarnet, *CDV* cidofovir, EC_{50} concentration of antiviral that reduces HCMV replication in cultured cells by 50 % compared to the control (without drug) determined in phenotypic assay (Adapted from Kotton et al. 2013)

to higher doses (10 mg/kg twice daily, adjusted for renal function), and drug-resistance mutations should be looked for in the *UL54* gene. If a mutation conferring cross-resistance to GCV and CDV is detected in the *UL54* gene, a switch to IV FOS therapy is recommended (or IV FOS should be kept).

The viral load is typically monitored once weekly by quantitative PCR during the period covering an episode of symptomatic HCMV disease. If there is no improvement in the viral load and a persistence of HCMV disease after a period of 3 weeks, genotypic testing should be repeated to assess the emergence of drug-resistance mutations in both the *UL97* and *UL54* genes. It is not recommended to switch to IV CDV for the treatment of GCV-resistant HCMV disease before obtaining the results of genotypic testing of the *UL54* gene because of the high frequency of cross-resistance between GCV and CDV. If a mutation conferring cross-resistance to GCV and CDV is detected, a switch to IV FOS is recommended (or IV FOS should be kept). If a resistance mutation to FOS is detected, a combination of high-dose IV GCV (10 mg/kg twice daily, adjusted for renal function) with IV FOS or CDV should be considered. Antiviral therapy is typically continued until viremia is no longer detectable. In case of multidrug-resistant HCMV disease, alternative or experimental therapies should also be considered (see below).

Several nonconventional interventions have been described for the treatment of multidrug-resistant HCMV diseases, although their clinical utility has not been adequately evaluated (Le Page et al. 2013). Artesunate, an antimalarial drug with activity against HCMV in vitro and in vivo (Kaptein et al. 2006), was shown to be effective in the treatment of a HSCT recipient with multidrug-resistant HCMV infections (Shapira et al. 2008). Leflunomide, an immunosuppressive agent used for rheumatoid arthritis, possesses anti-HCMV activity including against GCV-resistant isolates by acting on virion assembly (Waldman et al. 1999; Chong et al. 2006). Thus, no cross-resistance is expected with the current antiviral agents. The efficacy of leflunomide in the treatment of HCMV infection has been reported in a HSCT recipient failing to respond to all available antiviral agents (Avery et al. 2004). Leflunomide alone or in combination with standard antiviral agents has shown some efficacy in transplant recipients refractory to current therapy (Avery et al. 2010; Dunn et al. 2013; Verkaik et al. 2013). The combination of GCV and the immunosuppressive agent sirolimus for the treatment of GCV-resistant HCMV infections has led to a favorable outcome with respect to clinical status and graft rejection in kidney and kidney-pancreas recipients (Ozaki et al. 2007).

Conclusions

Drug-resistant HSV, VZV, and HCMV mutants may cause severe and chronic infections as well as increased mortality in immunocompromised patients. The number of patients with an immunocompromised status is currently increasing and the emergence of drug-resistant herpesvirus infections is not expected to fade. The development of fast and efficient methods for detecting viral mutant sequences directly in clinical specimens such as pyrosequencing (Kampmann et al. 2011) and ultra-deep pyrosequencing (Gorzer et al. 2010; Sahoo et al. 2013) will improve the diagnosis of drug-resistant herpesvirus infections. The use of more powerful recombinant phenotyping techniques (Drouot et al. 2013) and the availability of an Internet database (Chevillotte et al. 2010) to link individual mutations to their drug-susceptibility phenotypes should result in more rational therapeutic strategies.

As all currently available antiviral agents target the viral DNA polymerase, the development of new antiherpetic compounds with different mechanisms of action retaining efficacy against nucleoside/nucleotide analogue- and FOS-resistant isolates and with adequate safety profiles is an important priority. In that regard, some promising compounds are currently in clinical trials. The orally bioavailable lipid ester prodrug of CDV (i.e., hexadecyloxypropyl-cidofovir; CMX001) could avoid the dose-limiting renal toxicity of the parent drug and provide a safe alternative for ACV- and GCV-resistant herpesviruses in immunocompromised patients (Hostetler 2010). Treatment with oral CMX001 significantly reduced the incidence of HCMV events in HSCT recipients (Marty et al. 2013). Maribavir is a competitive inhibitor of the UL97 kinase (Biron et al. 2002). Surprisingly, mutations arising after in vitro selection with this drug most often map to the *UL27* gene and, less frequently, to the *UL97* gene. Of note, mutations found in the *UL97* gene are distinct from those described in GCV-resistant strains (Chou et al. 2012) and some have been detected outside the conserved kinase domains (Chou 2008). Thus, maribavir retains activity against GCV-resistant mutants. The emergence of resistance to this drug has been reported in some cases (Strasfeld et al. 2010; Schubert et al. 2013). Recently, maribavir faced some limitations in phase III clinical studies (Marty et al. 2011) but new trials using higher doses are in progress. Letermovir targets the terminase complex of HCMV and interferes with viral DNA concatemer maturation (Lischka et al. 2010; Goldner et al. 2011). Accordingly, mutations conferring resistance to letermovir map to the *UL56* gene (Goldner et al. 2011, 2014). Successful treatment of a multidrug-resistant HCMV infection with letermovir has been reported in a lung transplant recipient (Kaul et al. 2011). The preemptive treatment of HCMV infection with letermovir in kidney transplant recipients was recently investigated in a phase IIa trial (Stoelben et al. 2014). Novel classes of antiviral agents targeting the ribonucleotide reductase, the helicase-primase complex, and the process of viral DNA encapsidation are at earlier stages of development (Greco et al. 2007).

Acknowledgments G. B. is the holder of the Canada Research Chair on emerging viruses and antiviral resistance.

References

Ahmed AM, Brantley JS, Madkan V et al (2007) Managing herpes zoster in immunocompromised patients. Herpes 14:32–36

Allice T, Busca A, Locatelli F et al (2009) Valganciclovir as pre-emptive therapy for cytomegalovirus infection post-allogenic stem cell transplantation: implications for the emergence of drug-resistant cytomegalovirus. J Antimicrob Chemother 63:600–608

Alvarez-McLeod A, Havlik J, Drew KE (1999) Foscarnet treatment of genital infection due to acyclovir-resistant herpes simplex virus type 2 in a pregnant patient with AIDS: case report. Clin Infect Dis 29:937–938

Andrei G, Snoeck R (2013) Herpes simplex virus drug-resistance: new mutations and insights. Curr Opin Infect Dis 26:551–560

Andrei G, Fiten P, Froeyen M et al (2007) DNA polymerase mutations in drug-resistant herpes simplex virus mutants determine in vivo neurovirulence and drug-enzyme interactions. Antivir Ther 12:719–732

Andrei G, de Clercq E, Snoeck R (2009) Viral genome replication. In: Cameron CE, Gotte M, Raney K (eds) Viral DNA polymerase inhibitors. Springer, New York

Andrei G, Topalis D, Fiten P et al (2012) In vitro-selected drug-resistant varicella-zoster virus mutants in the thymidine kinase and DNA polymerase genes yield novel phenotype-genotype associations and highlight differences between antiherpesvirus drugs. J Virol 86:2641–2652

Asberg A, Humar A, Rollag H et al (2007) Oral valganciclovir is noninferior to intravenous ganciclovir for the treatment of cytomegalovirus disease in solid organ transplant recipients. Am J Transplant 7:2106–2113

Asberg A, Humar A, Jardine AG et al (2009) Long-term outcomes of CMV disease treatment with valganciclovir versus IV ganciclovir in solid organ transplant recipients. Am J Transplant 9:1205–1213

Avery RK, Bolwell BJ, Yen-Lieberman B et al (2004) Use of leflunomide in an allogeneic bone marrow transplant recipient with refractory cytomegalovirus infection. Bone Marrow Transplant 34:1071–1075

Avery RK, Mossad SB, Poggio E et al (2010) Utility of leflunomide in the treatment of complex cytomegalovirus syndromes. Transplantation 90:419–426

Bacon TH, Boon RJ, Schultz M et al (2002) Surveillance for antiviral-agent-resistant herpes simplex virus in the general population with recurrent herpes labialis. Antimicrob Agents Chemother 46:3042–3044

Bacon TH, Levin MJ, Leary JJ et al (2003) Herpes simplex virus resistance to acyclovir and penciclovir after two decades of antiviral therapy. Clin Microbiol Rev 16:114–128

Balasubramaniam NK, Veerisetty V, Gentry GA (1990) Herpesviral deoxythymidine kinases contain a site analogous to the phosphoryl-binding arginine-rich region of porcine adenylate kinase; comparison of secondary structure predictions and conservation. J Gen Virol 71 (Pt 12):2979–2987

Baldanti F, Underwood MR, Stanat SC et al (1996) Single amino acid changes in the DNA polymerase confer foscarnet resistance and slow-growth phenotype, while mutations in the UL97-encoded phosphotransferase confer ganciclovir resistance in three double-resistant human cytomegalovirus strains recovered from patients with AIDS. J Virol 70:1390–1395

Bernstein DI, Ireland J, Bourne N (2000) Pathogenesis of acyclovir-resistant herpes simplex type 2 isolates in animal models of genital herpes: models for antiviral evaluations. Antiviral Res 47:159–169

Besecker MI, Furness CL, Coen DM et al (2007) Expression of extremely low levels of thymidine kinase from an acyclovir-resistant herpes simplex virus mutant supports reactivation from latently infected mouse trigeminal ganglia. J Virol 81:8356–8360

Bestman-Smith J, Boivin G (2002) Herpes simplex virus isolates with reduced adefovir susceptibility selected in vivo by foscarnet therapy. J Med Virol 67:88–91

Bestman-Smith J, Boivin G (2003) Drug resistance patterns of recombinant herpes simplex virus DNA polymerase mutants generated with a set of overlapping cosmids and plasmids. J Virol 77:7820–7829

Bhorade SM, Lurain NS, Jordan A et al (2002) Emergence of ganciclovir-resistant cytomegalovirus in lung transplant recipients. J Heart Lung Transplant 21:1274–1282

Biron KK, Stanat SC, Sorrell JB et al (1985) Metabolic activation of the nucleoside analog 9-[(2-hydroxy-1-(hydroxymethyl)ethoxy]methyl)guanine in human diploid fibroblasts infected with human cytomegalovirus. Proc Natl Acad Sci U S A 82:2473–2477

Biron KK, Harvey RJ, Chamberlain SC et al (2002) Potent and selective inhibition of human cytomegalovirus replication by 1263 W94, a benzimidazole L-riboside with a unique mode of action. Antimicrob Agents Chemother 46:2365–2372

Boeckh M, Huang M, Ferrenberg J et al (2004) Optimization of quantitative detection of cytomegalovirus DNA in plasma by real-time PCR. J Clin Microbiol 42:1142–1148

Bohn K, Zell R, Schacke M et al (2011) Gene polymorphism of thymidine kinase and DNA polymerase in clinical strains of herpes simplex virus. Antivir Ther 16:989–997

Boivin G, Edelman CK, Pedneault L et al (1994) Phenotypic and genotypic characterization of acyclovir-resistant varicella-zoster viruses isolated from persons with AIDS. J Infect Dis 170:68–75

Boivin G, Gilbert C, Gaudreau A et al (2001) Rate of emergence of cytomegalovirus (CMV) mutations in leukocytes of patients with acquired immunodeficiency syndrome who are receiving valganciclovir as induction and maintenance therapy for CMV retinitis. J Infect Dis 184:1598–1602

Boivin G, Goyette N, Gilbert C et al (2004) Absence of cytomegalovirus-resistance mutations after valganciclovir prophylaxis, in a prospective multicenter study of solid-organ transplant recipients. J Infect Dis 189:1615–1618

Boivin G, Goyette N, Gilbert C et al (2005a) Analysis of cytomegalovirus DNA polymerase (UL54) mutations in solid organ transplant patients receiving valganciclovir or ganciclovir prophylaxis. J Med Virol 77:425–429

Boivin G, Goyette N, Gilbert C et al (2005b) Clinical impact of ganciclovir-resistant cytomegalovirus infections in solid organ transplant patients. Transpl Infect Dis 7:166–170

Boivin G, Goyette N, Rollag H et al (2009) Cytomegalovirus resistance in solid organ transplant recipients treated with intravenous ganciclovir or oral valganciclovir. Antivir Ther 14:697–704

Boivin G, Goyette N, Farhan M et al (2012) Incidence of cytomegalovirus UL97 and UL54 amino acid substitutions detected after 100 or 200 days of valganciclovir prophylaxis. J Clin Virol 53:208–213

Boon RJ, Bacon TH, Robey HL et al (2000) Antiviral susceptibilities of herpes simplex virus from immunocompetent subjects with recurrent herpes labialis: a UK-based survey. J Antimicrob Chemother 46:324–325

Boutolleau D, Burrel S, Agut H (2011) Genotypic characterization of human cytomegalovirus UL97 phosphotransferase natural polymorphism in the era of ganciclovir and maribavir. Antiviral Res 91:32–35

Breton G, Fillet AM, Katlama C et al (1998) Acyclovir-resistant herpes zoster in human immunodeficiency virus-infected patients: results of foscarnet therapy. Clin Infect Dis 27:1525–1527

Brink AA, van Gelder M, Wolffs PF et al (2011) Compartmentalization of acyclovir-resistant varicella zoster virus: implications for sampling in molecular diagnostics. Clin Infect Dis 52:982–987

Bryan CJ, Prichard MN, Daily S et al (2008) Acyclovir-resistant chronic verrucous vaccine strain varicella in a patient with neuroblastoma. Pediatr Infect Dis J 27:946–948

Burrel S, Deback C, Agut H et al (2010) Genotypic characterization of UL23 thymidine kinase and UL30 DNA polymerase of clinical isolates of herpes simplex virus: natural polymorphism and mutations associated with resistance to antivirals. Antimicrob Agents Chemother 54:4833–4842

Burrel S, Bonnafous P, Hubacek P et al (2012) Impact of novel mutations of herpes simplex virus 1 and 2 thymidine kinases on acyclovir phosphorylation activity. Antiviral Res 96:386–390

Burrel S, Aime C, Hermet L et al (2013a) Surveillance of herpes simplex virus resistance to antivirals: a 4-year survey. Antiviral Res 100:365–372

Burrel S, Boutolleau D, Azar G et al (2013b) Phenotypic and genotypic characterization of acyclovir-resistant corneal HSV-1 isolates from immunocompetent patients with recurrent herpetic keratitis. J Clin Virol 58:321–324

Castelo-Soccio L, Bernardin R, Stern J et al (2010) Successful treatment of acyclovir-resistant herpes simplex virus with intralesional cidofovir. Arch Dermatol 146:124–126

Chakrabarti S, Pillay D, Ratcliffe D et al (2000) Resistance to antiviral drugs in herpes simplex virus infections among allogeneic stem cell transplant recipients: risk factors and prognostic significance. J Infect Dis 181:2055–2058
Chatis PA, Miller CH, Schrager LE et al (1989) Successful treatment with foscarnet of an acyclovir-resistant mucocutaneous infection with herpes simplex virus in a patient with acquired immunodeficiency syndrome. N Engl J Med 320:297–300
Chen SH, Cook WJ, Grove KL et al (1998) Human thymidine kinase can functionally replace herpes simplex virus type 1 thymidine kinase for viral replication in mouse sensory ganglia and reactivation from latency upon explant. J Virol 72:6710–6715
Chen Y, Scieux C, Garrait V et al (2000) Resistant herpes simplex virus type 1 infection: an emerging concern after allogeneic stem cell transplantation. Clin Infect Dis 31:927–935
Chen SH, Pearson A, Coen DM et al (2004) Failure of thymidine kinase-negative herpes simplex virus to reactivate from latency following efficient establishment. J Virol 78:520–523
Chevillotte M, von Einem J, Meier BM et al (2010) A new tool linking human cytomegalovirus drug resistance mutations to resistance phenotypes. Antiviral Res 85:318–327
Chibo D, Druce J, Sasadeusz J et al (2004) Molecular analysis of clinical isolates of acyclovir resistant herpes simplex virus. Antiviral Res 61:83–91
Chilukuri S, Rosen T (2003) Management of acyclovir-resistant herpes simplex virus. Dermatol Clin 21:311–320
Chong AS, Zeng H, Knight DA et al (2006) Concurrent antiviral and immunosuppressive activities of leflunomide in vivo. Am J Transplant 6:69–75
Chou S (2008) Cytomegalovirus UL97 mutations in the era of ganciclovir and maribavir. Rev Med Virol 18:233–246
Chou S (2010) Recombinant phenotyping of cytomegalovirus UL97 kinase sequence variants for ganciclovir resistance. Antimicrob Agents Chemother 54:2371–2378
Chou S, Meichsner CL (2000) A nine-codon deletion mutation in the cytomegalovirus UL97 phosphotransferase gene confers resistance to ganciclovir. Antimicrob Agents Chemother 44:183–185
Chou S, Erice A, Jordan MC et al (1995a) Analysis of the UL97 phosphotransferase coding sequence in clinical cytomegalovirus isolates and identification of mutations conferring ganciclovir resistance. J Infect Dis 171:576–583
Chou S, Guentzel S, Michels KR et al (1995b) Frequency of UL97 phosphotransferase mutations related to ganciclovir resistance in clinical cytomegalovirus isolates. J Infect Dis 172:239–242
Chou S, Marousek G, Guentzel S et al (1997) Evolution of mutations conferring multidrug resistance during prophylaxis and therapy for cytomegalovirus disease. J Infect Dis 176:786–789
Chou S, Lurain NS, Weinberg A et al (1999) Interstrain variation in the human cytomegalovirus DNA polymerase sequence and its effect on genotypic diagnosis of antiviral drug resistance. Adult AIDS Clinical Trials Group CMV Laboratories. Antimicrob Agents Chemother 43:1500–1502
Chou S, Miner RC, Drew WL (2000) A deletion mutation in region V of the cytomegalovirus DNA polymerase sequence confers multidrug resistance. J Infect Dis 182:1765–1768
Chou S, Waldemer RH, Senters AE et al (2002) Cytomegalovirus UL97 phosphotransferase mutations that affect susceptibility to ganciclovir. J Infect Dis 185:162–169
Chou S, Lurain NS, Thompson KD et al (2003) Viral DNA polymerase mutations associated with drug resistance in human cytomegalovirus. J Infect Dis 188:32–39
Chou S, Marousek GI, Van Wechel LC et al (2007a) Growth and drug resistance phenotypes resulting from cytomegalovirus DNA polymerase region III mutations observed in clinical specimens. Antimicrob Agents Chemother 51:4160–4162
Chou S, Wechel LC, Marousek GI (2007b) Cytomegalovirus UL97 kinase mutations that confer maribavir resistance. J Infect Dis 196:91–94

Chou S, Marousek G, Li S et al (2008) Contrasting drug resistance phenotypes resulting from cytomegalovirus DNA polymerase mutations at the same exonuclease locus. J Clin Virol 43:107–109

Chou S, Hakki M, Villano S (2012) Effects on maribavir susceptibility of cytomegalovirus UL97 kinase ATP binding region mutations detected after drug exposure in vitro and in vivo. Antiviral Res 95:88–92

Christophers J, Clayton J, Craske J et al (1998) Survey of resistance of herpes simplex virus to acyclovir in northwest England. Antimicrob Agents Chemother 42:868–872

Cihlar T, Fuller MD, Cherrington JM (1998a) Characterization of drug resistance-associated mutations in the human cytomegalovirus DNA polymerase gene by using recombinant mutant viruses generated from overlapping DNA fragments. J Virol 72:5927–5936

Cihlar T, Fuller MD, Mulato AS et al (1998b) A point mutation in the human cytomegalovirus DNA polymerase gene selected in vitro by cidofovir confers a slow replication phenotype in cell culture. Virology 248:382–393

Coen DM (1994) Acyclovir-resistant, pathogenic herpesviruses. Trends Microbiol 2:481–485

Coen DM, Kosz-Vnenchak M, Jacobson JG et al (1989) Thymidine kinase-negative herpes simplex virus mutants establish latency in mouse trigeminal ganglia but do not reactivate. Proc Natl Acad Sci U S A 86:4736–4740

Collins P, Ellis MN (1993) Sensitivity monitoring of clinical isolates of herpes simplex virus to acyclovir. J Med Virol Suppl 1:58–66

Couzi L, Helou S, Bachelet T et al (2012) High incidence of anticytomegalovirus drug resistance among D + R- kidney transplant recipients receiving preemptive therapy. Am J Transplant 12:202–209

Crassard N, Souillet AL, Morfin F et al (2000) Acyclovir-resistant varicella infection with atypical lesions in a non-HIV leukemic infant. Acta Paediatr 89:1497–1499

Dambrosi S, Martin M, Yim K et al (2010) Neurovirulence and latency of drug-resistant clinical herpes simplex viruses in animal models. J Med Virol 82:1000–1006

Danve-Szatanek C, Aymard M, Thouvenot D et al (2004) Surveillance network for herpes simplex virus resistance to antiviral drugs: 3-year follow-up. J Clin Microbiol 42:242–249

Drew WL (2006) Is combination antiviral therapy for CMV superior to monotherapy? J Clin Virol 35:485–488

Drew WL, Miner RC, Busch DF et al (1991) Prevalence of resistance in patients receiving ganciclovir for serious cytomegalovirus infection. J Infect Dis 163:716–719

Drew WL, Miner R, Saleh E (1993) Antiviral susceptibility testing of cytomegalovirus: criteria for detecting resistance to antivirals. Clin Diagn Virol 1:179–185

Drouot E, Piret J, Boivin G (2013) Novel method based on "en passant" mutagenesis coupled with a Gaussia luciferase reporter assay for studying the combined effects of human cytomegalovirus mutations. J Clin Microbiol 51:3216–3224

Duan R, de Vries RD, Osterhaus AD et al (2008) Acyclovir-resistant corneal HSV-1 isolates from patients with herpetic keratitis. J Infect Dis 198:659–663

Duan R, de Vries RD, van Dun JM et al (2009) Acyclovir susceptibility and genetic characteristics of sequential herpes simplex virus type 1 corneal isolates from patients with recurrent herpetic keratitis. J Infect Dis 200:1402–1414

Dunn JH, Weinberg A, Chan LK et al (2013) Long-term suppression of multidrug-resistant cytomegalovirus retinitis with systemically administered leflunomide. JAMA Ophthalmol 131:958–960

Efstathiou S, Kemp S, Darby G et al (1989) The role of herpes simplex virus type 1 thymidine kinase in pathogenesis. J Gen Virol 70(Pt 4):869–879

Eid AJ, Arthurs SK, Deziel PJ et al (2008) Emergence of drug-resistant cytomegalovirus in the era of valganciclovir prophylaxis: therapeutic implications and outcomes. Clin Transplant 22:162–170

Emery VC, Cope AV, Bowen EF et al (1999) The dynamics of human cytomegalovirus replication in vivo. J Exp Med 190:177–182

Engel JP, Englund JA, Fletcher CV et al (1990) Treatment of resistant herpes simplex virus with continuous-infusion acyclovir. JAMA 263:1662–1664
Englund JA, Zimmerman ME, Swierkosz EM et al (1990) Herpes simplex virus resistant to acyclovir. A study in a tertiary care center. Ann Intern Med 112:416–422
Erard V, Wald A, Corey L et al (2007) Use of long-term suppressive acyclovir after hematopoietic stem-cell transplantation: impact on herpes simplex virus (HSV) disease and drug-resistant HSV disease. J Infect Dis 196:266–270
Erice A (1999) Resistance of human cytomegalovirus to antiviral drugs. Clin Microbiol Rev 12:286–297
Erlich KS, Jacobson MA, Koehler JE et al (1989) Foscarnet therapy for severe acyclovir-resistant herpes simplex virus type-2 infections in patients with the acquired immunodeficiency syndrome (AIDS). An uncontrolled trial. Ann Intern Med 110:710–713
Evans JS, Lock KP, Levine BA et al (1998) Herpesviral thymidine kinases: laxity and resistance by design. J Gen Virol 79(Pt 9):2083–2092
Evans KG, Morrissey KA, Goldstein SC et al (2011) Chronic acyclovir-resistant HSV-2 ulcer in an immunosuppressed patient treated with topical cidofovir. Arch Dermatol 147:1462–1463
Field HJ, Coen DM (1986) Pathogenicity of herpes simplex virus mutants containing drug resistance mutations in the viral DNA polymerase gene. J Virol 60:286–289
Fillet AM, Visse B, Caumes E et al (1995) Foscarnet-resistant multidermatomal zoster in a patient with AIDS. Clin Infect Dis 21:1348–1349
Fillet AM, Dumont B, Caumes E et al (1998) Acyclovir-resistant varicella-zoster virus: phenotypic and genetic characterization. J Med Virol 55:250–254
Fillet AM, Auray L, Alain S et al (2004) Natural polymorphism of cytomegalovirus DNA polymerase lies in two nonconserved regions located between domains delta-C and II and between domains III and I. Antimicrob Agents Chemother 48:1865–1868
Frangoul H, Wills M, Crossno C et al (2007) Acyclovir-resistant herpes simplex virus pneumonia post-unrelated stem cell transplantation: a word of caution. Pediatr Transplant 11:942–944
Frobert E, Thouvenot D, Lina B et al (2007) Genotyping diagnosis of acyclovir resistant herpes simplex virus. Pathol Biol (Paris) 55:504–511
Frobert E, Cortay JC, Ooka T et al (2008) Genotypic detection of acyclovir-resistant HSV-1: characterization of 67 ACV-sensitive and 14 ACV-resistant viruses. Antiviral Res 79:28–36
Gateley A, Gander RM, Johnson PC et al (1990) Herpes simplex virus type 2 meningoencephalitis resistant to acyclovir in a patient with AIDS. J Infect Dis 161:711–715
Gaudreau A, Hill E, Balfour HH Jr et al (1998) Phenotypic and genotypic characterization of acyclovir-resistant herpes simplex viruses from immunocompromised patients. J Infect Dis 178:297–303
Gilbert C, Boivin G (2005) Human cytomegalovirus resistance to antiviral drugs. Antimicrob Agents Chemother 49:873–883
Gilbert C, Roy J, Belanger R et al (2001) Lack of emergence of cytomegalovirus UL97 mutations conferring ganciclovir (GCV) resistance following preemptive GCV therapy in allogeneic stem cell transplant recipients. Antimicrob Agents Chemother 45:3669–3671
Gilbert C, Bestman-Smith J, Boivin G (2002) Resistance of herpesviruses to antiviral drugs: clinical impacts and molecular mechanisms. Drug Resist Updat 5:88–114
Gill RB, Frederick SL, Hartline CB et al (2009) Conserved retinoblastoma protein-binding motif in human cytomegalovirus UL97 kinase minimally impacts viral replication but affects susceptibility to maribavir. Virol J 6:9
Gimeno C, Solano C, Latorre JC et al (2008) Quantification of DNA in plasma by an automated real-time PCR assay (cytomegalovirus PCR kit) for surveillance of active cytomegalovirus infection and guidance of preemptive therapy for allogeneic hematopoietic stem cell transplant recipients. J Clin Microbiol 46:3311–3318
Goldner T, Hewlett G, Ettischer N et al (2011) The novel anticytomegalovirus compound AIC246 (Letermovir) inhibits human cytomegalovirus replication through a specific antiviral mechanism that involves the viral terminase. J Virol 85:10884–10893

Goldner T, Hempel C, Ruebsamen-Schaeff H et al (2014) Geno- and phenotypic characterization of human cytomegalovirus mutants selected in vitro after letermovir (AIC246) exposure. Antimicrob Agents Chemother 58:610–613

Gorzer I, Guelly C, Trajanoski S et al (2010) Deep sequencing reveals highly complex dynamics of human cytomegalovirus genotypes in transplant patients over time. J Virol 84:7195–7203

Greco A, Diaz JJ, Thouvenot D et al (2007) Novel targets for the development of anti-herpes compounds. Infect Disord Drug Targets 7:11–18

Hall JD, Orth KL, Sander KL et al (1995) Mutations within conserved motifs in the 3′–5′ exonuclease domain of herpes simplex virus DNA polymerase. J Gen Virol 76 (Pt 12):2999–3008

Hamprecht K, Eckle T, Prix L et al (2003) Ganciclovir-resistant cytomegalovirus disease after allogeneic stem cell transplantation: pitfalls of phenotypic diagnosis by in vitro selection of an UL97 mutant strain. J Infect Dis 187:139–143

Hanks SK, Quinn AM, Hunter T (1988) The protein kinase family: conserved features and deduced phylogeny of the catalytic domains. Science 241:42–52

Hantz S, Garnier-Geoffroy F, Mazeron MC et al (2010) Drug-resistant cytomegalovirus in transplant recipients: a French cohort study. J Antimicrob Chemother 65:2628–2640

Hostetler KY (2010) Synthesis and early development of hexadecyloxypropylcidofovir: an oral antipoxvirus nucleoside phosphonate. Viruses 2:2213–2225

Humar A, Kumar D, Preiksaitis J et al (2005) A trial of valganciclovir prophylaxis for cytomegalovirus prevention in lung transplant recipients. Am J Transplant 5:1462–1468

Hwang CB, Ruffner KL, Coen DM (1992) A point mutation within a distinct conserved region of the herpes simplex virus DNA polymerase gene confers drug resistance. J Virol 66:1774–1776

Jabs DA (1995) Ocular manifestations of HIV infection. Trans Am Ophthalmol Soc 93:623–683

Jabs DA, Enger C, Dunn JP et al (1998a) Cytomegalovirus retinitis and viral resistance: ganciclovir resistance. J Infect Dis 177:770–773

Jabs DA, Enger C, Forman M et al (1998b) Incidence of foscarnet resistance and cidofovir resistance in patients treated for cytomegalovirus retinitis. The Cytomegalovirus Retinitis and Viral Resistance Study Group. Antimicrob Agents Chemother 42:2240–2244

James SH, Prichard MN (2011) The genetic basis of human cytomegalovirus resistance and current trends in antiviral resistance analysis. Infect Disord Drug Targets 11:504–513

James SH, Prichard MN (2013) A possible pitfall in acyclovir prophylaxis for recurrent herpetic keratitis? J Infect Dis 208:1353–1355

Javaly K, Wohlfeiler M, Kalayjian R et al (1999) Treatment of mucocutaneous herpes simplex virus infections unresponsive to acyclovir with topical foscarnet cream in AIDS patients: a phase I/II study. J Acquir Immune Defic Syndr 21:301–306

Jeong TD, Sung H, Choi SH et al (2012) Cytomegalovirus ventriculoencephalitis with compartmentalization of antiviral-resistant cytomegalovirus in a T cell-depleted haploidentical peripheral blood stem cell transplant recipient. Diagn Microbiol Infect Dis 74:307–310

Kamiyama T, Kurokawa M, Shiraki K (2001) Characterization of the DNA polymerase gene of varicella-zoster viruses resistant to acyclovir. J Gen Virol 82:2761–2765

Kampmann SE, Schindele B, Apelt L et al (2011) Pyrosequencing allows the detection of emergent ganciclovir resistance mutations after HCMV infection. Med Microbiol Immunol 200:109–113

Kaptein SJ, Efferth T, Leis M et al (2006) The anti-malaria drug artesunate inhibits replication of cytomegalovirus in vitro and in vivo. Antiviral Res 69:60–69

Kaul DR, Stoelben S, Cober E et al (2011) First report of successful treatment of multidrug-resistant cytomegalovirus disease with the novel anti-CMV compound AIC246. Am J Transplant 11:1079–1084

Kim JH, Schaenman JM, Ho DY et al (2011) Treatment of acyclovir-resistant herpes simplex virus with continuous infusion of high-dose acyclovir in hematopoietic cell transplant patients. Biol Blood Marrow Transplant 17:259–264

Komatsu TE, Pikis A, Naeger LK et al (2014) Resistance of human cytomegalovirus to ganciclovir/valganciclovir: a comprehensive review of putative resistance pathways. Antiviral Res 101:12–25

Kopp T, Geusau A, Rieger A et al (2002) Successful treatment of an aciclovir-resistant herpes simplex type 2 infection with cidofovir in an AIDS patient. Br J Dermatol 147:134–138

Kotton CN, Kumar D, Caliendo AM et al (2013) Updated international consensus guidelines on the management of cytomegalovirus in solid-organ transplantation. Transplantation 96:333–360

Lalezari J, Schacker T, Feinberg J et al (1997) A randomized, double-blind, placebo-controlled trial of cidofovir gel for the treatment of acyclovir-unresponsive mucocutaneous herpes simplex virus infection in patients with AIDS. J Infect Dis 176:892–898

Landry ML, Stanat S, Biron K et al (2000) A standardized plaque reduction assay for determination of drug susceptibilities of cytomegalovirus clinical isolates. Antimicrob Agents Chemother 44:688–692

Langston AA, Redei I, Caliendo AM et al (2002) Development of drug-resistant herpes simplex virus infection after haploidentical hematopoietic progenitor cell transplantation. Blood 99:1085–1088

Lascaux AS, Caumes E, Deback C et al (2012) Successful treatment of aciclovir and foscarnet resistant Herpes simplex virus lesions with topical imiquimod in patients infected with human immunodeficiency virus type 1. J Med Virol 84:194–197

Le Page AK, Jager MM, Iwasenko JM et al (2013) Clinical aspects of cytomegalovirus antiviral resistance in solid organ transplant recipients. Clin Infect Dis 56:1018–1029

Levin MJ, Dahl KM, Weinberg A et al (2003) Development of resistance to acyclovir during chronic infection with the Oka vaccine strain of varicella-zoster virus, in an immunosuppressed child. J Infect Dis 188:954–959

Levin MJ, Bacon TH, Leary JJ (2004) Resistance of herpes simplex virus infections to nucleoside analogues in HIV-infected patients. Clin Infect Dis 39(Suppl 5):S248–S257

Limaye AP (2002) Ganciclovir-resistant cytomegalovirus in organ transplant recipients. Clin Infect Dis 35:866–872

Limaye AP, Corey L, Koelle DM et al (2000) Emergence of ganciclovir-resistant cytomegalovirus disease among recipients of solid-organ transplants. Lancet 356:645–649

Limaye AP, Raghu G, Koelle DM et al (2002) High incidence of ganciclovir-resistant cytomegalovirus infection among lung transplant recipients receiving preemptive therapy. J Infect Dis 185:20–27

Lisboa LF, Asberg A, Kumar D et al (2011) The clinical utility of whole blood versus plasma cytomegalovirus viral load assays for monitoring therapeutic response. Transplantation 91:231–236

Lischka P, Hewlett G, Wunberg T et al (2010) In vitro and in vivo activities of the novel anticytomegalovirus compound AIC246. Antimicrob Agents Chemother 54:1290–1297

Liu S, Homa FL (2009) Viral genome replication. In: Cameron CE, Gotte M, Raney K (eds) Atomic structure of the herpes simplex virus 1 DNA polymerase. Springer, New York

Ljungman P, Ellis MN, Hackman RC et al (1990) Acyclovir-resistant herpes simplex virus causing pneumonia after marrow transplantation. J Infect Dis 162:244–248

Lolis MS, Gonzalez L, Cohen PJ et al (2008) Drug-resistant herpes simplex virus in HIV infected patients. Acta Dermatovenerol Croat 16:204–208

LoPresti AE, Levine JF, Munk GB et al (1998) Successful treatment of an acyclovir- and foscarnet-resistant herpes simplex virus type 1 lesion with intravenous cidofovir. Clin Infect Dis 26:512–513

Lurain NS, Chou S (2010) Antiviral drug resistance of human cytomegalovirus. Clin Microbiol Rev 23:689–712

Lurain NS, Spafford LE, Thompson KD (1994) Mutation in the UL97 open reading frame of human cytomegalovirus strains resistant to ganciclovir. J Virol 68:4427–4431

Lurain NS, Bhorade SM, Pursell KJ et al (2002) Analysis and characterization of antiviral drug-resistant cytomegalovirus isolates from solid organ transplant recipients. J Infect Dis 186:760–768
Malartre N, Boulieu R, Falah N et al (2012) Effects of mutations on herpes simplex virus 1 thymidine kinase functionality: an in vitro assay based on detection of monophosphate forms of acyclovir and thymidine using HPLC/DAD. Antiviral Res 95:224–228
Malvy D, Treilhaud M, Bouee S et al (2005) A retrospective, case–control study of acyclovir resistance in herpes simplex virus. Clin Infect Dis 41:320–326
Marfori JE, Exner MM, Marousek GI et al (2007) Development of new cytomegalovirus UL97 and DNA polymerase mutations conferring drug resistance after valganciclovir therapy in allogeneic stem cell recipients. J Clin Virol 38:120–125
Martin BK, Ricks MO, Forman MS et al (2007) Change over time in incidence of ganciclovir resistance in patients with cytomegalovirus retinitis. Clin Infect Dis 44:1001–1008
Martin M, Goyette N, Boivin G (2010a) Contrasting effects on ganciclovir susceptibility and replicative capacity of two mutations at codon 466 of the human cytomegalovirus UL97 gene. J Clin Virol 49:296–298
Martin M, Goyette N, Ives J et al (2010b) Incidence and characterization of cytomegalovirus resistance mutations among pediatric solid organ transplant patients who received valganciclovir prophylaxis. J Clin Virol 47:321–324
Marty FM, Ljungman P, Papanicolaou GA et al (2011) Maribavir prophylaxis for prevention of cytomegalovirus disease in recipients of allogeneic stem-cell transplants: a phase 3, double-blind, placebo-controlled, randomised trial. Lancet Infect Dis 11:284–292
Marty FM, Winston DJ, Rowley SD et al (2013) CMX001 to prevent cytomegalovirus disease in hematopoietic-cell transplantation. N Engl J Med 369:1227–1236
Morfin F, Thouvenot D (2003) Herpes simplex virus resistance to antiviral drugs. J Clin Virol 26:29–37
Morfin F, Thouvenot D, De Turenne-Tessier M et al (1999) Phenotypic and genetic characterization of thymidine kinase from clinical strains of varicella-zoster virus resistant to acyclovir. Antimicrob Agents Chemother 43:2412–2416
Morfin F, Souillet G, Bilger K et al (2000) Genetic characterization of thymidine kinase from acyclovir-resistant and -susceptible herpes simplex virus type 1 isolated from bone marrow transplant recipients. J Infect Dis 182:290–293
Morfin F, Bilger K, Boucher A et al (2004) HSV excretion after bone marrow transplantation: a 4-year survey. J Clin Virol 30:341–345
Myhre HA, Haug Dorenberg D, Kristiansen KI et al (2011) Incidence and outcomes of ganciclovir-resistant cytomegalovirus infections in 1244 kidney transplant recipients. Transplantation 92:217–223
Nichols WG, Corey L, Gooley T et al (2001) Rising pp 65 antigenemia during preemptive anticytomegalovirus therapy after allogeneic hematopoietic stem cell transplantation: risk factors, correlation with DNA load, and outcomes. Blood 97:867–874
Nichols WG, Boeckh M, Carter RA et al (2003) Transferred herpes simplex virus immunity after stem-cell transplantation: clinical implications. J Infect Dis 187:801–808
Nugier F, Colin JN, Aymard M et al (1992) Occurrence and characterization of acyclovir-resistant herpes simplex virus isolates: report on a two-year sensitivity screening survey. J Med Virol 36:1–12
Oberg B (1989) Antiviral effects of phosphonoformate (PFA, foscarnet sodium). Pharmacol Ther 40:213–285
Ozaki KS, Camara NO, Nogueira E et al (2007) The use of sirolimus in ganciclovir-resistant cytomegalovirus infections in renal transplant recipients. Clin Transplant 21:675–680
Pan D, Kaye SB, Hopkins M et al (2014) Common and new acyclovir resistant herpes simplex virus-1 mutants causing bilateral recurrent herpetic keratitis in an immunocompetent patient. J Infect Dis 209:345–349

Paya C, Humar A, Dominguez E et al (2004) Efficacy and safety of valganciclovir vs. oral ganciclovir for prevention of cytomegalovirus disease in solid organ transplant recipients. Am J Transplant 4:611–620

Pechere M, Wunderli W, Trellu-Toutous L et al (1998) Treatment of acyclovir-resistant herpetic ulceration with topical foscarnet and antiviral sensitivity analysis. Dermatology 197:278–280

Pelosi E, Rozenberg F, Coen DM et al (1998) A herpes simplex virus DNA polymerase mutation that specifically attenuates neurovirulence in mice. Virology 252:364–372

Pescovitz MD, Rabkin J, Merion RM et al (2000) Valganciclovir results in improved oral absorption of ganciclovir in liver transplant recipients. Antimicrob Agents Chemother 44:2811–2815

Piiparinen H, Hockerstedt K, Gronhagen-Riska C et al (2004) Comparison of two quantitative CMV PCR tests, Cobas Amplicor CMV Monitor and TaqMan assay, and pp 65-antigenemia assay in the determination of viral loads from peripheral blood of organ transplant patients. J Clin Virol 30:258–266

Piret J, Boivin G (2011) Resistance of herpes simplex viruses to nucleoside analogues: mechanisms, prevalence, and management. Antimicrob Agents Chemother 55:459–472

Piret J, Boivin G (2014) Antiviral drug resistance in herpesviruses other than cytomegalovirus. Rev Med Virol 24:186–218

Pottage JC, Kessler HA (1995) Herpes simplex virus resistance to acyclovir: clinical relevance. Infect Agents Dis 4:115–124

Prichard MN, Gao N, Jairath S et al (1999) A recombinant human cytomegalovirus with a large deletion in UL97 has a severe replication deficiency. J Virol 73:5663–5670

Reardon JE, Spector T (1989) Herpes simplex virus type 1 DNA polymerase. Mechanism of inhibition by acyclovir triphosphate. J Biol Chem 264:7405–7411

Reusser P, Cordonnier C, Einsele H et al (1996) European survey of herpesvirus resistance to antiviral drugs in bone marrow transplant recipients. Infectious diseases working party of the European Group for Blood and Marrow Transplantation (EBMT). Bone Marrow Transplant 17:813–817

Reyes M, Shaik NS, Graber JM et al (2003) Acyclovir-resistant genital herpes among persons attending sexually transmitted disease and human immunodeficiency virus clinics. Arch Intern Med 163:76–80

Roberts GB, Fyfe JA, Gaillard RK et al (1991) Mutant varicella-zoster virus thymidine kinase: correlation of clinical resistance and enzyme impairment. J Virol 65:6407–6413

Sacks SL, Shafran SD, Diaz-Mitoma F et al (1998) A multicenter phase I/II dose escalation study of single-dose cidofovir gel for treatment of recurrent genital herpes. Antimicrob Agents Chemother 42:2996–2999

Safrin S, Assaykeen T, Follansbee S et al (1990) Foscarnet therapy for acyclovir-resistant mucocutaneous herpes simplex virus infection in 26 AIDS patients: preliminary data. J Infect Dis 161:1078–1084

Safrin S, Berger TG, Gilson I et al (1991) Foscarnet therapy in five patients with AIDS and acyclovir-resistant varicella-zoster virus infection. Ann Intern Med 115:19–21

Safrin S, Elbeik T, Phan L et al (1994a) Correlation between response to acyclovir and foscarnet therapy and in vitro susceptibility result for isolates of herpes simplex virus from human immunodeficiency virus-infected patients. Antimicrob Agents Chemother 38:1246–1250

Safrin S, Kemmerly S, Plotkin B et al (1994b) Foscarnet-resistant herpes simplex virus infection in patients with AIDS. J Infect Dis 169:193–196

Sahoo MK, Lefterova MI, Yamamoto F et al (2013) Detection of cytomegalovirus drug resistance mutations by next-generation sequencing. J Clin Microbiol 51:3700–3710

Saijo M, Yasuda Y, Yabe H et al (2002) Bone marrow transplantation in a child with Wiskott-Aldrich syndrome latently infected with acyclovir-resistant (ACV(r)) herpes simplex virus type 1: emergence of foscarnet-resistant virus originating from the ACV(r) virus. J Med Virol 68:99–104

Saint-Leger E, Caumes E, Breton G et al (2001) Clinical and virologic characterization of acyclovir-resistant varicella-zoster viruses isolated from 11 patients with acquired immunodeficiency syndrome. Clin Infect Dis 33:2061–2067

Sarisky RT, Bacon T, Boon R et al (2002) Penciclovir susceptibilities of herpes simplex virus isolates from patients using penciclovir cream for treatment of recurrent herpes labialis. Antimicrob Agents Chemother 46:2848–2853

Sarisky RT, Bacon TH, Boon RJ et al (2003) Profiling penciclovir susceptibility and prevalence of resistance of herpes simplex virus isolates across eleven clinical trials. Arch Virol 148:1757–1769

Sasadeusz JJ, Tufaro F, Safrin S et al (1997) Homopolymer mutational hot spots mediate herpes simplex virus resistance to acyclovir. J Virol 71:3872–3878

Sauerbrei A, Eichhorn U, Schacke M et al (1999) Laboratory diagnosis of herpes zoster. J Clin Virol 14:31–36

Sauerbrei A, Deinhardt S, Zell R et al (2010) Phenotypic and genotypic characterization of acyclovir-resistant clinical isolates of herpes simplex virus. Antiviral Res 86:246–252

Sauerbrei A, Bohn K, Heim A et al (2011a) Novel resistance-associated mutations of thymidine kinase and DNA polymerase genes of herpes simplex virus type 1 and type 2. Antivir Ther 16:1297–1308

Sauerbrei A, Taut J, Zell R et al (2011b) Resistance testing of clinical varicella-zoster virus strains. Antiviral Res 90:242–247

Sauerbrei A, Liermann K, Bohn K et al (2012) Significance of amino acid substitutions in the thymidine kinase gene of herpes simplex virus type 1 for resistance. Antiviral Res 96:105–107

Sauerbrei A, Vodisch S, Bohn K et al (2013) Screening of herpes simplex virus type 1 isolates for acyclovir resistance using DiviTum^{R} assay. J Virol Methods 188:70–72

Sawyer MH, Inchauspe G, Biron KK et al (1988) Molecular analysis of the pyrimidine deoxyribonucleoside kinase gene of wild-type and acyclovir-resistant strains of varicella-zoster virus. J Gen Virol 69(Pt 10):2585–2593

Schliefer K, Gumbel HO, Rockstroh JK et al (1999) Management of progressive outer retinal necrosis with cidofovir in a human immunodeficiency virus-infected patient. Clin Infect Dis 29:684–685

Schmit I, Boivin G (1999) Characterization of the DNA polymerase and thymidine kinase genes of herpes simplex virus isolates from AIDS patients in whom acyclovir and foscarnet therapy sequentially failed. J Infect Dis 180:487–490

Schubert A, Ehlert K, Schuler-Luettmann S et al (2013) Fast selection of maribavir resistant cytomegalovirus in a bone marrow transplant recipient. BMC Infect Dis 13:330

Schulte EC, Sauerbrei A, Hoffmann D et al (2010) Acyclovir resistance in herpes simplex encephalitis. Ann Neurol 67:830–833

Schuurman R, Demeter L, Reichelderfer P et al (1999) Worldwide evaluation of DNA sequencing approaches for identification of drug resistance mutations in the human immunodeficiency virus type 1 reverse transcriptase. J Clin Microbiol 37:2291–2296

Scott GM, Weinberg A, Rawlinson WD et al (2007) Multidrug resistance conferred by novel DNA polymerase mutations in human cytomegalovirus isolates. Antimicrob Agents Chemother 51:89–94

Sergerie Y, Boivin G (2006) Thymidine kinase mutations conferring acyclovir resistance in herpes simplex type 1 recombinant viruses. Antimicrob Agents Chemother 50:3889–3892

Shapira MY, Resnick IB, Chou S et al (2008) Artesunate as a potent antiviral agent in a patient with late drug-resistant cytomegalovirus infection after hematopoietic stem cell transplantation. Clin Infect Dis 46:1455–1457

Shin YK, Weinberg A, Spruance S et al (2003) Susceptibility of herpes simplex virus isolates to nucleoside analogues and the proportion of nucleoside-resistant variants after repeated topical application of penciclovir to recurrent herpes labialis. J Infect Dis 187:1241–1245

Shmueli E, Or R, Shapira MY et al (2014) High rate of cytomegalovirus drug resistance among patients receiving preemptive antiviral treatment after haploidentical stem cell transplantation. J Infect Dis 209:557–561

Sims CR, Thompson K, Chemaly RF et al (2007) Oral topical cidofovir: novel route of drug delivery in a severely immunosuppressed patient with refractory multidrug-resistant herpes simplex virus infection. Transpl Infect Dis 9:256–259

Snoeck R, Andrei G, Gerard M et al (1994) Successful treatment of progressive mucocutaneous infection due to acyclovir- and foscarnet-resistant herpes simplex virus with (S)-1-(3-hydroxy-2-phosphonylmethoxypropyl)cytosine (HPMPC). Clin Infect Dis 18:570–578

Stoelben S, Arns W, Renders L et al (2014) Preemptive treatment of Cytomegalovirus infection in kidney transplant recipients with letermovir: results of a Phase 2a study. Transpl Int 27:77–86

Stranska R, van Loon AM, Bredius RG et al (2004a) Sequential switching of DNA polymerase and thymidine kinase-mediated HSV-1 drug resistance in an immunocompromised child. Antivir Ther 9:97–104

Stranska R, van Loon AM, Polman M et al (2004b) Genotypic and phenotypic characterization of acyclovir-resistant herpes simplex viruses isolated from haematopoietic stem cell transplant recipients. Antivir Ther 9:565–575

Stranska R, Schuurman R, Nienhuis E et al (2005) Survey of acyclovir-resistant herpes simplex virus in the Netherlands: prevalence and characterization. J Clin Virol 32:7–18

Strasfeld L, Lee I, Tatarowicz W et al (2010) Virologic characterization of multidrug-resistant cytomegalovirus infection in 2 transplant recipients treated with maribavir. J Infect Dis 202:104–108

Sugar EA, Jabs DA, Ahuja A et al (2012) Incidence of cytomegalovirus retinitis in the era of highly active antiretroviral therapy. Am J Ophthalmol 153(1016–1024):e1015

Sullivan V, Biron KK, Talarico C et al (1993) A point mutation in the human cytomegalovirus DNA polymerase gene confers resistance to ganciclovir and phosphonylmethoxyalkyl derivatives. Antimicrob Agents Chemother 37:19–25

Suzutani T, Ishioka K, De Clercq E et al (2003) Differential mutation patterns in thymidine kinase and DNA polymerase genes of herpes simplex virus type 1 clones passaged in the presence of acyclovir or penciclovir. Antimicrob Agents Chemother 47:1707–1713

Swierkosz EM, Hodinka RL, Moore BM et al (2004) Antiviral susceptibility testing: herpes simplex virus by plaque reduction assay; approved standard. Clinical and Laboratory Standards Institute, Wayne

Talarico CL, Phelps WC, Biron KK (1993) Analysis of the thymidine kinase genes from acyclovir-resistant mutants of varicella-zoster virus isolated from patients with AIDS. J Virol 67:1024–1033

van der Beek MT, Marijt EW, Vossen AC et al (2012) Failure of pre-emptive treatment of cytomegalovirus infections and antiviral resistance in stem cell transplant recipients. Antivir Ther 17:45–51

van der Beek MT, Vermont CL, Bredius RG et al (2013) Persistence and antiviral resistance of VZV in hematological patients. Clin Infect Dis 56:335–343

van Velzen M, van Loenen FB, Meesters RJ et al (2012) Latent acyclovir-resistant herpes simplex virus type 1 in trigeminal ganglia of immunocompetent individuals. J Infect Dis 205:1539–1543

van Velzen M, van de Vijver DA, van Loenen FB et al (2013) Acyclovir prophylaxis predisposes to antiviral-resistant recurrent herpetic keratitis. J Infect Dis 208:1359–1365

Verdonck LF, Cornelissen JJ, Smit J et al (1993) Successful foscarnet therapy for acyclovir-resistant mucocutaneous infection with herpes simplex virus in a recipient of allogeneic BMT. Bone Marrow Transplant 11:177–179

Verkaik NJ, Hoek RA, van Bergeijk H et al (2013) Leflunomide as part of the treatment for multidrug-resistant cytomegalovirus disease after lung transplantation: case report and review of the literature. Transpl Infect Dis 15:E243–E249

Visse B, Dumont B, Huraux JM et al (1998) Single amino acid change in DNA polymerase is associated with foscarnet resistance in a varicella-zoster virus strain recovered from a patient with AIDS. J Infect Dis 178(Suppl 1):S55–S57

Visse B, Huraux JM, Fillet AM (1999) Point mutations in the varicella-zoster virus DNA polymerase gene confers resistance to foscarnet and slow growth phenotype. J Med Virol 59:84–90

Wade JC, McLaren C, Meyers JD (1983) Frequency and significance of acyclovir-resistant herpes simplex virus isolated from marrow transplant patients receiving multiple courses of treatment with acyclovir. J Infect Dis 148:1077–1082

Waldman WJ, Knight DA, Lurain NS et al (1999) Novel mechanism of inhibition of cytomegalovirus by the experimental immunosuppressive agent leflunomide. Transplantation 68:814–825

Weinberg A, Jabs DA, Chou S et al (2003) Mutations conferring foscarnet resistance in a cohort of patients with acquired immunodeficiency syndrome and cytomegalovirus retinitis. J Infect Dis 187:777–784

Wolf DG, Lee DJ, Spector SA (1995a) Detection of human cytomegalovirus mutations associated with ganciclovir resistance in cerebrospinal fluid of AIDS patients with central nervous system disease. Antimicrob Agents Chemother 39:2552–2554

Wolf DG, Smith IL, Lee DJ et al (1995b) Mutations in human cytomegalovirus UL97 gene confer clinical resistance to ganciclovir and can be detected directly in patient plasma. J Clin Invest 95:257–263

Wong SW, Wahl AF, Yuan PM et al (1988) Human DNA polymerase alpha gene expression is cell proliferation dependent and its primary structure is similar to both prokaryotic and eukaryotic replicative DNA polymerases. Embo J 7:37–47

Xiong X, Smith JL, Chen MS (1997) Effect of incorporation of cidofovir into DNA by human cytomegalovirus DNA polymerase on DNA elongation. Antimicrob Agents Chemother 41:594–599

Zhang J, Chung DW, Tan CK et al (1991) Primary structure of the catalytic subunit of calf thymus DNA polymerase delta: sequence similarities with other DNA polymerases. Biochemistry 30:11742–11750

Ziyaeyan M, Alborzi A, Japoni A et al (2007) Frequency of acyclovir-resistant herpes simplex viruses isolated from the general immunocompetent population and patients with acquired immunodeficiency syndrome. Int J Dermatol 46:1263–1266

Quasispecies and Drug Resistance

Celia Perales, Ana M. Ortega-Prieto, Nathan M. Beach, Julie Sheldon, Luis Menéndez-Arias, and Esteban Domingo

Contents

C. Perales (✉) • E. Domingo
Centro de Biología Molecular "Severo Ochoa" (CSIC-UAM), Consejo Superior de Investigaciones Científicas (CSIC), Madrid, Spain

Centro de Investigación Biomédica en Red de Enfermedades Hepáticas y Digestivas (CIBERehd), Barcelona, Spain
e-mail: cperales@cbm.csic.es; edomingo@cbm.uam.es

A.M. Ortega-Prieto • N.M. Beach • L. Menéndez-Arias
Centro de Biología Molecular "Severo Ochoa" (CSIC-UAM), Consejo Superior de Investigaciones Científicas (CSIC), Madrid, Spain
e-mail: ana.ortega.prieto@gmail.com; beachnm@gmail.com; lmenendez@cbm.csic.es

J. Sheldon
Centro de Biología Molecular "Severo Ochoa" (CSIC-UAM), Consejo Superior de Investigaciones Científicas (CSIC), Madrid, Spain

Division of Experimental Virology, Twincore, Centre for Experimental and Clinical Infection Research, a joint venture between Medical School Hannover and Helmholtz Centre for Infection Research, Hannover, Germany
e-mail: julie.sheldon@twincore.de

M. Gotte et al. (eds.), *Handbook of Antimicrobial Resistance*,
DOI 10.1007/978-1-4939-0694-9_1

Abstract
Mutant spectra of viral quasispecies are complex reservoirs of genetic and phenotypic variants, including drug-resistant mutants. Here we review basic features of RNA viral quasispecies such as internal interactions within mutant spectra and the effect of population size and bottleneck events as they affect the frequency of inhibitor-escape mutants. Genetic barriers to resistance and fitness cost of specific amino acid substitutions involved in resistance are discussed, with specific examples for human immunodeficiency virus type 1 (HIV-1) and hepatitis C virus (HCV). Prospects for new antiviral designs aimed at counteracting the adaptive potential of viral quasispecies are presented.

Keywords
Antiviral therapy • Drug resistance • Genetic barrier • Hepatitis C virus (HCV) • Human immunodeficiency virus type 1 (HIV-1) • Mutant spectrum • Replication rate • Viral fitness • Viral load • Viral quasispecies

Introduction: Relevance of Quasispecies in Virus Biology

Viral quasispecies are mutant distributions (also termed mutant spectra, clouds, or swarms) that characterize genome populations of RNA viruses and at least some DNA viruses (Fig. 1). Both clonal analyses by classic nucleotide sequencing techniques and bulk population analyses by ultra-deep sequencing have documented that mutant distributions are extremely complex with many minority mutations occurring at low frequency (1 % which is the present standard cutoff value for reliable mutant frequency determination and probably lower according to studies that achieved lower cutoff values). From all evidence, mutant spectra originate from high mutation rates in RNA (and some DNA) viruses, which have been estimated in 10^{-3} to 10^{-5} mutations introduced per nucleotide copied, together with competition and intrapopulation interactions among genomes [reviewed in (Domingo et al. 2012)]. Viral quasispecies took its name from a theory of the origin of life developed by M. Eigen, P. Schuster, and their colleagues (Eigen and Schuster 1979). Theoretical studies on quasispecies have paralleled experimental investigations with RNA viruses, reaching a considerable degree of conceptual cross-fertilization (Eigen 2013; Holland 2006; Mas et al. 2010; Ojosnegros et al. 2011).

The biological behavior of viral quasispecies is not equivalent to that of sets of identical genomes undergoing only occasional mutations for two main reasons. One is that mutant spectra constitute vast reservoirs of genetic and phenotypic variants, including, notably, drug-, antibody-, or cytotoxic T-cell (CTL)-escape mutants. The second reason is that the variant genomes which dynamically arise, persist, increase, or decrease in frequency or are eliminated (transiently or irreversibly) do not act independently. Variants can complement each other to give rise to a new phenotype (Cao et al. 2014; Shirogane et al. 2012), to trigger large evolutionary transitions such as genome segmentation (Moreno et al. 2014), or to maintain a higher average fitness of the mutant ensemble relative to its individual components (Domingo et al. 1978, 2012;

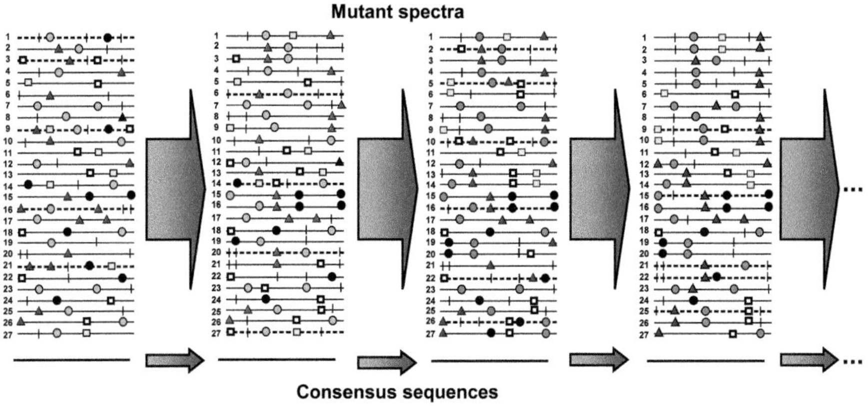

Fig. 1 **Schematic representation of quasispecies evolution**. The four successive populations (*lines* represent genomes and symbols on lines mutations) evolve by modification of the mutant spectrum while the consensus sequence remains invariant. In the simplified dynamics depicted here, genomes that acquire five or more mutations (genomes with discontinuous lines) do not survive. In reality, viral populations (even single replicative units in a replication complex) consist of hundreds or thousands genomes subjected to the dynamics of mutant generation, competition, and selection. (Figure reproduced from Domingo et al. (2012) with permission from ASM)

Duarte et al. 1994). A specific high-fidelity mutant of poliovirus that displayed limited mutant spectrum complexity was attenuated and could not adapt to complex environments or reach the central nervous system in a mouse model (Pfeiffer and Kirkegaard 2005a; Vignuzzi et al. 2006). However, an accompanying mutant spectrum allowed the mutant to reach its target organ *in vivo* (Vignuzzi and Andino 2010; Vignuzzi et al. 2006). Thus, mutant spectrum complexity is relevant to viral pathogenesis, and the control of replication fidelity may serve to engineer attenuated virus vaccines (Vignuzzi et al. 2008).

Quasispecies swarms can have an effect opposite to complementation: the suppression of individual viral mutant progeny which in isolation displays superior fitness than the parental quasispecies (de la Torre and Holland 1990). Theoretical quasispecies predicts that the behavior of any individual component may be modulated by the mutant spectrum that surrounds it. In one of the computer simulations, near an error threshold (preceding a second and final threshold where no genomes can be maintained), a slightly inferior mutant was strongly favored by virtue of its better mutant environment [(Swetina and Schuster 1982), reviewed in Eigen and Biebricher (1988)]. In the case of viruses, the suppressive effect of a mutant ensemble on particular variants is exerted through different biological mechanisms, derived from the biochemical reactions during genome replication and the effect of *trans*-acting proteins. Specifically, in poliovirus, four mechanisms of mutant-mediated interference were identified (Crowder and Kirkegaard 2005). Some capsid and polymerase mutants produced dominant negative phenotypes, attributed to the fact that these proteins function as oligomers. Mutations in *cis*-regulatory element (CRE) and VPg protein indicated that nonproductive priming of initiation of viral RNA replication is inhibitory. The authors confirmed that, as anticipated, a drug-sensitive poliovirus inhibited the intracellular growth of a drug-resistant mutant (Crowder and Kirkegaard 2005). In line with these findings, a mutagenized, preextinction foot-and-mouth disease virus (FMDV) population interfered with replication of the standard virus (González-López et al. 2004). The accumulation of defective, mutated genomes in the heavily mutagenized FMDV population produced an interfering swarm, an event that was shown to participate in viral extinction by lethal mutagenesis (Grande-Pérez et al. 2005). A study with specific FMDV capsid and polymerase mutants confirmed their interfering activity on wild-type virus and showed that the mutants had to be competent in RNA replication to be inhibitory (Perales et al. 2007). This requirement is one of the factors that contribute to an advantage of sequential inhibitor-mutagen treatment over the corresponding combination, to prevent the selection of inhibitor-escape mutants and favor virus extinction (Iranzo et al. 2011; Moreno et al. 2012; Perales et al. 2009, 2012).

Modulating effects of mutant spectra have been observed also *in vivo*. Virulent poliovirus can have its phenotype suppressed by attenuated virus in the population (Chumakov et al. 1991). A growth hormone deficiency syndrome induced by lymphocytic choriomeningitis virus can be suppressed by disease-negative variants (Teng et al. 1996) [reviewed in (Domingo et al. 2012)].

Major Factors in the Generation and Dominance of Drug Resistance in Viruses

Drug-resistant mutants are those present in quasispecies that can replicate more efficiently than other components of the mutant swarm in the presence of the drug. Their selection and maintenance in a viral population is conditional upon two events which are influenced by different parameters: (i) mutant generation and (ii) the efficiency of mutant replication relative to other components of the same population. Mutant generation depends on the genetic barrier to resistance, defined as the number and types of mutations required to reach the resistance phenotype. Telaprevir resistance in hepatitis C virus (HCV) can be achieved by amino acid substitution R155K in NS3. In HCV genotype 1a, these substitutions can be attained by a single nucleotide transition (AGA → AAA). In contrast, in genotype 1b, by virtue of the R codon being CGA, the same amino acid substitution requires two mutations: a transversion and a transition (CGA → AAA). Since the probability of occurrence of two independent mutations is the product of probabilities of occurrence of the individual mutations, and transversions are usually less frequent than transitions, the HCV genetic barrier to telaprevir resistance is higher for HCV genotype 1b than 1a. There is no molecular or evolutionary reason to exclude that genetic variations that modify the genetic barrier to a drug can occur among viruses of the same genotype or among components of a mutant spectrum. Obviously, the genetic barrier will be increased when two or more amino acid substitutions (each requiring at least one mutation) are needed to reach the drug-resistance phenotype. In general terms, requirements of multiple mutations (excessive number of steps in sequence space) are what preclude viruses of surviving in some environments. This is the main reason

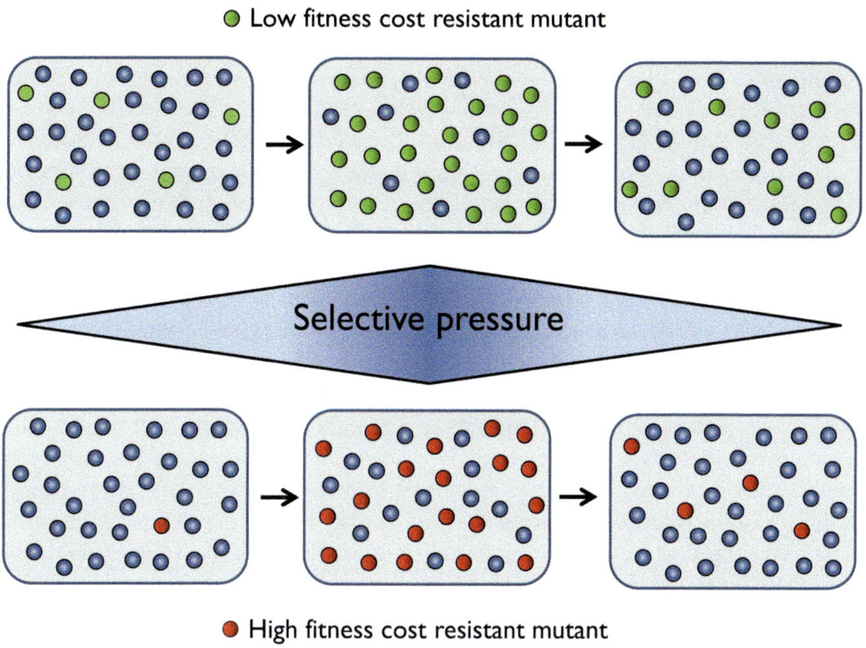

Fig. 2 Phenotypic barrier or fitness cost to overcome a selective pressure. The escape mutants that experience a low fitness cost (depicted as *green circles* in the upper three successive populations) may preexist with considerable frequency before the selective pressure is exerted; they can reach high proportions in the presence of the selective pressure and remain at elevated levels even when the selective pressure is removed (*upper right population*). The escape mutants that experience a high fitness cost (depicted as *red circles* in the bottom three successive populations) will be present at low frequency before the selective pressure is exerted; they can reach high proportions in the presence of the selective pressure and return to low levels when the selective pressure is removed (*bottom right population*)

of the advantages of combination therapies over monotherapy, with the exceptions discussed in section "Conclusions and New Prospects for Antiviral Therapy".

Once the genetic barrier has been overcome and the resistant mutant has been generated, a second barrier, termed phenotypic barrier or fitness cost, intervenes. If the relevant amino acid substitution, in addition to conferring drug resistance, impairs any step in the viral life cycle, the proportion of the mutant in the viral quasispecies will decrease. The higher the fitness cost, the lower the proportion of the mutant in the mutant spectrum. Two possible outcomes can be anticipated: either the fitness cost does not allow the mutant to become dominant or compensatory mutations (that counteract the fitness cost of the drug-resistance mutations without significantly altering the resistance level) occur that allow dominance of the resistant mutant. Fitness effects apply to viruses escaping any type of selective pressure (drugs, immune responses, tropism, host range changes, etc.). The consequence of fitness cost of a drug-resistance mutation has been schematically represented in Fig. 2, in which the frequency of the relevant escape mutant (green circles in the upper population and red circles in the bottom population) is fitness-dependent. If the fitness cost is severe (even more than implied in the bottom panels of Fig. 2), the relevant escape mutant may not preexist in the population. With 10^{-3} to 10^{-5} mutations introduced per nucleotide copied (Domingo et al. 2012), a type of arms race is established between the occurrence of the relevant mutation and the opportunity of the genome harboring it to replicate sufficiently in the presence of the drug. These conflicting requirements may allow the virus to improve replication through compensatory mutations and evolve towards dominance or be irreversibly lost in the mutant spectrum. Studies of deep sequencing of viral populations that are confronted with a strong selective pressure [e.g., in human immunodeficiency virus type 1 (HIV-1)-infected patients treated with vicriviroc (Tsibris et al. 2009)] suggest that viral quasispecies screen multiple escape routes, and only a subset of those are successful. Drug-escape mutants are present at high frequencies in populations of many important pathogenic viruses such as HIV-1, hepatitis B virus, HCV, or influenza virus, and such mutants can dramatically lead to treatment failure. Yet, what the experimental studies on quasispecies dynamics suggest is that the observed drug-resistance mutations recorded are only a minor subset of all possible resistance mutations that would be found if fitness effects did not intervene.

To complicate matters even further, as noted in the Introduction, fitness levels are not only a property of individual viral genomes. Rather, the frequency of a given mutant can be influenced by the surrounding quasispecies. Specifically, the presence of a complex mutant spectrum can suppress a drug-resistant mutant to avoid or delay its dominance (see Introduction for references).

Effect of Variations in Population Size and Viral Load

The virus population size often varies during the course of the natural infectious cycle of viruses. It generally increases from the initial infecting dose to a viremic state, and it may decrease again if persistence or chronicity is established. During an acute infection, subsets of viruses may invade new cells, tissues, or organs, and such invasions may involve reductions of population size (bottleneck events). Since viral populations consist of mutant swarms, the viral population size that is transmitted (from host to host, organ to organ, or cell to cell) will determine the numbers and types of mutants that can continue replicating (Fig. 3). Drug-resistant mutants may be generated in an infected host subjected to therapy with the drug (e.g., the mutants depicted as yellow stars in Fig. 3). This mutant will not contribute directly to drug resistance in a recipient virus-naïve individual unless the transmitted population reaches a critical size. The term primary resistance was coined during the AIDS epidemics to denote infections by HIV-1 which harbored an antiretroviral resistance mutation selected prior to transmission.

Not only fluctuations of population size and bottleneck events are important to understand quasispecies evolution, the total population size (viral load) is also relevant. We have previously emphasized the connections between four parameters in virus survival: viral load, replication rate, genetic heterogeneity, and viral

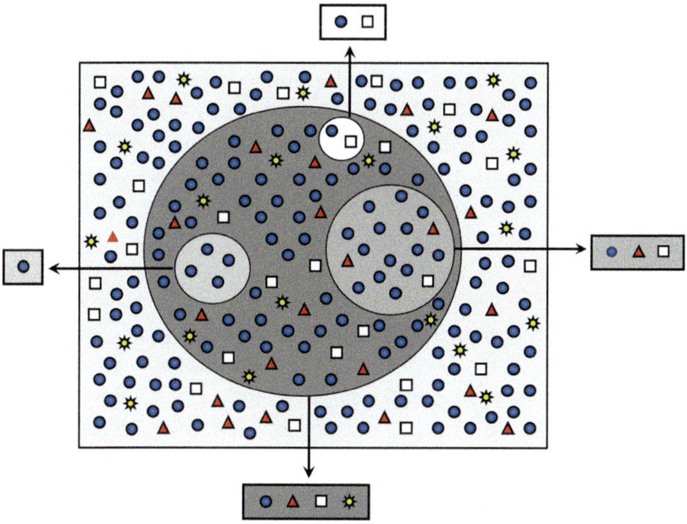

Fig. 3 The effect of population size in a mutant repertoire. The *large square* represents a viral quasispecies, in which four types of genomes are present. Small sample sizes will result in detection of only the highest frequency genomes (*small gray circle*) but may randomly fluctuate based on chance detection (*small white circle*). Greater diversity will be detected in larger sample sizes, represented by larger *gray circles* (Figure modified from Domingo et al. (2012) with permission from ASM)

fitness. As explained elsewhere (Domingo et al. 2012), potent replication which is a key component of fitness values tends to produce elevated viral loads. When endowed with the adequate diversity (mutant spectrum amplitude), high viral loads will contribute to adaptedness and survival. Several lines of evidence suggest that these four interconnected parameters are linked to disease progression, again emphasizing the relevance of quasispecies for viral pathogenesis (Domingo et al. 2012).

Clinical Impact of Drug-Resistant Viral Mutants

Escape mutants have been reported ever since the first controlled studies with viral populations subjected to antiviral inhibitors were performed (Eggers and Tamm 1965; Melnick et al. 1961). Many examples, both historical and current, have been periodically reviewed [Domingo (1989), Domingo et al. (2012), Richman (1996) and references therein]. Several data banks offer updated information on drug resistance of important viral pathogens.

Here we review, as specific examples, drug-resistance mutations of some clinically relevant viruses such as HIV-1 and HCV.

HIV Variability and Antiretroviral Therapy

HIV is a retrovirus that causes the acquired immunodeficiency syndrome (AIDS) in humans. Currently, there are around 34 million people worldwide infected with HIV. Although HIV-1 strains are responsible for most of the global AIDS pandemic, there are about 1–2 million people infected with HIV type 2 (HIV-2). Genetic variability is one of the hallmarks of HIV. These viruses have high mutation rates (around 10^{-4} to 10^{-5} mutations per nucleotide and replication cycle) and high recombination frequencies (reviewed in (Menéndez-Arias 2009)). This is partly due to the relatively low fidelity of the viral reverse transcriptase that like other polymerases found in RNA viruses is devoid of proofreading activity. In addition, it has been estimated that the minimum duration of the HIV life cycle *in vivo* is only 1.2 days, while the average number of virions produced per day in an infected individual is 1.03×10^{10} (Perelson et al. 1996). These characteristics of the HIV infection are responsible for the generation of complex quasispecies that facilitate the selection of strains resistant to antiretroviral drugs, as discussed in sections "Introduction: Relevance of Quasispecies in Virus Biology" to "Effect of Variations in Population Size and Viral Load".

Six years after the first clinical observation of AIDS in the United States (Centers for Disease Control [CDC] 1981), AZT (3′-azido-3′-deoxythymidine; zidovudine) became the first drug approved for treatment of HIV-1 infection (Fig. 4). AZT is a prodrug that in its triphosphate form is incorporated into the viral genome by the reverse transcriptase, while blocking DNA synthesis due to the absence of a 3′-OH in its ribose ring. For several years, AZT was administered to patients in monotherapy, leading to the selection of resistant HIV-1 strains with amino acid substitutions such as M41L, D67N, K70R, L210W, T215F or T215Y, and K219E or K219Q in the reverse transcriptase [(Larder et al. 1989); reviewed in Menéndez-Arias (2008)]. Other nucleoside analogs (e.g., didanosine, zalcitabine, stavudine, and lamivudine) were approved in the following years, and very often these drugs were prescribed alone after failure of AZT monotherapy due to the emergence of drug-resistant HIV-1. Sequential treatments facilitated the selection of multidrug-resistant viral strains due to accumulation of resistance mutations specific for each drug. On the other hand, the combined use of AZT and didanosine or zalcitabine in untreated patients facilitated the selection of multidrug-resistant HIV-1 variants containing a different set of mutations including A62V, V75I, F77L, F116Y, and Q151M (Shirasaka et al. 1995).

A remarkable breakthrough in the antiretroviral treatment was achieved in 1995 when the first HIV-1 protease inhibitor (i.e., saquinavir) was approved. Highly active antiretroviral therapy (HAART) was then introduced as a combination of two nucleoside analogs (e.g., AZT, lamivudine, etc.) and a protease inhibitor (Gulick et al. 1997; Hammer et al. 1997). By targeting two different steps in the HIV life cycle (i.e., viral genome replication and maturation), it was possible to decrease viral loads below the limits of detection and minimize the impact and emergence of drug resistance. In the following years, the approval of nonnucleoside analog inhibitors of

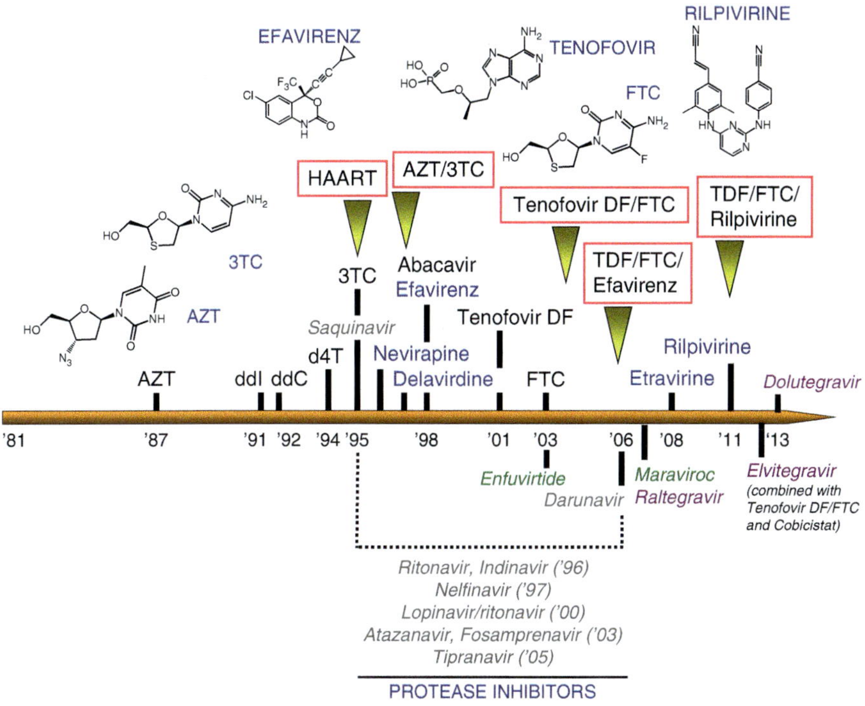

Fig. 4 Timeline for approval of antiretroviral drugs. Nucleoside reverse transcriptase inhibitors are shown in *black*, nonnucleoside reverse transcriptase inhibitors in *blue*, protease inhibitors in *gray*, integrase inhibitors in *purple*, and entry inhibitors in *green*. Abbreviations: 3TC (lamivudine), β-L-(−)-2′,3′-dideoxy-3′-thiacytidine; AZT (zidovudine), β-D-(+)-3′-azido-3′-deoxythymidine; d4T (stavudine), β-D-(+)-2′,3′-didehydro-2′,3′-dideoxythymidine; ddC (zalcitabine), β-D-(+)-2′,3-′-dideoxycytidine; ddI (didanosine), β-D-(+)-2′,3′-dideoxyinosine; FTC (emtricitabine), β-L-(−)-2′,3′-dideoxy-5-fluoro-3′-thiacytidine; HAART, highly active antiretroviral therapy; tenofovir DF, tenofovir disoproxil fumarate

HIV-1 reverse transcriptase increased the number of available HAART regimens by allowing novel drug combinations acting on different HIV targets.

Effective Combination Therapies for HIV-1 Infection

Despite their impressive success in reducing AIDS mortality, combination therapies developed in the late 1990s were still problematic due to the poor pharmacokinetic properties of HIV protease inhibitors (very high doses and a large number of pills were needed) and the low genetic barrier to resistance of nevirapine and other nonnucleoside reverse transcriptase inhibitors. In 2006, the introduction of Atripla®, a combination of two nucleoside analogs (tenofovir disoproxil fumarate and emtricitabine) and the nonnucleoside reverse transcriptase inhibitor efavirenz, constituted a significant accomplishment as it became the standard of care for therapy-naïve patients. With one pill a day, its dosage is optimal and facilitates adherence to antiretroviral therapy. Based on the same principles, other recently approved combinations include a single tablet tenofovir disoproxil fumarate and emtricitabine either with rilpivirine (a nonnucleoside reverse transcriptase inhibitor) or with elvitegravir (an integrase inhibitor which is administered together with cobicistat). Cobicistat is an inhibitor of cytochrome P450 3A enzymes that boosts blood levels of elvitegravir.

The Molecular Basis of Drug Resistance in HIV-1

In addition to the simplification of dosing regiments, drugs used today are more potent and have longer half-lives than compounds used 15 years ago. Furthermore, current regimens have less toxicity and are more tolerable over time. At present, viral suppression using combination therapies is effective and emergence of resistance has been significantly reduced in the clinical setting. However, there are still patients infected with drug-resistant strains that were selected after successive treatments with different antiretroviral drugs or individuals that were infected with drug-resistant HIV-1 (i.e., transmitted drug resistance). In addition, natural resistance to various antiretroviral drugs has been observed in several HIV-1 clades, as well as in HIV-2 (Menéndez-Arias and Álvarez 2014). Therefore, in this scenario, compounds targeting different steps of the virus life cycle are still needed. Currently licensed drugs target (i) viral entry (e.g., maraviroc and enfuvirtide), (ii) reverse transcription (nucleoside and nonnucleoside reverse transcriptase inhibitors), (iii) integration (integrase inhibitors, such as raltegravir, elvitegravir, and dolutegravir), and (iv) viral maturation (protease inhibitors) [reviewed in (Menéndez-Arias 2013)]. A list of amino acid substitutions associated with resistance to antiretroviral drugs is given in Table 1.

Nucleoside reverse transcriptase inhibitors are the backbone of current antiretroviral therapies. Some of those drugs have a relatively low genetic barrier (section "Major Factors in the Generation and Dominance of Drug Resistance in Viruses"). For example, high-level resistance to lamivudine and emtricitabine is conferred by single mutations generating the amino acid substitutions M184I or M184V. These amino acid changes reduce the ability of the reverse transcriptase to incorporate the inhibitor relative to its natural substrates (i.e., dNTPs) [reviewed in Menéndez-Arias (2008)]. On the other hand, at least 2–3 mutations are needed to produce an AZT-resistant HIV-1 strain. The relevant thymidine analog resistance mutations (e.g., M41L, D67N, T215Y, etc.) facilitate the excision of AZT-monophosphate, stavudine-monophosphate, or tenofovir from the 3′ end of blocked DNA primers, in a reaction mediated by ATP and other pyrophosphate donors (Meyer et al. 1999; Tu et al. 2010). The same molecular mechanism operates for HIV variants having reverse transcriptases that contain a dipeptide insertion between codons 69 and 70 and thymidine analog resistance mutations such as M41L or T215Y [reviewed

Table 1 Amino acid substitutions associated with HIV-1 resistance to antiretroviral drugs

Drugs	Amino acid substitutions associated with drug resistance
Nucleoside analog reverse transcriptase inhibitors	
Zidovudine (AZT)	M41L, D67N, K70R, V118I, L210W, **T215F/Y**, K219E/Q
Didanosine (ddI)	K65R, L74V, M184V
Lamivudine (3TC)	(E44D/V118I), K65R, **M184I/V**
Stavudine (d4T)	M41L, D67N, K70R, V118I, L210W, T215F/Y, K219E/Q
Abacavir	K65R, L74V, Y115F, M184V (M41L, D67N, K70R, L210W, T215F/Y, K219E/Q)
Emtricitabine (FTC)	(K65R/Q151M), **M184I/V**
Tenofovir	**K65R**, K70E
Combinations of mutations that confer resistance to various nucleoside analogs	
	(i) M41L, D67N, K70R, L210W, T215F/Y, K219E/Q; (ii) A62V, V75I, F77L, F116Y, Q151M; (iii) insertions between codons 69–70 (i.e., T69SSS or T69SSG or T69SSA), M41L, A62V, K70R, L210W, T215F/Y
Nonnucleoside reverse transcriptase inhibitors	
Nevirapine	L100I, K101P, K103N/S, V106A/M, V108I, Y181C/I, Y188C/L/H, G190A/C/E/Q/S/T
Delavirdine	K103H/N/T, V106M, Y181C, Y188L, G190E, P236L
Efavirenz	L100I, K101P, K103H/N, V106M, V108I, Y188L, G190A/S/T, P225H, M230L
Etravirine	V90I, A98G, L100I, K101E/H/P/Q, V106I, **E138A**/G/K/**Q**/**R**/S, **V179**D/**F**/**I**/**L**, Y181C/I/V, G190A/S, F227C, M230L, T386A, E399D
Rilpivirine	V90I, K101E/P, **E138**A/G/**K**/Q/**R** (±M184I/V), V179F/I/L, Y181C/I/V, Y188L, V189I, H221Y, F227C, M230I/L
Combinations of mutations that confer cross-resistance to nevirapine, delavirdine and efavirenz	
	(i) K103N alone; (ii) V106M alone; (iii) Y188L alone; (iv) two or more amino acid changes of the group: L100I, V106A, Y181C/I, G190A/S, M230L, and Y318F
Protease inhibitors	
Saquinavir	L10I/R/V, **G48V**, I54L/V, A71T/V, G73S, V77I, V82A, I84V, **L90M**, and A431V [in the Gag polyprotein cleavage site p7(NC)/p1)]
Ritonavir	L10I/R/V, K20M/R, V32I, L33F, M36I, M46I/L, I54L/V, A71T/V, V77I, **V82A/F/S/T**, **I84V**, L90M, and A431V [in the Gag polyprotein cleavage site p7(NC)/p1)]
Indinavir	L10I/R/V, K20M/R, L24I, V32I, M36I, **M46I/L**, I54V, A71T/V, G73A/S, V77I, **V82A/F/S/T**, **I84V**, L90M, and in the Gag cleavage sites: A431V [in p7(NC)/p1)] and L449F [in p1/p6]
Nelfinavir	L10F/I, **D30N**, M36I, M46I/L, A71T/V, V77I, V82A/F/S/T, I84V, N88D/S, **L90M**, and in the Gag cleavage sites L449F and P453L [in p1/p6]
Amprenavir (fosamprenavir)	L10F/I/R/V, V32I, M46I/L, I47V, **I50V**, I54V/M, **I84V**, L90M, and Gag cleavage sites L449F and P453L [in p1/p6]

(continued)

Table 1 (continued)

Drugs	Amino acid substitutions associated with drug resistance
Lopinavir	L10F/I/R/V, G16E, K20I/M/R, L24I, **V32I**, L33F, E34Q, K43T, M36I/L, **M46I**/L, **I47A**/V, G48M/V, I50V, **I54L/V**/A/M/S/T, Q58E, I62V, L63T, A71T, G73T, T74S, **L76V**, **V82A**/F/S/T, I84V, L89I/M, L90M, and A431V [in the Gag polyprotein cleavage site p7(NC)/p1)]
Atazanavir	L10F/I/V, K20I/M/R, L24I, L33F/I/V, M36I/L/V, M46I/L, G48V, **I50L**, I54L/V, L63P, A71I/T/V, G73A/C/S/T, V82A/F/S/T, **I84V**, **N88S**, L90M
Tipranavir	L10I/S/V, I13V, K20M/R, **L33F/I/V**, E35G, M36I/L/V, K43T, M46L, I47V, I54A/M/V, Q58E, H69K, T74P, **V82L/T**, N83D, **I84V**, L89I/M/V, L90M
Darunavir	V11I, V32I, L33F, I47V, **I50V**, I54L/M, T74P, L76V, V82F, I84V, L89V, and in the Gag cleavage sites A431V [in p7(NC)/p1)] and S451T and R452S [in p1/p6]
Combinations that confer resistance to multiple protease inhibitors	
	L10F/I/R/V, **M46I/L**, I54L/M/V, **V82A/F/T/S**, **I84V**, **L90M**[a]
Fusion inhibitors	
Enfuvirtide	G36D/E/S, I37T/N/V, V38A/E/M, Q40H, N42T, N43D/K/S (all in gp41)
Integrase inhibitors	
Raltegravir	G140S, **Y143C/R**, **Q148H/K/R**, **N155H**
Elvitegravir	T66A/I/K, L74M, E92Q/V, **Q148H/K/R**, V151L, **N155H**
Dolutegravir	F121Y, E138A/K, G140A/S, Q148H, R263K
CCR5 antagonists	
Maraviroc	Resistance usually develops through the selection of viruses that use the CXCR4 (X4) coreceptor. In addition, maraviroc resistance mutations have been selected in vitro in the V2, V3, and V4 loops of gp120 (Westby et al. 2007)

For additional information, see Clotet et al. (2014), Wensing et al. (2014), and the websites of the International Antiviral Society–USA (http://www.iasusa.org) and the Stanford University HIV Drug Resistance Database (http://hivdb.stanford.edu)
Major resistance mutations are shown in *bold*. Most protease inhibitors are usually prescribed in combination with a low dose of ritonavir that has a boosting effect on the protease inhibitor concentration in plasma
[a]Multiple protease inhibitor resistance can be achieved through the accumulation of four or five mutations of those indicated in the list

in (Menéndez-Arias et al. 2006)]. The substitution of Gln^{151} by Met, considered as the initial step in the Q151M pathway, requires two nucleotide changes. Q151M and accompanying mutations confer resistance by reducing the viral polymerase ability to incorporate nucleoside analogs in the DNA chain.

Classical nonnucleoside reverse transcriptase inhibitors (e.g., nevirapine, delavirdine, and efavirenz) have a very low genetic barrier. Single nucleotide changes occurring at several codons in the reverse transcriptase-coding region can individually confer high-level resistance to those drugs. Interestingly, some of them (notably, K103N) confer cross-resistance to all three drugs. Next-generation inhibitors such as etravirine and rilpivirine are more potent and show a higher genetic barrier to resistance. However, E138K and other substitutions at this position are sufficient to confer partial resistance to these drugs (Asahchop et al. 2013). Nevertheless, unlike in the case of nevirapine, delavirdine, or efavirenz, two amino acid substitutions are needed to attain high-level resistance in vitro (Azijn et al. 2010; Javanbakht et al. 2010). Rilpivirine is now substituting efavirenz in the most effective antiretroviral drug combinations.

Resistance to HIV protease inhibitors is relatively complex, since for most drugs in this class, high-level resistance involves a relatively large number of amino acid substitutions [for a recent review, see Menéndez-Arias (2013)]. Major mutations associated with resistance map within the substrate/inhibitor binding site (e.g., D30N, G48V, V82A, I84V, etc.). These amino acid changes usually have a significant impact on the viral replication capacity. Secondary mutations that are selected later during treatment increase viral fitness and usually locate out of the substrate binding site. In some cases, these amino acid substitutions have an impact on protease stability (e.g., L10I or A71V) (Chang and Torbett 2011). Further viral fitness recovery during treatment can be facilitated by mutations occurring at the viral polypeptide substrates cleaved by the HIV protease (e.g., at Gag cleavage sites NC/p1 and p1/p6). These mutations facilitate viral polyprotein processing by improving Gag susceptibility to protease cleavage.

Approved integrase inhibitors bind to the catalytic domain of the enzyme blocking its strand transfer activity. Resistance to raltegravir and elvitegravir is associated with single amino acid substitutions (usually Q148K/R/H, but also N155H). Integrase inhibitors have been recently combined with nucleoside analogs in HAART regimens. Interestingly, the latest integrase inhibitor approved for treatment (i.e., dolutegravir) shows a surprisingly high genetic barrier. In phase III clinical trials, approximately 88 % of the patients treated with dolutegravir and two nucleoside reverse transcriptase inhibitors attained viral load suppression to <50 copies of RNA/ml, without developing drug-resistance-associated mutations after 48 weeks of treatment (Raffi et al. 2013; Wainberg et al. 2013). It is possible that development of dolutegravir resistance mutations may result in viruses with greatly diminished replicative capacity, thereby constituting a major barrier towards the development of resistance.

Other drugs used in antiretroviral rescue therapy include entry inhibitors targeting either the step involving the recognition of the viral coreceptor (CCR5 antagonists) or fusion inhibitors (enfuvirtide). Enfuvirtide is a largely helical polypeptide that interferes with the packaging of HIV-1 gp41 α-helical segments required for the fusion of the viral envelope and the cell membrane. Resistance is achieved by mutations in gp41 that encode amino acid changes that disrupt interactions between α-helices in the transmembrane protein and enfuvirtide (Greenberg and Cammack 2004). On the other hand, maraviroc is a CCR5 antagonist. This drug binds to a pocket in the chemokine receptor and makes it unavailable for the HIV-1 surface glycoprotein gp120. Viral strains resistant to maraviroc may still infect the host by using other chemokine receptors (e.g., CXCR4) (Westby et al. 2006). In addition, resistance to maraviroc mediated by specific amino acid substitutions in the V3 loop of gp120 allows HIV-1 to continue using CCR5 coreceptors, even in the presence of bound maraviroc (Westby et al. 2007). This use of a drug-bound coreceptor illustrates that viruses have multiple resources to overcome a selective pressure intended to limit their replication and that even drugs that target a cellular function are not free of the problem of selection of virus-escape mutants (see section "Conclusions and New Prospects for Antiviral Therapy").

HCV Variability and Current Therapy

HCV is a member of the *Flaviviridae* family affecting approximately 170 million individuals worldwide. HCV shows a very high variability which is mainly due to the absence of proofreading activity of the RNA polymerase and very high rate of virion production, approximately 10^{12} per infected individual per day (Neumann et al. 1998). For over ten years, the standard of care treatment for HCV infection was a combination of pegylated interferon-α (IFN-α) and ribavirin, which achieved viral eradication in 40–50 % of patients infected with HCV genotype 1 and 80 % in those infected with genotypes 2 and 3 (Quer et al. 2008; Shiffman 2008). Unfortunately, the use of IFN-α and ribavirin results in moderate to severe side effects in many patients. The approval of telaprevir and boceprevir in 2011 for the treatment of chronic HCV infection was a major breakthrough in the field of anti-HCV therapy. Therapy consisting of a protease inhibitor combined with IFN-α and ribavirin for HCV genotype 1 patients significantly increased sustained virological response (SVR) rates compared with IFN-α and ribavirin treatment alone and reduced the rate of selection of resistant variants (Bacon et al. 2011; Jacobson et al. 2011; Poordad et al. 2011; Zeuzem et al. 2011). There are currently several new compounds targeting various HCV proteins that have been or will soon be added to the arsenal of drugs available for new combination therapies, that might render possible the implementation of IFN-free regimens (deLemos and Chung 2014; Lange and Zeuzem 2013). The newest direct-acting antiviral agents (DAAs) are candidates to be included in these regimens, such as second-generation NS3, NS5A, and viral polymerase (NS5B) inhibitors. However, appropriate combinations of these inhibitors must be selected to avoid cross-resistance and overcome problems associated with low barrier of resistance to individual drugs.

Resistance to Interferon-α and to Ribavirin

The administration of exogenous IFN-α exerts antiviral effects via activation of innate immunity. It is not clear why some patients respond differently to IFN–αbased treatments, though several host factors (gender, age, ethnicity, obesity, etc.) have been implicated. Sequence polymorphisms within the IL28B locus (IFN-λ3) have been linked to variations in the virological response to IFN-α-based therapy (Ge et al. 2009). Particularly difficult cases are null responders to previous treatment with IFN-α and ribavirin, those infected by certain HCV genotypes, patients coinfected with HIV-1, or those with advanced liver fibrosis (Lange and Zeuzem 2013). The number of escape routes that a virus may use to avoid suppression by antivirals depends on the complexity of the response exerted by the drugs. For DAAs that target specific viral proteins, resistance often depends on one or a few key amino acid substitutions. In contrast, the pluricomponent antiviral response exerted by IFN-α affects multiple cell signaling pathways, which may explain why IFN-α resistance has been linked to several HCV genes (Kozuka et al. 2012; Perales et al. 2013, 2014; Serre et al. 2013). Among other examples, the viral protease NS3/4A cleaves mitochondrial antiviral signaling (MAVS) and TIR-domain-containing adaptor-inducing interferon-β (TRIF), interrupting signal transduction via retinoic acid-inducible gene-I (RIG-I), toll-like receptor 3 (TLR3), and protein kinase R (PKR) response pathways. Additionally, HCV core protein has been linked to decreased signaling via Jak-STAT, resulting in decreased expression of interferon-stimulated genes (ISGs) (Horner and Gale 2013).

Another unsettled issue is whether resistant variants with IFN-α-specific mutations are directly responsible for treatment failure. Though sequence analysis of HCV from patients failing treatment with IFN-α and ribavirin has been performed, no consensus amino acid changes have been associated with genotype-specific IFN-α response. However, variations detected in broad regions of core, E2, and NS5A have been correlated with treatment outcome (Chayama and Hayes 2011; Enomoto et al. 1996; Pawlotsky et al. 1998). This is consistent with the results of *in vitro* studies, where HCV passaged in the presence of IFN-α has selected multiple substitutions throughout the viral genome (Perales et al. 2013, 2014; Serre et al. 2013). Interestingly, the mutations seen in patients failing therapy are not the same as those observed after *in vitro* selection in the presence of IFN-α (Kozuka et al. 2012; Perales et al. 2013, 2014).

There seems to be a strong link between enhanced fitness and IFN-α resistance *in vitro*, making it more difficult to distinguish *bona fide* IFN resistance from cell culture adaptation. Thus, the need of HCV to cope with multiple ISG proteins renders IFN-α resistance a far more complex issue than resistance to standard antiviral inhibitors that target a specific viral protein (Perales et al. 2014). In the serial passages of HCV to select IFN-α-resistant mutants, it was observed that virus that had been passaged in human hepatoma Huh-7.5 cells in the absence of IFN-α also acquired partial resistance to IFN-α (Perales et al. 2013). Further studies with the multiply passaged populations documented that the partial resistance extended to several DAAs and ribavirin, despite the virus not having been exposed to the drugs. Mutant spectrum analyses and the kinetics of progeny production by serially diluted populations and by individual clones excluded that drug resistance was associated with the presence of drug-escape mutants in the multiply passaged populations. The results established viral fitness as a multidrug-resistance factor in HCV (Sheldon et al. 2014).

The inclusion of ribavirin in combination therapies increased the rates of SVR compared with treatment using IFN-α alone, though the mechanism is not fully understood (Sostegni et al. 1998). Several antiviral mechanisms of ribavirin have been described: (i) immunomodulation and enhancement of the Th1 antiviral immune response, (ii) upregulation of genes involved in IFN signaling, (iii) inhibition of viral RNA-dependent RNA polymerases, (iv) depletion of intracellular GTP levels, (v) inhibition of mRNA cap formation, and (vi) lethal mutagenesis. Although the precise mechanism (or combination of mechanisms) of ribavirin-mediated viral inhibition during anti-HCV therapy has not been elucidated, several lines of evidence suggest that lethal mutagenesis is involved (Asahina et al. 2005; Cuevas et al. 2009; Dietz et al. 2013; Dixit et al. 2004; Lutchman et al. 2007). The ribavirin-induced bias in the mutant spectrum (an excess of G-A and C-U transitions), which reflects the mutagenic activity of ribavirin, has been observed both *in vivo* (Dietz et al. 2013) and in cell culture (Ortega-Prieto et al. 2013). In general, resistance mutations against a mutagen are less frequent than for classical inhibitors. The first identification of a ribavirin-resistance mutation (F415Y in NS5B) in HCV was during ribavirin monotherapy in patients (Young et al. 2003). Experiments with HCV replicon containing cell lines showed that ribavirin resistance occurred by changes in the cell lines (the resistant cell lines were defective in ribavirin import) or from mutations in NS5A (G404S and E442G) (Ibarra and Pfeiffer 2009; Pfeiffer and Kirkegaard 2005b). Additionally, serial passage of a genotype 2a replicon in the presence of ribavirin resulted in reduced sensitivity to the drug, and NS5B mutation Y33H was determined to be responsible, presumably due to a decrease in replicative fitness (Hmwe et al. 2010). Passage of infectious J6/JFH1 of HCV in the presence of ribavirin yielded a resistant virus with many mutations, but the responsible mutation was not identified (Feigelstock et al. 2011).

Resistance to Directly Acting Antiviral Agents (DAAs)

The number of HCV antiviral drugs under development has increased greatly over the past few years, with many drugs now approved by the US Food and Drug Administration and more in late-phase clinical trials. These DAAs are taking a more central role in therapy, with the aim of shortening treatment duration and avoiding IFN in standard of care therapy.

Telaprevir and boceprevir were the first two DAAs to be approved for use in anti-HCV therapy. However, despite their exceptionally potent antiviral activity, use of these first-generation inhibitors of the NS3/4A protease results in the rapid selection of resistance mutations and viral "breakthrough" of monotherapy (Sarrazin et al. 2007; Susser et al. 2009). *In vitro* studies have identified many single amino acid changes associated with reduced sensitivity to protease inhibitors, indicating a low barrier to resistance that has also been evidenced in clinical trials (Lange and Zeuzem 2013; Thompson et al. 2011). The ease of crossing the resistance barrier can be partly explained by the structural characteristics of the NS3/4A protease active site. Only a few side-chain interactions are needed for the binding of inhibitors to the greatly exposed protease active site (Romano et al. 2010). There are mutations at key positions in NS3 (Arg^{155}, Ala^{156}, and Asp^{168}) that make HCV resistant to nearly all protease inhibitors (Sarrazin and Zeuzem 2010; Thompson et al. 2011; Wyles 2013). Some newer protease inhibitors, such as MK-5172, have shown increased potency against variants containing Arg^{155} mutations (Summa et al. 2012). Most of the protease inhibitors currently in use were developed to target the NS3 protease domain of genotype 1 HCV. Due to differences in NS3 amino acid sequence, the efficacy of protease inhibitors in genotypes 2–6 is decreased (Lange et al. 2010). As mentioned in section "Major Factors in the Generation and Dominance of Drug Resistance in Viruses" above, there is also a difference in susceptibility to NS3/4A inhibitors based on HCV subtype, due to differences in nucleotide sequence at key amino acid-coding positions (McCown et al. 2009).

Daclatasvir was the first NS5A inhibitor to be used in clinical trials. NS5A inhibitors show a very potent antiviral activity across all genotypes due to conservation of targeted domains, but the barrier to resistance is relatively low, as for protease inhibitors. Substitutions at positions Met^{28}, Gln^{30}, Leu^{31}, Pro^{32}, and Tyr^{93} are frequently selected by this class of inhibitor (Gao 2013; Halfon and Sarrazin 2012; Nakamoto et al. 2014; Nettles et al. 2011). Similar to protease inhibitors, the viral genotype was found to influence the rate of resistant mutant selection, with virus from patients infected with genotype 1b being less likely to acquire resistance than virus from genotype 1a-infected patients (Fridell et al. 2011; Nettles et al. 2011).

In contrast, nucleoside analog NS5B inhibitors display high antiviral activity, broad genotype coverage, and relatively high barrier to resistance. Nucleoside inhibitors of NS5B are analogs of the polymerase substrates and bind directly to the NS5B active site. Importantly, because the active site of NS5B is highly conserved, nucleoside analogs have similar efficacy across all HCV genotypes. While amino acid substitutions resulting in weak resistance to nucleoside analog are readily selected, the resulting loss of replicative fitness limits breakthrough (McCown et al. 2008; Sarrazin and Zeuzem 2010). This contrasts with substitutions selected by NS3/4A protease and nonnucleoside inhibitors, which have greater resistance and do not profoundly affect replication capacity (Pawlotsky 2009). Sofosbuvir is an approved pyrimidine-derived nucleoside analog NS5B inhibitor that may be of great importance in future IFN-free treatment regimens. The barrier to resistance is relatively high, as only a few NS5B mutations have been confirmed to confer resistance [S282T (Sofia et al. 2010); L159F/L320F (Tong et al. 2014; Donaldson et al. 2014)].

Ongoing clinical trials with newly approved DAAs aim at finding effective, IFN-free combinations applicable to all HCV genotypes, which is challenging due to the continuing diversification of HCV in nature and the many escape routes that viruses find to combat drugs. To avoid rapid selection of cross-resistant mutant populations of HCV, combinations of inhibitors should be directed against several viral genes simultaneously (Lange and Zeuzem 2013). This concept is supported by the known sensitivity of viruses with protease inhibitor-resistance mutations to other classes of DAAs (such as NS5A, NS5B, and cyclophilin inhibitors) (Thompson et al. 2011) and the accumulated experience with treatments against HIV-1 infections (section "Effective Combination Therapies for HIV-1 Infection"). In a study where treatment-naïve HCV genotype 1a and 1b patients were treated with mericitabine, danoprevir (NS3/4A inhibitor), and ribavirin, viral breakthrough was mainly associated with NS3/4A resistance mutants while specific resistance mutations in NS5B were obtained in a single patient (Lange and Zeuzem 2013). In clinical trials with patients infected by genotype 1 HCV treated with a combination of the NS5A inhibitor ledipasvir and sofosbuvir, high rates of SVR were achieved (>94 %), regardless of prior treatment history (Afdhal et al. 2014a, b). Combination therapy using the NS5A inhibitor daclatasvir with sofosbuvir resulted in SVR rates of 98 %, 92 %, and 89 % in patients infected by genotypes 1, 2, and 3, respectively (Sulkowski et al. 2014). Resistance mutations present in patients were limited to known NS5A resistant variants, and no sofosbuvir-specific mutations were observed. Thus, the combination of inhibitors used in IFN-free therapies must be chosen carefully in order to minimize risk of breakthrough resistance. It is difficult to anticipate to what extent a wider use of IFN-free treatments will affect HCV evolution and select for new drug-resistance mutations that will acquire epidemiological relevance (as was the case with HIV-1). It will largely depend on the administration of the new combinations to poorly responding patients, who provide environments that are prone to select for escape mutants, and also on the fitness and frequency of transmission of the newly generated mutants.

Due to the high basal mutation frequency in natural HCV populations, it may be important to evaluate the presence of preexisting resistance mutations within patient HCV quasispecies. Presence of a naturally occurring variant of genotype 1a (Q80K) has been associated with decreased SVR after simeprevir-based triple therapy (Forns et al. 2014). When resistant mutants emerge after treatment failure, it is not well known how long they remain in the population and whether they can impact future therapy. Studies using population sequencing techniques have revealed a rapid loss of detection of resistant variants (Mauss et al. 2014) although in other studies, sequencing detected resistant variants even several years after treatment with telaprevir or boceprevir (Susser et al. 2011). Furthermore, increased failure of simeprevir-based triple therapy was observed after re-treatment of patients who had developed simeprevir resistance previously during monotherapy, likely an effect of persistent resistance variants within the viral population (Lenz et al. 2012). The analysis of resistance mutations within the quasispecies both at baseline and after failure of IFN-free regimens will guide future selection of inhibitor combinations to be used.

Conclusions and New Prospects for Antiviral Therapy

High mutation rates and quasispecies dynamics confer to RNA viruses an adaptive potential that may be counteracted using five main strategies: (i) combination therapy (i.e., HAART for AIDS, as has been described in section "HIV Variability and Antiretroviral Therapy"), (ii) splitting of the treatment into a first induction regimen (to decrease the number of viral mutants and viral load) and a second maintenance regimen (to maintain a viral load sufficiently low) (von Kleist et al. 2011), (iii) targeting of cellular proteins (taking advantage of viral reliance on host cell functions) (Geller et al. 2007; Hopkins et al. 2010; Kumar et al. 2011), (iv) combined use of immunotherapy and chemotherapy (in order to stimulate a broad adaptive immune response) (Li et al. 2005; Seiler et al. 2000; Webster et al. 1986), and (v) lethal mutagenesis [Domingo et al. (2012) and references therein].

It has been proposed that the targeting of cellular functions should limit selection of viral escape mutants. This is not necessarily the case, as evidenced by selection of mutations in NS5A that were associated with resistance to cyclosporine A (Chatterji et al. 2010; Delang et al. 2011) and maraviroc-resistant HIV-1 mutants (section "The Molecular Basis of Drug Resistance in HIV-1"). Moreover, such agents may produce side effects derived from the perturbation of cellular functions. However, the ability of these compounds to simultaneously inhibit the replication of multiple virus types may increase their therapeutic potential (Pawlotsky 2014).

Lethal mutagenesis aims at extinguishing viruses by increasing mutation rates via administration of mutagenic agents. Population behavior of RNA viruses is strongly influenced by interactions among viral genomes within the mutant spectra. Thus, the generation of defective viral genomes (as a consequence of increased mutagenesis) and the collapse of the whole ensemble due to interfering interactions with the replication of the standard virus are consistent with the features of viral quasispecies (Grande-Pérez et al. 2005; Perales et al. 2007). A first clinical trial using a mutagenic nucleoside analog was conducted against HIV-1 in AIDS patients, showing that lethal mutagenesis could be effective *in vivo* (Mullins et al. 2011). Therapies involving inhibitors and mutagenic agents should consider the mechanism of action of both drugs due mainly to two reasons: (i) defective mutants (generated by the mutagen) should be replication-competent to exert their interfering activity and this is impeded in the presence of an inhibitor and (ii) due to the mutagen-induced error rate, the selection of inhibitor-escape mutants could be favored when both drugs are administered simultaneously, and this probability will increase with the viral load (Iranzo et al. 2011; Perales et al. 2009, 2012). In light of this, sequential therapies with a first phase of viral load reduction (via a combination of inhibitors) followed by a second phase of increased mutagenesis deserve further investigation. From a general perspective, such explorations of new treatment designs will become even more justified if, as can be anticipated, the new combinations fail to eradicate current and emerging pathogenic viruses worldwide.

Acknowledgments Work at Centro de Biología Molecular Severo Ochoa (CSIC-UAM) supported by grant BFU2011-23604 and Fundación Ramón Areces. N.M.B. is supported by a JAE-DOC contract from Consejo Superior de Investigaciones Científicas (CSIC) and J.S. by a Juan de la Cierva contract from CSIC. CIBERehd is funded by Instituto de Salud Carlos III. Work in the lab of Dr. Menéndez-Arias was supported in part by grants of the Spanish Ministries of Economy and Competitiveness (BIO2010/15542 and BIO2013-48788-C2-1-R) and Health, Social Services and Equality (EC11-025).

References

Afdhal N, Reddy KR, Nelson DR et al (2014a) Ledipasvir and sofosbuvir for previously treated HCV genotype 1 infection. N Engl J Med 370:1483–1493

Afdhal N, Zeuzem S, Kwo P et al (2014b) Ledipasvir and sofosbuvir for untreated HCV genotype 1 infection. N Engl J Med 370(20):1889–1898. doi:10.1056/NEJMoa1402454

Asahchop EL, Wainberg MA, Oliveira M et al (2013) Distinct resistance patterns to etravirine and rilpivirine in viruses containing nonnucleoside reverse transcriptase inhibitor mutations at baseline. Aids 27:879–887
Asahina Y, Izumi N, Enomoto N et al (2005) Mutagenic effects of ribavirin and response to interferon/ribavirin combination therapy in chronic hepatitis C. J Hepatol 43:623–629
Azijn H, Tirry I, Vingerhoets J et al (2010) TMC278, a next-generation nonnucleoside reverse transcriptase inhibitor (NNRTI), active against wild-type and NNRTI-resistant HIV-1. Antimicrob Agents Chemother 54:718–727
Bacon BR, Gordon SC, Lawitz E et al (2011) Boceprevir for previously treated chronic HCV genotype 1 infection. N Engl J Med 364:1207–1217
Cao L, Wu C, Shi H et al (2014) Coexistence of hepatitis B virus quasispecies enhances viral replication and the ability to induce host antibody and cellular immune responses. J Virol 88:8656–8666
Centers for Disease Control (1981) Pneumocystis pneumonia–Los Angeles. MMWR Morb Mortal Wkly Rep 30:250–252
Chang MW, Torbett BE (2011) Accessory mutations maintain stability in drug-resistant HIV-1 protease. J Mol Biol 410:756–760
Chatterji U, Lim P, Bobardt MD et al (2010) HCV resistance to cyclosporin A does not correlate with a resistance of the NS5A-cyclophilin A interaction to cyclophilin inhibitors. J Hepatol 53:50–56
Chayama K, Hayes CN (2011) Hepatitis C virus: how genetic variability affects pathobiology of disease. J Gastroenterol Hepatol 26(Suppl 1):83–95
Chumakov KM, Powers LB, Noonan KE et al (1991) Correlation between amount of virus with altered nucleotide sequence and the monkey test for acceptability of oral poliovirus vaccine. Proc Natl Acad Sci U S A 88:199–203
Clotet B, Menéndez-Arias L, Schapiro JM et al (2014) The HIV & hepatitis drug resistance and PK guide, 13th edn. Fundació de Lluita contra la SIDA, Barcelona, 706 pp
Crowder S, Kirkegaard K (2005) Trans-dominant inhibition of RNA viral replication can slow growth of drug-resistant viruses. Nat Genet 37:701–709
Cuevas JM, Gonzalez-Candelas F, Moya A et al (2009) Effect of ribavirin on the mutation rate and spectrum of hepatitis C virus in vivo. J Virol 83:5760–5764
de la Torre JC, Holland JJ (1990) RNA virus quasispecies populations can suppress vastly superior mutant progeny. J Virol 64:6278–6281
Delang L, Vliegen I, Froeyen M et al (2011) Comparative study of the genetic barriers and pathways towards resistance of selective inhibitors of hepatitis C virus replication. Antimicrob Agents Chemother 55:4103–4113
deLemos AS, Chung RT (2014) Hepatitis C treatment: an incipient therapeutic revolution. Trends Mol Med 20:315–321
Dietz J, Schelhorn SE, Fitting D et al (2013) Deep sequencing reveals mutagenic effects of ribavirin during monotherapy of hepatitis C virus genotype 1-infected patients. J Virol 87:6172–6181
Dixit NM, Layden-Almer JE, Layden TJ et al (2004) Modelling how ribavirin improves interferon response rates in hepatitis C virus infection. Nature 432:922–924
Domingo E (1989) RNA virus evolution and the control of viral disease. Prog Drug Res 33:93–133
Domingo E, Sabo D, Taniguchi T et al (1978) Nucleotide sequence heterogeneity of an RNA phage population. Cell 13:735–744
Domingo E, Sheldon J, Perales C (2012) Viral quasispecies evolution. Microbiol Mol Biol Rev 76:159–216
Donaldson EF, Harrington PR, O'Rear JJ et al (2014) Clinical evidence and bioinformatics characterization of potential hepatitis C virus resistance pathways for sofosbuvir. Hepatology (in press)
Duarte EA, Novella IS, Ledesma S et al (1994) Subclonal components of consensus fitness in an RNA virus clone. J Virol 68:4295–4301

Eggers HJ, Tamm I (1965) Coxsackie A9 virus: mutation from drug dependence to drug independence. Science 148:97–98
Eigen M (2013) From strange simplicity to complex familiarity. Oxford University Press, Oxford
Eigen M, Biebricher CK (1988) Sequence space and quasispecies distribution. In: Domingo E, Ahlquist P, Holland JJ (eds) RNA genetics. CRC Press, Boca Raton, pp 211–245
Eigen M, Schuster P (1979) The hypercycle. A principle of natural self-organization. Springer, Berlin
Enomoto N, Sakuma I, Asahina Y et al (1996) Mutations in the nonstructural protein 5A gene and response to interferon in patients with chronic hepatitis C virus 1b infection. N Engl J Med 334:77–81
Feigelstock DA, Mihalik KB, Feinstone SM (2011) Selection of hepatitis C virus resistant to ribavirin. Virol J 8:402
Forns X, Lawitz E, Zeuzem S et al (2014) Simeprevir with peginterferon and ribavirin leads to high rates of SVR in patients with HCV genotype 1 who relapsed after previous therapy: a phase 3 trial. Gastroenterology. doi:10.1053/j.gastro.2014.02.051
Fridell RA, Wang C, Sun JH et al (2011) Genotypic and phenotypic analysis of variants resistant to hepatitis C virus nonstructural protein 5A replication complex inhibitor BMS-790052 in humans: in vitro and in vivo correlations. Hepatology 54:1924–1935
Gao M (2013) Antiviral activity and resistance of HCV NS5A replication complex inhibitors. Curr Opin Virol 3:514–520
Ge D, Fellay J, Thompson AJ et al (2009) Genetic variation in IL28B predicts hepatitis C treatment-induced viral clearance. Nature 461:399–401
Geller R, Vignuzzi M, Andino R et al (2007) Evolutionary constraints on chaperone-mediated folding provide an antiviral approach refractory to development of drug resistance. Genes Dev 21:195–205
González-López C, Arias A, Pariente N et al (2004) Preextinction viral RNA can interfere with infectivity. J Virol 78:3319–3324
Grande-Pérez A, Lázaro E, Lowenstein P et al (2005) Suppression of viral infectivity through lethal defection. Proc Natl Acad Sci U S A 102:4448–4452
Greenberg ML, Cammack N (2004) Resistance to enfuvirtide, the first HIV fusion inhibitor. J Antimicrob Chemother 54:333–340
Gulick RM, Mellors JW, Havlir D et al (1997) Treatment with indinavir, zidovudine, and lamivudine in adults with human immunodeficiency virus infection and prior antiretroviral therapy. N Engl J Med 337:734–739
Halfon P, Sarrazin C (2012) Future treatment of chronic hepatitis C with direct acting antivirals: is resistance important? Liver Int 32(Suppl 1):79–87
Hammer SM, Squires KE, Hughes MD et al (1997) A controlled trial of two nucleoside analogues plus indinavir in persons with human immunodeficiency virus infection and CD4 cell counts of 200 per cubic millimeter or less. AIDS Clinical Trials Group 320 Study Team. N Engl J Med 337:725–733
Hmwe SS, Aizaki H, Date T et al (2010) Identification of hepatitis C virus genotype 2a replicon variants with reduced susceptibility to ribavirin. Antiviral Res 85:520–524
Holland JJ (2006) Transitions in understanding of RNA viruses: an historical perspective. Curr Top Microbiol Immunol 299:371–401
Hopkins S, Scorneaux B, Huang Z et al (2010) SCY-635, a novel nonimmunosuppressive analog of cyclosporine that exhibits potent inhibition of hepatitis C virus RNA replication in vitro. Antimicrob Agents Chemother 54:660–672
Horner SM, Gale M Jr (2013) Regulation of hepatic innate immunity by hepatitis C virus. Nat Med 19:879–888
Ibarra KD, Pfeiffer JK (2009) Reduced ribavirin antiviral efficacy via nucleoside transporter-mediated drug resistance. J Virol 83:4538–4547
Iranzo J, Perales C, Domingo E et al (2011) Tempo and mode of inhibitor-mutagen antiviral therapies: a multidisciplinary approach. Proc Natl Acad Sci U S A 108:16008–16013

Jacobson IM, McHutchison JG, Dusheiko G et al (2011) Telaprevir for previously untreated chronic hepatitis C virus infection. N Engl J Med 364:2405–2416
Javanbakht H, Ptak RG, Chow E et al (2010) In vitro resistance development for RO-0335, a novel diphenylether nonnucleoside reverse transcriptase inhibitor. Antiviral Res 86:212–219
Kozuka R, Enomoto M, Hai H et al (2012) Changes in sequences of core region, interferon sensitivity-determining region and interferon and ribavirin resistance-determining region of hepatitis C virus genotype 1 during interferon-alpha and ribavirin therapy, and efficacy of retreatment. Hepatol Res 42:1157–1167
Kumar N, Liang Y, Parslow TG et al (2011) Receptor tyrosine kinase inhibitors block multiple steps of influenza a virus replication. J Virol 85:2818–2827
Lange CM, Zeuzem S (2013) Perspectives and challenges of interferon-free therapy for chronic hepatitis C. J Hepatol 58:583–592
Lange CM, Sarrazin C, Zeuzem S (2010) Review article: specifically targeted anti-viral therapy for hepatitis C – a new era in therapy. Aliment Pharmacol Ther 32:14–28
Larder BA, Darby G, Richman DD (1989) HIV with reduced sensitivity to zidovudine (AZT) isolated during prolonged therapy. Science 243:1731–1734
Lenz O, de Bruijne J, Vijgen L et al (2012) Efficacy of re-treatment with TMC435 as combination therapy in hepatitis C virus-infected patients following TMC435 monotherapy. Gastroenterology 143(1176–1178):e1171–e1176
Li MJ, Kim J, Li S et al (2005) Long-term inhibition of HIV-1 infection in primary hematopoietic cells by lentiviral vector delivery of a triple combination of anti-HIV shRNA, anti-CCR5 ribozyme, and a nucleolar-localizing TAR decoy. Mol Ther 12:900–909
Lutchman G, Danehower S, Song BC et al (2007) Mutation rate of the hepatitis C virus NS5B in patients undergoing treatment with ribavirin monotherapy. Gastroenterology 132:1757–1766
Mas A, Lopez-Galíndez C, Cacho I et al (2010) Unfinished stories on viral quasispecies and Darwinian views of evolution. J Mol Biol 397:865–877
Mauss S, Berg T, Rockstroh J et al (2014) Short guide to hepatitis C. Flying Publisher & Kamps, Germany
McCown MF, Rajyaguru S, Le Pogam S et al (2008) The hepatitis C virus replicon presents a higher barrier to resistance to nucleoside analogs than to nonnucleoside polymerase or protease inhibitors. Antimicrob Agents Chemother 52:1604–1612
McCown MF, Rajyaguru S, Kular S et al (2009) GT-1a or GT-1b subtype-specific resistance profiles for hepatitis C virus inhibitors telaprevir and HCV-796. Antimicrob Agents Chemother 53:2129–2132
Melnick JL, Crowther D, Barrera-Oro J (1961) Rapid development of drug-resistant mutants of poliovirus. Science 134:557
Menéndez-Arias L (2008) Mechanisms of resistance to nucleoside analogue inhibitors of HIV-1 reverse transcriptase. Virus Res 134:124–146
Menéndez-Arias L (2009) Mutation rates and intrinsic fidelity of retroviral reverse transcriptases. Viruses 1:1137–1165
Menéndez-Arias L (2013) Molecular basis of human immunodeficiency virus type 1 drug resistance: overview and recent developments. Antiviral Res 98:93–120
Menéndez-Arias L, Álvarez M (2014) Antiretroviral therapy and drug resistance in human immunodeficiency virus type 2 infection. Antiviral Res 102:70–86
Menéndez-Arias L, Matamoros T, Cases-González CE (2006) Insertions and deletions in HIV-1 reverse transcriptase: consequences for drug resistance and viral fitness. Curr Pharm Des 12:1811–1825
Meyer PR, Matsuura SE, Mian AM et al (1999) A mechanism of AZT resistance: an increase in nucleotide-dependent primer unblocking by mutant HIV-1 reverse transcriptase. Mol Cell 4:35–43
Moreno H, Grande-Pérez A, Domingo E et al (2012) Arenaviruses and lethal mutagenesis. Prospects for new ribavirin-based interventions. Viruses 4:2786–2805

Moreno E, Ojosnegros S, García-Arriaza J et al (2014) Exploration of sequence space as the basis of viral RNA genome segmentation. Proc Natl Acad Sci U S A 111:6678–6683

Mullins JI, Heath L, Hughes JP et al (2011) Mutation of HIV-1 genomes in a clinical population treated with the mutagenic nucleoside KP1461. PLoS One 6:e15135

Nakamoto S, Kanda T, Wu S et al (2014) Hepatitis C virus NS5A inhibitors and drug resistance mutations. World J Gastroenterol 20:2902–2912

Nettles RE, Gao M, Bifano M et al (2011) Multiple ascending dose study of BMS-790052, a nonstructural protein 5A replication complex inhibitor, in patients infected with hepatitis C virus genotype 1. Hepatology 54:1956–1965

Neumann AU, Lam NP, Dahari H et al (1998) Hepatitis C viral dynamics in vivo and the antiviral efficacy of interferon-alpha therapy. Science 282:103–107

Ojosnegros S, Perales C, Mas A et al (2011) Quasispecies as a matter of fact: viruses and beyond. Virus Res 162:203–215

Ortega-Prieto AM, Sheldon J, Grande-Pérez A et al (2013) Extinction of hepatitis C virus by ribavirin in hepatoma cells involves lethal mutagenesis. PLoS One 8:e71039

Pawlotsky JM (2009) Therapeutic implications of hepatitis C virus resistance to antiviral drugs. Therap Adv Gastroenterol 2:205–219

Pawlotsky JM (2014) What are the pros and cons of the use of host-targeted agents against hepatitis C? Antiviral Res 105:22–25

Pawlotsky JM, Germanidis G, Neumann AU et al (1998) Interferon resistance of hepatitis C virus genotype 1b: relationship to nonstructural 5A gene quasispecies mutations. J Virol 72:2795–2805

Perales C, Mateo R, Mateu MG et al (2007) Insights into RNA virus mutant spectrum and lethal mutagenesis events: replicative interference and complementation by multiple point mutants. J Mol Biol 369:985–1000

Perales C, Agudo R, Tejero H et al (2009) Potential benefits of sequential inhibitor-mutagen treatments of RNA virus infections. PLoS Pathog 5:e1000658

Perales C, Iranzo J, Manrubia SC et al (2012) The impact of quasispecies dynamics on the use of therapeutics. Trends Microbiol 20:595–603

Perales C, Beach NM, Gallego I et al (2013) Response of hepatitis C virus to long-term passage in the presence of alpha interferon: multiple mutations and a common phenotype. J Virol 87:7593–7607

Perales C, Beach NM, Sheldon J et al (2014) Molecular basis of interferon resistance in hepatitis C virus. Curr Opin Virol 8C:38–44

Perelson AS, Neumann AU, Markowitz M et al (1996) HIV-1 dynamics in vivo: virion clearance rate, infected cell life-span, and viral generation time. Science 271:1582–1586

Pfeiffer JK, Kirkegaard K (2005a) Increased fidelity reduces poliovirus fitness under selective pressure in mice. PLoS Pathog 1:102–110

Pfeiffer JK, Kirkegaard K (2005b) Ribavirin resistance in hepatitis C virus replicon-containing cell lines conferred by changes in the cell line or mutations in the replicon RNA. J Virol 79:2346–2355

Poordad F, McCone J Jr, Bacon BR et al (2011) Boceprevir for untreated chronic HCV genotype 1 infection. N Engl J Med 364:1195–1206

Quer J, Martell A, Rodríguez R et al (2008) The impact of rapid evolution of hepatitis viruses. In: Domingo E, Parrish C, Holland JJ (eds) Origin and evolution of viruses. Elsevier, Oxford, pp 303–350

Raffi F, Rachlis A, Stellbrink HJ et al (2013) Once-daily dolutegravir versus raltegravir in antiretroviral-naive adults with HIV-1 infection: 48 week results from the randomised, double-blind, non-inferiority SPRING-2 study. Lancet 381:735–743

Richman DD (1996) Antiviral drug resistance. Wiley, New York

Romano KP, Ali A, Royer WE et al (2010) Drug resistance against HCV NS3/4A inhibitors is defined by the balance of substrate recognition versus inhibitor binding. Proc Natl Acad Sci U S A 107:20986–20991

Sarrazin C, Zeuzem S (2010) Resistance to direct antiviral agents in patients with hepatitis C virus infection. Gastroenterology 138:447–462

Sarrazin C, Kieffer TL, Bartels D et al (2007) Dynamic hepatitis C virus genotypic and phenotypic changes in patients treated with the protease inhibitor telaprevir. Gastroenterology 132:1767–1777

Seiler P, Senn BM, Klenerman P et al (2000) Additive effect of neutralizing antibody and antiviral drug treatment in preventing virus escape and persistence. J Virol 74:5896–5901

Serre SB, Krarup HB, Bukh J et al (2013) Identification of alpha interferon-induced envelope mutations of hepatitis C virus in vitro associated with increased viral fitness and interferon resistance. J Virol 87:12776–12793

Sheldon J, Beach NM, Moreno E et al (2014) Increased replicative fitness can lead to decreased drug sensitivity of hepatitis C virus. J Virol 88:12098–12111

Shiffman ML (2008) Optimizing the current therapy for chronic hepatitis C virus: peginterferon and ribavirin dosing and the utility of growth factors. Clin Liver Dis 12:487–505, vii

Shirasaka T, Kavlick MF, Ueno T et al (1995) Emergence of human immunodeficiency virus type 1 variants with resistance to multiple dideoxynucleosides in patients receiving therapy with dideoxynucleosides. Proc Natl Acad Sci U S A 92:2398–2402

Shirogane Y, Watanabe S, Yanagi Y (2012) Cooperation between different RNA virus genomes produces a new phenotype. Nat Commun 3:1235

Sofia MJ, Bao D, Chang W et al (2010) Discovery of a beta-D-2'-deoxy-2'-alpha-fluoro-2'-beta-C-methyluridine nucleotide prodrug (PSI-7977) for the treatment of hepatitis C virus. J Med Chem 53:7202–7218

Sostegni R, Ghisetti V, Pittaluga F et al (1998) Sequential versus concomitant administration of ribavirin and interferon alfa-n3 in patients with chronic hepatitis C not responding to interferon alone: results of a randomized, controlled trial. Hepatology 28:341–346

Sulkowski MS, Gardiner DF, Rodriguez-Torres M et al (2014) Daclatasvir plus sofosbuvir for previously treated or untreated chronic HCV infection. N Engl J Med 370:211–221

Summa V, Ludmerer SW, McCauley JA et al (2012) MK-5172, a selective inhibitor of hepatitis C virus NS3/4a protease with broad activity across genotypes and resistant variants. Antimicrob Agents Chemother 56:4161–4167

Susser S, Welsch C, Wang Y et al (2009) Characterization of resistance to the protease inhibitor boceprevir in hepatitis C virus-infected patients. Hepatology 50:1709–1718

Susser S, Vermehren J, Forestier N et al (2011) Analysis of long-term persistence of resistance mutations within the hepatitis C virus NS3 protease after treatment with telaprevir or boceprevir. J Clin Virol 52:321–327

Swetina J, Schuster P (1982) Self-replication with errors. A model for polynucleotide replication. Biophys Chem 16:329–345

Teng MN, Oldstone MB, de la Torre JC (1996) Suppression of lymphocytic choriomeningitis virus-induced growth hormone deficiency syndrome by disease-negative virus variants. Virology 223:113–119

Thompson AJ, Locarnini SA, Beard MR (2011) Resistance to anti-HCV protease inhibitors. Curr Opin Virol 1:599–606

Tong X, Le Pogam S, Li L et al (2014) In vivo emergence of a novel mutant L159F/L320F in the NS5B polymerase confers low-level resistance to the HCV polymerase inhibitors mericitabine and sofosbuvir. J Infect Dis 209:668–675

Tsibris AM, Korber B, Arnaout R et al (2009) Quantitative deep sequencing reveals dynamic HIV-1 escape and large population shifts during CCR5 antagonist therapy in vivo. PLoS One 4:e5683

Tu X, Das K, Han Q et al (2010) Structural basis of HIV-1 resistance to AZT by excision. Nat Struct Mol Biol 17:1202–1209

Vignuzzi M, Andino R (2010) Biological implications of picornavirus fidelity mutants. In: Ehrenfeld E, Domingo E, Roos RP (eds) The picornaviruses. ASM Press, Washington, DC, pp 213–228

Vignuzzi M, Stone JK, Arnold JJ et al (2006) Quasispecies diversity determines pathogenesis through cooperative interactions in a viral population. Nature 439:344–348
Vignuzzi M, Wendt E, Andino R (2008) Engineering attenuated virus vaccines by controlling replication fidelity. Nat Med 14:154–161
von Kleist M, Menz S, Stocker H et al (2011) HIV quasispecies dynamics during pro-active treatment switching: impact on multi-drug resistance and resistance archiving in latent reservoirs. PLoS One 6:e18204
Wainberg MA, Mesplede T, Raffi F (2013) What if HIV were unable to develop resistance against a new therapeutic agent? BMC Med 11:249
Webster RG, Kawaoka Y, Bean WJ (1986) Vaccination as a strategy to reduce the emergence of amantadine- and rimantadine-resistant strains of A/Chick/Pennsylvania/83 (H5N2) influenza virus. J Antimicrob Chemother 18:157–164
Wensing AM, Calvez V, Günthard HF et al (2014) 2014 Update of the drug resistance mutations in HIV-1. Top Antivir Med 22:642–650
Westby M, Lewis M, Whitcomb J et al (2006) Emergence of CXCR4-using human immunodeficiency virus type 1 (HIV-1) variants in a minority of HIV-1-infected patients following treatment with the CCR5 antagonist maraviroc is from a pretreatment CXCR4-using virus reservoir. J Virol 80:4909–4920
Westby M, Smith-Burchnell C, Mori J et al (2007) Reduced maximal inhibition in phenotypic susceptibility assays indicates that viral strains resistant to the CCR5 antagonist maraviroc utilize inhibitor-bound receptor for entry. J Virol 81:2359–2371
Wyles DL (2013) Antiviral resistance and the future landscape of hepatitis C virus infection therapy. J Infect Dis 207(Suppl 1):S33–S39
Young KC, Lindsay KL, Lee KJ et al (2003) Identification of a ribavirin-resistant NS5B mutation of hepatitis C virus during ribavirin monotherapy. Hepatology 38:869–878
Zeuzem S, Andreone P, Pol S et al (2011) Telaprevir for retreatment of HCV infection. N Engl J Med 364:2417–2428

Substrate-Envelope-Guided Design of Drugs with a High Barrier to the Evolution of Resistance

Ayşegül Özen and Celia A. Schiffer

Contents

Abstract

Drug resistance is a major problem in quickly evolving diseases. One way for drug resistance to emerge is through mutations in the drug target under the selective pressure of therapy. Antiviral drug targets especially have a high mutational plasticity due to the diverse genetic viral population. An ideal antiviral inhibitor should be robust against these quasispecies. Fortunately, a therapeutic target can be evolutionarily constrained by the biological function, which limits the mutational space. Taking advantage of this evolutionary constraint, the substrate-envelope hypothesis quantitatively defines the balance between natural substrate recognition and inhibitor binding and provides a framework to design robust inhibitors that retain potency against mutational ensemble of quasispecies of the target. The Substrate envelope hypothesis, based on structural studies on

A. Özen • C.A. Schiffer (✉)
Department of Biochemistry and Molecular Pharmacology, University of Massachusetts Medical School, Worcester, MA, USA
e-mail: aysegul.ozen@umassmed.edu; celia.schiffer@umassmed.edu

M. Gotte et al. (eds.), *Handbook of Antimicrobial Resistance*,
DOI 10.1007/978-1-4939-0694-9_9

the proteases of HIV-1 and hepatitis C, provides a structural basis for the specificity of natural substrate recognition and mechanisms for the resistance mutations in the active site.

Keywords
Antiviral • HCV NS3/4A • HIV-1 protease • Crystallography • Molecular dynamics • Substrate envelope • Structure-based drug design

Introduction

Antiviral drug targets are prone to mutations under the selective pressure of drug therapies. These mutations contribute to drug resistance by reducing the activity of inhibitors while allowing the drug-resistant variant of the target to function on the native substrates. The delicate balance between inhibitor binding and substrate recognition is effectively altered by drug resistance mutations at the expense of the inhibitor. The substrate-envelope hypothesis provides the structural basis for this alteration. This review provides a general background on the evolution of drug resistance in viral proteases, specifically in human immunodeficiency viral protease and hepatitis c viral protease, NS3/4A. The general applicability of the substrate-envelope hypothesis to other systems is discussed and a framework for substrate-envelope-guided drug design is outlined to minimize the probability of drug resistance in the design of new inhibitors.

Evolution of Resistance Against Anti-HIV Drugs

Human immunodeficiency virus (HIV) is a lentivirus of the Retroviridae family that infects the human immune system and causes the acquired immunodeficiency syndrome (HIV/AIDS). HIV is a quickly evolving disease that, without effective treatment, results in serious medical, social, and economic burden. UNAIDS reports that 35.3 million people were living with HIV globally with 2.3 million new infections and 1.6 million people died from AIDS-related causes by the end of 2012 (Global report: UNAIDS report on the global AIDS epidemic 2013). HIV has two types and several clades within each type with distinct patterns of spread and progression to AIDS (Santos and Soares 2010). HIV type 1 (HIV-1) is responsible for the pandemic. Because HIV-1 cannot be cured, suppressing viral replication and maintaining viral load at low to undetectable levels have become critical goals in the field of HIV-1 research. Highly active antiretroviral therapy (HAART) has been a successful strategy in providing long, quality life for infected individuals and is the current global standard of care for HIV/AIDS patients (Palella et al. 1998; Hoggs et al. 1998). As a part of HAART, the US Food and Drug Administration (FDA) has approved more than 30 drugs that target various stages of viral replication cycle including fusion and entry, reverse transcription, and integration and proteolytic processing of viral polyproteins. However, a high frequency of random nucleotide misincorporation by the error-prone reverse transcriptase (about three mutations per virion per round of replication) and a huge reservoir of replicating virus (10^{10} infected cells in an average patient) diversify the viral population (Coffin 1995). The selective pressure of therapy, especially combined with low drug adherence, facilitates the emergence of drug resistance viral variants (Ali et al. 2010).

HIV-1 Protease: A Virally Encoded Protease as a Drug Target

Viral genome is translated as polyproteins, which are proteolytically processed by the virally encoded protease to yield functional and structural proteins. Due to this crucial role in the viral life cycle, HIV-1 protease has been a key drug target in the treatment of HIV/AIDS (Kohl et al. 1988). HIV-1 protease is an aspartyl protease and a symmetric homodimer of 99 amino acids each (Fig. 1a). Each monomer contains a flap comprising two antiparallel β-strands connected by a β-turn and situated on top of the catalytic site. Dimeric enzyme is stabilized by four antiparallel β-strands, two from each subunit, which form an interdigitated β-sheet. Substrates are hydrolyzed at the dimer interface. The active site is typically considered as the residues 25–32, 47–53, and 80–84 with each monomer contributing a catalytic triad (Asp-25/Thr-26/Gly-27). Accurate and precise processing of the viral polyproteins is critical for virion assembly and maturation; therefore, HIV-1 protease cleaves the Gag and Gag-Pol polyproteins at twelve known sites in a highly specific order. While hydrophobic residues are favored at P1/P1′ residues, between which the scissile bond is hydrolyzed, in general, the cleavage sites are nonhomologous in sequence and asymmetric in size and charge (Fig. 1b). The fact that the protease is symmetric and the cleavage sites are diverse and asymmetric has challenged complete understanding of the specificity determinants of substrate recognition using a sequence-based approach.

Development of HIV-1 PIs is regarded as a major success of structure-based rational drug design. Nine protease inhibitors (PIs) have been so far approved for clinical use: saquinavir (SQV) (Roberts et al. 1990), indinavir (IDV) (Dorsey et al. 1994), ritonavir (RTV) (Kempf et al. 1995), nelfinavir (NFV) (Kaldor et al. 1997), amprenavir (APV) (Kim et al. 1995), lopinavir (LPV) (Sham et al. 1998), atazanavir (ATV) (Robinson et al. 2000a), tipranavir (TPV) (Turner et al. 1998), and darunavir (DRV) (Fig. 1d) (De Meyer et al. 2005; Koh et al. 2003; Surleraux et al. 2005). All PIs, except for TPV, are peptidomimetics. These PIs were rationally designed to bind to the protease with the flaps of the enzyme tightly closed over the active site, mimicking the transition state between substrate binding and cleavage reaction and thereby effectively inactivating the enzyme.

As PIs are an essential component of HAART (Gulick et al. 2000, Bartless et al. 2001), drug resistance to PIs has become an issue in the failure of HAART. Mutations at almost half of the protease residues are selected in different combinations with drug treatment and some combinations confer drug resistance (Wu et al. 2003; Rhee et al. 2003) (Figure 1c). Primary mutations in the active site

a

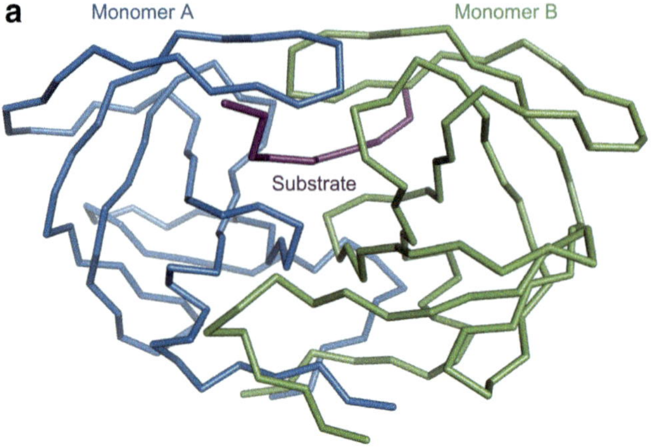

b

	P4	P3	P2	P1	*	P1′	P2′	P3′	P4′
MA-CA	S	Q	N	F	*	P	I	V	Q
CA-p2	A	R	V	L	*	A	E	A	M
p2-NC	A	T	I	M	*	M	Q	R	G
NC-p1	R	Q	A	N	*	F	L	G	K
p1-p6	P	G	N	F	*	L	Q	S	K
NC-Tr	R	Q	A	N	*	F	L	R	E
Tr-p6pol	D	L	A	F	*	L	Q	G	K
p6pol-Pr	S	F	N	F	*	P	Q	I	T
AutoPr	Q	I	T	L	*	W	Q	R	P
Pr-RT	T	L	N	F	*	P	I	S	P
RT-RH	A	E	T	F	*	Y	V	D	G
RH-IN	R	R	I	L	*	F	L	D	G

c

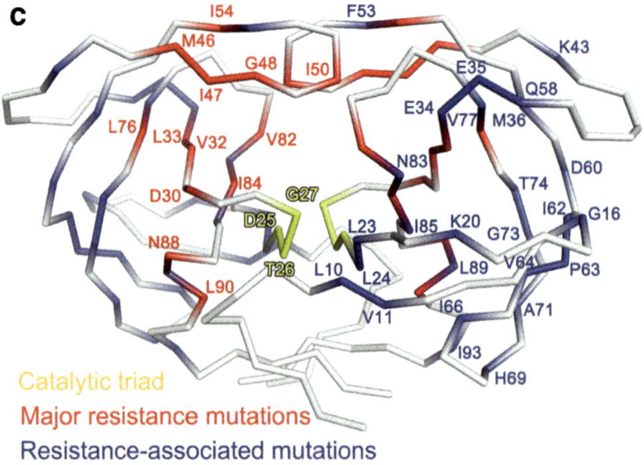

Fig. 1 (continued)

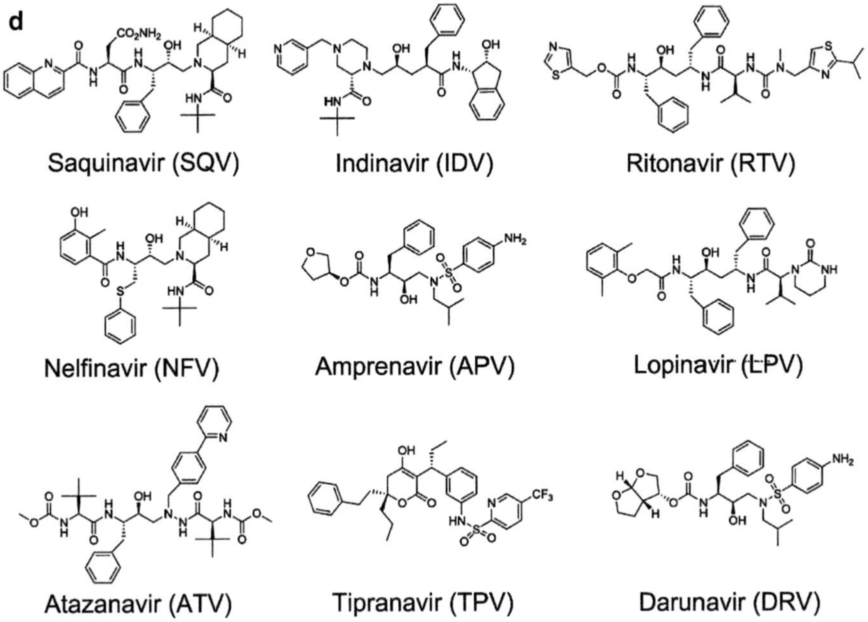

Fig. 1 (**a**) HIV-1 protease is a homodimeric aspartyl protease, shown in ribbon. Identical monomers A and B are colored in *blue* and *green*. Substrate-binding region is located at the dimer interface, and a bound-substrate peptide is colored in magenta. (**b**) HIV-1 protease recognizes 12 sites on Gag and Gag-Pol polyproteins and cleaves the scissile bond between P1 and P1' residues. (**c**) More than half of the protease gene mutates under the selective pressure of protease inhibitor involving therapies. Major drug resistance mutations and resistance-associated mutations are colored *red* and *dark blue*, respectively. Major drug resistance mutations are labeled on monomer A, while resistance-associated mutations are labeled on monomer B. The catalytic triad, at the dimeric interface, is colored *yellow*. (**d**) FDA-approved drugs targeting HIV-1 protease

reduce both protease catalytic efficiency and viral replicative capacity (Martinez-Picado et al. 2000, 1999; Croteau et al. 1997; Bleiber et al. 2001). Major PI resistance mutations occur at residues 30, 32, 33, 46, 47, 48, 50, 54, 76, 82, 84, 88, and 90, while mutations at residues 10, 11, 16, 20, 23, 24, 34, 35, 36, 43, 53, 58, 60, 62, 63, 64, 66, 69, 71, 73, 74, 77, 83, 85, 89, and 93 were reported to be selected in PI-treated patients, and some were shown to contribute to resistance (HIV Databases; Johnson et al. 2013). Among the major resistance-causing mutations, D30N, V32I, I47V/A, G48V/M, I50V/L, V82A/F/T/S/L, and I84V are located in the active site, while L33F, M46I/L, I54V/T/A/L/M, L76V, N88S/D, and L90M are non-active site mutations.

Mutations in HIV-1 protease, either within or outside the active site, can contribute to drug resistance directly by impacting inhibitor binding or indirectly in an interdependent and cooperative manner. Most primary mutations in the active site reduce binding affinity of PIs. On the contrary, some non-active site mutations are located in the hydrophobic core of the protein (13, 24, 33, 36, 62, 66, 77, 85, 90, 93) and contribute to resistance by altering the exchange dynamics of the hydrophobic interactions within the core (Foulkes-Murzycki et al. 2007; Mittal et al. 2012). While certain primary resistance mutations are a signature of particular PIs, cross-resistance is an issue in HIV-1 PIs. For example, D30N is a nonpolymorphic NFV-selected mutation which confers phenotypic and clinical resistance to NFV (Rhee et al. 2003; Patick et al. 1998); however, I50L is selected with ATV treatment and confers high-level ATV resistance while significantly increasing susceptibility to the rest of the PIs (Colonno et al. 2004). On the contrary, I50V is selected in APV-, LPV-, and DRV-treated patients and reduces the efficacy of these PIs while increasing TPV efficacy (HIV Databases). V82A is selected primarily by IDV and LPV (Condra et al. 1996; Kantor et al. 2005). In addition to decreasing susceptibility to IDV and LPV, V82A also confers cross-resistance to ATV and NFV and is associated with decreased susceptibility to SQV and APV in combination with other mutations (Condra et al. 1996; Kempf et al. 2001). I84V is a very severe mutation that is selected by each of the available PIs and cause cross-resistance to most PIs (Rhee et al. 2003; HIV Databases). Similarly, G48V is a primary resistance mutation selected by SQV and less often IDV and LPV conferring high-level resistance to SQV, intermediate resistance to ATV, and low-level resistance to NFV, IDV, and LPV (Rhee et al. 2003; Kantor et al. 2002; Schapiro et al. 1996; Rhee et al. 2010). Mutations have been selected at either single or a combination of sites. The mechanisms by which resistance is conferred via these mutations are very complex and interdependent. Nevertheless, in addition to the accumulation of resistance mutations within the active site, mutations also develop in non-active site protease residues and within the substrate cleavage sites, predominantly at NC-p1 and p1-p6 sites, altering the susceptibility to various PIs (Zhang et al. 1997; Bally et al. 2000; Mammano et al. 1998; Maguire et al. 2002; Kolli et al. 2009). Evolution of mutations within the cleavage sites leads to not only improved viral fitness compared to the viral variants carrying protease resistance mutations (Zhang et al. 1997; Mammano et al. 1998; Doyon et al. 1996; Robinson et al. 2000b) but also often increased resistance (Kolli et al. 2009). The vast number of mutation sites in both the protease and substrates with several possibilities of amino acid substitutions at each site in combination with cross-resistance has proven drug resistance a very complex problem.

The Substrate-Envelope Hypothesis

HIV-1 protease is a structurally well-studied drug target with more than 600 entries in the Protein Databank as of December 2013 (Berman et al. 2000). A vast majority of these entries are co-crystal structures of small-molecule inhibitors with HIV-1 protease variants including drug-resistant forms. These structural studies shed light on the molecular mechanisms by which protease mutations render inhibitors less effective; however, investigating only the inhibitor complexes has not been sufficient as a rational drug design strategy to minimize the likelihood of emerging resistance mutations.

Resistance to available drugs occurs when the balance in molecular recognition is subtly altered. Drug-resistant variants of HIV-1 protease are no longer effectively blocked by the competitive inhibitors but are still active against the natural substrates efficient enough for viral survival. This observation leads to the assumption that the native function of the protease imposes an evolutionary constraint under the selective pressure of drug therapy. To discover robust drugs that can resist drug resistance, the balance between natural substrate recognition and inhibitor binding needed to be characterized at the molecular level.

The substrate-envelope hypothesis, which was established on the basis of crystallographic studies on HIV-1 protease and later shown to be valid for HCV NS3/4A protease, provides a structural explanation for the specificity determinants of natural substrate recognition and drug resistance upon primary mutations in the protease active site. According to the substrate-envelope hypothesis, the inhibitors that are better at mimicking the natural substrate-binding features are less susceptible to the rapidly emerging mutations populated upon drug treatment. In this section, crystallographic studies that lead to the substrate-envelope hypothesis are described in detail, focusing on the substrate specificity and drug resistance in HIV-1 protease. In addition, parallels in the molecular basis of resistance against HIV-1 and HCV NS3/4A protease inhibitors are highlighted, and the up-to-date evidence suggesting that mutational ensembles of NS3/4A protease can also be targeted rationally taking a substrate-envelope-based drug design approach.

Structural Basis of Substrate Specificity and Drug Resistance

HIV-1 protease, a symmetric enzyme, specifically recognizes diverse asymmetric sequences on the Gag and GagProPol (Prabu-Jeyabalan et al. 2000). Amino acid sequence alone is not the specificity determinant for asymmetric substrate recognition, but the substrates share a binding mode in an extended conformation (Prabu-Jeyabalan et al. 2002). Co-crystal structures of decameric peptides corresponding to the cleavage sites showed that HIV-1 protease recognizes a consensus shape in substrates, not necessarily a consensus sequence (Prabu-Jeyabalan et al. 2002). This consensus shape is defined by the volume adopted by the majority of the substrates within the protease active site and has been defined as the *substrate envelope* (Fig. 2a). According to the substrate-envelope hypothesis, the substrate envelope is the recognition motif for HIV-1 protease, and the cleavage sites within Gag that are able to adopt this shape are likely to be processed.

HIV-1 PIs that have been approved for clinical use are all low-molecular-weight compounds with fairly similar three-dimensional shape and electrostatic character, and they all have large, hydrophobic moieties that interact with the mainly hydrophobic S2-S2′ pockets in the binding site. In the co-crystal structures, most HIV-1 PIs adopt a very similar binding mode interacting with a common set of protease residues in the active site. The inhibitors were shown to occupy a consensus inhibitor volume within the binding site, termed the *inhibitor envelope* (Fig. 2) (King et al. 2004a). Based on the structural comparison of the inhibitor and substrate

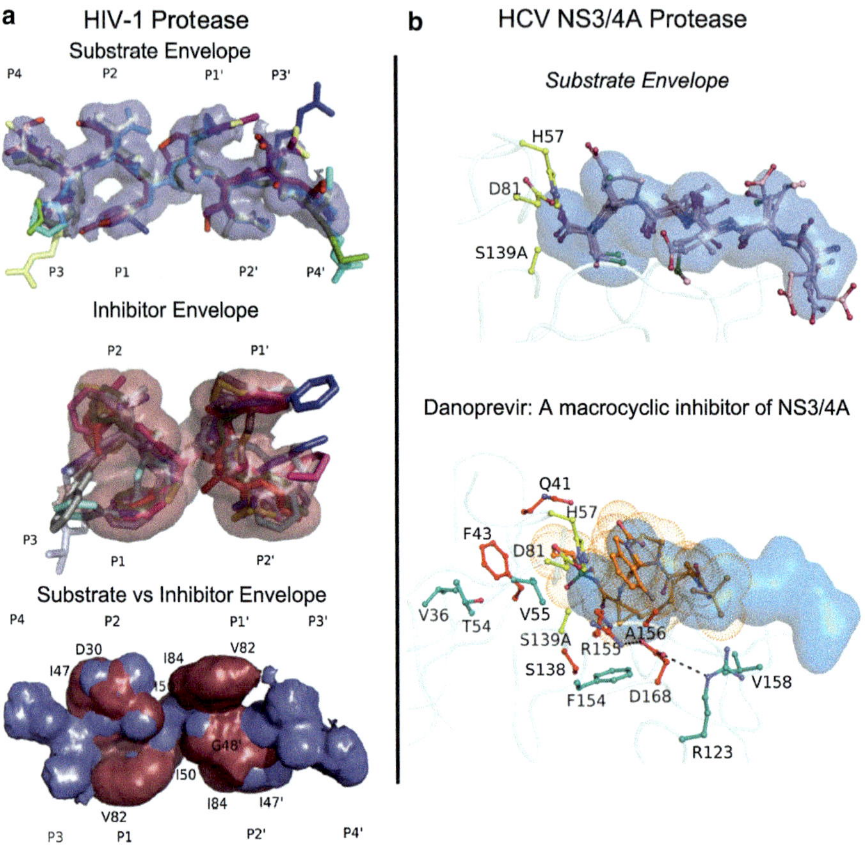

Fig. 2 (**a**) HIV-1 protease-substrate and inhibitor envelopes are colored *blue* and *red*, respectively. The two envelopes were superimposed to highlight the regions where inhibitors protrude beyond the substrate to make more extensive contacts with the protease residues that correspond to the previously known sites of drug resistance (Figure modified from King et al. (2004a)). (**b**) Hepatitis C virus NS3/4A protease-substrate envelope (*blue*) and a small-molecule inhibitor of NS3/4A protease, danoprevir, are shown in comparison along with the binding site residues (Figure modified Romano et al. (2010))

envelopes, the inhibitors were shown to protrude beyond the substrate envelope and make favorable contacts with certain protease residues of the wild-type protease. Because these protease residues interact more favorably with the inhibitors than the natural substrates, these protease residues are more important for inhibitor binding than substrate recognition. Strikingly, the protease residues contacted by inhibitors outside the substrate envelope corresponded to the previously known drug resistance mutation sites. Mutations at these sites would specifically impact inhibitor binding, while substrate recognition and cleavage would be less affected. Most sites of drug-resistant mutations in the active site do not contact the substrates, which led to the hypothesis that the inhibitors that fit well within the substrate envelope would be less susceptible to drug resistance, because a mutation that affects inhibitor binding would simultaneously impact the recognition and processing of the majority of the substrates (King et al. 2004a). As a retrospective validation, of the currently prescribed inhibitors, the most efficacious is DRV, and although not designed using the substrate-envelope constraint, DRV fits well within this volume (King et al. 2004b; Lefebvre and Schiffer 2008).

Sequence diversification in the protease is not the only mechanism for the virus to develop resistance to PIs. Occasionally, secondary mutations in the cleavage sites are also seen in patients who have failed PI-containing regimens. Crystallographic studies coupled with molecular dynamics simulations on wild-type and coevolved substrate complexes have revealed the structural rationale for why certain cleavage sites are more susceptible to resistance than others and how the cleavage site mutations compensate for the substrate processing efficiency lost upon protease mutations. The substrate-envelope hypothesis allowed quantitative assessment of the fit of each substrate within the substrate envelope. These studies, first, showed that some substrates are less in consensus with the majority of the substrates in terms of the shape adopted within the binding site, including NC-p1 and p1-p6 cleavage sites (Ozen et al. 2011). These substrates, along with inhibitors, interact favorably with a small subset of resistance mutation sites in the protease, e.g., D30, I50, and V82 (King et al. 2004a; Ozen et al. 2011). Strikingly, the outlier substrates, NC-p1 and p1-p6, correspond to the cleavage sites at which mutations were observed in patients who failed PI-containing regimens (Kolli et al. 2009, 2006). The substrate-envelope hypothesis, based on structural evidence, suggests that these substrates protrude beyond the substrate envelope and contact the sites of drug resistance mutations in the protease, leading to impaired substrate recognition and cleavage. This results in coevolution of compensatory mutations within the protease cleavage sites but often at other positions within the cleavage site (King et al. 2004a).

Emergence of D30N/N88D mutations in the protease in a correlated manner with the L449F Gag mutation on the p1-p6 cleavage site is a good example demonstrating that the protease-substrate coevolution validates the substrate envelope as the recognition motif for HIV-1 protease. D30N, a nelfinavir-signature protease mutation, is selected with high frequency in nelfinavir-treated HIV-infected individuals. From co-crystal structures, nelfinavir is known to pick up critical interactions with D30 at one monomer of the protease, which makes nelfinavir hypersusceptible to D30N mutation. Residue 88, on the contrary, does not directly interact with nelfinavir, but the N88D mutation is thought to maintain the overall local charge in the D30N background because 88 is in close proximity of 30 (Kolli et al. 2006).

However, the resistance mechanism through L449F Gag mutation in p1-p6 cleavage site is not obvious from the nelfinavir-bound crystal structures. A complete understanding of resistance against nelfinavir requires special attention to the substrate specificity and the mechanisms by which substrate specificity is maintained by the drug-resistant virus. Evidently, p1-p6 interacts with D30 on the other monomer outside the substrate envelope (i.e., p1-p6 interacts with D30 on the other monomer more than the majority of the substrates). Therefore, D30N mutation interferes with both nelfinavir-binding and p1-p6 processing with likely minimal detrimental effects on the recognition of other substrates. Substituting the wild-type leucine with bulkier phenylalanine at Gag 449, corresponding to S1′ pocket of the binding site, compensates the loss of interactions with the D30N/N88D protease filling the substrate envelope much more efficiently (Ozen et al. 2012). As a result, drug therapy selects for the cleavage site mutations, which are able to restore the loss of fit within the substrate envelope and bring the cleavage site more in consensus with the majority of the substrates. In conclusion, coevolved mutations within the cleavage sites play a key role in the development of resistance and affect the virological response during therapy. The substrate-envelope hypothesis, in addition to specificity of the substrates, explains the development of resistance to various PIs and substrate coevolution.

Substrate-Envelope-Guided Drug Design

The substrate envelope can guide the development of robust PIs that retain potency against severely resistant HIV-1 protease variants. Based on the substrate-envelope hypothesis, the optimum strategy to minimize resistance is to design inhibitors that fit within the substrate envelope (Fig. 3). In retrospect, where the five drugs in clinical use specifically protrude outside, the substrate envelope correlates with the loss of affinity to drug-resistant proteases (Chellappan et al. 2007a). Meanwhile, DRV, the most potent of the currently prescribed inhibitors, fits well within the substrate envelope although not designed using the substrate envelope as a constraint (King et al. 2004a; Lefebvre and Schiffer 2008). Retrospective correlation of the substrate envelope with resistance mutations promoted the design of new inhibitors with substrate-envelope constraints (Nalam and Schiffer 2008; Altman et al. 2008; Nalam et al. 2010; Ali et al. 2006; Chellappan et al. 2007b).

To validate the substrate-envelope hypothesis, various groups designed new HIV-1 PIs on the hydroxyethylamine scaffold taking different approaches. Two computational methods incorporated the substrate envelope as an a priori constraint during the design stage of the inhibitors, while the third method employed a structure-activity relationship (SAR) that does not include the substrate-envelope constraint explicitly. The first computational design, based on optimized docking, resulted in two good candidates exhibiting flat affinity profiles against multidrug-resistant mutants, although the binding affinity of these candidates were in the nM range (Chellappan et al. 2007b). The second computational design systematically explored the combinatorial space for three constituent R groups on the same scaffold in two rounds of computational design, chemical synthesis, biochemical testing, and crystallographic analysis. The second round resulted in low nM–pM range compounds, the majority of which have flatter resistance profiles against a wide range of drug-resistant viral variants (Altman et al. 2008). As a negative control, the inhibitors designed with the SAR approach resulted in pM inhibitors; however, they were

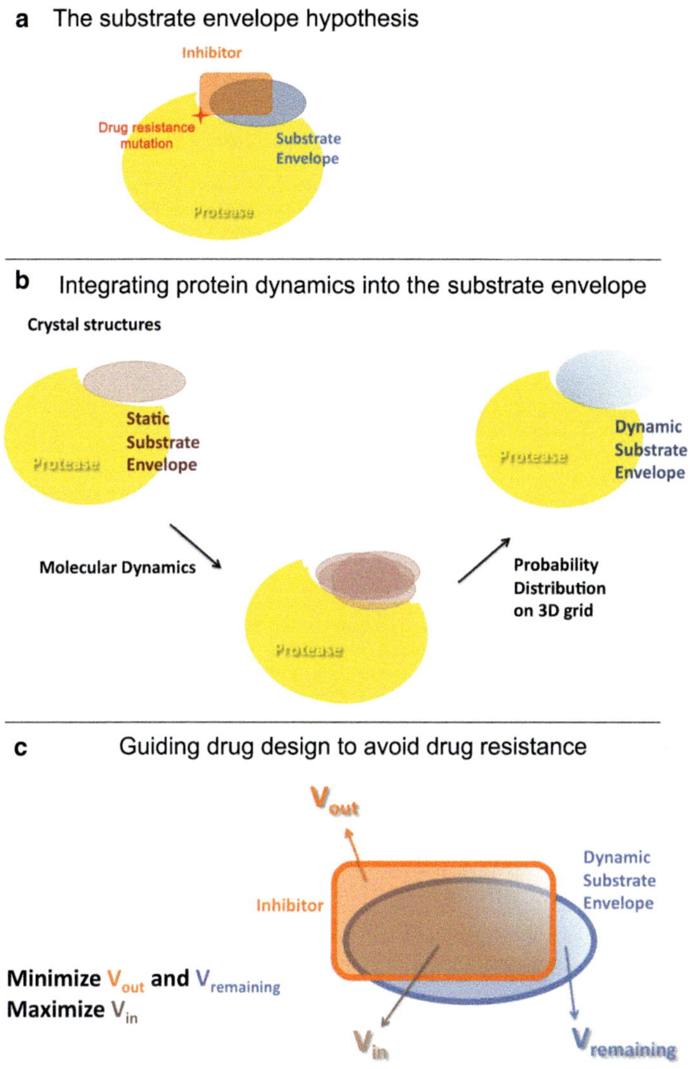

Fig. 3 Substrate-envelope-based drug design. (**a**) Most severe resistance mutations (*red*) occur at sites contacted by competitive inhibitors (*orange*) outside the substrate envelope (*blue*). (**b**) Dynamic substrate envelope can be defined as a probability distribution of the consensus substrate shape within the binding site by combining molecular dynamics simulations and three-dimensional grid-based volume calculations. (**c**) Dynamic substrate envelope can be integrated into structure-based design of robust drugs by systematically optimizing two metrics: (1) V_{out}, the probabilistic volume of an inhibitor falling outside the dynamic substrate envelope, and (2) $V_{remanining}$, the portion of the dynamic substrate envelope that is not fully occupied and, therefore, can be better utilized by an inhibitor

significantly less potent against the resistant variants (Ali et al. 2006). These studies successfully validated the substrate-envelope constraint as a robust design strategy for HIV-1 PIs with improved susceptibility to resistance and yielded several leads for potential new drugs (Nalam et al. 2010).

When the designed inhibitors effectively mimic the wild-type substrate-binding features, a larger number of mutations in the protease and cleavage sites will be needed to alter the balance between the substrate recognition and inhibitor binding in favor of substrate recognition to achieve drug resistance. Using the substrate envelope as a constraint not only improves the efficacy of the new inhibitors against the known resistant variants of HIV-1 protease but also likely minimizes the chances of potential compensatory mutations in the cleavage sites.

Generality of the Substrate-Envelope Hypothesis

Crystal structures typically capture a static image of the native state. To test the general applicability of the crystallography-based substrate envelope, the effect of substrate dynamics in the bound state was assessed by molecular dynamics simulations. In addition, drug targets other than HIV-1 protease were assessed in retrospect for the correlation of the substrate envelope with the mutational sensitivity.

Effect of Protein Dynamics on the Substrate Envelope: Dynamic Substrate Envelope

Protein dynamics is often neglected in drug design. Conformational ensembles of the native state are not readily accessible experimentally at atomistic level in a high-throughput manner. Computational methods can aid to estimate conformational dynamics at the expense of computational time. While the force field describing the molecular interactions can still benefit from improvements, the advancements in parallel computing architectures and algorithms have tremendously revolutionized the molecular dynamics field and increased the ability to simulate wider timescales and larger systems. The earlier simulations of an ~900 atom protein lasted 9 ps (McCammon et al. 1977), while protein-folding simulations as long as 1 ms (Lindorff-Larsen et al. 2011) or 50 ns simulation of an intact virion of one million atoms (Freddolino et al. 2006) can now be performed.

Taking advantage of these advancements, the substrate-envelope model was recently extended by considering the role of protein dynamics in the interactions of HIV-1 protease with its substrates. The *dynamic substrate envelope*, which was defined based on thousands of substrate conformers from molecular dynamics simulations, has turned out as a more accurate representation of protease-substrate interactions and better defined the substrate specificity for HIV-1 protease (Ozen et al. 2011). The dynamic substrate envelope, being a more realistic model, reproduced the essentials of the static substrate envelope, which was based on the crystal structures, validating the substrate envelope as a valid and realistic hypothesis but not a crystallographic artifact (Fig. 3b).

In addition, characterization of structural dynamics of a series of substrates provided insights into the interdependent nature of substrate recognition, which was not immediately evident in crystal structures. HIV-1 protease substrates all need to be recognized and processed by the same enzyme; however, the polyprotein processing is tightly regulated and premature/imprecise processing leads to noninfectious virions. Molecular dynamics studies showed that the substrates all possess common properties that allow the recognition by the protease, but also subtle differences in the interactions with the protease result in preferential recognition. The balance between the shape commonality (i.e., *consensus volume*) and sequence diversity of the substrates is maintained by interdependence within individual substrates in terms of conformational and sequence preferences. In conclusion, the interplay between the conserved and varied properties of the cleavage sites enables the preferential substrate recognition and regulation of substrate processing.

Application of the Substrate-Envelope Hypothesis to Other Drug Targets

Applicability of the substrate-envelope hypothesis has been tested for five prospective drug targets from a diverse set of diseases: Abl kinase, chitinase, thymidylate synthase, dihydrofolate reductase, and neuraminidase (Kairys et al. 2009). The volume of inhibitors protruding beyond the native substrate envelope trended with average mutational sensitivity, suggesting that inhibitor design would benefit from a similar reverse engineering strategy for these enzymes. Similarly, the two reverse transcriptase inhibitors, AZT and 3TC, have elements protruding beyond the native substrate envelope formed by deoxyribonucleotides. These elements create an opportunity for the reverse transcriptase to develop resistant mutations at the deoxyribonucleotide binding site. However, tenofovir, a reverse transcriptase inhibitor designed with the substrate-envelope constraints, lacks such protrusions and is relatively effective against AZT-resistant HIV variants (Tuske et al. 2004). Finally, the substrate envelope rationalized drug resistance against hepatitis C viral serine protease NS3/4A inhibitors (Romano et al. 2010). NS3/4A is described below as an emerging candidate to target with the substrate-envelope approach.

Substrate Envelope of Hepatitis C Viral Serine Protease NS3/4A

Hepatitis C is a liver disease with significant global impact, which is also caused by an RNA virus of Flaviviridae family. The hepatitis C virus (HCV) infection can lead to liver cirrhosis and hepatocellular sarcoma and is the most common reason for liver transplants in the United States (US). The World Health Organization estimates 150 million people worldwide are infected with HCV and 3–4 million new infections coming up every year with more than 350,000 cases of death from HCV-related liver diseases (Lesage et al. 2009). Similar to HIV, HCV is also genetically highly diverse. So far, six major HCV genotypes and several subtypes within each genotype have been identified (Simmonds et al. 2005). High viral replication rate combined with the error-prone RNA-dependent RNA polymerase causes large inter-patient genetic diversity as well as viral diversity within a single infected individual (Bukh et al. 1995a, b). Genetic heterogeneity of the virus across and within patients has greatly challenged the development of robust direct-acting antiviral agents (DAAs) that retain efficacy against multiple genotypes and drug-resistant variants of these genotypes since the discovery of HCV in 1989 as the cause of the hepatitis C (Choo et al. 1989; Kuo et al. 1989). Until 2011, the standard of care for HCV was weekly injections of pegylated interferon α combined with ribavirin (Peg-IFN/RBV), which can result in undetectable levels of HCV in 70–80 % of people with genotypes 2 and 3 but only 40–50 % of people with genotype 1 (Lesage et al. 2009). Genotype 1, the most difficult genotype to treat, is also the most common form of HCV in the US accounting for about 75–80 % of the cases (Alter et al. 1999; Blatt et al. 2000). In 2011, two DAAs, telaprevir and boceprevir, were approved by FDA for clinical use in combination with Peg-IFN/RBV for the treatment of genotype 1 patients. In addition to the problem of drug resistance, the severe side effect profile of this combination therapy amplifies the need to develop widely effective and better-tolerated DAAs.

Among the drug targets against HCV is the nonstructural protein 3 (NS3), which is a 631-amino acid bifunctional protein, with a serine protease domain located in the N-terminal one-third and an NTPase/RNA helicase domain in the C-terminal two-third (Fig. 4a). The reason for the protease and helicase domains to be physically linked is not fully understood. Although their interplay has been reported (Beran and Pyle 2008; Beran et al. 2007, 2009; Frick et al. 2004), both domains fold independently and are active in the absence of the other (Beran and Pyle 2008; Frick et al. 2004; Beran et al. 2007; Lam et al. 2003; Gallinari et al. 1998). NS3/4A protease adopts a chymotrypsin-like fold with two β-barrel domains. The catalytic triad is formed by His-57, Asp-81, and Ser-139 and is located in a cleft separating the two domains. The structure is stabilized by a Zn^{+2} ion that is coordinated by Cys-97, Cys-99, Cys-145, and His-149. The most efficient proteolytic activity of NS3 requires a cofactor NS4A, a 54-amino acid peptide that is tightly associated with the protease (Lesage et al. 2009). NS4A aids in the proper folding of NS3; the central 11 amino acids of NS4A inserts as a β-strand to the N-terminal β-barrel of NS3. The HCV genome encodes a single polyprotein of ~3,000 acids, which is processed by a series of host and viral proteases into at least 10 structural and nonstructural proteins. The viral NS3/4A hydrolyzes the polyprotein precursor at four cleavage sites (3-4A, 4A-4B, 4B-5A, 5A-5B), yielding nonstructural proteins essential for viral maturation. The first proteolytic event occurs at 3-4A junction in cis as a unimolecular reaction, while processing of the remaining junctions 4A-4B, 4B-5A, and 5A-5B occurs bimolecularly in *trans* (Bartenschlager et al. 1994). Similar to HIV, the cleavage sites of NS3/4A protease are nonhomologous except for an Asp/Glu at P6, Cys/Thr at P1, and Ser/Ala at P1′ (Fig. 4b). NS3/4A also confounds the innate immune response to viral infection by cleaving the human cellular targets TRIF and

a

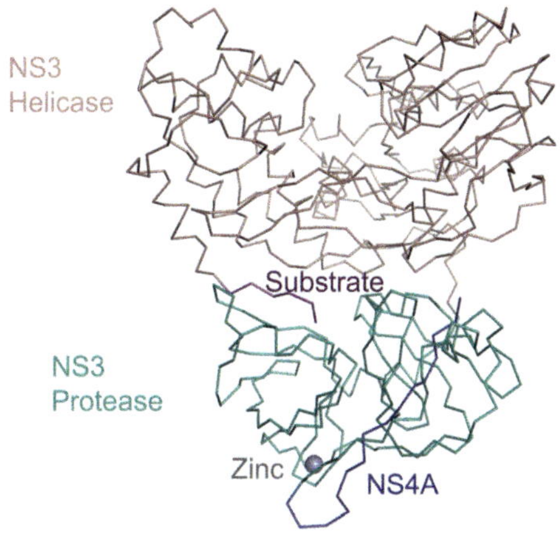

b

	P6	P5	P4	P3	P2	P1	*	P1′	P2′	P3′	P4′
3-4A	D	L	E	V	V	T	*	S	T	W	V
4A-4B	D	E	M	E	E	C	*	S	Q	W	L
4B-5A	E	C	T	T	P	C	*	S	G	S	W
5A-5B	E	D	V	V	C	C	*	S	M	S	Y
TRIF*	P	S	S	T	P	C	*	S	A	H	L
MAVS*	E	R	E	V	P	C	*	H	R	P	S
TC-PTP*	K	E	S	V	K	C	*	A	Q	Y	W
TC-PTP*	P	A	V	I	H	C	*	S	A	G	I
DDB1*	G	Q	L	V	T	C	*	S	G	A	F

*Host cellular targets of NS3/4A protease.

c

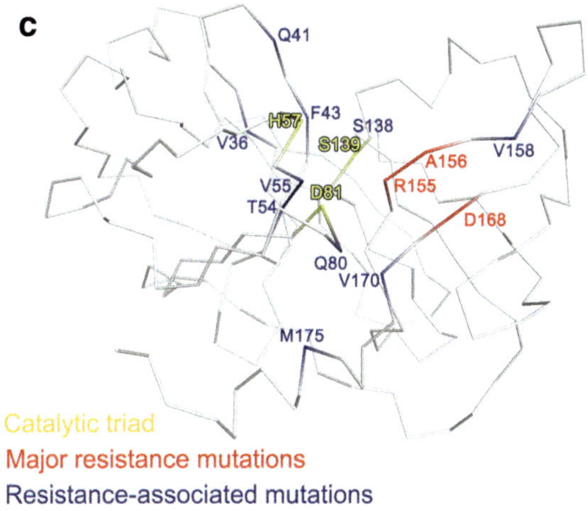

Fig. 4 (continued)

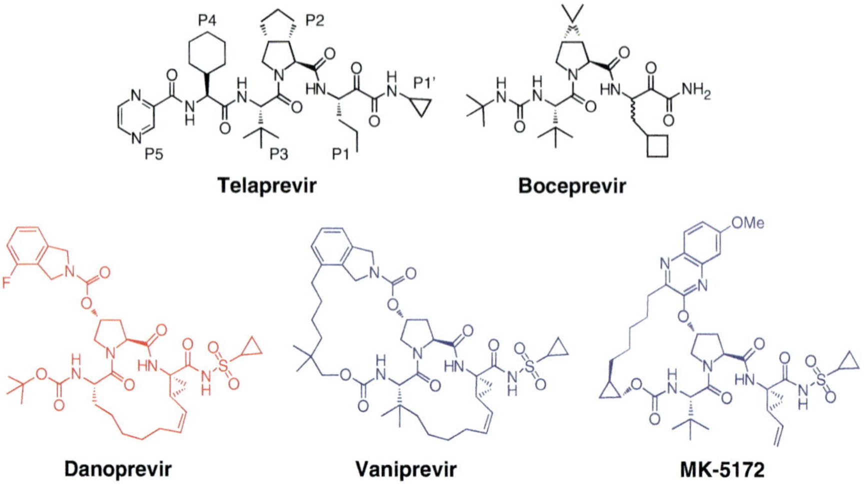

Fig. 4 (**a**) Hepatitis C viral NS3 is a bifunctional protein with helicase and protease domains, shown in ribbon. Helicase and protease are colored in *light pink* and *teal*, respectively. A cleaved substrate product is shown in *magenta*. (**b**) NS3/4A proteases recognized four sites on the ~3,000-amino acid viral polyprotein and a series of host cellular proteins. (**c**) Major drug resistance mutations and resistance-associated mutations are labeled *red* and *dark blue*, respectively. The catalytic triad is colored *yellow*. (**d**) NS3/4A protease inhibitors targeting NS3/4A protease, telaprevir and boceprevir, were approved in May 2011. Three of the macrocyclic NS3/4A inhibitors in development were shown as examples

MAVS and to block toll-like receptor three signaling and RIG-I signaling, respectively (Chen et al. 2007; Heim 2013; Li et al. 2005a, b). Cleavage of another cellular target, TC-PTP, at two separate sites enhances EGF signaling and basal Akt activity (Brenndorfer et al. 2009). Very recently, DDB1, a core subunit of the Cul4-based ubiquitin ligase complex, was reported to play a critical role in HCV replication and get cleaved by NS3/4A (Kang et al. 2013). Thus, in addition to blocking the viral maturation, effective inhibition of the proteolytic activity of the NS3/4A may also exert indirect antiviral effects, further interfering with viral replication.

The very shallow binding site of HCV NS3/4A protease has presented a big challenge to develop high-affinity and low-molecular-weight inhibitors because engineering small-molecule inhibitors to pick up tight interactions at the shallow surface was not straightforward. However, product inhibition by the N-termini of the trans-cleavage sites formed the basis for the development and optimization of peptidomimetic inhibitors of the NS3/4A protease (Steinkuhler et al. 1998; Llinas-Brunet et al. 1998; De Francesco and Migliaccio 2005). The proof of concept for antiviral efficacy was first demonstrated in 2002 with the macrocyclic inhibitor BILN-2061 (ciluprevir), which was later discontinued due to concerns about its cardiotoxicity (Lamarre et al. 2003; Hinrichsen et al. 2004; Vanwolleghem et al. 2007).

Telaprevir and boceprevir, the FDA-approved NS3/4A inhibitors, were developed by Vertex and Schering-Plough, respectively (Fig. 4d). Both telaprevir (Perni et al. 2006; Kwong et al. 2011) and boceprevir (Malcolm et al. 2006) are acyclic ketoamide inhibitors that associate with the protease through a reversible, covalent bond with the catalytic serine (S139) as well as short-range molecular interactions with the binding site. In addition, several non-covalent inhibitors, including macrocyclic compounds, are currently at various stages of clinical development. The non-covalent acylsulfonamide inhibitors contain a macrocycle connecting either P1 and P3 groups (ITMN-191 or danoprevir (Seiwert et al. 2011)) or alternatively P2 and P4 groups (MK-5172 (Harper et al. 2012), MK-7009, or vaniprevir (Liverton et al. 2010)), reducing the entropic cost associated with binding the shallow surface on the protease. In addition to the reported resistance in replicon studies, HCV quickly evolves to confer resistance to these protease inhibitors even at early stages of clinical trials compromising their high efficacy (He et al. 2008; Kieffer et al. 2007; Lin et al. 2005; Sarrazin et al. 2007; Tong et al. 2008, 2006). Despite the subnanomolar potency, the macrocyclic inhibitors also select for drug resistance mutations in clinic. Most PIs, in clinic or development, are susceptible to a common set of protease mutations, which raises the issue of cross-resistance. However, level of susceptibility to different mutations varies with drug. For example, R155K, A156T, and D168A are three mutations that are observed in patients treated with both linear and macrocyclic inhibitors, but the macrocyclic inhibitors appear to be more susceptible to R155K than linear compounds (Fig. 4c) (Romano et al. 2012).

Limitation of the current drugs to a single genotype and their susceptibility to quickly emerging resistance mutations pushes the research for developing inhibitors with broader activity. The substrate-envelope hypothesis has aided in elucidating the mechanism by which the protease mutations confer resistance to the current inhibitors.

High-resolution co-crystal structures have been determined for the wild-type NS3/4A protease domain with the cleavage products as well as inhibitors, including telaprevir, boceprevir, simeprevir, danoprevir, MK-5172, and vaniprevir (Romano et al. 2010, 2012). In these structures, the products, despite the low sequence homology, adopted a consensus volume at P6 to P1 residues, *the substrate envelope*. Similar to HIV, the most severe resistance mutations occur at protease residues that are contacted by the inhibitors outside the substrate envelope.

Crystal structures of the resistant protease variants bound to telaprevir and three macrocyclic inhibitors in development, danoprevir, vaniprevir, and MK-5172, revealed the structural basis of the three major active site resistance mutations, R155K, A156T, and D168A (Romano et al. 2010, 2012). The protease residue 155 is contacted much more favorably by the carbamate-linked bulky isoindoline groups of vaniprevir and danoprevir outside the substrate envelope compared to telaprevir, boceprevir, and MK-5172. Therefore, a mutation at this residue renders the isoindoline-containing compounds less effective, while MK-5172 retains reasonable affinity against R155K protease since MK-5172 has an ether-linked quinoxaline group that packs against the conserved catalytic His-57.

However, the fold change in affinity against R155K protease varies with inhibitor. The wild-type Arg-155 participates in an electrostatic network of hydrogen bonds along the binding surface. This network involves residues His-57, Arg-155, Asp-168, and Arg-123. Substituting the arginine at 155, which can make two hydrogen bonds, with a lysine, which can make only one hydrogen bond, disrupts this electrostatic network and compromises the stability of the binding surface.

Although both danoprevir and vaniprevir have favorable interactions with R155, mutation has more detrimental effect on the binding affinity of vaniprevir than danoprevir because vaniprevir has a linker connecting the bulky P2 isoindoline to P4, whereas danoprevir lacks this linker. Molecular dynamics simulations, in consistent with the crystallographic temperature factors and the inhibitor conformations in multiple molecules in the asymmetric unit, suggest that the lack of this linker renders the P2 group to be locally flexible without altering the binding mode of the inhibitor core. This local flexibility likely tolerates the instabilization of the binding surface due to R155K, while vaniprevir, constrained with P2-P4 macrocycle, cannot escape from the destabilizing effects of R155K. As a result, a 4.5 fold change is observed in the loss of affinity against the R155K protease between danoprevir and vaniprevir (Ozen et al. 2013).

Although the flat binding surface of NS3/4A is difficult to target, the comparative analysis of substrates and chemically diverse small-molecule inhibitors supports that a substrate-envelope-based design approach has the potential to result in more robust novel inhibitors. Taking this approach, considering conformational dynamics is probably even more critical than HIV because even the bound compounds have unique flexibilities, which have critical implications for drug resistance.

Conclusions and Future Perspective

Drug resistance will occur anytime rapid growth and evolution exists under the selective pressure of drug treatment but the growth is not completely inhibited by the drug. This widespread problem is in everything from invasive cancers and pathogenic microbes such as bacteria, malaria, fungi, tuberculosis, and viruses. The mechanisms by which resistance can emerge include point mutations in the target protein. To overcome drug resistance, resistance should be predicted before it happens, and drugs should be designed accordingly to avoid the accurately predicted resistance mutations. To achieve this goal, target identification is critical. The enzymes with multiple substrates that cannot easily tolerate mutations and maintain function are potentially good candidates.

Crystallography is extremely informative to provide insights into the most probable molecular interactions in the native state. However, proteins are dynamic and exist in conformational ensembles even in native state. Depending on the inherent structural and dynamic properties of the drug target, ignoring protein dynamics may delay the successful discovery of novel drugs that have high potency, good selectivity, and low toxicity and are also robust against the evolution of resistance. Developing these robust drugs, experimental techniques and computational methods should be used in concert, each according to its particular strengths. Dynamic substrate envelope is a useful tool to systematically incorporate the protein dynamics and evolution into structure-based rational drug design. Substrate-envelope-guided drug design necessitates constant partnering of multiple disciplines such as chemical synthesis, thermodynamics and enzyme kinetics, crystallography, NMR, molecular modeling and dynamics simulations, deep sequencing, and virology.

The current understanding of the structure and dynamics of substrate recognition and drug resistance in HIV and HCV proteases will serve as a useful guide for the rational design of future generation drugs that remain active against diverse populations of drug targets. Combating quickly evolving diseases, all drug targets should be viewed as evolutionarily dynamic, and inhibitors should be designed as evolutionarily constrained as possible. The target is moving and robust drug design requires hitting multiple targets at a time.

Acknowledgments The research described in this review supported by a combination of the following NIH grants P01 GM109767, R01 AI085051, P01 GM66524, R01 GM65347.

References

Ali A, Reddy GS, Cao H, Anjum SG, Nalam MN, Schiffer CA, Rana TM (2006) Discovery of HIV-1 protease inhibitors with picomolar affinities incorporating *N*-aryl-oxazolidinone-5-carboxamides as novel P2 ligands. J Med Chem 49(25):7342–7356

Ali A, Bandaranayake RM, Cai Y, King NM, Kolli M, Mittal S, Murzycki JF, Nalam MN, Nalivaika EA, Ozen A, Prabu-Jeyabalan MM, Thayer K, Schiffer CA (2010) Molecular basis for drug resistance in HIV-1 protease. Viruses 2(11):2509–2535

Alter MJ, Kruszon-Moran D, Nainan OV, McQuillan GM, Gao F, Moyer LA, Kaslow RA, Margolis HS (1999) The prevalence of hepatitis C virus infection in the United States, 1988 through 1994. N Engl J Med 341(8):556–562

Altman MD, Ali A, Reddy GS, Nalam MN, Anjum SG, Cao H, Chellappan S, Kairys V, Fernandes MX, Gilson MK, Schiffer CA, Rana TM, Tidor B (2008) HIV-1 protease inhibitors from inverse design in the substrate envelope exhibit subnanomolar binding to drug-resistant variants. J Am Chem Soc 130(19):6099–6113

Bally F, Martinez R, Peters S, Sudre P, Telenti A (2000) Polymorphism of HIV type 1 gag p7/p1 and p1/p6 cleavage sites: clinical significance and implications for resistance to protease. AIDS Res Hum Retroviruses 16(13):1209–1213

Bartenschlager R, Ahlborn-Laake L, Mous J, Jacobsen H (1994) Kinetic and structural analyses of hepatitis C virus polyprotein processing. J Virol 68(8):5045–5055

Bartless JA, DeMasi R, Quinn J, Moxham C, Rousseau F (2001) Overview of the effectiveness of triple combination therapy in antiretroviral-naive HIV-1 infected adults. AIDS 15 (11):1369–1377

Beran RK, Pyle AM (2008) Hepatitis C viral NS3-4A protease activity is enhanced by the NS3 helicase. J Biol Chem 283(44):29929–29937

Beran RK, Serebrov V, Pyle AM (2007) The serine protease domain of hepatitis C viral NS3 activates RNA helicase activity by promoting the binding of RNA substrate. J Biol Chem 282 (48):34913–34920

Beran RK, Lindenbach BD, Pyle AM (2009) The NS4A protein of hepatitis C virus promotes RNA-coupled ATP hydrolysis by the NS3 helicase. J Virol 83(7):3268–3275

Berman HM, Westbrook J, Feng Z, Gilliland G, Bhat TN, Weissig H, Shindyalov IN, Bourne PE (2000) The protein data bank. Nucleic Acids Res 28(1):235–242

Blatt LM, Mutchnick MG, Tong MJ, Klion FM, Lebovics E, Freilich B, Bach N, Smith C, Herrera J, Tobias H, Conrad A, Schmid P, McHutchison JG (2000) Assessment of hepatitis C virus RNA and genotype from 6807 patients with chronic hepatitis C in the United States. J Viral Hepat 7 (3):196–202

Bleiber G, Munoz M, Ciuffi A, Meylan P, Telenti A (2001) Individual contributions of mutant protease and reverse transcriptase to viral infectivity, replication, and protein maturation of antiretroviral drug-resistant human immunodeficiency virus type 1. J Virol 75(7):3291–3300

Brenndorfer ED, Karthe J, Frelin L, Cebula P, Erhardt A, Schulte am Esch J, Hengel H, Bartenschlager R, Sallberg M, Haussinger D, Bode JG (2009) Nonstructural 3/4A protease of hepatitis C virus activates epithelial growth factor-induced signal transduction by cleavage of the T-cell protein tyrosine phosphatase. Hepatology 49(6):1810–1820

Bukh J, Miller RH, Purcell RH (1995a) Biology and genetic heterogeneity of hepatitis C virus. Clin Exp Rheumatol 13(Suppl 13):S3–S7

Bukh J, Miller RH, Purcell RH (1995b) Genetic heterogeneity of hepatitis C virus: quasispecies and genotypes. Semin Liver Dis 15(1):41–63

Chellappan S, Kairys V, Fernandes MX, Schiffer C, Gilson MK (2007a) Evaluation of the substrate envelope hypothesis for inhibitors of HIV-1 protease. Proteins 68(2):561–567

Chellappan S, Kiran Kumar Reddy GS, Ali A, Nalam MN, Anjum SG, Cao H, Kairys V, Fernandes MX, Altman MD, Tidor B, Rana TM, Schiffer CA, Gilson MK (2007b) Design of mutation-resistant HIV protease inhibitors with the substrate envelope hypothesis. Chem Biol Drug Des 69(5):298–313

Chen Z, Benureau Y, Rijnbrand R, Yi J, Wang T, Warter L, Lanford RE, Weinman SA, Lemon SM, Martin A, Li K (2007) GB virus B disrupts RIG-I signaling by NS3/4A-mediated cleavage of the adaptor protein MAVS. J Virol 81(2):964–976

Choo QL, Kuo G, Weiner AJ, Overby LR, Bradley DW, Houghton M (1989) Isolation of a cDNA clone derived from a blood-borne non-A, non-B viral hepatitis genome. Science 244 (4902):359–362

Coffin JM (1995) HIV population dynamics in vivo: implications for genetic variation, pathogenesis, and therapy. Science 267(5197):483–489

Colonno R, Rose R, McLaren C, Thiry A, Parkin N, Friborg J (2004) Identification of I50L as the signature atazanavir (ATV)-resistance mutation in treatment-naive HIV-1-infected patients receiving ATV-containing regimens. J Infect Dis 189(10):1802–1810

Condra JH, Holder DJ, Schleif WA, Blahy OM, Danovich RM, Gabryelski LJ, Graham DJ, Laird D, Quintero JC, Rhodes A, Robbins HL, Roth E, Shivaprakash M, Yang T, Chodakewitz JA, Deutsch PJ, Leavitt RY, Massari FE, Mellors JW, Squires KE, Steigbigel RT, Teppler H, Emini EA (1996) Genetic correlates of in vivo viral resistance to indinavir, a human immunodeficiency virus type 1 protease inhibitor. J Virol 70:8270–8276

Croteau G, Doyon L, Thibeault D, McKercher G, Pilote L, Lamarre D (1997) Impaired fitness of human immunodeficiency virus type 1 variants with high-level resistance to protease inhibitors. J Virol 71(2):1089–1096

De Francesco R, Migliaccio G (2005) Challenges and successes in developing new therapies for hepatitis C. Nature 436(7053):953–960

De Meyer S, Azijn H, Surleraux D, Jochmans D, Tahri A, Pauwels R, Wigerinck P, de Bethune MP (2005) TMC114, a novel human immunodeficiency virus type 1 protease inhibitor active against protease inhibitor-resistant viruses, including a broad range of clinical isolates. Antimicrob Agents Chemother 49(6):2314–2321

Dorsey BD, Levin RB, McDaniel SL, Vacca JP, Guare JP, Darke PL, Zugay JA, Emini EA, Schleif WA, Quintero JC et al (1994) L-735,524: the design of a potent and orally bioavailable HIV protease inhibitor. J Med Chem 37(21):3443–3451

Doyon L, Croteau G, Thibeault D, Poulin F, Pilote L, Lamarre D (1996) Second locus involved in human immunodeficiency virus type 1 resistance to protease inhibitors. J Virol 70 (6):3763–3769

Foulkes-Murzycki JE, Scott WR, Schiffer CA (2007) Hydrophobic sliding: a possible mechanism for drug resistance in human immunodeficiency virus type 1 protease. Structure 15 (2):225–233

Freddolino PL, Arkhipov AS, Larson SB, McPherson A, Schulten K (2006) Molecular dynamics simulations of the complete satellite tobacco mosaic virus. Structure 14(3):437–449

Frick DN, Rypma RS, Lam AM, Gu B (2004) The nonstructural protein 3 protease/helicase requires an intact protease domain to unwind duplex RNA efficiently. J Biol Chem 279(2):1269–1280

Gallinari P, Brennan D, Nardi C, Brunetti M, Tomei L, Steinkuhler C, De Francesco R (1998) Multiple enzymatic activities associated with recombinant NS3 protein of hepatitis C virus. J Virol 72(8):6758–6769
Joint United Nations Programme on HIV/AIDS (UNAIDS) Global report: UNAIDS report on the global AIDS epidemic 2013. Geneva, UNAIDS/JC2502/1/E, UNAIDS
Gulick RM, Mellors JW, Havlir D, Eron JJ, Meibohm A, Condra JH, Valentine FT, McMahon D, Gonzalez C, Jonas L, Emini EA, Chodakewitz JA, Isaacs R, Richman DD (2000) 3-year suppression of HIV viremia with indinavir, zidovudine, and lamivudine. Ann Intern Med 133 (1):35–39
Harper S, McCauley JA, Rudd MT, Ferrara M, DiFilippo M, Crescenzi B, Koch U, Petrocchi A, Holloway MK, Butcher JW, Romano JJ, Bush KJ, Gilbert KF, McIntyre CJ, Nguyen KT, Nizi E, Carroll SS, Ludmerer SW, Burlein C, DiMuzio JM, Graham DJ, McHale CM, Stahlhut MW, Olsen DB, Monteagudo E, Cianetti S, Giuliano C, Pucci V, Trainor N, Fandozzi CM, Rowley M, Coleman PJ, Vacca JP, Summa V, Liverton NJ (2012) Discovery of MK-5172, a Macrocyclic Hepatitis C Virus NS3/4a Protease Inhibitor. ACS Med Chem Lett 3(4):332–336
He Y, King MS, Kempf DJ, Lu L, Lim HB, Krishnan P, Kati W, Middleton T, Molla A (2008) Relative replication capacity and selective advantage profiles of protease inhibitor-resistant hepatitis C virus (HCV) NS3 protease mutants in the HCV genotype 1b replicon system. Antimicrob Agents Chemother 52(3):1101–1110
Heim MH (2013) Innate immunity and HCV. J Hepatol 58(3):564–574
Hinrichsen H, Benhamou Y, Wedemeyer H, Reiser M, Sentjens RE, Calleja JL, Forns X, Erhardt A, Cronlein J, Chaves RL, Yong CL, Nehmiz G, Steinmann GG (2004) Short-term antiviral efficacy of BILN 2061, a hepatitis C virus serine protease inhibitor, in hepatitis C genotype 1 patients. Gastroenterology 127(5):1347–1355
Hoggs RS, Heath KV, Yip B et al (1998) Improved survival among HIV-infected individuals following initiation of antiretroviral therapy. J Am Med Assoc 279:450–454
Johnson VA, Calvez V, Gunthard HF, Paredes R, Pillay D, Shafer RW, Wensing AM, Richman DD (2013) Update of the drug resistance mutations in HIV-1: March 2013. Top Antivir Med 21 (1):6–14
Kairys V, Gilson MK, Lather V, Schiffer CA, Fernandes MX (2009) Toward the design of mutation-resistant enzyme inhibitors: further evaluation of the substrate envelope hypothesis. Chem Biol Drug Des 74(3):234–245
Kaldor SW, Kalish VJ, Davies JN, Shetty BV, Fritz JE, Appelt K, Burgess JA, Campanale KM, Chirgadze NY, Clawson DK, Dressman BA, Hatch SD, Khalil DA, Kosa MB, Lubbehusen PP, Muesing MA, Patick AK, Reich SH, Su KS, Tatlock JH (1997) Viracept (nelfinavir mesylate, AG1343): a potent, orally bioavailable inhibitor of HIV-1 protease. J Med Chem 40 (24):3979–3985
Kang X, Chen X, He Y, Guo D, Guo L, Zhong J, Shu HB (2013) DDB1 is a cellular substrate of NS3/4A protease and required for hepatitis C virus replication. Virology 435(2):385–394
Kantor R, Fessel WJ, Zolopa AR, Israelski D, Shulman N, Montoya JG, Harbour M, Schapiro JM, Shafer RW (2002) Evolution of primary protease inhibitor resistance mutations during protease inhibitor salvage therapy. Antimicrob Agents Chemother 46(4):1086–1092
Kantor R, Katzenstein DA, Efron B, Carvalho AP, Wynhoven B, Cane P, Clarke J, Sirivichayakul S, Soares MA, Snoeck J, Pillay C, Rudich H, Rodrigues R, Holguin A, Ariyoshi K, Bouzas MB, Cahn P, Sugiura W, Soriano V, Brigido LF, Grossman Z, Morris L, Vandamme AM, Tanuri A, Phanuphak P, Weber JN, Pillay D, Harrigan PR, Camacho R, Schapiro JM, Shafer RW (2005) Impact of HIV-1 subtype and antiretroviral therapy on protease and reverse transcriptase genotype: results of a global collaboration. PLoS Med 2(4):e112
Kempf DJ, Marsh KC, Denissen JF, McDonald E, Vasavanonda S, Flentge CA, Green BE, Fino L, Park CH, Kong XP et al (1995) ABT-538 is a potent inhibitor of human immunodeficiency virus protease and has high oral bioavailability in humans. Proc Natl Acad Sci U S A 92 (7):2484–2488

Kempf DJ, Isaacson JD, King MS, Brun SC, Xu Y, Real K, Bernstein BM, Japour AJ, Sun E, Rode RA (2001) Identification of genotypic changes in human immunodeficiency virus protease that correlate with reduced susceptibility to the protease inhibitor lopinavir among viral isolates from protease inhibitor-experienced patients. J Virol 75(16):7462–7469

Kieffer TL, Sarrazin C, Miller JS, Welker MW, Forestier N, Reesink HW, Kwong AD, Zeuzem S (2007) Telaprevir and pegylated interferon-alpha-2a inhibit wild-type and resistant genotype 1 hepatitis C virus replication in patients. Hepatology 46(3):631–639

Kim EE, Baker CT, Dwyer MD, Murcko MA et al (1995) Crystal structure of HIV-1 protease in complex with vx-478, a potent and orally bioavailable inhibitor of the enzyme. J Am Chem Soc 117:1181–1182

King NM, Prabu-Jeyabalan M, Nalivaika EA, Schiffer CA (2004a) Combating susceptibility to drug resistance: lessons from HIV-1 protease. Chem Biol 11(10):1333–1338

King NM, Prabu-Jeyabalan M, Nalivaika EA, Wigerinck P, de Bethune MP, Schiffer CA (2004b) Structural and thermodynamic basis for the binding of TMC114, a next-generation human immunodeficiency virus type 1 protease inhibitor. J Virol 78(21):12012–12021

Koh Y, Nakata H, Maeda K, Ogata H, Bilcer G, Devasamudram T, Kincaid JF, Boross P, Wang YF, Tie Y, Volarath P, Gaddis L, Harrison RW, Weber IT, Ghosh AK, Mitsuya H (2003) Novel bis-tetrahydrofuranylurethane-containing nonpeptidic protease inhibitor (PI) UIC-94017 (TMC114) with potent activity against multi-PI-resistant human immunodeficiency virus in vitro. Antimicrob Agents Chemother 47(10):3123–3129

Kohl NE, Emini EA, Schleif WA, Davis LJ, Heimbach JC, Dixon RA, Scolnick EM, Sigal IS (1988) Active human immunodeficiency virus protease is required for viral infectivity. Proc Natl Acad Sci U S A 85(13):4686–4690

Kolli M, Lastere S, Schiffer CA (2006) Co-evolution of nelfinavir-resistant HIV-1 protease and the p1-p6 substrate. Virology 347(2):405–409

Kolli M, Stawiski E, Chappey C, Schiffer CA (2009) Human immunodeficiency virus type 1 protease-correlated cleavage site mutations enhance inhibitor resistance. J Virol 83 (21):11027–11042

Kuo G, Choo QL, Alter HJ, Gitnick GL, Redeker AG, Purcell RH, Miyamura T, Dienstag JL, Alter MJ, Stevens CE et al (1989) An assay for circulating antibodies to a major etiologic virus of human non-A, non-B hepatitis. Science 244(4902):362–364

Kwong AD, Kauffman RS, Hurter P, Mueller P (2011) Discovery and development of telaprevir: an NS3-4A protease inhibitor for treating genotype 1 chronic hepatitis C virus. Nat Biotechnol 29 (11):993–1003

Lam AM, Keeney D, Eckert PQ, Frick DN (2003) Hepatitis C virus NS3 ATPases/helicases from different genotypes exhibit variations in enzymatic properties. J Virol 77(7):3950–3961

Lamarre D, Anderson PC, Bailey M, Beaulieu P, Bolger G, Bonneau P, Bos M, Cameron DR, Cartier M, Cordingley MG, Faucher AM, Goudreau N, Kawai SH, Kukolj G, Lagace L, LaPlante SR, Narjes H, Poupart MA, Rancourt J, Sentjens RE, St George R, Simoneau B, Steinmann G, Thibeault D, Tsantrizos YS, Weldon SM, Yong CL, Llinas-Brunet M (2003) An NS3 protease inhibitor with antiviral effects in humans infected with hepatitis C virus. Nature 426(6963):186–189

Lefebvre E, Schiffer CA (2008) Resilience to resistance of HIV-1 protease inhibitors: profile of darunavir. AIDS Rev 10(3):131–142

Lesage S, Condroyer C, Lannuzel A, Lohmann E, Troiano A, Tison F, Damier P, Thobois S, Ouvrard-Hernandez AM, Rivaud-Pechoux S, Brefel-Courbon C, Destee A, Tranchant C, Romana M, Leclere L, Durr A, Brice A (2009) Molecular analyses of the LRRK2 gene in European and North African autosomal dominant Parkinson's disease. J Med Genet 46 (7):458–464

Li XD, Sun L, Seth RB, Pineda G, Chen ZJ (2005a) Hepatitis C virus protease NS3/4A cleaves mitochondrial antiviral signaling protein off the mitochondria to evade innate immunity. Proc Natl Acad Sci U S A 102(49):17717–17722

Li K, Foy E, Ferreon JC, Nakamura M, Ferreon AC, Ikeda M, Ray SC, Gale M Jr, Lemon SM (2005b) Immune evasion by hepatitis C virus NS3/4A protease-mediated cleavage of the Toll-like receptor 3 adaptor protein TRIF. Proc Natl Acad Sci U S A 102(8):2992–2997

Lin C, Gates CA, Rao BG, Brennan DL, Fulghum JR, Luong YP, Frantz JD, Lin K, Ma S, Wei YY, Perni RB, Kwong AD (2005) In vitro studies of cross-resistance mutations against two hepatitis C virus serine protease inhibitors, VX-950 and BILN 2061. J Biol Chem 280(44):36784–36791

Lindorff-Larsen K, Piana S, Dror RO, Shaw DE (2011) How fast-folding proteins fold. Science 334 (6055):517–520

Liverton NJ, Carroll SS, Dimuzio J, Fandozzi C, Graham DJ, Hazuda D, Holloway MK, Ludmerer SW, McCauley JA, McIntyre CJ, Olsen DB, Rudd MT, Stahlhut M, Vacca JP (2010) MK-7009, a potent and selective inhibitor of hepatitis C virus NS3/4A protease. Antimicrob Agents Chemother 54(1):305–311

Llinas-Brunet M, Bailey M, Fazal G, Goulet S, Halmos T, Laplante S, Maurice R, Poirier M, Poupart MA, Thibeault D, Wernic D, Lamarre D (1998) Peptide-based inhibitors of the hepatitis C virus serine protease. Bioorg Med Chem Lett 8(13):1713–1718

Maguire MF, Guinea R, Griffin P, Macmanus S, Elston RC, Wolfram J, Richards N, Hanlon MH, Porter DJ, Wrin T, Parkin N, Tisdale M, Furfine E, Petropoulos C, Snowden BW, Kleim JP (2002) Changes in human immunodeficiency virus type 1 Gag at positions L449 and P453 are linked to I50V protease mutants in vivo and cause reduction of sensitivity to amprenavir and improved viral fitness in vitro. J Virol 76(15):7398–7406

Malcolm BA, Liu R, Lahser F, Agrawal S, Belanger B, Butkiewicz N, Chase R, Gheyas F, Hart A, Hesk D, Ingravallo P, Jiang C, Kong R, Lu J, Pichardo J, Prongay A, Skelton A, Tong X, Venkatraman S, Xia E, Girijavallabhan V, Njoroge FG (2006) SCH 503034, a mechanism-based inhibitor of hepatitis C virus NS3 protease, suppresses polyprotein maturation and enhances the antiviral activity of alpha interferon in replicon cells. Antimicrob Agents Chemother 50 (3):1013–1020

Mammano F, Petit C, Clavel F (1998) Resistance-associated loss of viral fitness in human immunodeficiency virus type 1: phenotypic analysis of protease and gag coevolution in protease inhibitor-treated patients. J Virol 72(9):7632–7637

Martinez-Picado J, Savara AV, Sutton L, D'Aquila RT (1999) Replicative fitness of protease inhibitor-resistant mutants of human immunodeficiency virus type 1. J Virol 73(5):3744–3752

Martinez-Picado J, Savara AV, Shi L, Sutton L, D'Aquila RT (2000) Fitness of human immunodeficiency virus type 1 protease inhibitor-selected single mutants. Virology 275(2):318–322

McCammon JA, Gelin BR, Karplus M (1977) Dynamics of folded proteins. Nature 267 (5612):585–590

Mittal S, Cai Y, Nalam MN, Bolon DN, Schiffer CA (2012) Hydrophobic core flexibility modulates enzyme activity in HIV-1 protease. J Am Chem Soc 134(9):4163–4168

Nalam MN, Schiffer CA (2008) New approaches to HIV protease inhibitor drug design II: testing the substrate envelope hypothesis to avoid drug resistance and discover robust inhibitors. Curr Opin HIV AIDS 3(6):642–646

Nalam MN, Ali A, Altman MD, Reddy GS, Chellappan S, Kairys V, Ozen A, Cao H, Gilson MK, Tidor B, Rana TM, Schiffer CA (2010) Evaluating the substrate-envelope hypothesis: structural analysis of novel HIV-1 protease inhibitors designed to be robust against drug resistance. J Virol 84(10):5368–5378

Ozen A, Haliloglu T, Schiffer CA (2011) Dynamics of preferential substrate recognition in HIV-1 protease: redefining the substrate envelope. J Mol Biol 410(4):726–744

Ozen A, Haliloglu T, Schiffer CA (2012) HIV-1 protease and substrate coevolution validates the substrate envelope as the recognition pattern. J Chem Theory Comput 8:703–714

Ozen A, Sherman W, Schiffer CA (2013) Improving the resistance profile of hepatitis C NS3/4A inhibitors: dynamic substrate envelope guided design. J Chem Theory Comput 9:5693–5705

Palella FJ Jr, Delaney KM, Moorman AC, Loveless MO, Fuhrer J, Satten GA, Aschman DJ, Holmberg SD (1998) Declining morbidity and mortality among patients with advanced human

immunodeficiency virus infection. HIV outpatient study investigators. N Engl J Med 338 (13):853–860
Patick AK, Duran M, Cao Y, Shugarts D, Keller MR, Mazabel E, Knowles M, Chapman S, Kuritzkes DR, Markowitz M (1998) Genotypic and phenotypic characterization of human immunodeficiency virus type 1 variants isolated from patients treated with the protease inhibitor nelfinavir. Antimicrob Agents Chemother 42(10):2637–2644
Perni RB, Almquist SJ, Byrn RA, Chandorkar G, Chaturvedi PR, Courtney LF, Decker CJ, Dinehart K, Gates CA, Harbeson SL, Heiser A, Kalkeri G, Kolaczkowski E, Lin K, Luong YP, Rao BG, Taylor WP, Thomson JA, Tung RD, Wei Y, Kwong AD, Lin C (2006) Preclinical profile of VX-950, a potent, selective, and orally bioavailable inhibitor of hepatitis C virus NS3-4A serine protease. Antimicrob Agents Chemother 50(3):899–909
Prabu-Jeyabalan M, Nalivaika E, Schiffer CA (2000) How does a symmetric dimer recognize an asymmetric substrate? A substrate complex of HIV-1 protease. J Mol Biol 301(5):1207–1220
Prabu-Jeyabalan M, Nalivaika E, Schiffer CA (2002) Substrate shape determines specificity of recognition for HIV-1 protease: analysis of crystal structures of six substrate complexes. Structure 10(3):369–381
Rhee SY, Gonzales MJ, Kantor R, Betts BJ, Ravela J, Shafer RW (2003) Human immunodeficiency virus reverse transcriptase and protease sequence database. Nucleic Acids Res 31(1):298–303
Rhee SY, Taylor J, Fessel WJ, Kaufman D, Towner W, Troia P, Ruane P, Hellinger J, Shirvani V, Zolopa A, Shafer RW (2010) HIV-1 protease mutations and protease inhibitor cross-resistance. Antimicrob Agents Chemother 54(10):4253–4261
Roberts NA, Martin JA, Kinchington D, Broadhurst AV, Craig JC, Duncan IB, Galpin SA, Handa BK, Kay J, Krohn A et al (1990) Rational design of peptide-based HIV proteinase inhibitors. Science 248(4953):358–361
Robinson BS, Riccardi KA, Gong YF, Guo Q, Stock DA, Blair WS, Terry BJ, Deminie CA, Djang F, Colonno RJ, Lin PF (2000a) BMS-232632, a highly potent human immunodeficiency virus protease inhibitor that can be used in combination with other available antiretroviral agents. Antimicrob Agents Chemother 44(8):2093–2099
Robinson LH, Myers RE, Snowden BW, Tisdale M, Blair ED (2000b) HIV type 1 protease cleavage site mutations and viral fitness: implications for drug susceptibility phenotyping assays. AIDS Res Hum Retroviruses 16:1149–1156
Romano KP, Ali A, Royer WE, Schiffer CA (2010) Drug resistance against HCV NS3/4A inhibitors is defined by the balance of substrate recognition versus inhibitor binding. Proc Natl Acad Sci U S A 107(49):20986–20991
Romano KP, Ali A, Aydin C, Soumana D, Ozen A, Deveau LM, Silver C, Cao H, Newton A, Petropoulos CJ, Huang W, Schiffer CA (2012) The molecular basis of drug resistance against hepatitis C virus NS3/4A protease inhibitors. PLoS Pathog 8(7):e1002832
Santos AF, Soares MA (2010) HIV genetic diversity and drug resistance. Viruses 2(2):503–531
Sarrazin C, Rouzier R, Wagner F, Forestier N, Larrey D, Gupta SK, Hussain M, Shah A, Cutler D, Zhang J, Zeuzem S (2007) SCH 503034, a novel hepatitis C virus protease inhibitor, plus pegylated interferon alpha-2b for genotype 1 nonresponders. Gastroenterology 132 (4):1270–1278
Schapiro JM, Winters MA, Stewart F, Efron B, Norris J, Kozal MJ, Merigan TC (1996) The effect of high-dose saquinavir on viral load and CD4+ T-cell counts in HIV-infected patients. Ann Intern Med 124(12):1039–1050
Seiwert SD, Kossen K, Pan L, Liu J, Buckman BO (2011) Discovery and development of the HCV NS3/4A protease inhibitor danoprevir (ITMN-191/RG7227). In: Antiviral drugs. Wiley, Hoboken, New Jersey, pp 257–271
Sham HL, Kempf DJ, Molla A, Marsh KC, Kumar GN, Chen C-M, Kati W, Stewart K, Lal R, Hsu A, Betebenner D, Korneyeva M, Vasavanonda S, McDonald E, Saldivar A, Wideburg N, Chen X, Niu P, Park C, Jayanti V, Grabowski B, Granneman GR, Sun E, Japour AJ, Leonard JM, Plattner JJ, Norbeck DW (1998) ABT-378, a highly potent inhibitor of human immunodeficiency virus protease. Antimicrob Agents Chemother 42(12):3218–3224

Simmonds P, Bukh J, Combet C, Deleage G, Enomoto N, Feinstone S, Halfon P, Inchauspe G, Kuiken C, Maertens G, Mizokami M, Murphy DG, Okamoto H, Pawlotsky JM, Penin F, Sablon E, Shin IT, Stuyver LJ, Thiel HJ, Viazov S, Weiner AJ, Widell A (2005) Consensus proposals for a unified system of nomenclature of hepatitis C virus genotypes. Hepatology 42 (4):962–973

Soo-Yon Rhee, Matthew J. Gonzales, Rami Kantor, Bradley J. Betts, Jaideep Ravela, and Robert W. Shafer (2003) Human immunodeficiency virus reverse transcriptase and protease sequence database. Nucleic Acids Research, 31(1), 298–303

Steinkuhler C, Biasiol G, Brunetti M, Urbani A, Koch U, Cortese R, Pessi A, De Francesco R (1998) Product inhibition of the hepatitis C virus NS3 protease. Biochemistry 37 (25):8899–8905

Surleraux DL, Tahri A, Verschueren WG, Pille GM, de Kock HA, Jonckers TH, Peeters A, De Meyer S, Azijn H, Pauwels R, de Bethune MP, King NM, Prabu-Jeyabalan M, Schiffer CA, Wigerinck PB (2005) Discovery and selection of TMC114, a next generation HIV-1 protease inhibitor. J Med Chem 48(6):1813–1822

Tong X, Chase R, Skelton A, Chen T, Wright-Minogue J, Malcolm BA (2006) Identification and analysis of fitness of resistance mutations against the HCV protease inhibitor SCH 503034. Antiviral Res 70(2):28–38

Tong X, Bogen S, Chase R, Girijavallabhan V, Guo Z, Njoroge FG, Prongay A, Saksena A, Skelton A, Xia E, Ralston R (2008) Characterization of resistance mutations against HCV ketoamide protease inhibitors. Antiviral Res 77(3):177–185

Turner SR, Strohbach JW, Tommasi RA, Aristoff PA, Johnson PD, Skulnick HI, Dolak LA, Seest EP, Tomich PK, Bohanon MJ, Horng MM, Lynn JC, Chong KT, Hinshaw RR, Watenpaugh KD, Janakiraman MN, Thaisrivongs S (1998) Tipranavir (PNU-140690): a potent, orally bioavailable nonpeptidic HIV protease inhibitor of the 5,6-dihydro-4-hydroxy-2-pyrone sulfonamide class. J Med Chem 41(18):3467–3476

Tuske S, Sarafianos SG, Clark AD Jr, Ding J, Naeger LK, White KL, Miller MD, Gibbs CS, Boyer PL, Clark P, Wang G, Gaffney BL, Jones RA, Jerina DM, Hughes SH, Arnold E (2004) Structures of HIV-1 RT-DNA complexes before and after incorporation of the anti-AIDS drug tenofovir. Nat Struct Mol Biol 11(5):469–474

Vanwolleghem T, Meuleman P, Libbrecht L, Roskams T, De Vos R, Leroux-Roels G (2007) Ultra-rapid cardiotoxicity of the hepatitis C virus protease inhibitor BILN 2061 in the urokinase-type plasminogen activator mouse. Gastroenterology 133(4):1144–1155

Wu TD, Schiffer CA, Gonzales M, Kantor R, Chou S, Israelski D, Zolopa A, Fessel J, Shafer RW (2003) Mutation patterns and structural correlates in HIV-1 protease following varying degrees of protease inhibitor treatment. J Virol 77:4836–4847

Zhang YM, Imamichi H, Imamichi T, Lane HC, Falloon J, Vasudevachari MB, Salzman NP (1997) Drug resistance during indinavir therapy is caused by mutations in the protease gene and in its Gag substrate cleavage sites. J Virol 71(9):6662–6670

Part II

Bacteriology

The Mechanisms of Resistance to β-Lactam Antibiotics

Dustin T. King, Solmaz Sobhanifar, and Natalie C. J. Strynadka

Contents

Abstract

Bacterial diseases have had an enormous impact on human health and continue to be a major focus in modern medicine. The most widespread class of human antibacterials is the β-lactams that target the transpeptidase enzymes, which are responsible for cross-linking the peptidoglycan cell wall. There are over 34 FDA-approved β-lactams which together constitute ~50 % of all antibiotic prescriptions worldwide (Tahlan K and Jensen SE, J Antibiot (Tokyo) 66:401–410, 2013). However, bacteria have gained resistance mechanisms to overcome all major classes of β-lactam antibiotics to date. In this chapter, we will address the major mechanisms of bacterial resistance to the β-lactams and highlight some of the recent advances in circumventing this resistance.

D.T. King • S. Sobhanifar • N.C.J. Strynadka (✉)
Department of Biochemistry and Molecular Biology and Center for Blood Research, University of British Columbia, Vancouver, BC, Canada
e-mail: dustin@byron.biochem.ubc.ca; sobhanifar9@gmail.com; ncjs@mail.ubc.ca

M. Gotte et al. (eds.), *Handbook of Antimicrobial Resistance*,
DOI 10.1007/978-1-4939-0694-9_10

Keywords
β-Lactams • β-Lactamase • Antibiotic resistance • Efflux pump • Penicillin-binding proteins

Introduction

Sir Alexander Fleming's discovery of penicillin in the late 1920s initiated interest in deciphering the molecular mechanism of β-lactam action. Subsequent observations in the 1940s revealed that upon treatment with penicillin, bacteria adopt a filamentous morphology and that radioactive penicillin G localized to the membrane leading to the conclusion that β-lactams were affecting the synthesis of some key cell surface structure (Duguid 1946; Waxman and Strominger 1983). However, further target identification had to wait a further 20 years for elucidation of the peptidoglycan (PG) chemical architecture and biosynthetic pathway (for a detailed review on PG synthesis, please see (Lovering et al. 2012)). The bacterial PG is a vast glycan mesh that envelops the entire bacterial cell and imparts the rigidity necessary to define cell shape and morphogenesis as well as protect the cell from osmotic rupture (Typas et al. 2011). PG is made up of long linear polysaccharide chains of alternating *N*-acetylglucosamine and *N*-acetylmuramic acid pentapeptide. The pentapeptide group (or stem peptide) in Gram-negative bacteria is typically comprised of L-alanine-γ-D-glutamate-diaminopimelate(meso-DAP)-D-alanine-D-alanine. In Gram-positive organisms, the stem peptide is typically comprised of L-alanine-γ-D-glutamate-L-lysine-D-alanine-D-alanine with a pentaglycine branch protruding from the L-lysine residue. In the mid-1960s, the stem peptide cross-linking PG transpeptidases (TPs) were identified as the lethal target of the β-lactams, and the complexity of β-lactam action was attributed to the multiple penicillin-binding proteins (PBPs) that are targeted by them (Wise and Park 1965; Tipper and Strominger 1965). The PBP TPs typically catalyze a two-step reaction in which the position 3 amino group of an acceptor strand attacks the peptide bond of the terminal D-alanine-D-alanine of a donor strand, releasing the D-alanine leaving group and forming a peptide cross-link (Sauvage et al. 2008; Macheboeuf et al. 2006). The inhibition of PBPs ultimately results in reduced PG stem peptide cross-links and deregulation of PG degradation, which causes the accumulation of sacculus defects. These localized PG defects ultimately result in the inability of the cell wall to withstand the osmotic turgor pressure of the cytoplasmic membrane resulting in outer membrane encased balloon-like structures on the surface of the bacterial cell that eventually rupture leading to cell death (Yao et al. 2012).

β-Lactams

β-Lactam-Mediated Inhibition of PG Transpeptidase

The β-lactam antibiotics act as covalent substrate analogues of the D-alanine-D-alanine portion of the acceptor stem peptide. All PBP TP domains contain three highly conserved active site sequence motifs: (i) the SXXK motif (that includes the catalytic serine nucleophile and general base lysine), (ii) the SXN triad, and (iii) the KTG(T/S) motif (Sauvage et al. 2008). The mechanism of TP inhibition is initiated by deprotonation of the motif in catalytic S70 by the concerted general base K73 facilitating nucleophilic attack on the β-lactam amide carbonyl carbon resulting in the formation of a tetrahedral intermediate (Fig. 1a). This transiently formed intermediate is stabilized by hydrogen bonding to conserved residues in the oxyanion hole (comprised of main chain hydrogens of motifs i and iii). Subsequently, the tetrahedral intermediate collapses to expel the negatively charged nitrogen leaving group which is presumably stabilized by protonation via S120 (motif ii), thereby forming an acyl-enzyme intermediate. The stable species is resistant to hydrolysis, presumably due to steric blockage of a requisite deacylating water by the nitrogen of the former β-lactam ring (Fig. 1b; reviewed in Sauvage et al. (2008); Macheboeuf et al. (2006)).

Major Classes of β-Lactams

Since the initial discovery of benzylpenicillin, numerous other β-lactam classes have been developed, expanding our antibiotic arsenal to combat resistance. β-Lactams fall into four distinct structural classes that all have the four-membered lactam core moiety in common (penicillins, cephalosporins, carbapenems, and monobactams). Taken together, the multiple β-lactams constitute a comprehensive and structurally diverse set of compounds that display different pharmacological properties and are used for unique clinical indications.

Penicillins

The penicillins were initially derived from *Penicillium* fungi and represent the oldest "pure" antibiotic concoction used by man. The clinical testing of Fleming's purified penicillin extract in the early 1940s was met with unparalleled success and marked a seminal advancement in medical history (Keefer et al. 1943). The penicillin core consists of a five-membered thiazolidine ring fused at the 2′ and 3′ positions to the β-lactam ring (Fig. 2). Today, there are four major penicillin subclasses: (i) natural penicillins, (ii) penicillinase-resistant penicillins, (iii) aminopenicillins, and (iv) extended-spectrum penicillins (Miller 2002). The evolution of bacterial resistance to natural product penicillins stimulated a renaissance in the development of novel semisynthetic derivatives, which are made using the 6-aminopenicillanic acid (6-APA) precursor molecule (Rolinson and Geddes 2007). Although the penicillin family continues to be an important cornerstone in modern medicine, the emergence of widespread bacterial resistance has led to decreased efficacy in recent decades driving development of alternative β-lactams.

Cephalosporins

The cephalosporins (the first of which, cephalosporin C, was isolated from the fungi *Cephalosporium acremonium* in 1948) have a six-membered dihydrothiazine ring attached to the lactam core (Fig. 2). Interest in the clinical development of

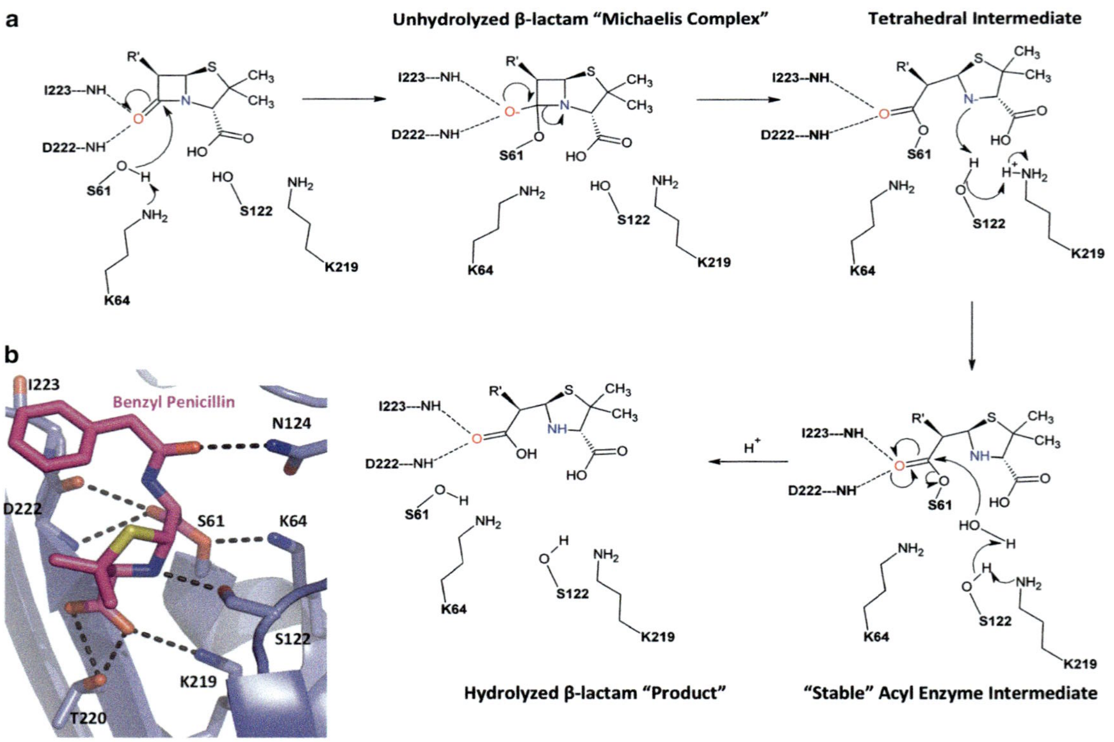

Fig. 1 β-Lactam-mediated inhibition of PBP TPase. (**a**) Mechanism of PBP-mediated β-lactam acylation and eventual hydrolysis. (**b**) Active site close-up of benzylpenicillin-bound *Thermosynechococcus elongatus* PBPA. The benzylpenicillin-bound PBPA active site (PDB ID: 2JBF) is depicted as a blue cartoon with selected active site residues shown as *blue* sticks with atoms colored by type (N, *blue*; O, *red*; S, *yellow*). The acylated benzylpenicillin is depicted as *pink* sticks with atoms colored by type. Hydrogen bonding and electrostatic interactions are shown as *black dashes*

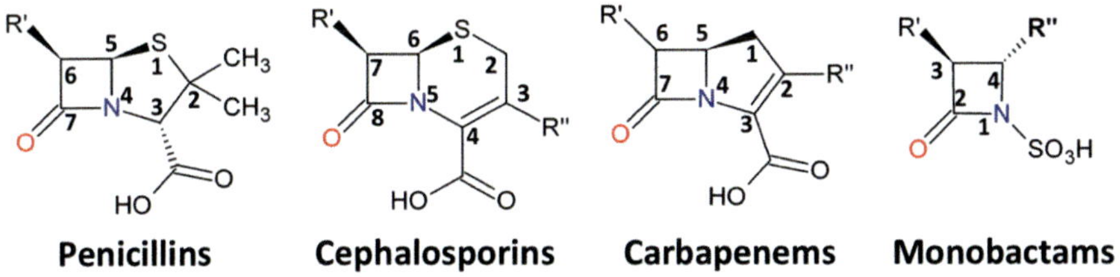

Fig. 2 Chemical structure of β-lactam antibiotic classes that are in current clinical use

cephalosporins stemmed from their resistance to hydrolysis by penicillinases (Neu 1982). The side chains used in the development of semisynthetic penicillins were incorporated into the cephalosporin core scaffold (Page 2012). However, in contrast to the penicillins, the cephalosporin core offers an additional site of variation at the C3 position (Fig. 2), giving rise to a breadth of structural diversity. The cephalosporins are generally grouped into four distinct generations based upon several features of antimicrobial activity (reviewed in Page 2012). The most recent cephalosporins in development either display antipseudomonal activity or are effective against methicillin-resistant *Staphylococcus aureus* (MRSA) (i.e., ceftobiprole) (Bush and Macielag 2010).

Carbapenems

The carbapenems (the first of which, thienamycin, was discovered in the mid-1980s as a metabolic product of *Streptomyces cattleya* (Birnbaum et al. 1985)) have a five-membered 2,3 unsaturated system with a C1 carbon rather than sulfur 4,5 fused to the lactam core. In place of the acylamino group seen at the R1 position in penicillins and cephalosporins, the carbapenems have a hydroxyethyl side chain that is important for resisting β-lactamase-mediated hydrolysis (Fig. 2) (Maveyraud et al. 1998). Remarkably, carbapenems have overall broader antimicrobial activity than the penicillins, cephalosporins, and other β-lactam/β-lactamase inhibitor combinations (Papp-Wallace et al. 2011). A key attribute of the carbapenems is their ability to bind indiscriminately to multiple PBPs and resist hydrolysis or inhibit many β-lactamases (Queenan et al. 2009; Bonfiglio et al. 2002). Today, carbapenems are often our last line of defense against multidrug-resistant Gram-negative pathogens. However, clinically available carbapenems have low oral bioavailability and thus do not readily penetrate gastrointestinal tissues and are typically administered intravenously (Papp-Wallace et al. 2011).

Monobactams

Monobactams are predominantly synthetic monocyclic β-lactams with variable organic groups at positions C2 and C4 as well as a sulfonic acid moiety attached to the N1 nitrogen (Fig. 2). The sulfonic acid group is thought to activate the β-lactam ring assisting the acylation of transpeptidases (Finberg and Guharoy 2012). Aztreonam is currently the only clinically approved monobactam. Aztreonam binds to PBP3 of susceptible Gram-negative pathogens with high affinity, yet displays very poor acylation of Gram-positive PBPs resulting in its inability to treat Gram-positive infections. Due to its relatively narrow spectrum of activity, aztreonam is generally used as part of antibiotic combination therapies (such as aztreonam-vancomycin) (Ellis-Grosse et al. 2005). However, there is substantial interest in developing new monobactams given that they are stable to the emerging metallo-β-lactamase (MBL) enzymes (King and Strynadka 2012).

β-Lactam Resistance

Major Resistance Mechanisms

Even before penicillin was commercialized in the early 1940s, penicillin-resistant β-lactamase expressing strains of *E. coli* were identified (Abraham and Chain 1988). The identification of β-lactam resistance led to the development of extended-spectrum antibiotics such as ceftazidime, cefotaxime, and the carbapenems as well as β-lactam-based serine β-lactamase inhibitors such as tazobactam, sulbactam, and clavulanic acid (Page 2000). However, extensive use of these compounds both in medicine and in the agricultural industry has placed a tremendous selective pressure on bacteria, such that currently no single β-lactam is free from resistance. It is now commonplace for individual bacteria to have multiple different resistance genes that function in concert to confer extended-spectrum resistance. The three main mechanisms of bacterial resistance to the β-lactam antibiotics are (i) enzymatic degradation by β-lactamases, (ii) target modification of the PBPs resulting in a lack of β-lactam binding, and (iii) regulation of β-lactam entry and efflux.

Enzymatic Degradation

The single most prominent mechanism of bacterial resistance to the β-lactams is the expression of hydrolytic enzymes called β-lactamases. These enzymes specifically recognize and hydrolyze the four-membered β-lactam ring leading to an inactivated product that is no longer effective at inhibiting TPs. Most frequently, resistance is conferred by mutation of preexisting β-lactamase enzymes resulting in an enhanced spectrum or targeted specificity of their hydrolytic properties against the various β-lactam classes listed above. Many β-lactamases are encoded on mobile genetic elements leading to increased transmission and spread such that it is now commonplace to find bacterial strains harboring as many as eight different β-lactamases each tailored to inactivate a unique subset of antibiotics (Bush 2013). β-Lactamases themselves are typically grouped into four distinct classes based upon DNA sequence similarity (molecular classes A–D). Molecular classes A, C, and D evolved from TPs and utilize an active site serine to initiate bond hydrolysis and are thereby referred to as serine β-lactamases (SBLs). In contrast, the unique molecular class B enzymes are metallo-β-lactamases (MBLs) that use active site zinc ions to coordinate a nucleophilic hydroxide to mediate ring opening. The class B enzymes are further categorized into the subclasses B1, B2, and B3 based upon DNA sequence similarities. Collectively, these enzymes are capable of hydrolyzing every clinically available β-lactam.

Class A (SBLs)

The class A penicillinase TEM (or RTEM) was the first clinically relevant plasmid-encoded β-lactamase identified in Gram-negative bacteria (*E. coli* and *Salmonella enterica*) in the early 1960s (reviewed in Bush 2012). By the late 1970s and early 1980s, broad-spectrum TEM and SHV were the most common plasmid-encoded β-lactamases in Gram-negative isolates. Their apparent abundance and location on mobile genetic elements provided a rich environment for the evolution of these enzymes in response to the introduction of new β-lactams (Turner 2005). Class A extended-spectrum β-lactamases (ESBLs) of the TEM, SHV, and CTX-M families are currently among the most clinically significant β-lactamases and have evolved to not only hydrolyze the penicillins but also broad-spectrum cephalosporins and monobactams (Bush 2012). Today, the CTX-M family of class A β-lactamase is the most prominent set of ESBL enzymes globally and has the ability to readily hydrolyze extended-spectrum cephalosporins such as cefotaxime (Delmas et al. 2010). KPC-2 is the most frequently reported class A carbapenemase to date and has been found as the causative agent in numerous carbapenem-resistant outbreaks worldwide (Nordmann et al. 2009).

The active site of class A β-lactamases contains four distinct motifs that are important for substrate binding and catalysis: (i) S70XXK, (ii) S130XN, (iii) K234-T/SG, and (iv) the Ω loop (Fig. 3a). The general mechanism of class A β-lactamase hydrolysis begins with the activation of S70 by deprotonation. There are currently two proposed mechanisms for S70 activation: (i) K73 acts as a general base to deprotonate the catalytic S70 (Swaren et al. 1995; Strynadka et al. 1992), and (ii) E166 activates a water molecule which subsequently deprotonates S70 (Hermann et al. 2005). Once activated, S70 attacks the β-lactam amide bond resulting in the formation of a tetrahedral intermediate that is stabilized by the oxyanion hole of the enzyme (Strynadka et al. 1996). Subsequently, the tetrahedral intermediate breaks down to expel the N4 nitrogen leaving group, which is subsequently protonated by S130 resulting in the formation of the transient acyl-enzyme intermediate. K73 is thought to shuttle a proton to S130 for leaving group protonation during this process (Hermann et al. 2005). Deacylation is generally thought to proceed through activation of a nucleophilic water molecule by E166, resulting in the hydrolysis of the acyl bond with concomitant back donation of a proton, likely through a concerted shuttle via K73, to the catalytic S70 and release of the de-activated product from the active site.

Class B (MBLs)

The first discovered class B enzyme was the *Bacillus cereus* metallo-β-lactamase (MBL) BcII in 1966 by Sabath and Abraham (Sabath and Abraham 1966). By 1989, only four MBL enzymes had been discovered, and each appeared to be chromosomally encoded and species specific. For the following two decades, the MBLs were seen as interesting, yet clinically insignificant. However, in 1991, the discovery of plasmid-encoded IMP-1 from *Pseudomonas aeruginosa* in Japan launched a

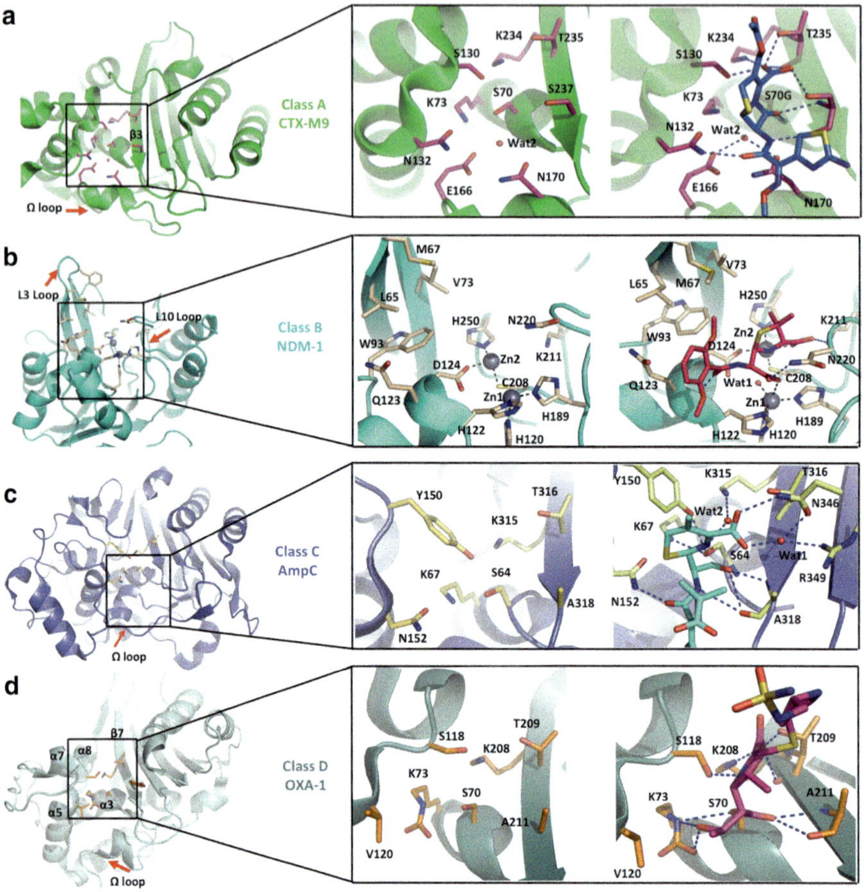

Fig. 3 Structural comparison of β-lactamase enzymes. (**a**) Overall structure and active site close-up of the class A β-lactamase CTX-M9 (PDB ID: 3HLW). The CTX-M9 protein is depicted as a *green* cartoon with selected active site residues shown as *pink* sticks. Acylated cefotaxime is depicted as *blue* sticks. (**b**) Overall structure and active site close-up of the class B1 β-lactamase NDM-1 (PDB ID: 4EY2). The NDM-1 protein is depicted as a *cyan* cartoon with selected active site residues shown as *beige* sticks with atoms colored by type. Hydrolyzed methicillin is depicted as *pink* sticks. (**c**) Overall structure and active site close-up of the class C β-lactamase AmpC (PDB ID: 1IEL). The AmpC protein is depicted in *blue* cartoon representation with selected active site residues shown as *gold* sticks with atoms colored by type. Acylated ceftazidime is shown as *cyan* sticks. (**d**) Overall structure and active site close-up of the class D β-lactamase OXA-1 (PDB ID: 3ISG). The OXA-1 protein is depicted in *dark teal* cartoon representation with selected active site residues shown as *orange* sticks with atoms colored by type. Acylated doripenem is shown as *pink* sticks. In (**a**–**d**), a close-up of the apo (*left*) and acylated (*right*) enzyme is depicted. In all panels, hydrogen bonding and electrostatic interactions are shown as *blue dashes*, and all non-carbon ligand and residue atoms are colored by type

renaissance in the discovery and characterization of new MBLs (Bebrone 2007). MBL-mediated resistance in nosocomial infections has gained traction in many multidrug-resistant Gram-negative pathogens including *P. aeruginosa*, *E. coli*, *Klebsiella pneumoniae*, *Bacteroides fragilis*, and *Aeromonas hydrophila* (Bebrone 2007). Today, MBLs are predominantly plasmid encoded as part of mobile genetic cassettes, which facilitates their transmission throughout microbial populations (Walsh et al. 2005). Furthermore, MBLs are known for their promiscuous nature and ability to hydrolyze nearly all β-lactams with the exception of the monobactams. Furthermore, MBLs constitute the most molecularly diverse class of carbapenemases (Walsh 2010). Recent years have seen the development of MBLs such as the New Delhi metallo-β-lactamase that can confer enteric pathogens such as *E. coli* and *K. pneumoniae* with nearly complete resistance to all β-lactams including the carbapenems (Yong et al. 2009). Additionally, bacteria co-expressing SBLs and MBLs are often capable of hydrolyzing the clinically relevant monobactam aztreonam (Nordmann et al. 2011). Despite vast research efforts, and due in part to the lack of a covalently bound adduct during hydrolysis, the development of a clinically useful MBL inhibitor is yet to materialize.

Despite having divergent sequences, the MBL enzymes have a remarkably conserved fold, which is characterized by an internal β-sandwich flanked on its outer face by five solvent-exposed α-helices (Fig. 3b). The zinc-containing active site is localized to one face of the β-sandwich in a broad, yet shallow groove (King and Strynadka 2012). Although MBLs are generally homovalent zinc-dependent hydrolases, several have nevertheless been found to bind cobalt and cadmium in addition to zinc, with varying degrees of hydrolytic efficiency (de Seny et al. 2001). The MBLs are either monovalent or divalent depending upon the particular enzyme subclass being considered. The B1 and B3 enzymes utilize a divalent zinc center to mediate hydrolysis, while the B2 MBLs are monovalent enzymes that are inhibited by the presence of a second active site zinc ion and display high specificity for carbapenem hydrolysis (Bebrone et al. 2009; Hernandez Valladares et al. 1997).

For the subclass B1 and B3 MBLs (for which the mechanism has been more extensively studied), the β-lactam carbonyl is coordinated by Zn1 in the precatalytic complex. The C3 carboxylate of the substrate interacts electrostatically with the conserved K224 (Fig. 3b). Binding by the electropositive zinc ions maintains the bridging catalytic hydroxide at a measured pKa of 5–6 (Wang et al. 1999). Nucleophilic attack by this hydroxide on the activated carbonyl results in the formation of a tetrahedral intermediate, which is stabilized by a predicted oxyanion hole (consisting of Zn1 and potentially the amide side chain nitrogen of N220). The tetrahedral intermediate then breaks down to expel the negatively charged nitrogen, which is proposed to be protonated by bulk solvent (Page and Badarau 2008). The product is subsequently released from the active site, and the nucleophilic hydroxide is reloaded between the zinc ions for another round of catalysis. For a more complete analysis of the MBL catalytic mechanism, please refer to the following reviews (Page and Badarau 2008; Xu et al. 2006).

Class C (SBLs)

The class C β-lactamases or AmpC enzymes originally evolved to hydrolyze cephalosporin antibiotics. However, today many of these enzymes show high catalytic efficiency toward the penicillins. These enzymes are typically chromosomally encoded carbapenemases that are often under inducible expression. However, several class C enzymes have now been found localized on high copy number mobile plasmids (Philippon et al. 2002). The class C enzymes are predominantly found in Gram-negative organisms such as *E. coli* and *K. pneumoniae* (Fenollar-Ferrer et al. 2008). Typically, AmpC enzymes are nonsusceptible to the clinically approved β-lactamase inhibitors; however, some remain susceptible to sulbactam and tazobactam (Jacoby 2009).

The four active site motifs that define the class C enzymes are (i) the S64XXK, (ii) Y150AN, (iii) K314TG, and (iv) the Ω loop. The Ω loop occupies a unique position when compared to the class A enzymes, leaving room for more bulky cephalosporin β-lactam side chains (Fig. 3c) (Jacoby 2009). The general mechanism of catalysis for AmpC β-lactamases is assumed to be quite similar to the class A enzymes. However, the unique Y150 (motif ii) is ideally positioned to act as a potential proton donor to the β-lactam nitrogen leaving group following acylation, and it is generally accepted that this residue has a vital role in catalysis for the class C enzymes (Fenollar-Ferrer et al. 2008).

Class D (SBLs)

The class D β-lactamases are the most structurally divergent of the SBL subclasses, and DNA sequence similarity to the class A and C enzymes is restricted to distinct active site regions. These β-lactamases are predominantly known as OXA enzymes, which are named due to their ability to hydrolyze oxacillin (Majiduddin et al. 2002). The class D genes are typically plasmid encoded and are often localized to gene cassettes in integron regions. Similar to class A enzymes, the class D β-lactamases were originally identified as penicillinases, which have subsequently evolved the ability to hydrolyze a specific subset of cephalosporins and carbapenems (Majiduddin et al. 2002). Recently, the carbapenem-hydrolyzing OXA-48 enzyme has gained attention due to its broad specificity and large clinical prevalence (Poirel et al. 2012). Several class D SBLs have been found to exist as a dimer in solution, and the dimer-monomer equilibrium appears to be an important factor governing the kinetics of β-lactam hydrolysis (Paetzel et al. 2000; Vercheval et al. 2010). It is disquieting that this emerging class of enzymes cannot be efficiently inhibited by any of the clinically approved β-lactamase inhibitors and is developing hydrolytic activity toward the heralded carbapenems (Szarecka et al. 2011).

Class D enzymes have a truncated sequence between helices α3 and α5, as well as between α8 and strand β7, resulting in a dramatically larger active site cleft (Fig. 3d). As for other SBLs, the class D enzymes contain four key active site sequence motifs, (i) S67XXK, (ii) S115XXV, (iii) the K205-T/S-G motif, and (iv) the Ω loop (Paetzel et al. 2000). When compared to the class A enzymes, the Ω loop is more compact and further from the active site core, which results in a more open substrate-binding cleft. In addition, the (motif i) K70 is *N*-carboxylated to a varying extent depending on the particular OXA enzyme in question (Majiduddin et al. 2002). As in other SBLs, S67 (motif i) acts as a nucleophile to attack the β-lactam amide. However, it is thought that the role of carboxylation is to increase the basicity of K70 so as to serve as a more potent base to abstract a proton directly from S67 (Docquier et al. 2009). Furthermore, it is thought that the carboxylated K70 is positioned ideally to activate the deacylating water during hydrolysis (Golemi et al. 2001). The class D active site has significant hydrophobic character in proximity to K70, an environment that likely favors the free base form of lysine, promoting its carboxylation in the presence of carbon dioxide.

β-Lactamase Inhibitors

The identification of plasmid-borne TEM β-lactamase in gonococci in the late 1960s stimulated pharmaceutical companies to focus on the development of TEM-stable β-lactams and to discover inhibitors that could be used as part of a combination therapy to potentiate the activity of previously ineffective β-lactams. These efforts resulted in the development of β-lactam-based β-lactamase inhibitors (clavulanic acid, sulbactam, and tazobactam) (Payne et al. 1994). Initially, these compounds provided excellent antimicrobial properties against common Gram-negative pathogens harboring TEM-1 and SHV-1 type β-lactamases as well as penicillinases from the Gram-positive *S. aureus*. However, almost immediately after their introduction into clinical practice, bacteria began to produce new β-lactamase variants that were immune to inhibition by these compounds. Currently, there are several SBL inhibitors, both β-lactam and non-β-lactam, in clinical development. As this topic is beyond the scope of this chapter, we refer you to recent reviews on SBL inhibitors in current clinical development and MBL inhibitors in preclinical development (King and Strynadka 2012; Buynak 2013).

Target Modification

A common method by which bacteria avoid the action of antibiotics is via alteration of the intended target. Indeed, this mechanism is so successful that it can be found for every class of antibiotic, regardless of mechanism. These target alterations generally occur as a result of genetic mutations upon selective pressures in the presence of antibiotics. In other cases, however, modified targets may be acquired by way of genetic exchange. There are many examples of target modification among the PBPs from several bacterial types (reviewed in Lambert 2005). One of the best studied examples is the *S. aureus* PBP2a, responsible for high-level resistance in MRSA (Fig. 4). The encoding gene of PBP2a, mecA, resides on a large mobile genetic element called the staphylococcal chromosomal cassette (SCCmec), believed to have been acquired by horizontal transfer from a coagulase-negative staphylococcus species (reviewed in Shore and Coleman 2013). PBP2a is a high molecular weight class B D,D-transpeptidase that catalyzes the formation of cross-bridges in bacterial PG and is effectively resistant to most β-lactams at clinical concentrations. Together, with the transglycosylase activities of other PBPs, it is capable of maintaining the biosynthesis of PG and securing bacterial survival in the presence of β-lactams (Kim et al. 2012; Pinho et al. 2001). Kinetic studies performed with several β-lactams (including penicillins, cephalosporins, and carbapenems) suggest that a combination of decreased noncovalent binding of these drugs to the active site, as well as reduced subsequent acylation may be responsible for the lower sensitivity of PBP2a (Fuda et al. 2004). The structure of PBP2a furthermore suggests that poor acylation may result from a β-strand alteration, resulting in a distorted active site, which must undergo energetically unfavorable conformational changes for acylation to occur (Lim and Strynadka 2002). It is also suggested that an allosteric mechanism involving binding of nascent PG may participate in rearrangements that facilitate preferential active site binding to substrates rather than inhibitors (Fuda et al. 2005; Otero et al. 2013), allowing MRSA to survive during antibiotic treatment. Modified PBPs are however not always acquired, but in many cases are derived from recombination or mutation events. For example, the PBP1a and PBP2× of *Streptococcus pneumoniae* (Pernot et al. 2004; Dowson et al. 1994) and the PBP2 of *Neisseria meningitidis* (Bowler et al. 1994) possess mosaic structures derived from recombination of PBP genes with those acquired from closely related species. Mutation-derived low-affinity PBPs are also encountered in the *Helicobacter pylori* PBP1 (Okamoto et al. 2002), the *Neisseria gonorrhoeae* PBP2 (Brannigan et al. 1990) and PBP1 (Ropp et al. 2002), and the *Haemophilus influenzae* PBP3 (Dabernat et al. 2002). Enterococci on the other hand possess intrinsically low-affinity PBPs. Interestingly, the crystal structure of the *Enterococcus faecium* PBP5fm reveals a loop residing on the edge of the catalytic cavity that confers increased rigidity and restricted access to the active site, a feature observed in other low-affinity PBPs such as the *S. aureus* PBP2a (Sauvage et al. 2002).

Signaling Pathways Involved in β-Lactam Sensing

Bacteria have developed intricate systems of sensing the presence of β-lactams in their surroundings and responding by regulating the expression of β-lactamases and β-lactam-resistant PBPs. Indeed, both Gram-negative and Gram-positive bacteria sense and orchestrate a response to β-lactam antibiotics in a process intimately linked to the PG recycling pathway.

Sensor-/Transducer-Mediated Regulation of β-lactam Resistance

Although biologically distinct, the expression of β-lactamases and nonsensitive PBPs (i.e., PBP2a) is regulated in a very similar fashion. In staphylococci and certain Gram-positive species such as *Bacillus licheniformis*, β-lactamase expression is controlled by the concerted action of the repressor BlaI and the sensor/transducer protein BlaR1. The genes encoding β-lactamase (*blaZ*), BlaI (*blaI*), and BlaR1 (*blaR1*) are organized on a single divergon, with the expression of all three under the control of the BlaI repressor, occupying a palindromic promoter region (Fig. 4). On exposure, BlaR1 acts as a sentinel by covalently binding the β-lactam antibiotic,

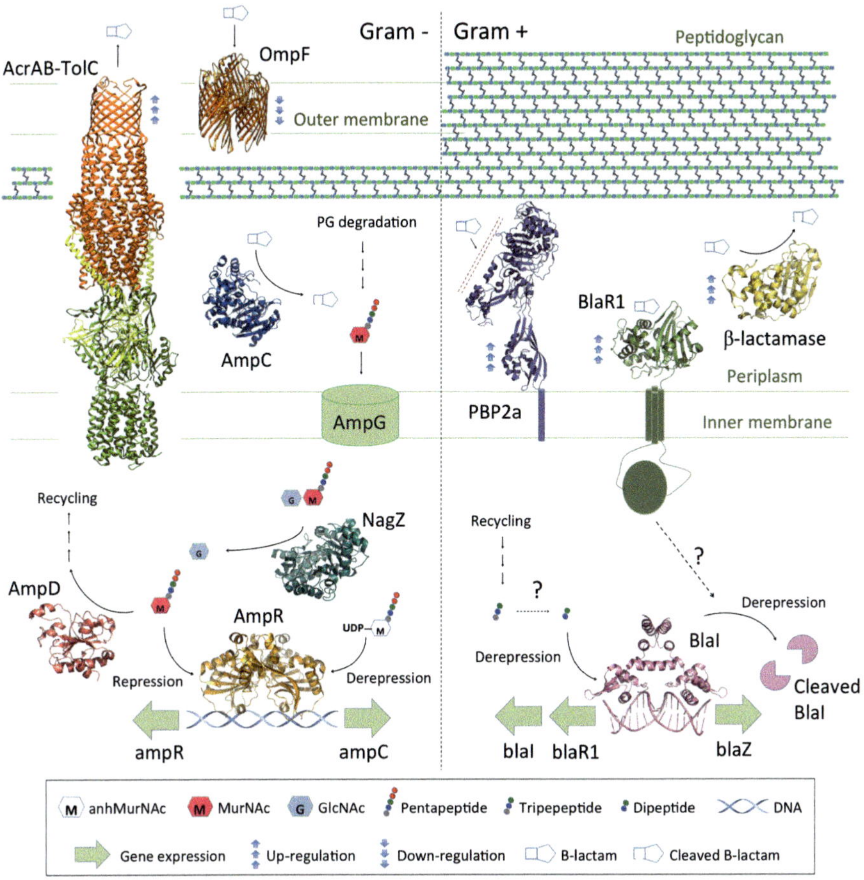

Fig. 4 Major mechanisms involved in β-lactam resistance. Reduced porin entry (e.g., OmpF, PDB ID: 2ZFG), increased efflux (e.g., AcrAB-TolC, PDB ID: 2F1M, 1OYE, 1EK9), β-lactam hydrolysis (e.g., AmpC, PDB ID: IKE4; β-lactamase, PDB ID: 1BLC), target modification (e.g., PBP2a, PDB ID: 1MWU), sensor-transducer signaling (e.g., BlaR1 sensor domain, PDB ID: 1XA7; BlaI, PDB ID: 1XSD), and murein recycling (AmpG; NagZ, PDB ID: 1TR9; AmpD, PDB ID: 2Y28; AmpR, PDB ID: 3KOS; BlaR1 sensor domain, PDB ID: 1XA7; BlaI, PDB ID: 1XSD) all play a part in resistance to β-lactams. Porin and efflux pump regulation and modification play important roles in Gram-negative resistance, whereas Gram-positive bacteria that lack an outer membrane rely heavily on β-lactamase-mediated β-lactam inactivation and PBP target modification

the ultimate consequence of which is the release and cleavage of the BlaI repressor (Hackbarth and Chambers 1993). The BlaR1 signal/transducer is a bi-modular protein consisting of an extracellular sensor domain linked via a transmembrane four-helix bundle to a cytoplasmic protease domain. The sensor domain of BlaR1 (BlaRs) shares the greatest structural homology and mechanistic similarity with the class D β-lactamases (Figs. 3d and 4; Birck et al. 2004; Wilke et al. 2004). Upon contact with β-lactams, BlaRs is irreversibly acylated at its active site serine, concurrent with cleavage of the β-lactam ring. Much like the class D β-lactamases, this acylation event is proposed to be mediated by an adjacent *N*-carboxylated lysine that deprotonates the nucleophilic serine (Golemi et al. 2001). However, unlike the class D β-lactamases, the carboxylated lysine of BlaR1 is proposed to be unstable and is rapidly decarboxylated following serine acylation, such that it is no longer able to activate a water molecule for subsequent deacylation (Cha and Mobashery 2007). In this manner, the stability of the carboxylated lysine may have been decisive in the evolution of the respective β-lactamase vs. β-lactam sensor functions. The cytosolic protease domain of BlaR1 (BlaRp) harbors the signature HEXXH and EXXXD motifs common to the gluzincin family of zinc metalloproteases and is believed to be in a zymogenic state until activated by auto-cleavage (Zhang et al. 2001). This cleavage event is believed to be initiated by the β-lactam acylation of BlaRs, resulting in conformational changes in the transmembrane bundle that carry the signal across the bilayer (Zhang et al. 2001). Although the ultimate result of BlaRp activation is the cleavage of BlaI, it is not yet certain whether BlaI is the direct substrate of BlaRp or the end result of a proteolytic relay (Llarrull and Mobashery 2012; Amoroso et al. 2012).

Interestingly, the *mec* operon of MRSA strains has analogous molecular players to that of bla operon, yet is involved in the regulation of PBP2a expression. Here, genes encoding the signal/transducer MecR1 (mecR1), PBP2a (mecA), and the transcriptional repressor MecI (mecI) are similarly organized on a single divergon under control of a repressor (either MecI or BlaI, as is discussed below). The MecR sensor domain (MecRs) displays a similar overall fold to BlaRs and likewise forms acylated β-lactam intermediates via the active site serine (Marrero et al. 2006). MecR1 also possesses a four transmembrane helical bundle as well as a cytoplasmic metalloprotease domain. Although most of the data concerning the mechanism of signal transduction described above has been obtained from the bla pathway, the many parallels in the mec system suggest strongly that it also adopts a similar induction mechanism. Indeed, in *Macrococcus caseolyticus*, a bacteria whose genus is closely related to that of staphylococci, the mec divergon takes a peculiar form: instead of the mecA-mecR1-mecI present in SCCmec, the divergon is composed of blaZ-mecA-mecR1-mecI. This structure is considered the ancestral form of the mec gene complex that is thought to have been generated by the integration of the mecA gene into the bla divergon, blaZ-blaR1-blaI (Baba et al. 2009; Tsubakishita et al. 2010). Indeed, BlaI and MecI have been shown to be interchangeable as repressors of both the bla and mec divergons (McKinney et al. 2001), an observation in agreement with their similar overall structures and active site composition. BlaR1 and MecR1 are, however, only specific for their cognate repressors and display distinct kinetics, where BlaR1 induces β-lactamase in a matter of minutes in contrast to MecR1 which requires hours for PBP2a induction (McKinney et al. 2001). MecI is a stronger repressor of mecA as compared to BlaI (McKinney et al. 2001), while MecR1 is much less efficient than BlaR1 in sensing β-lactams (Cha et al. 2007). It is perhaps for this reason that certain highly resistant MRSA strains have evolved to rely on the efficient bla system for the expression of PBP2a rather than the mec machinery which in these strains is defective or altogether absent (Archer et al. 1994; Ryffel et al. 1992; Milheirico et al. 2011).

PG Recycling and Regulation of β-Lactam Resistance

In Gram-negative bacteria, radiolabelling experiments have revealed that a surprisingly small amount of labeled PG is lost per generation and is instead recycled and reincorporated into new PG(Goodell 1985). We are now beginning to understand the importance of PG recycling to β-lactam resistance, where fluctuations in the cytoplasmic pool of broken-down PG fragments allow bacteria to gage the state of the cell wall, alerting them to the possible presence of β-lactams. In *E. coli*, the major recycling pathway involves the cytoplasmic transport of anhydro-muropeptides. These PG fragments are generated by the lytic transglycosylases and require the permease AmpG for delivery to the cytoplasm (Jacobs et al. 1994), where they are further hydrolyzed by the glucosaminidase NagZ to anhydro-MurNAc peptides and subsequently by the amidase AmpD to precursors for recycling (Fig. 4) (reviewed in Johnson et al. 2012). In the presence of β-lactams, there is an increase in the cytoplasmic pool of anhydro-MurNAc peptides that compete for binding to the transcriptional activator, AmpR. This leads to the induction of the β-lactamase, AmpC, and the subsequent breakdown of the antibiotic. Although the recycling pathway in Gram-positive bacteria is far less understood, it appears that these bacteria rely on lysozyme-like muramidases rather than lytic transglycosylases to produce MurNAc-containing muropeptides. These peptides and their breakdown products are postulated to be transported to the cytoplasm via conserved ABC transporters or the phosphotransferase system for recycling (Reith and Mayer 2011). Recently, it has been demonstrated that in *B. Licheniformis*, a cell-wall-derived dipeptide fragment, γ-D-Glu-m-DAP, is capable of binding the BlaI (MecI) repressor, leading to its dissociation from the bla operon and subsequent induction of the β-lactamase, BlaP (Amoroso et al. 2012). Although the exact pathway for the generation of the dipeptide has not yet been discerned, this finding draws an interesting parallel between recycling and antibiotic resistance in Gram-positive and Gram-negative bacteria.

Regulation of β-Lactam Entry and Efflux

β-Lactams are among the few drugs effective against both Gram-positive and Gram-negative strains, facilitated by the accessibility of the PBP targets that reside on the outer leaflet of the cytoplasmic membrane. Nevertheless, some Gram negatives such as *P. aeruginosa* are notorious for their resistance to β-lactams and other drugs, using cell wall modifications and changes to outer membrane architecture to create a near-impenetrable barrier. The two most well-understood mechanisms that regulate this drug-resistance phenomenon at the Gram-negative outer membrane are the restricted entry of drugs via the alteration or loss of porins and their active expulsion via efflux pumps.

Porin-Mediated Resistance

Porins are the most abundant proteins in the outer membrane of bacteria and act as selective permeable barriers that facilitate the uptake of nutrients and confer protection against harmful compounds. These water-filled channels act as molecular sieves that allow hydrophilic molecules below a specific exclusion limit to enter as determined by the channel diameter. High-resolution structures of porins have revealed a large similarity in architecture, with small variations in loop topology and surface charge. Porins lack a classic hydrophobic region and instead consist of transmembrane antiparallel β-strands with alternating hydrophobic and hydrophilic residues that, respectively, line the membrane- and water-exposed surfaces of the β-barrel. In general, the higher strand number β-barrel porins act as channels, often in a stable trimeric form, with those consisting of 18 β-strands often classified as substrate-specific porins and the 16 β-strand variants acting as general porins with typically less stringent substrate specificity. In Gram negatives, general porins are believed to be the primary route of entry for many antibiotics including small hydrophilic drugs such as β-lactams, tetracycline, chloramphenicol, and fluoroquinolones (reviewed in Galdiero et al. 2013). With pore exclusion limits close to the size of many antibiotics, general porins can act to promote or limit the diffusion rate of these compounds. Dependent on the bacterial species, the number and type of porins can also dictate the degree of susceptibility and intrinsic resistance of the organism (pseudomonas is a prominent example). Bacteria can limit porin-mediated drug entry either by adaptive or mutational means. In the first instance, porin expression can be modified upon antibiotic exposure by responsive regulatory elements (Farra et al. 2008). In the second instance, disruptive mutations in the porin-encoding gene can lead to either loss or defect in the porin, and mutations in the promoter region or regulatory elements can likewise decrease porin levels (Doumith et al. 2009). For example, the loss of OmpF (Harder et al. 1981) or mutations in OmpC around the point of pore "constriction" (Lou et al. 2011) is involved in β-lactam resistance in *E. coli*, and resistance to carbapenems in *P. aeruginosa* has been linked to a combination of pore-modulating loop mutations or complete loss of the general porin OprD (Huang and Hancock 1996), as well as regulatory mutations involving the MexT transcriptional repressor (Ochs et al. 1999) (reviewed in Fernandez and Hancock 2012).

Antibiotic Efflux

Bacterial efflux pumps may be categorized as primary or secondary transporters, the first type being driven by ATP hydrolysis and the second by proton motive force. These pumps are further categorized into five major superfamilies: the major facilitator superfamily (MFS), the ATP-binding cassette superfamily (ABC), the small multidrug-resistance family (SMR), the resistance-nodulation-cell division superfamily (RND), and the multi-antimicrobial extrusion protein family (MATE). Of these, only ABC family members are primary transporters, all others being secondary transporters using proton (MFS, RND, SMR, MATE) or sodium (MATE) antiport (Brown et al. 1999). Efflux pumps are often capable of recognizing multiple substrates, since affinity tends to be based on physiochemical characteristics such as hydrophobicity, aromaticity, or charge rather than a distinct structural chemistry. This can account for the prevalence of multidrug-resistance (MDR) efflux pumps, found in all five major superfamilies, which can capture and expel many structurally diverse antibiotics, in addition to nonantibiotic compounds (reviewed in Lewis (1994), Lomovskaya et al. (2007)). In Gram-positive bacteria, MSF efflux systems, such as the *S. aureus* NorA (Deng et al. 2012), are mainly responsible for MDR efflux. In Gram-negative bacteria, the MDR phenotype is largely conferred by RND efflux systems such as MexAB-OprM and AcrAB-TolC, contributing to the intrinsic resistance of *P. aeruginosa* and *E. coli*, respectively, to β-lactams and other antibiotics.

RND pump complexes are assembled as tripartite membrane machineries, composed of the RND pump located in the cytoplasmic membrane and two accessory proteins: a periplasmic adaptor protein of the membrane fusion protein (MFP) family and an outer membrane channel belonging to the outer membrane factor (OMF) family. As such, this complex is able to expel substrates across the entire cellular envelope and out of the cell. Interestingly, it has been found that dianionic β-lactams such as carbenicillin which are not able to cross into the cytoplasm are nevertheless expelled from the cell, suggesting that the RND complex is able to capture these substrates from the periplasm or from the periplasmic-cytoplasm interface (Li et al. 1994a; Nikaido and Takatsuka 2009). Although no structure currently exists for the intact tripartite complex, the atomic structures of each of the three pump components are available along with proposed composite models (Symmons et al. 2009; Su et al. 2011). The RND pump is typically trimeric with a total of 12 transmembrane helices and two large periplasmic loops (Murakami et al. 2002). The pump appears to function in a rotatory manner driven by alternate protonation of individual subunits in a process that results in substrate capture and subsequent release (Pos 2009; Murakami et al. 2006; Seeger et al. 2006). The periplasmic MFP adaptor protein is proposed to stabilize weak interactions between the RND and OMF and consists of an extended β-barrel connected by a lipoyl domain to a long periplasmic α-helical hairpin (Higgins et al. 2004; Mikolosko et al. 2006). The OMF channel protein consists of a trimeric arrangement that collectively forms a 12-stranded β-barrel inserted into the outer membrane, attached to an extended ~100 Å coiled-coil α-helical domain that protrudes into the periplasm (Koronakis et al. 2000), providing an iris-like mechanism to regulate access of small-molecule substrates (Andersen et al. 2002; Bavro et al. 2008) (Fig. 4). These observations are based on a wealth of structural information, reviewed in Hinchliffe et al. (2013).

In Gram-negative bacteria, MDR efflux pumps can form a near-impenetrable barrier against antimicrobial agents. Certain species of Gram-negative bacteria such *P. aeruginosa* and *Acinetobacter* spp. are notorious for efflux-mediated β-lactam resistance. For example, in *P. aeruginosa*, upregulation of the MexAB-OprM (RND) combined with the organisms low outer membrane permeability can contribute to increased resistance to penicillins and cephalosporins (Li et al. 1994b), and the overexpression of the RND-type efflux pump AdeABC in *Acinetobacter baumannii* can contribute to a higher level of resistance to most β-lactams including carbapenems (Heritier et al. 2005). It has also been demonstrated that AcrAB-TolC

(RND) efflux plays a key role in β-lactam uptake and susceptibility in *H. influenzae* (Kaczmarek et al. 2004) and *K. pneumoniae* (Pages et al. 2009).

Future Perspectives

Antibiotic resistance is a constant threat that must be challenged with the same innovation and ingenuity by which it emerges. This ongoing struggle will likely rely on various combined strategies, some of which are touched upon here. Given that porin loss or downregulation is an effective way of limiting antibiotic entry, clever attempts are being made to avoid this form of resistance by taking advantage of other bacterial uptake machinery. For example, as many bacteria are heavily reliant upon iron for their survival, they secrete iron-chelating molecules known as siderophores that upon iron binding are transported back into the bacteria (reviewed in Saha et al. 2012). By fusing β-lactam and other drugs to siderophores, it is possible to bypass the need for porins to cross the bacterial outer membrane (reviewed in Mollmann et al. 2009). A promising example of this is the siderophore sulfactam BAL30072, currently in phase 1 clinical study (Landman et al. 2014). Similarly, inhibition of bacterial efflux systems is an appealing anti-resistance strategy, although past efforts with promising drugs have often faced in vivo toxicity related to cross inhibition of efflux pumps in human cells. However, certain phenothiazines, some of which are previously approved antipsychotic drugs, have recently been used for the successful efflux-targeted treatment of extremely drug-resistant mycobacterium tuberculosis (Abbate et al. 2011; Amaral and Molnar 2012; Amaral et al. 2008). Another approach is the development of new β-lactam and β-lactamase inhibitor combinations. Indeed, several examples of these are in phase 3 clinical trials, including ceftaroline-avibactam (Castanheira et al. 2014), ceftazidime-avibactam (Keepers et al. 2014), and ceftolozane-tazobactam (Sader et al. 2014). In addition, synergistic combinations of β-lactams and glycopeptides in overcoming resistance in strains such as VRSA have proven useful both in vitro and in animal models and may provide a viable option for patient treatment (Fox et al. 2006; McConeghy et al. 2013). Other non-β-lactam-related strategies are also being explored in the fight against resistance, including the use of the peptide antibiotics, vaccination, and phage therapy, to name a few (reviewed in Jovetic et al. 2010).

Conclusion

Fleming's fortuitous and triumphant discovery of the "miracle drug," penicillin, was shortly followed by the sobering observation that the improper use of the drug led to rapid bacterial resistance in the clinic and community. Indeed, resistance is a natural consequence of general antibiotic use against microorganisms that are exquisitely designed to persist against threats to their survival. As it is imperative to keep pace with continuing resistance by way of new antibiotic design, it is likewise increasingly necessary to understand resistance processes in order to expose strengths and weaknesses that may be exploited. It is furthermore of the utmost importance that we use our already present antibiotic artillery wisely and conscientiously, particularly with regard to the precious β-lactams that arguably distinguish themselves as the most valuable drugs in human history.

Acknowledgements We gratefully acknowledge the following funding agencies for supporting this work: Canadian Institute of Health Research (to SS, DTK, and NCJS), Howard Hughes Medical Institute (to NCJS), Canada Foundation for Innovation (to NCJS), British Columbia Knowledge Development Fund (to NCJS), and Michael Smith Foundation for Health Research (to SS).

References

Abbate E et al (2011) Successful alternative treatment of extensively drug-resistant tuberculosis in Argentina with a combination of linezolid, moxifloxacin and thioridazine. J Antimicrob Chemother 67:473–477

Abraham EP, Chain E (1988) An enzyme from bacteria able to destroy penicillin. 1940. Rev Infect Dis 10:677–678

Amaral L, Molnar J (2012) Potential therapy of multidrug-resistant and extremely drug-resistant tuberculosis with thioridazine. In Vivo 26:231–236

Amaral L, Martins M, Viveiros M, Molnar J, Kristiansen JE (2008) Promising therapy of XDR-TB/MDR-TB with thioridazine an inhibitor of bacterial efflux pumps. Curr Drug Targets 9:816–819

Amoroso A et al (2012) A peptidoglycan fragment triggers beta-lactam resistance in Bacillus licheniformis. PLoS Pathog 8:e1002571

Andersen C et al (2002) Transition to the open state of the TolC periplasmic tunnel entrance. Proc Natl Acad Sci U S A 99:11103–11108

Archer GL, Niemeyer DM, Thanassi JA, Pucci MJ (1994) Dissemination among staphylococci of DNA sequences associated with methicillin resistance. Antimicrob Agents Chemother 38:447–454

Baba T et al (2009) Complete genome sequence of Macrococcus caseolyticus strain JCSCS5402, [corrected] reflecting the ancestral genome of the human-pathogenic staphylococci. J Bacteriol 191:1180–1190

Bavro VN et al (2008) Assembly and channel opening in a bacterial drug efflux machine. Mol Cell 30:114–121

Bebrone C (2007) Metallo-beta-lactamases (classification, activity, genetic organization, structure, zinc coordination) and their superfamily. Biochem Pharmacol 74:1686–1701

Bebrone C et al (2009) The structure of the dizinc subclass B2 metallo-beta-lactamase CphA reveals that the second inhibitory zinc ion binds in the histidine site. Antimicrob Agents Chemother 53:4464–4471

Birck C et al (2004) X-ray crystal structure of the acylated beta-lactam sensor domain of BlaR1 from *Staphylococcus aureus* and the mechanism of receptor activation for signal transduction. J Am Chem Soc 126:13945–13947

Birnbaum J, Kahan FM, Kropp H, MacDonald JS (1985) Carbapenems, a new class of beta-lactam antibiotics. Discovery and development of imipenem/cilastatin. Am J Med 78:3–21

Bonfiglio G, Russo G, Nicoletti G (2002) Recent developments in carbapenems. Expert Opin Investig Drugs 11:529–544

Bowler LD, Zhang QY, Riou JY, Spratt BG (1994) Interspecies recombination between the penA genes of *Neisseria meningitidis* and commensal Neisseria species during the emergence of penicillin resistance in *N. meningitidis*: natural events and laboratory simulation. J Bacteriol 176:333–337

Brannigan JA, Tirodimos IA, Zhang QY, Dowson CG, Spratt BG (1990) Insertion of an extra amino acid is the main cause of the low affinity of penicillin-binding protein 2 in penicillin-resistant strains of *Neisseria gonorrhoeae*. Mol Microbiol 4:913–919

Brown MH, Paulsen IT, Skurray RA (1999) The multidrug efflux protein NorM is a prototype of a new family of transporters. Mol Microbiol 31:394–395

Bush K (2012) Evolution of beta-lactamases: past, present, and future. In: Dougherty TJ and Pucci MJ (ed) Antibiotic discovery and development. Springer, New York, pp 427–453

Bush K (2013) Proliferation and significance of clinically relevant beta-lactamases. Ann N Y Acad Sci 1277:84–90

Bush K, Macielag MJ (2010) New beta-lactam antibiotics and beta-lactamase inhibitors. Expert Opin Ther Pat 20:1277–1293

Buynak JD (2013) beta-Lactamase inhibitors: a review of the patent literature (2010–2013). Expert Opin Ther Pat 23:1469–1481

Castanheira M, Williams G, Jones RN, Sader HS (2014) Activity of ceftaroline-avibactam tested against contemporary Enterobacteriaceae isolates carrying beta-lactamases prevalent in the United States. Microb Drug Resist 20:436–440

Cha J, Mobashery S (2007) Lysine N(zeta)-decarboxylation in the BlaR1 protein from *Staphylococcus aureus* at the root of its function as an antibiotic sensor. J Am Chem Soc 129:3834–3835

Cha J, Vakulenko SB, Mobashery S (2007) Characterization of the beta-lactam antibiotic sensor domain of the MecR1 signal sensor/transducer protein from methicillin-resistant *Staphylococcus aureus*. Biochemistry 46:7822–7831

Dabernat H et al (2002) Diversity of beta-lactam resistance-conferring amino acid substitutions in penicillin-binding protein 3 of *Haemophilus influenzae*. Antimicrob Agents Chemother 46:2208–2218

de Seny D et al (2001) Metal ion binding and coordination geometry for wild type and mutants of metallo-beta -lactamase from Bacillus cereus 569/H/9 (BcII): a combined thermodynamic, kinetic, and spectroscopic approach. J Biol Chem 276:45065–45078

Delmas J et al (2010) Structural insights into substrate recognition and product expulsion in CTX-M enzymes. J Mol Biol 400:108–120

Deng X et al (2012) Expression of multidrug resistance efflux pump gene norA is iron responsive in *Staphylococcus aureus*. J Bacteriol 194:1753–1762

Docquier JD et al (2009) Crystal structure of the OXA-48 beta-lactamase reveals mechanistic diversity among class D carbapenemases. Chem Biol 16:540–547

Doumith M, Ellington MJ, Livermore DM, Woodford N (2009) Molecular mechanisms disrupting porin expression in ertapenem-resistant Klebsiella and Enterobacter spp. clinical isolates from the UK. J Antimicrob Chemother 63:659–667

Dowson CG, Coffey TJ, Spratt BG (1994) Origin and molecular epidemiology of penicillin-binding-protein-mediated resistance to beta-lactam antibiotics. Trends Microbiol 2:361–366

Duguid JP (1946) The sensitivity of bacteria to the action of penicillin. Edinb Med J 53:401–412

Ellis-Grosse EJ, Babinchak T, Dartois N, Rose G, Loh E (2005) The efficacy and safety of tigecycline in the treatment of skin and skin-structure infections: results of 2 double-blind phase 3 comparison studies with vancomycin-aztreonam. Clin Infect Dis 41(Suppl 5): S341–S353

Farra A, Islam S, Stralfors A, Sorberg M, Wretlind B (2008) Role of outer membrane protein OprD and penicillin-binding proteins in resistance of *Pseudomonas aeruginosa* to imipenem and meropenem. Int J Antimicrob Agents 31:427–433

Fenollar-Ferrer C, Donoso J, MuÃ ± oz F, Frau J (2008) Evolution of class C Î^{2}-lactamases: factors influencing their hydrolysis and recognition mechanisms. Theor Chem Accounts 121:209–218

Fernandez L, Hancock RE (2012) Adaptive and mutational resistance: role of porins and efflux pumps in drug resistance. Clin Microbiol Rev Springer, New York 25:661–681

Finberg RW, Guharoy R (2012) Monobactams. In: Clinical use of anti-infective agents Springer, New York pp 37–39

Fox PM, Lampen RJ, Stumpf KS, Archer GL, Climo MW (2006) Successful therapy of experimental endocarditis caused by vancomycin-resistant *Staphylococcus aureus* with a combination of vancomycin and beta-lactam antibiotics. Antimicrob Agents Chemother 50:2951–2956

Fuda C, Suvorov M, Vakulenko SB, Mobashery S (2004) The basis for resistance to beta-lactam antibiotics by penicillin-binding protein 2a of methicillin-resistant *Staphylococcus aureus*. J Biol Chem 279:40802–40806

Fuda C et al (2005) Activation for catalysis of penicillin-binding protein 2a from methicillin-resistant *Staphylococcus aureus* by bacterial cell wall. J Am Chem Soc 127:2056–2057

Galdiero S et al (2013) Microbe-host interactions: structure and role of Gram-negative bacterial porins. Curr Protein Pept Sci 13:843–854

Golemi D, Maveyraud L, Vakulenko S, Samama JP, Mobashery S (2001) Critical involvement of a carbamylated lysine in catalytic function of class D beta-lactamases. Proc Natl Acad Sci U S A 98:14280–14285

Goodell EW (1985) Recycling of murein by *Escherichia coli*. J Bacteriol 163:305–310

Hackbarth CJ, Chambers HF (1993) blaI and blaR1 regulate beta-lactamase and PBP 2a production in methicillin-resistant *Staphylococcus aureus*. Antimicrob Agents Chemother 37:1144–1149

Harder KJ, Nikaido H, Matsuhashi M (1981) Mutants of *Escherichia coli* that are resistant to certain beta-lactam compounds lack the ompF porin. Antimicrob Agents Chemother 20:549–552

Heritier C, Poirel L, Lambert T, Nordmann P (2005) Contribution of acquired carbapenem-hydrolyzing oxacillinases to carbapenem resistance in *Acinetobacter baumannii*. Antimicrob Agents Chemother 49:3198–3202

Hermann JC, Hensen C, Ridder L, Mulholland AJ, Holtje HD (2005) Mechanisms of antibiotic resistance: QM/MM modeling of the acylation reaction of a class A beta-lactamase with benzylpenicillin. J Am Chem Soc 127:4454–4465

Hernandez Valladares M et al (1997) Zn(II) dependence of the *Aeromonas hydrophila* AE036 metallo-beta-lactamase activity and stability. Biochemistry 36:11534–11541

Higgins MK, Bokma E, Koronakis E, Hughes C, Koronakis V (2004) Structure of the periplasmic component of a bacterial drug efflux pump. Proc Natl Acad Sci U S A 101:9994–9999

Hinchliffe P, Symmons MF, Hughes C, Koronakis V (2013) Structure and operation of bacterial tripartite pumps. Annu Rev Microbiol 67:221–242

Huang H, Hancock RE (1996) The role of specific surface loop regions in determining the function of the imipenem-specific pore protein OprD of *Pseudomonas aeruginosa*. J Bacteriol 178:3085–3090

Jacobs C, Huang LJ, Bartowsky E, Normark S, Park JT (1994) Bacterial cell wall recycling provides cytosolic muropeptides as effectors for beta-lactamase induction. EMBO J 13:4684–4694

Jacoby GA (2009) AmpC beta-lactamases. Clin Microbiol Rev 22:161–182, Table of Contents

Johnson JW, Fisher JF, Mobashery S (2012) Bacterial cell-wall recycling. Ann N Y Acad Sci 1277:54–75

Jovetic S, Zhu Y, Marcone GL, Marinelli F, Tramper J (2010) beta-Lactam and glycopeptide antibiotics: first and last line of defense? Trends Biotechnol 28:596–604

Kaczmarek FS et al (2004) Genetic and molecular characterization of beta-lactamase-negative ampicillin-resistant *Haemophilus influenzae* with unusually high resistance to ampicillin. Antimicrob Agents Chemother 48:1630–1639

Keefer CS, Blake FG, Marshall EK, Lockwood JS, Wood WB (1943) Penicillin in the treatment of infections. J Am Med Assoc 122:1217–1224

Keepers TR, Gomez M, Celeri C, Nichols WW, Krause KM (2014) Bactericidal activity, absence of serum effect, and time-kill kinetics of ceftazidime-avibactam against beta-lactamase-producing Enterobacteriaceae and *Pseudomonas aeruginosa*. Antimicrob Agents Chemother 58:5297–5305

Kim C et al (2012) Properties of a novel PBP2A protein homolog from *Staphylococcus aureus* strain LGA251 and its contribution to the beta-lactam-resistant phenotype. J Biol Chem 287:36854–36863

King DT, Strynadka NC (2012) Targeting metallo-beta-lactamase enzymes in antibiotic resistance. Future Med Chem 5:1243–1263

Koronakis V, Sharff A, Koronakis E, Luisi B, Hughes C (2000) Crystal structure of the bacterial membrane protein TolC central to multidrug efflux and protein export. Nature 405:914–919

Lambert PA (2005) Bacterial resistance to antibiotics: modified target sites. Adv Drug Deliv Rev 57:1471–1485

Landman D et al (2014) In vitro activity of the siderophore monosulfactam BAL30072 against contemporary Gram-negative pathogens from New York City, including multidrug-resistant isolates. Int J Antimicrob Agents 43:527–532

Lewis K (1994) Multidrug resistance pumps in bacteria: variations on a theme. Trends Biochem Sci 19:119–123

Li XZ, Ma D, Livermore DM, Nikaido H (1994a) Role of efflux pump(s) in intrinsic resistance of *Pseudomonas aeruginosa*: active efflux as a contributing factor to beta-lactam resistance. Antimicrob Agents Chemother 38:1742–1752

Li XZ, Livermore DM, Nikaido H (1994b) Role of efflux pump(s) in intrinsic resistance of *Pseudomonas aeruginosa*: resistance to tetracycline, chloramphenicol, and norfloxacin. Antimicrob Agents Chemother 38:1732–1741

Lim D, Strynadka NC (2002) Structural basis for the beta lactam resistance of PBP2a from methicillin-resistant *Staphylococcus aureus*. Nat Struct Biol 9:870–876

Llarrull LI, Mobashery S (2012) Dissection of events in the resistance to beta-lactam antibiotics mediated by the protein BlaR1 from *Staphylococcus aureus*. Biochemistry 51:4642–4649

Lomovskaya O, Zgurskaya HI, Totrov M, Watkins WJ (2007) Waltzing transporters and 'the dance macabre' between humans and bacteria. Nat Rev Drug Discov 6:56–65

Lou H et al (2011) Altered antibiotic transport in OmpC mutants isolated from a series of clinical strains of multi-drug resistant *E. coli*. PLoS One 6(e25825)

Lovering AL, Safadi SS, Strynadka NC (2012) Structural perspective of peptidoglycan biosynthesis and assembly. Annu Rev Biochem 81:451–478

Macheboeuf P, Contreras-Martel C, Job V, Dideberg O, Dessen A (2006) Penicillin binding proteins: key players in bacterial cell cycle and drug resistance processes. FEMS Microbiol Rev 30:673–691

Majiduddin FK, Materon IC, Palzkill TG (2002) Molecular analysis of beta-lactamase structure and function. Int J Med Microbiol 292:127–137

Marrero A, Mallorqui-Fernandez G, Guevara T, Garcia-Castellanos R, Gomis-Ruth FX (2006) Unbound and acylated structures of the MecR1 extracellular antibiotic-sensor domain provide insights into the signal-transduction system that triggers methicillin resistance. J Mol Biol 361:506–521

Maveyraud L et al (1998) Structural basis for clinical longevity of carbapenem antibiotics in the face of challenge by the common class A Î^2-lactamases from the antibiotic-resistant bacteria. J Am Chem Soc 120:9748–9752

McConeghy KW, Bleasdale SC, Rodvold KA (2013) The empirical combination of vancomycin and a beta-lactam for Staphylococcal bacteremia. Clin Infect Dis 57:1760–1765

McKinney TK, Sharma VK, Craig WA, Archer GL (2001) Transcription of the gene mediating methicillin resistance in *Staphylococcus aureus* (mecA) is corepressed but not coinduced by cognate mecA and beta-lactamase regulators. J Bacteriol 183:6862–6868

Mikolosko J, Bobyk K, Zgurskaya HI, Ghosh P (2006) Conformational flexibility in the multidrug efflux system protein AcrA. Structure 14:577–587

Milheirico C, Portelinha A, Krippahl L, de Lencastre H, Oliveira DC (2011) Evidence for a purifying selection acting on the beta-lactamase locus in epidemic clones of methicillin-resistant *Staphylococcus aureus*. BMC Microbiol 11:76

Miller EL (2002) The penicillins: a review and update. J Midwifery Women's Health 47:426–434

Mollmann U, Heinisch L, Bauernfeind A, Kohler T, Ankel-Fuchs D (2009) Siderophores as drug delivery agents: application of the "Trojan Horse" strategy. Biometals 22:615–624

Murakami S, Nakashima R, Yamashita E, Yamaguchi A (2002) Crystal structure of bacterial multidrug efflux transporter AcrB. Nature 419:587–593
Murakami S, Nakashima R, Yamashita E, Matsumoto T, Yamaguchi A (2006) Crystal structures of a multidrug transporter reveal a functionally rotating mechanism. Nature 443:173–179
Neu HC (1982) The new beta-lactamase-stable cephalosporins. Ann Intern Med 97:408–419
Nikaido H, Takatsuka Y (2009) Mechanisms of RND multidrug efflux pumps. Biochim Biophys Acta 1794:769–781
Nordmann P, Cuzon G, Naas T (2009) The real threat of Klebsiella pneumoniae carbapenemase-producing bacteria. Lancet Infect Dis 9:228–236
Nordmann P, Poirel L, Walsh TR, Livermore DM (2011) The emerging NDM carbapenemases. Trends Microbiol 19:588–595
Ochs MM, McCusker MP, Bains M, Hancock RE (1999) Negative regulation of the *Pseudomonas aeruginosa* outer membrane porin OprD selective for imipenem and basic amino acids. Antimicrob Agents Chemother 43:1085–1090
Okamoto T et al (2002) A change in PBP1 is involved in amoxicillin resistance of clinical isolates of *Helicobacter pylori*. J Antimicrob Chemother 50:849–856
Otero LH et al (2013) How allosteric control of *Staphylococcus aureus* penicillin binding protein 2a enables methicillin resistance and physiological function. Proc Natl Acad Sci U S A 110:16808–16813
Paetzel M et al (2000) Crystal structure of the class D beta-lactamase OXA-10. Nat Struct Biol 7:918–925
Page MGP (2000) Beta-lactamase inhibitors. Drug Resist Updat 3:109–125
Page MGP (2012) β-lactam antibiotics. In: Dougherty TJ and Pucci MJ (ed) Antibiot Discov Dev Springer, New York, 79–117
Page MI, Badarau A (2008) The mechanisms of catalysis by metallo beta-lactamases. Bioinorg Chem Appl 576297 10.1155/2008/576297
Pages JM et al (2009) Efflux pump, the masked side of beta-lactam resistance in *Klebsiella pneumoniae* clinical isolates. PLoS One 4:e4817
Papp-Wallace KM, Endimiani A, Taracila MA, Bonomo RA (2011) Carbapenems: past, present, and future. Antimicrob Agents Chemother 55:4943–4960
Payne DJ, Cramp R, Winstanley DJ, Knowles DJ (1994) Comparative activities of clavulanic acid, sulbactam, and tazobactam against clinically important beta-lactamases. Antimicrob Agents Chemother 38:767–772
Pernot L et al (2004) A PBP2x from a clinical isolate of *Streptococcus pneumoniae* exhibits an alternative mechanism for reduction of susceptibility to beta-lactam antibiotics. J Biol Chem 279:16463–16470
Philippon A, Arlet G, Jacoby GA (2002) Plasmid-determined AmpC-type beta-lactamases. Antimicrob Agents Chemother 46:1–11
Pinho MG, de Lencastre H, Tomasz A (2001) An acquired and a native penicillin-binding protein cooperate in building the cell wall of drug-resistant staphylococci. Proc Natl Acad Sci U S A 98:10886–10891
Poirel L, Potron A, Nordmann P (2012) OXA-48-like carbapenemases: the phantom menace. J Antimicrob Chemother 67:1597–1606
Pos KM (2009) Drug transport mechanism of the AcrB efflux pump. Biochim Biophys Acta 1794:782–793
Queenan AM, Shang W, Flamm R, Bush K (2009) Hydrolysis and inhibition profiles of beta-lactamases from molecular classes A to D with doripenem, imipenem, and meropenem. Antimicrob Agents Chemother 54:565–569
Reith J, Mayer C (2011) Peptidoglycan turnover and recycling in Gram-positive bacteria. Appl Microbiol Biotechnol 92:1–11
Rolinson GN, Geddes AM (2007) The 50th anniversary of the discovery of 6-aminopenicillanic acid (6-APA). Int J Antimicrob Agents 29:3–8

Ropp PA, Hu M, Olesky M, Nicholas RA (2002) Mutations in ponA, the gene encoding penicillin-binding protein 1, and a novel locus, penC, are required for high-level chromosomally mediated penicillin resistance in *Neisseria gonorrhoeae*. Antimicrob Agents Chemother 46:769–777

Ryffel C, Kayser FH, Berger-Bachi B (1992) Correlation between regulation of mecA transcription and expression of methicillin resistance in staphylococci. Antimicrob Agents Chemother 36:25–31

Sabath LD, Abraham EP (1966) Zinc as a cofactor for cephalosporinase from Bacillus cereus 569. Biochem J 98:11C–13C

Sader HS, Farrell DJ, Castanheira M, Flamm RK, Jones RN (2014) Antimicrobial activity of ceftolozane/tazobactam tested against *Pseudomonas aeruginosa* and Enterobacteriaceae with various resistance patterns isolated in European hospitals (2011–12). J Antimicrob Chemother 69:2713–2722

Saha R, Saha N, Donofrio RS, Bestervelt LL (2012) Microbial siderophores: a mini review. J Basic Microbiol 53:303–317

Sauvage E et al (2002) The 2.4-A crystal structure of the penicillin-resistant penicillin-binding protein PBP5fm from *Enterococcus faecium* in complex with benzylpenicillin. Cell Mol Life Sci 59:1223–1232

Sauvage E, Kerff F, Terrak M, Ayala JA, Charlier P (2008) The penicillin-binding proteins: structure and role in peptidoglycan biosynthesis. FEMS Microbiol Rev 32:234–258

Seeger MA et al (2006) Structural asymmetry of AcrB trimer suggests a peristaltic pump mechanism. Science 313:1295–1298

Shore AC, Coleman DC (2013) Staphylococcal cassette chromosome mec: recent advances and new insights. Int J Med Microbiol 303:350–359

Strynadka NC et al (1992) Molecular structure of the acyl-enzyme intermediate in beta-lactam hydrolysis at 1.7 A resolution. Nature 359:700–705

Strynadka NC, Martin R, Jensen SE, Gold M, Jones JB (1996) Structure-based design of a potent transition state analogue for TEM-1 beta-lactamase. Nat Struct Biol 3:688–695

Su CC et al (2011) Crystal structure of the CusBA heavy-metal efflux complex of *Escherichia coli*. Nature 470:558–562

Swaren P et al (1995) Electrostatic analysis of TEM1 beta-lactamase: effect of substrate binding, steep potential gradients and consequences of site-directed mutations. Structure 3:603–613

Symmons MF, Bokma E, Koronakis E, Hughes C, Koronakis V (2009) The assembled structure of a complete tripartite bacterial multidrug efflux pump. Proc Natl Acad Sci U S A 106:7173–7178

Szarecka A, Lesnock KR, Ramirez-Mondragon CA, Nicholas HB Jr, Wymore T (2011) The Class D beta-lactamase family: residues governing the maintenance and diversity of function. Protein Eng Des Sel 24:801–809

Tipper DJ, Strominger JL (1965) Mechanism of action of penicillins: a proposal based on their structural similarity to acyl-D-alanyl-D-alanine. Proc Natl Acad Sci U S A 54:1133–1141

Tsubakishita S, Kuwahara-Arai K, Baba T, Hiramatsu K (2010) Staphylococcal cassette chromosome mec-like element in Macrococcus caseolyticus. Antimicrob Agents Chemother 54:1469–1475

Turner PJ (2005) Extended-spectrum beta-lactamases. Clin Infect Dis 41(Suppl 4):S273–S275

Typas A, Banzhaf M, Gross CA, Vollmer W (2011) From the regulation of peptidoglycan synthesis to bacterial growth and morphology. Nat Rev Microbiol 10:123–136

Vercheval L et al (2010) Three factors that modulate the activity of class D beta-lactamases and interfere with the post-translational carboxylation of Lys70. Biochem J 432:495–504

Walsh TR (2010) Emerging carbapenemases: a global perspective. Int J Antimicrob Agents 36 (Suppl 3):S8–S14

Walsh TR, Toleman MA, Poirel L, Nordmann P (2005) Metallo-beta-lactamases: the quiet before the storm? Clin Microbiol Rev 18:306–325

Wang Z, Fast W, Valentine AM, Benkovic SJ (1999) Metallo-beta-lactamase: structure and mechanism. Curr Opin Chem Biol 3:614–622

Waxman DJ, Strominger JL (1983) Penicillin-binding proteins and the mechanism of action of beta-lactam antibiotics. Annu Rev Biochem 52:825–869

Wilke MS, Hills TL, Zhang HZ, Chambers HF, Strynadka NC (2004) Crystal structures of the Apo and penicillin-acylated forms of the BlaR1 beta-lactam sensor of *Staphylococcus aureus*. J Biol Chem 279:47278–47287

Wise EM Jr, Park JT (1965) Penicillin: its basic site of action as an inhibitor of a peptide cross-linking reaction in cell wall mucopeptide synthesis. Proc Natl Acad Sci U S A 54:75–81

Xu D, Xie D, Guo H (2006) Catalytic mechanism of class B2 metallo-beta-lactamase. J Biol Chem 281:8740–8747

Yao Z, Kahne D, Kishony R (2012) Distinct single-cell morphological dynamics under beta-lactam antibiotics. Mol Cell 48:705–712

Yong D et al (2009) Characterization of a new metallo-beta-lactamase gene, bla(NDM-1), and a novel erythromycin esterase gene carried on a unique genetic structure in Klebsiella pneumoniae sequence type 14 from India. Antimicrob Agents Chemother 53:5046–5054

Zhang HZ, Hackbarth CJ, Chansky KM, Chambers HF (2001) A proteolytic transmembrane signaling pathway and resistance to beta-lactams in staphylococci. Science 291:1962–1965

Antibiotic Resistance and Tolerance in Bacterial Biofilms

Geoffrey McKay and Dao Nguyen

Contents

G. McKay (✉)
Department of Medicine, McGill University, Montreal, QC, Canada
e-mail: geoffrey.mckay@mail.mcgill.ca

D. Nguyen
Department of Medicine, McGill University, Montreal, QC, Canada

Research Institute of McGill University Health Centre, Montreal, QC, Canada
e-mail: dao.nguyen@mcgill.ca

M. Gotte et al. (eds.), *Handbook of Antimicrobial Resistance*,
DOI 10.1007/978-1-4939-0694-9_11

Abstract

Bacteria can grow as multicellular communities called biofilms, and this sessile lifestyle is distinct from planktonic growth. While microbial biofilms are ubiquitous in the natural and industrial environment, their importance in human infections has only been fully recognized in the past few decades. Biofilm-associated bacteria typically cause subacute and chronic infections. Many bacterial pathogens, such as *Staphylococcus aureus,* readily form biofilms, and *Pseudomonas aeruginosa,* which causes chronic airway infections in patients with cystic fibrosis, is an important model organism for biofilm studies. They are clinically significant due to their persistence despite sustained antimicrobial treatments and adequate host defenses. Biofilm bacteria are highly resistant to a wide range of antimicrobial compounds and disinfectants, and the mechanisms underlying this resistance are likely multifactorial. This chapter will review the cellular processes and pathways implicated in antibiotic resistance and tolerance of bacterial biofilms.

Keywords

Biofilms • Antibiotic • Resistance • Tolerance • Infections • Pseudomonas aeruginosa

Introduction

Bacteria can grow as multicellular communities called biofilms, and this sessile lifestyle is distinct from planktonic growth. While microbial biofilms are ubiquitous in the natural and industrial environment, their importance in human infections has only been fully recognized in the past few decades (Potera 1999; Costerton et al. 1999; Parsek and Singh 2003). Biofilm-associated bacteria cause many subacute and chronic infections, ranging from periodontitis to chronic wound infections, endocarditis, chronic otitis media, osteomyelitis, recurrent urinary tract infection, medical device and indwelling catheter infections, and cystic fibrosis-associated airway infections. They are clinically significant due to their persistence despite sustained antimicrobial treatments and adequate host defenses. Many bacterial pathogens, such as *Staphylococcus aureus,* readily form biofilms, and *Pseudomonas aeruginosa,* which causes chronic airway infections in patients with cystic fibrosis, is an important model organism for biofilm studies. Biofilms are also often polymicrobial communities composed of multiple bacterial species.

Biofilms: Multicellular Communities Distinct from Unicellular Planktonic Organisms

Biofilms are multicellular aggregates, in which cells are encased in an extracellular polymeric matrix. In many natural and *in vivo* conditions, as well as in laboratory models, biofilm aggregates are adherent to a surface. For example, biofilms can grow attached to indwelling medical devices or dental surfaces. Biofilm aggregates can also be suspended at the air-liquid interface or within a semisolid environment, such as in the viscous sputum of cystic fibrosis patients (Ude et al. 2006; Alhede et al. 2011; Staudinger et al. 2014). Biofilm structures allow bacteria to grow at high-cell density and in close proximity, in contrast to planktonic bacteria growing as free-living individual cells in a liquid environment. The biofilm environment facilitates cell-cell communication (Parsek and Greenberg 2000) and horizontal transfer of virulence traits (Hausner and Wuertz 1999). In polymicrobial communities, the close proximity also promotes interspecies communication, metabolic and functional cooperation, or competition between different species. These complex interactions have implications on disease pathogenesis, host-pathogen relationships, as well as resistance to antibiotics and host defense mechanisms.

Biofilms differ significantly from planktonic bacteria on many levels. Global transcriptomic or proteomic studies have shown wide-ranging changes, with hundreds of genes and as much as 50 % of the proteome being differentially expressed during biofilm growth (Whiteley et al. 2001; Beenken et al. 2004; Folsom et al. 2010; Dotsch et al. 2012; Waite et al. 2005; Southey-Pillig et al. 2005; Sauer et al. 2002). It is important to note that laboratory biofilm models vary significantly, from continuous flow systems, 96-well plates, to colonies on agar surfaces or membranes, and such diverse experimental conditions have generated conflicting results on the differences between planktonic and biofilm cells (Mikkelsen et al. 2007). Although there are no hallmark gene or cellular processes that define biofilm bacteria, they typically have reduced motility, have increased production of extracellular polysaccharides, and can express specific protective factors not present during planktonic growth (Whiteley et al. 2001; Sauer et al. 2002).

In many bacterial species, the transition to biofilm growth is also associated with the downregulation of acute virulence factors, and this contributes to the persistence and chronic nature of biofilm infections. Biofilm bacteria are less invasive, causing less tissue destruction, and expression of key ligands recognized by the immune system, such as flagella, is repressed (Whiteley et al. 2001). Many studies have described the transition from planktonic to biofilm growth as an ordered process, starting with surface attachment, leading to microcolony formation and maturation, and followed by dispersal of biofilm cells back to a planktonic state (Sauer et al. 2002; O'Toole et al. 2000). While some experimental systems support the notion that biofilm formation is the result of such a structured process, this is likely not necessary nor universal across different bacterial species and conditions (Alhede et al. 2011; Staudinger et al. 2014; Sriramulu et al. 2005). Much research has also investigated the role of cell signaling in biofilm formation. Quorum sensing is a cell-cell signaling system in many gram-negative and gram-positive bacteria that controls cell density-dependent gene expression via the secretion and detection of chemical signals that accumulate as cell density increases. While the chemical signals and genes under quorum sensing control differ between different bacterial species, quorum sensing allows bacteria to respond and coordinate their gene expression in response to population density (Waters and Bassler 2005). In *P. aeruginosa*, quorum sensing can alter biofilm formation through multiple different pathways: swarming (a form of surface motility), production of rhamnolipids (a surfactant that influences biofilm structures), LecA (a carbohydrate-binding lectin involved in surface adhesion), or the exopolysaccharide Psl (Shrout et al. 2011). In recent years, the second messenger cyclic-di-GMP (c-di-GMP) has emerged as a conserved signal that controls the switch between motile planktonic states and sessile biofilm formation in several bacterial species (Romling et al. 2013).

Biofilms: A Sheltered Lifestyle that Confers High Resistance and Tolerance to Antibiotics

Biofilm growth confers many advantages to bacteria, allowing them to better survive and adapt to diverse environmental stresses encountered in the natural and host environment. A hallmark of biofilm bacteria is their remarkable resistance and tolerance to a wide range of biocides, antibiotics, and host defenses, which play a key role in their persistence during chronic infections. Multiple mechanisms are at work, some regulated through biofilm-specific mechanisms, while others are physiological adaptions to the biofilm microenvironment.

Antibiotic resistance typically refers to an inheritable trait that allows bacteria to replicate at elevated concentrations of antibiotics and is defined by increased minimal inhibitory concentrations (MIC) of antibiotics. Such resistance mechanisms may be intrinsic or acquired and include antibiotic-modifying enzymes, genetic mutations of target molecules, low membrane permeability, or drug efflux pumps. While the term biofilm "resistance" is widely used in the literature, this term can be misleading as it often refers to tolerance (also variably called non-inherited resistance, drug indifference, or persistence), a phenotypic characteristic where bacteria are refractory to antibiotic or biocide killing in the absence of inheritable resistance mechanisms or genetic mutations. Distinct from resistant bacteria, tolerant ones remain viable but do not grow at elevated concentrations of antibiotics. This phenotypic tolerance is also reversible when biofilm bacteria resume a planktonic state (Anwar et al. 1989). This chapter will be focused on the mechanisms involved in both antibiotic resistance and tolerance of biofilms. While the concepts of resistance and tolerance are distinct, the contribution of specific mechanisms to one or the other is not always well defined, and many studies do not make this distinction. For this review, the term tolerance will be used whenever the studies specifically defined and addressed this phenotype.

Biofilm-Specific Mechanisms of Resistance

Matrix and Diffusion Barriers

Biofilm bacteria are embedded in a self-produced extracellular matrix (also termed extracellular polymeric substances or EPS) typically composed of extracellular polysaccharides, DNA, and proteins. The matrix can represent up to 90 % of the biofilm biomass, and its exact composition, while often poorly characterized, can vary considerably dependent on the strains, species, and growth conditions (such as nutrient source and shear forces) (Zogaj et al. 2001; Branda et al. 2005). The EPS provides mechanical structure to multicellular aggregates and promotes physical aggregation and surface adhesion. Due to its physicochemical properties, the EPS acts as a molecular sieve that can confer a protective barrier against some antimicrobial compounds, including disinfectants and antibiotics. While the diffusion barrier and limited penetration of antimicrobials were originally thought to play a primary role in biofilm resistance, more recent research suggests that its contribution to the overall biofilm resistance is more limited.

Extracellular Polymeric Substances (EPS)

Exopolysaccharides are a major component of the EPS in several bacterial species, such as *Bacillus subtilis, P. aeruginosa*, and *S. aureus* (Branda et al. 2005). These polymers are composed of different polysaccharides, from sucrose-derived glucans and fructans, cellulose, or mixtures of neutral and charged heteropolysaccharides. Their chemical composition and substituents determine the physicochemical properties of the EPS. Most known exopolysaccharides are polyanionic, but polycationic exopolysaccharides such as b-1,6-linked *N*-acetylglucosamine are found in staphylococcal biofilms, for example (Gotz 2002). The exopolysaccharide composition varies considerably from one species to another and even between strains of the same species.

Exopolysaccharides have been identified in biofilms from natural environments, laboratory experimental systems, as well as biofilms associated with human infections. Mutants lacking components of the EPS produce biofilms with altered morphology or reduced surface adhesion. While exopolysaccharides clearly have a role in the adhesion and structure of biofilms, their role in antibiotic resistance is still poorly defined. Exopolysaccharides may sequester charged molecules or indirectly alter the EPS structure. Across several studies comparing biofilm resistance to different antibiotics, the positively charged aminoglycosides appear to be most susceptible to the sequestering effect of exopolysaccharides.

Pseudomonas aeruginosa produces at least three chemically distinct polymers for its EPS: alginate, Pel, and Psl. Alginate is a polymer of uronic acids and among the best-studied exopolysaccharides. While alginate is not required for biofilm formation (Wozniak et al. 2003) and is not produced by all *P. aeruginosa* strains, it is overproduced by mucoid *P. aeruginosa* variants isolated from cystic fibrosis patients. In several laboratory biofilm models, alginate-overproducing strains formed biofilms more tolerant to aminoglycoside treatment than wild-type strains (Alkawash et al. 2006), and alginate can inhibit diffusion of aminoglycosides (Gordon et al. 1988), suggesting that alginate has a protective role against aminoglycosides. Studies with Pel-deficient mutants or Pel-overexpressing strains show a limited role in biofilm resistance to aminoglycosides and aztreonam, but the contribution of Pel is likely strain-specific and most significant in the Psl-negative strain PA14 (Colvin et al. 2011; Khan et al. 2010; Yu et al. 2012). Psl may also be involved in resistance to detergents, as Psl-deficient mutants form biofilms susceptible to polysorbate-80, while Psl overproduction confers resistance (Zegans et al. 2012). The mechanism of this resistance remains unknown.

Extracellular Proteins

Various extracellular proteins can accumulate within the biofilm EPS. Many enzymes are involved in the degradation of EPS constituents, while others nonenzymatic proteins are involved in EPS stability and structure, such as the carbohydrate-binding proteins (lectins) (Lynch et al. 2007; Diggle et al. 2006). Periplasmic beta-lactamases may be released in the EPS following cell death or by membrane vesicles, but their contribution to biofilm resistance to beta-lactams remains unclear (Ciofu et al. 2000).

Extracellular DNA

Extracellular DNA (eDNA) is passively or actively released by bacteria, and can be a major constituent of the EPS in certain bacterial species. eDNA primarily provides a structural role and enhances aggregation and stability of biofilms. Interestingly, exogenous eDNA can induce resistance to cationic antimicrobial peptides and aminoglycosides in *P. aeruginosa* by sequestering cations and inducing PhoPQ/PmrAB-mediated LPS modifications (Mulcahy et al. 2008). However, it remains unclear whether the eDNA in the biofilm EPS is sufficient to induce the PhoPQ/PmrAB systems (Pamp et al. 2008).

Diffusion of Antimicrobial Compounds

The biofilm EPS contains a mixture of charged or hydrophobic polymers that can sequester or limit the penetration of molecules. Although the protective barrier function of the EPS was initially proposed as a major mechanism of biofilm resistance, many studies now suggest that this diffusion limitation only plays a minor role. Biofilms grown on dialysis membranes retarded the diffusion of piperacillin, a weakly anionic beta-lactam, while high Ca^{2+} concentrations further reduced its diffusion (Hoyle et al. 1992). *Pseudomonas aeruginosa* biofilms sequestered and delayed the diffusion of tobramycin (a positively charged aminoglycoside) but not ciprofloxacin (a neutral fluoroquinolone) (Walters et al. 2003; Shigeta et al. 1997; Yasuda et al. 1993; Beloin et al. 2004). Kumon et al. examined the diffusion of antimicrobials through alginate: only aminoglycosides and polypeptides showed limited diffusion, while beta-lactams, fluoroquinolones, and macrolides did not (Kumon et al. 1994). Biocides such as hypochlorite also do now show any significant limitation in diffusion (Stewart et al. 2001). Taken together, these studies show that the diffusion rate and chemical structure of specific compounds do not correlate with their efficacy against biofilms. Among antibiotics, only aminoglycosides show a degree of limited penetration, and this likely does not fully account for the high tolerance of biofilms to these compounds (Vrany et al. 1997; Stewart 1996).

Other Biofilm-Specific Mechanisms

Liao et al. reported on BrlR, a Mer-like transcriptional regulator involved in both antibiotic tolerance and resistance to multiple antibiotics in *P. aeruginosa*. Inactivation of *brlR* reduced biofilm tolerance without altering susceptibility in planktonic bacteria (Liao and Sauer 2012). This is likely due to its high expression during biofilm but not planktonic growth. While the mechanism of BrlR is still unknown, MerR family members can activate the expression of multidrug efflux pumps. Since *brlR* is induced under oxygen-limiting conditions (Trunk et al. 2010), Liao et al. speculate that such conditions may lead to high *brlR* expression in biofilms.

Other examples of biofilm-specific mechanisms of antibiotic resistance include periplasmic glucans. In *P. aeruginosa*, *ndvB* encodes a glucosyltransferase required for the synthesis of periplasmic glucans, which is preferentially expressed during biofilm growth and may contribute to biofilm resistance by sequestering antibiotics (Mah et al. 2003).

Physiologic Heterogeneity

In contrast to well-mixed planktonic bacterial cultures, biofilms are bacterial aggregates where subpopulations encounter diverse microenvironments, leading to a physiologically heterogeneous population (Fig. 1). This heterogeneity is therefore a central characteristic of biofilm communities that confers antibiotic tolerance to biofilm bacteria through multiple different mechanisms (Stewart and Franklin 2008).

The heterogeneous physical environment, and the nutrient consumption and metabolism by spatially distinct bacterial subpopulations lead to gradients in nutrient and oxygen availability within biofilm aggregates (Stewart and Franklin 2008). The microenvironment within biofilms also changes over time, as the biofilm structure and surrounding physicochemical environment change during biofilm development and maturation. Different bacterial subpopulations therefore respond to their local

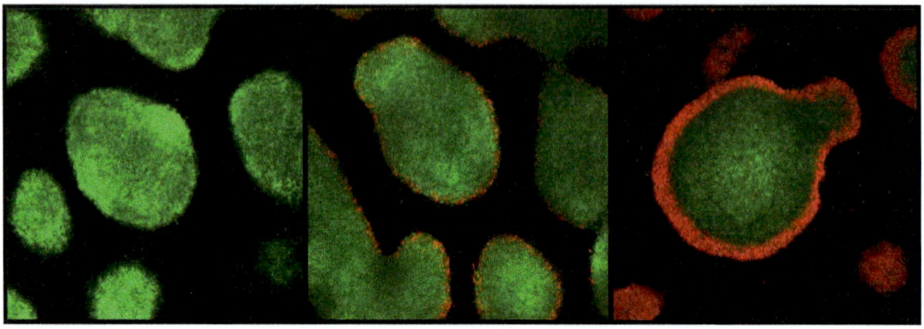

Fig. 1 Confocal microscopy images of *P. aeruginosa* biofilms grown in flow cell chambers. Mature biofilms are challenged with tobramycin for 0–24 h: bacterial killing occurs only in a subpopulation of biofilm cells located in the "outer layers" of biofilm aggregates. Viable bacteria are labeled with GFP (*green*) and dead cells are stained with propidium iodine (*red*) (Images were kindly provided by Pradeep Singh (U. Washington))

environments and express distinct biological activities, metabolic pathways, and stress responses. For example, biofilm bacteria may respond to microaerophilic or anaerobic conditions, pH stress, or nutrient limitation. Concentrations of solutes such as nitrate (Schramm et al. 1996), hydrogen peroxide (Lu et al. 1998), chlorine (De Beer et al. 1994a), or oxygen (Borriello et al. 2004) have been determined experimentally. This creates gradients in growth rate and metabolic activity and induces stress responses.

Several studies using reporter fusions (e.g., GFP, LacZ, alkaline phosphatase), dyes staining for nucleic acids or cell membrane permeability clearly demonstrated the physiological heterogeneity of biofilm communities (Stewart and Franklin 2008; Serra et al. 2013). Transcriptomic studies also support the importance of such environmental conditions on biofilm cells' physiology (Beenken et al. 2004; Folsom et al. 2010; Dotsch et al. 2012). However, it is worth noting that these global approaches, which typically analyze the bacterial population as an average, are not well suited to capture the heterogeneity present within biofilms (An and Parsek 2007). The total RNA abundance as well as the amount of specific RNA sequences can vary by over 100-fold in different biofilm subpopulations when measured by laser capture microdissection microscopy combined with qRT-PCR (Lenz et al. 2008; Pérez-Osorio et al. 2010).

Metabolic and Growth Rate

It has been long reported that the ability of antibiotics (such as β-lactams) to kill bacteria was linked to bacterial growth rate. Using chemostat systems where the rate of bacterial replication is controlled by the influx of nutrients, the killing rate of *Escherichia coli* by beta-lactam antibiotics was proportional to the bacterial generation time (Tuomanen et al. 1986; Cozens et al. 1986; Evans et al. 1991;

Brown et al. 1988). Thus, nongrowing cells are generally tolerant to antibiotics. Using an IPTG-inducible GFP reporter as an indicator of metabolic activity, Kim et al. sorted biofilm cells by flow cytometry based on their GFP fluorescence. By challenging the bright (active) and dim (dormant) cells with antibiotics or biocides, they determined that active cells were slightly more tolerant to tobramycin and silver ions but not ciprofloxacin (Kim et al. 2009). These results suggest that metabolic activity may determine tolerance to certain antibiotics (such as aminoglycosides) but not others (such as fluoroquinolones). The latter observation is not surprising, with others observing that fluoroquinolones are effective at killing non-replicating or stationary phase cells (Dalhoff et al. 1995; Zeiler 1985).

It has been frequently suggested that biofilm growth leads to steep gradients in growth rate and metabolic activity, and slow-growing or metabolically inactive subpopulations are thus more tolerant to antibiotic killing. For example, using an *rrnBP1*-GFP reporter where the growth rate-regulated *rrnBP1* promoter is fused to a short half-life GFP reporter, Sternberg et al. monitored the rates of rRNA synthesis in *E. coli* biofilms (Sternberg et al. 1999). With confocal microscopy imaging, they detected subpopulations in the center of biofilm aggregates showing reduced metabolic rate, while those in the outer layers of biofilm aggregates had high metabolic rate. Similar spatial patterns were observed by several others (Walters et al. 2003; Werner et al. 2004). While the use of GFP-based reporters provides elegant visualization of live biofilm cells over time and space without disrupting biofilm growth and structures, GFP does not mature under anaerobic conditions. These fluorescent reporters can thus pose a limitation in inferring metabolic or growth rate in the presence of oxygen gradients and anaerobic microenvironments within biofilms (as described in the next section).

Using laser capture microdissection microscopy combined with qRT-PCR, Lenz et al. and Perez-Osorio et al. demonstrated that mRNA levels for individual genes vary significantly across different biofilm sections in *P. aeruginosa*, using both drip flow biofilm and colony biofilm models (Lenz et al. 2008; Pérez-Osorio et al. 2010). These included housekeeping genes (*acpP*), quorum sensing (*rhlR*), and quorum sensing-regulated genes (*aprA, phzA1*) and the stationary phase sigma factor *rpoS*. Furthermore, Lenz et al. showed that the 16S rRNA to rDNA ratio varied across different biofilm layers, with the inner bacterial subpopulations showing rRNA/rDNA ratio similar to stationary phase cells and the outer layer subpopulations showing a higher rRNA/rDNA ratio closer to exponential phase cells (Lenz et al. 2008).

Oxygen Gradients

The oxygen gradient is primarily determined by the rate of consumption by the layers of cells first exposed to oxygen but also by the overall balance of diffusion. The role of oxygen availability in determining the local physiological responses has been well documented (Folsom et al. 2010; Xu et al. 1998). Significant oxygen gradients can be measured by microelectrodes in laboratory-grown biofilm structures formed by aerobic or facultative anaerobic bacteria (Walters et al. 2003; Borriello et al. 2004; de Beer et al. 1994b), with oxygen concentrations declining within the depths of biofilm structures. The presence of anaerobic microenvironments explains the growth of strict anaerobes within aerated biofilms, such as dental plaques (Kolenbrander 2000). Several transcriptomic studies show activation of genes involved in anaerobic metabolism during biofilm growth (Folsom et al. 2010; Phillips et al. 2012; Patell et al. 2010). Furthermore, the *P. aeruginosa* terminal oxidases required for growth under microaerophilic conditions are also required for optimal biofilm growth (Alvarez-Ortega and Harwood 2007). Xu et al. also used alkaline phosphatase activity as a physiological indicator of biofilm bacteria in phosphate-limiting conditions. They demonstrated a gradient of alkaline phosphatase activity, primarily determined by oxygen concentration (Xu et al. 1998).

Oxygen availability to biofilm subpopulations correlates with their antibiotic tolerance (Walters et al. 2003; Borriello et al. 2004; Werner et al. 2004; Tresse et al. 1995). Borriello et al. showed that bacterial subpopulations growing in oxygen replete biofilm regions were more readily killed by several classes of antibiotics compared to subpopulations growing in oxygen-limited regions (Borriello et al. 2004). Similarly, Werner showed that antibiotic-induced cell damage (filamentation, cell vacuolization, and lysis) were predominantly at the air-biofilm interface, within regions of high protein synthetic activity (as measured by IPTG-inducible GFP) (Werner et al. 2004). Antibiotic killing was also reduced when the biofilms were transferred to anaerobic conditions, an observation also reported by others (Field et al. 2005; Hill et al. 2005). Collectively, these studies suggest that oxygen-limited subpopulations exist within biofilms, and these are more tolerant to antibiotics. Whether the tolerance is directly due to oxygen depletion or anaerobic conditions per se, or whether it is caused by an indirect reduction in metabolic/growth rate, is still unclear. In the case of *P. aeruginosa*, a facultative anaerobe, growth stops under anaerobic conditions in the absence of an alternate electron acceptor (such as nitrate) or fermentation substrate (such as arginine). Borriello et al. thus investigated whether stimulating bacterial anaerobic metabolism could restore antibiotic susceptibility (Borriello et al. 2006). They showed that arginine and nitrate supplementation enhanced ciprofloxacin and tobramycin killing of *P. aeruginosa* biofilms grown under anaerobic conditions but not aerobic conditions. These findings support the idea that oxygen limitation confers a degree of antibiotic tolerance due to its effect on growth and metabolic rate.

Stress Responses

During biofilm growth, several stress responses are activated, which in turn can regulate cellular pathways that confer antibiotic resistance and tolerance. Such stress responses may be induced by the environmental cues that trigger the switch from planktonic to biofilm lifestyles or by the microenvironment created by biofilm growth. Interestingly, nonoptimal growth conditions can promote biofilm formation in many bacterial species. For example, biofilm formation is increased during growth in defined medium compared to rich medium (Castonguay et al. 2006; Wijman et al. 2007), and growth at reduced temperatures enhances surface adhesion and EPS production (Wijman et al. 2007; Perry et al. 2004; Sommerfeldt et al. 2009). Such stress may be environmental cues that promote cellular processes involved in both formation of biofilm structures as well as mechanisms of antibiotic resistance or tolerance.

Environmental and Nutrient Cues Affect Antibiotic Tolerance

Environmental and nutrient conditions have a significant impact on antibiotic tolerance and adaptive resistance, and biofilm growth creates nutrient gradients, with spatially distinct biofilm subpopulations experiencing nutrient limitation. While nutrient limitation may slow growth, it also induces specific stress responses that play an important protective role in antibiotic tolerance (Poole 2012). For example, cells in the central regions of *P. aeruginosa* biofilm aggregates are sufficiently limited for iron that expression of siderophores are induced as part of iron starvation responses (Kaneko et al. 2007; Banin et al. 2005). Iron limitation induces multidrug tolerance through several mechanisms. Importantly, intracellular iron homeostasis modulates the oxidative stress pathways that contribute to antibiotic killing (Kohanski et al. 2007; Frawley et al. 2013; Vinella et al. 2005; Yeom et al. 2010). Mg^{2+}, Ca^{2+}, and phosphate limitation also promote resistance to cationic antimicrobial peptides, and eDNA within the EPS matrix may chelate and limit Mg^{2+} and Ca^{2+} cations, as described in the section on eDNA (Macfarlane et al. 1999; Groisman et al. 1997). Finally, the carbon sources and transition can also affect antibiotic tolerance and the formation of persisters (Allison et al. 2011; Amato et al. 2013), suggesting that the nutrient environment within biofilms is an important determinant of antibiotic tolerance.

Stringent Response

The stringent response is a conserved bacterial stress response induced by amino acid, carbon, iron, and other nutrient limitation, as well as environmental stressors such as osmotic or temperature shifts (Cashel et al. 1996; Braeken et al. 2006). In response to stress, synthesis and accumulation of the signal (p)ppGpp (guanosine 5′-(tri) diphosphate, 3′-diphosphate), in cooperation with the action of DksA, trigger a widespread reorganization of cellular metabolism, macromolecule biosynthesis, and other protective cellular processes allowing stress adaptation and survival (Potrykus and Cashel 2008). (p)ppGpp likely promotes multidrug tolerance through multiple different mechanisms, from regulation of toxin-antitoxin modules and persister formation (Maisonneuve et al. 2011; Aizenman et al. 1996; Korch et al. 2003) to modulation of oxidative stress pathways (Khakimova et al. 2013; Nguyen et al. 2011). As a master regulator of the adaptive responses to nutrient and environmental stress, (p)ppGpp likely plays a central role in biofilm tolerance.

Nguyen et al. showed that *P. aeruginosa* and *E. coli* mutants lacking the (p)ppGpp synthetases RelA and SpoT, and thus unable to produce any (p)ppGpp, were profoundly susceptible to killing from multiple different classes of antibiotics, including quinolones, aminoglycosides, and antimicrobial peptides (Nguyen et al. 2011).

Oxidative Stress

Several observations support the idea that biofilms are an oxidative-stress-inducing environment. Oxidative DNA damage is increased and is associated with the increased genetic mutability in several species (Boles and Singh 2008; Ryder et al. 2012; Allegrucci and Sauer 2007) (Arce Miranda et al. 2011). Although discrepant results have been reported, several transcriptomic and proteomic studies reveal an upregulated response to oxidative stress and expression of antioxidant defenses (Resch et al. 2005; Patrauchan et al. 2007; van Alen et al. 2010; Kim et al. 2006; Tremoulet et al. 2002). This oxidative stress-rich environment can promote antibiotic resistance and tolerance to biofilm cells through several mechanisms. The increased genetic mutability promotes the emergence and selection of antibiotic-resistant mutants in biofilm bacterial populations (see section "Genetic Mutations and Horizontal Gene Transfer"). Oxidative stress induces multidrug efflux pumps (Chen et al. 2008; Fraud and Poole 2011; Miller and Sulavik 1996), and enhanced antioxidant defenses also contribute to antibiotic tolerance (Kohanski et al. 2007; Khakimova et al. 2013; Seneviratne et al. 2012). Finally, the SOS response and expression of *recA*, triggered by DNA damage, are also activated in *E. coli* biofilms and confer tolerance to quinolones (Beloin et al. 2004; Bernier et al. 2013; Dorr et al. 2010).

Envelope Stress and Other Stress Responses

Biofilm growth is associated with the activation of CpxA/CpxR stress responses (Beloin et al. 2004), a two-component regulatory system in *E. coli* that is triggered by various signals related to cell envelope stress (Dorel et al. 2006) and can mediate antibiotic resistance (Raivio et al. 2013). The role of the Cpx system in *E. coli* and AmgRS, a functionally similar system in *P. aeruginosa*, is discussed in the section "Two-Component Systems (TCS)."

RpoS (or σ^{38}), the stationary phase alternative sigma factor in γ- and β-proteobacteria (including *E. coli* and *P. aeruginosa*), controls many genes involved in a general stress response (Battesti et al. 2011; Potvin et al. 2008) and contributes to antibiotic tolerance (Hansen et al. 2008; Kayama et al. 2009). Since expression of RpoS or RpoS-regulated genes is induced in biofilms, this response may also contribute to biofilm antibiotic tolerance (Xu et al. 2001; Ito et al. 2009).

Persisters

Persisters are a subpopulation of bacteria that survive bactericidal antibiotics yet are genetically identical to susceptible bacteria. They show phenotypic multidrug tolerance and are often considered "dormant." Such cells replicate slowly and are metabolically inactive (Balaban et al. 2004; Shah et al. 2006; Wood et al. 2013). Persisters represent a very small fraction of exponentially growing planktonic cultures (approximately one in one million) but become more abundant in stationary phase planktonic cultures (Keren et al. 2004). Biofilm bacteria are also highly tolerant to multiple classes of antibiotics, and it has been proposed that biofilm growth gives rise to a greater fraction of multidrug tolerant persister cells (Wood et al. 2013; Lewis 2008).

What molecular pathways are involved in the persister phenotype and whether all persister cells are alike remain actively debated. Multiple mechanisms have been implicated in persister formation and have been extensively reviewed recently (Wood et al. 2013; Gerdes and Maisonneuve 2012; Balaban 2011; Kint et al. 2012; Cohen et al. 2013; Yamaguchi and Inouye 2011; Lewis 2010). A primary model for persister formation involves expression of toxin-antitoxin (TA) modules. TA systems are functionally redundant, with *E. coli* encoding at least 15 TA modules and *M. tuberculosis* encoding 88, for example. They typically include a stable toxin protein that disrupts an essential cellular process and a labile antitoxin (RNA or protein) that prevents toxicity. Degradation of antitoxins or overexpression of toxins in excess of their corresponding antitoxins induces a state of dormancy. Several studies have shown that persister formation and activation of TA systems require the stringent response alarmone (p)ppGpp (Maisonneuve et al. 2011; Aizenman et al. 1996; Korch et al. 2003). In particular, the Lon protease, which plays a major role in inactivating type II antitoxins in *E. coli*, is activated by (p)ppGpp levels (Maisonneuve et al. 2013). Persister formation may also be under stochastic control (Balaban et al. 2004; Fasani and Savageau 2013; Rotem et al. 2010), induced by the SOS response (Dorr et al. 2009), by specific carbon metabolism (Allison et al. 2011; Amato et al. 2013) or in response to a specific environmental cue (Vega et al. 2012).

Most studies on persisters have been done in planktonic bacteria. Whether persisters in biofilms arise from similar molecular mechanisms remains to be determined. Harrison et al. reported that deletion of the toxin-encoding gene *yafQ* reduced multidrug tolerance in *E. coli* biofilms but not stationary phase planktonic bacteria, and *yafQ* overexpression increases tolerance (Harrison et al. 2009). The persister phenotype presents many similarities with tolerant biofilm cells; it is thus compelling to infer that both tolerant populations share common mechanisms of tolerance. However, tolerant subpopulations in biofilms typically display distinct non-stochastic spatial patterns, in keeping with the physiological heterogeneity that arises from metabolic and stress gradients within biofilms. Such nutrient or environmental cues may signal or promote persister formation, including through activation of TA systems.

Cyclic Di-GMP (c-di-GMP)

C-di-GMP has emerged in recent years as an important intracellular secondary messenger in a wide range of bacteria, synthesized by GGDEF domain-containing diguanylate cyclases and hydrolyzed by EAL or HD-GYP domain-containing phosphodiesterases. C-di-GMP is implicated in biofilm formation, motility, virulence, and other cellular processes. Several recent reviews on c-di-GMP signaling and its function in bacteria were recently published (Romling et al. 2013; Romling 2012; Mills et al. 2011).

C-di-GMP plays a key role in the transition from the motile planktonic to sessile adherent biofilm lifestyle: through transcriptional, translational, and posttranslational mechanisms, c-di-GMP regulates multiple cellular functions required for biofilm growth. C-di-GMP downregulates bacterial motility, from flagellar (swimming and swarming) to type IV pilus surface (twitching) motility, thus promoting the initial transition from planktonic to biofilm growth and the detachment from biofilms back to planktonic growth. Furthermore, c-di-GMP can also regulate all components of the biofilm matrix, in particular EPS production, thus promoting bacterial surface adherence and biofilm formation.

Bacterial variants with increased c-di-GMP levels (such as small colony variants (SCV) described below) are associated with enhanced biofilm formation, surface adherence, and cell-cell aggregation. While such variants are associated with increased biofilm resistance, this is likely through indirect c-di-GMP-dependent regulation of EPS production (Starkey et al. 2009; Drenkard and Ausubel 2002), peptidoglycan cross-linking, and autolysin production (Luo and Helmann 2012).

Colony Variants

Small colony variants (SCV) are phenotypic variants that arise during biofilm growth and chronic infections, such as abscesses and cystic fibrosis airway infections. They can be observed in multiple bacterial species, including *S. aureus, P. aeruginosa, Streptococcus pneumonia, Salmonella enterica,* and *Vibrio cholerae* (Starkey et al. 2009; Proctor et al. 2006; Haussler et al. 2003; von Gotz et al. 2004; Allegrucci and Sauer 2008; Yildiz and Schoolnik 1999). They share a common colony morphology associated with slow growth and increased auto-aggregation that is attributed to the overexpression of exopolysaccharides (Starkey et al. 2009; Singh et al. 2010; Laham et al. 2007). SCV have an enhanced ability to form biofilms, can be more resistant to antibiotics, and are formed through several different genetic pathways (Proctor et al. 2006).

In *P. aeruginosa*, a subset of SCV have a rugose (or wrinkly) appearance, and mutations leading to increased intracellular levels of c-di-GMP levels are identified from rugose SCV (RSCV) isolated from both laboratory biofilms, as well as clinical isolates from cystic fibrosis patients (Starkey et al. 2009; Drenkard and Ausubel 2002; Meissner et al. 2007; Mikkelsen et al. 2009). Interestingly, environmental signals regulate the emergence of resistant RSCV, as their frequency increases during growth in the presence of NaCl, lower temperature, or minimal media (Drenkard and Ausubel 2002). SCV in *S. aureus* have also been extensively studied: different metabolic alterations in SCV cause their slow growth, and many SCV are deficient in electron transport (menadione or hemin auxotrophs) (Proctor et al. 2006). The latter likely is the cause of aminoglycoside resistance due to the loss of the proton motor force. *S. aureus* SCV overexpress the polysaccharide intercellular adhesin (PIA) (Singh et al. 2010).

While some of these variants share similar colony morphologies (e.g., SCV), the underlying genetic and molecular mechanisms are clearly varied. Similarly, the association between the SCV phenotype with increased antibiotic resistance during biofilm growth depends on the underlying molecular pathways involved.

Genetic Mutations and Horizontal Gene Transfer

Several studies have shown that biofilm growth leads to increased genetic diversification and horizontal gene transfer compared to planktonic growth, thus promoting the emergence of inheritable antibiotic resistance. Under antibiotic selective pressures, populations of antibiotic-resistant variants can expand (Molin and Tolker-Nielsen 2003; Driffield et al. 2008; Conibear et al. 2009; Król et al. 2011).

Genetic variants readily emerge during biofilm growth in different bacterial species (Boles and Singh 2008; Allegrucci and Sauer 2008; Boles et al. 2004; Koh et al. 2007), through genetic mutations or rearrangements (Drenkard and Ausubel 2002; McEllistrem et al. 2007). Genetic variants with altered colony morphology are readily recognized, with many sharing a common small and/or rugose colony morphology associated with increased EPS production (see section "SCV"). Antibiotic-resistant variants have been described in *P. aeruginosa* (Drenkard and Ausubel 2002; Boles et al. 2004) and *S. aureus* (Garcia et al. 2013) that overproduce EPS, while others may harbor other mutations unrelated to EPS production. For example, Boles et al. reported that the genetic diversification in biofilms not only led to many colony morphology variants but also a ~1,000 fold increase in the number of gentamicin-resistant bacteria (Boles et al. 2004).

Several studies have shown that the mutation frequency is greater in biofilm compared to planktonic bacteria (Ryder et al. 2012; Driffield et al. 2008; Conibear et al. 2009). Genetic mutations may be due to DNA damage and *recA*-mediated DNA repair from oxidative stress generated during biofilm growth (Boles and Singh 2008). However, genetic variants can represent more than 10 % of a biofilm population after only a few days of laboratory biofilm growth (Boles et al. 2004). Mutations, even a high frequency, are therefore unlikely to account for all variants observed, and variant subpopulations are likely enriched in the biofilm environment. For example, SCV overexpressing exopolysaccharides have enhanced surface adhesion and self-aggregate (Zogaj et al. 2001). Boles et al. proposed that this genetic diversity provided greater community stress resistance and sustainability through the "insurance effect," a benefit that is clear under antibiotic stress (Boles et al. 2004). Chromosomal rearrangements can also lead to genetic variants.

Adaptive Resistance Mechanisms

Adaptive resistance is induced by the antibiotics themselves or various environmental signals. The mechanisms presented below are typically not specific to biofilm growth and can also confer resistance to planktonic bacteria under certain conditions.

Efflux Pumps

Drug efflux is an important mechanism of antibiotic resistance, particularly in gram-negative bacteria. Species such as *P. aeruginosa* have a large number of multicomponent efflux pumps that can export many substrates into the extracellular environment. Among the different families of efflux pumps, resistance-nodulation division (RND) efflux systems are particularly relevant to antibiotic resistance because of their ability to extrude a wide array of compounds, including aminoglycosides, beta-lactams, fluoroquinolones, macrolides, and tetracyclines (Gotz 2002). The expression of these efflux pumps is highly regulated and typically low without inducing conditions.

While the contribution of efflux pumps to antibiotic resistance in planktonic cells is well established, their contribution to biofilm antibiotic resistance remains equivocal. For example, expression of *P. aeruginosa* multidrug efflux systems is low during biofilm growth (Folsom et al. 2010; De Kievit et al. 2001). Inactivation or overexpression of the MexAB-OprM and MexCD-OprJ systems has no or limited impact on biofilm antibiotic resistance, and the MexEF-OprN and MexXY systems do not appear to contribute to biofilm antibiotic resistance either (De Kievit et al. 2001; Brooun et al. 2000). However, MexCD-OprJ is induced by the antimicrobial peptide colistin, and MexCD-OprJ mutant biofilms are more susceptible to colistin during biofilm growth (Chiang et al. 2012). Gillis et al. reported that MexCD-OprJ is induced in biofilms by the macrolide azithromycin, and mutant biofilms lacking both MexCD-OprJ and MexAB-OprM are susceptible to azithromycin (Gillis et al. 2005). Interestingly, the expression of several RND efflux systems is modulated by oxygen concentration, raising the intriguing possibility that reduced oxygen levels within biofilms may induce drug efflux (Schaible et al. 2012).

Zhang et al. described a novel efflux system (PA1874-1877) in *P. aeruginosa* strain PA14 that contributes to biofilm-specific resistance toward tobramycin, gentamicin, and ciprofloxacin. The PA1874-1877 genes are more highly expressed in biofilms than in planktonic bacteria and encode a putative RND efflux and ABC transporter system that confer increased antibiotic resistance to biofilms but not planktonic bacteria (Zhang and Mah 2008). Liao et al. also recently identified a MerR-like transcriptional regulator BrlR only expressed in biofilms. BrlR appears to contribute to biofilm tolerance to aminoglycosides and colistin, partly by inducing the expression of the MexAB-OprM and MexEF-OprM efflux pumps (Liao et al. 2013) and by repressing *phoPQ* expression (Chambers and Sauer 2013).

In *E. coli*, AcrAB-TolC, an RND family efflux pump, is the most common efflux system and can export a wide range of antibiotics. Although its expression can be upregulated during biofilm growth, this does not correlate well with increased antibiotic resistance (Maira-Litran et al. 2000). On the other hand, many other genes encoding efflux pumps are upregulated in *E. coli* biofilms, and efflux pump inhibitors enhance tetracycline susceptibility of *E. coli* and *Klebsiella pneumoniae* biofilms (Kvist et al. 2008).

Determining the contribution of specific efflux systems is challenging because of their redundant functions and heterogeneous expression within biofilm structures (Pamp et al. 2008; Chiang et al. 2012). Furthermore, expression of the efflux systems can be induced by poorly characterized conditions or substrates. However, in most studies, drug efflux likely does not account for the profound antibiotic resistance of biofilms.

β-Lactamases

ampC is a chromosomally encoded β-lactamase, and it's expression and activity can be activity can be induced in mature biofilms, as well as biofilm subpopulations treated with beta-lactams (Bowler et al. 2012; Bagge et al. 2004). While this can lead to adaptive beta-lactam resistance, this is also unlikely to explain the high resistance of biofilm cells to this class of antibiotics, observed without prior beta-lactam exposure.

Two-Component Systems (TCS)

Two-component systems (TCS) are key signaling systems in bacteria, allowing them to sense their environment and elicit an appropriate response. They are typically made of a sensor kinase and a response regulator, although many are hybrid kinases or orphan response regulators. While many TCS contribute to biofilm formation, as well as antibiotic resistance in planktonic bacteria, their direct implication in antibiotic resistance of biofilms is less well characterized.

The CpxAR system in *E. coli* is a TCS that primarily responds to cell envelope stress, such as accumulation of misfolded proteins. This system controls many targets, including genes involved in motility and adhesion and transcription of several drug exporter genes and can confer resistance to aminoglycosides and antimicrobial peptides (Hirakawa et al. 2003). Cpx-regulated genes are induced at initial attachment and during biofilm growth in *E. coli* (Beloin et al. 2004; Dorel et al. 1999; Otto and Silhavy 2002), suggesting that the Cpx system may contribute to antibiotic resistance in biofilms. Interestingly, the AmgRS TCS in *P. aeruginosa*, although closest to the *E. coli* OmpR/EnvZ system by sequence homology, share several functional similarities with the *E. coli* Cpx system. It controls a conserved cell envelope stress response and nearly half of its target genes are homologous to Cpx-controlled genes (Lee et al. 2009). Lee et al. reported that mutations in *amgRS* increase tobramycin killing of tolerant biofilms and improved outcomes in lethal murine infections (Lee et al. 2009).

The PhoPQ and PmrAB TCS present in several gram-negative bacterial species (including *Salmonella* spp., *E. coli*, and *P. aeruginosa*) are activated by conditions limited for divalent cations (Mg^{2+} and Ca^{2+}) and confer resistance to cationic antimicrobial peptides (CAP) and aminoglycoside (Macfarlane et al. 1999; McPhee et al. 2003). Both TCS induce the *pmr(arn)BCADTEF-pmrE* operon responsible for amino-arabinose modification of lipopolysaccharide (LPS) molecules within the outer membrane. Such LPS modifications alter the charge interactions at the cell surface, leading to CAP and aminoglycoside resistance in planktonic bacteria. Whether these pathways contribute significantly to resistance in biofilm bacteria remains to be determined. In *P. aeruginosa*, the *pmr* genes are required for colistin (a CAP) tolerance in flow chamber-grown biofilms, but *pmr* expression in biofilms is low and only induced by colistin treatment (Pamp et al. 2008). Chambers et al. recently characterized BrlR, a transcriptional regulator that represses the PhoPQ system during biofilm growth, thus suppressing CAP resistance (Chambers and Sauer 2013).

Zhang et al. recently identified a putative TCS in *P. aeruginosa* encoded by PA0756-0757 that confers aminoglycoside resistance and is highly expressed in biofilms (Zhang et al. 2013). The unusual PrpAB TCS in *P. aeruginosa* is associated with enhanced biofilm formation when activated but reduced antibiotic resistance and attenuated virulence (de Bentzmann et al. 2012). Both these systems contribute to biofilm resistance through yet uncharacterized mechanisms.

Conclusion

Biofilm infections pose a great medical challenge, as conventional antimicrobial therapies do not effectively eradicate such bacterial infections. Our evolving understanding of the mechanisms of antibiotic resistance and tolerance in biofilm bacteria reveals multiple contributing cellular processes and pathways. Whether these mechanisms can be targeted to effectively overcome biofilms multidrug resistance and tolerance remains to be seen. Such strategies will undoubtedly have a major impact in our therapeutic arsenal against devastating infections such as the chronic *P. aeruginosa* airway infections of cystic fibrosis patients.

References

Aizenman E, Engelberg-Kulka H, Glaser G (1996) An *Escherichia coli* chromosomal "addiction module" regulated by guanosine [corrected] 3′,5′-bispyrophosphate: a model for programmed bacterial cell death. Proc Natl Acad Sci U S A 93(12):6059–6063

Alhede M, Kragh KN, Qvortrup K, Allesen-Holm M, van Gennip M, Christensen LD, Jensen P, Nielsen AK, Parsek M, Wozniak D, Molin SR, Tolker-Nielsen T, Høiby N, Givskov M, Bjarnsholt T (2011) Phenotypes of non-attached *Pseudomonas aeruginosa* aggregates resemble surface attached biofilm. PLoS One 6(11):e27943

Alkawash MA, Soothill JS, Schiller NL (2006) Alginate lyase enhances antibiotic killing of mucoid *Pseudomonas aeruginosa* in biofilms. APMIS 114(2):131–138, Epub 08 Mar 2006

Allegrucci M, Sauer K (2007) Characterization of colony morphology variants isolated from *Streptococcus pneumoniae* biofilms. J Bacteriol 189(5):2030–2038

Allegrucci M, Sauer K (2008) Formation of *Streptococcus pneumoniae* non-phase-variable colony variants is Due to increased mutation frequency present under biofilm growth conditions. J Bacteriol 190(19):6330–6339

Allison KR, Brynildsen MP, Collins JJ (2011) Metabolite-enabled eradication of bacterial persisters by aminoglycosides. Nature 473(7346):216–220

Alvarez-Ortega C, Harwood CS (2007) Responses of *Pseudomonas aeruginosa* to low oxygen indicate that growth in the cystic fibrosis lung is by aerobic respiration. Mol Microbiol 65 (1):153

Amato SM, Orman MA, Brynildsen MP (2013) Metabolic control of persister formation in *Escherichia coli*. Mol Cell 50(4):475–487

An D, Parsek MR (2007) The promise and peril of transcriptional profiling in biofilm communities. Curr Opin Microbiol 10(3):292–296

Anwar H, Dasgupta M, Lam K, Costerton JW (1989) Tobramycin resistance of mucoid *Pseudomonas aeruginosa* biofilm grown under iron limitation. J Antimicrob Chemother 24(5):647–655

Arce Miranda JE, Sotomayor CE, Albesa I, Paraje MG (2011) Oxidative and nitrosative stress in *Staphylococcus aureus* biofilm. FEMS Microbiol Lett 315(1):23–29

Bagge N, Schuster M, Hentzer M, Ciofu O, Givskov M, Greenberg EP, Hoiby N (2004) *Pseudomonas aeruginosa* biofilms exposed to imipenem exhibit changes in global gene expression and?-lactamase and alginate production. Antimicrob Agents Chemother 48(4):1175–1187

Balaban NQ (2011) Persistence: mechanisms for triggering and enhancing phenotypic variability. Curr Opin Genet Dev 21(6):768–775

Balaban NQ, Merrin J, Chait R, Kowalik L, Leibler S (2004) Bacterial persistence as a phenotypic switch. Science 305(5690):1622–1625, Epub 17 Aug 2004

Banin E, Vasil ML, Greenberg EP (2005) Iron and *Pseudomonas aeruginosa* biofilm formation. Proc Natl Acad Sci U S A 102(31):11076–11081

Battesti A, Majdalani N, Gottesman S (2011) The RpoS-mediated general stress response in *Escherichia coli**. Annu Rev Microbiol 65(1):189–213

Beenken KE, Dunman PM, McAleese F, Macapagal D, Murphy E, Projan SJ, Blevins JS, Smeltzer MS (2004) Global gene expression in *Staphylococcus aureus* biofilms. J Bacteriol 186 (14):4665–4684

Beloin C, Valle J, Latour-Lambert P, Faure P, Kzreminski M, Balestrino D, Haagensen JA, Molin S, Prensier G, Arbeille B, Ghigo JM (2004) Global impact of mature biofilm lifestyle on *Escherichia coli* K-12 gene expression. Mol Microbiol 51(3):659–674, Epub 21 Jan 2004

Bernier SP, Lebeaux D, DeFrancesco AS, Valomon A, Soubigou G, Coppe J-Y, Ghigo J-M, Beloin C (2013) Starvation, together with the SOS response, mediates high biofilm-specific tolerance to the fluoroquinolone ofloxacin. PLoS Genet 9(1):e1003144

Boles BR, Singh PK (2008) Endogenous oxidative stress produces diversity and adaptability in biofilm communities. Proc Natl Acad Sci 105(34):12503–12508

Boles BR, Thoendel M, Singh PK (2004) Self-generated diversity produces "insurance effects" in biofilm communities. Proc Natl Acad Sci U S A 101(47):16630–16635

Borriello G, Werner E, Roe F, Kim AM, Ehrlich GD, Stewart PS (2004) Oxygen limitation contributes to antibiotic tolerance of *Pseudomonas aeruginosa* in biofilms. Antimicrob Agents Chemother 48(7):2659–2664

Borriello G, Richards L, Ehrlich GD, Stewart PS (2006) Arginine or nitrate enhances antibiotic susceptibility of *Pseudomonas aeruginosa* in biofilms. Antimicrob Agents Chemother 50 (1):382–384

Bowler LL, Zhanel GG, Ball TB, Saward LL (2012) Mature *Pseudomonas aeruginosa* biofilms prevail compared to young biofilms in the presence of ceftazidime. Antimicrob Agents Chemother 56(9):4976–4979

Braeken K, Moris M, Daniels R, Vanderleyden J, Michiels J (2006) New horizons for (p)ppGpp in bacterial and plant physiology. Trends Microbiol 14(1):45–54

Branda SS, Vik Å, Friedman L, Kolter R (2005) Biofilms: the matrix revisited. Trends Microbiol 13 (1):20–26

Brooun A, Liu S, Lewis K (2000) A dose-response study of antibiotic resistance in *Pseudomonas aeruginosa* biofilms. Antimicrob Agents Chemother 44(3):640–646, Epub 19 Feb 2000

Brown MR, Allison DG, Gilbert P (1988) Resistance of bacterial biofilms to antibiotics: a growth-rate related effect? J Antimicrob Chemother 22(6):777–780, Epub 01 Dec 1988

Cashel M, Gentry DR, Hernandez VJ, Vinella D (1996) The stringent response. In: Neidhardt FC (ed) *Escherichia coli* and *Salmonella*, 2nd edn. ASM Press, Washington, DC, pp 1458–1496

Castonguay MH, van der Schaaf S, Koester W, Krooneman J, van der Meer W, Harmsen H, Landini P (2006) Biofilm formation by *Escherichia coli* is stimulated by synergistic interactions and co-adhesion mechanisms with adherence-proficient bacteria. Res Microbiol 157(5):471–478

Chambers JR, Sauer K (2013) The MerR-like regulator BrlR impairs *Pseudomonas aeruginosa* biofilm tolerance to colistin by repressing PhoPQ. J Bacteriol 195(20):4678–4688

Chen H, Hu J, Chen PR, Lan L, Li Z, Hicks LM, Dinner AR, He C (2008) The *Pseudomonas aeruginosa* multidrug efflux regulator MexR uses an oxidation-sensing mechanism. Proc Natl Acad Sci 105(36):13586–13591

Chiang W-C, Pamp SJ, Nilsson M, Givskov M, Tolker-Nielsen T (2012) The metabolically active subpopulation in *Pseudomonas aeruginosa* biofilms survives exposure to membrane-targeting antimicrobials via distinct molecular mechanisms. FEMS Immunol Med Microbiol 65(2):245

Ciofu O, Beveridge TJ, Kadurugamuwa J, Walther-Rasmussen J, Høiby N (2000) Chromosomal β-lactamase is packaged into membrane vesicles and secreted from *Pseudomonas aeruginosa*. J Antimicrob Chemother 45(1):9–13

Cohen NR, Lobritz MA, Collins JJ (2013) Microbial persistence and the road to drug resistance. Cell Host Microbe 13(6):632–642

Colvin KM, Gordon VD, Murakami K, Borlee BR, Wozniak DJ, Wong GCL, Parsek MR (2011) The Pel polysaccharide can serve a structural and protective role in the biofilm matrix of *Pseudomonas aeruginosa*. PLoS Pathog 7(1):e1001264

Conibear TCR, Collins SL, Webb JS (2009) Role of mutation in *Pseudomonas aeruginosa* biofilm development. PLoS One 4(7):e6289

Costerton JW, Stewart PS, Greenberg EP (1999) Bacterial biofilms: a common cause of persistent infections. Science 284(5418):1318–1322

Cozens RM, Tuomanen E, Tosch W, Zak O, Suter J, Tomasz A (1986) Evaluation of the bactericidal activity of beta-lactam antibiotics on slowly growing bacteria cultured in the chemostat. Antimicrob Agents Chemother 29(5):797–802

Dalhoff A, Matutat S, Ullmann U (1995) Effect of quinolones against slowly growing bacteria. Chemotherapy 41(2):92–99, Epub 01 Mar 1995

De Beer D, Srinivasan R, Stewart PS (1994a) Direct measurement of chlorine penetration into biofilms during disinfection. Appl Environ Microbiol 60(12):4339–4344, Epub 01 Dec 1994

de Beer D, Stoodley P, Roe F, Lewandowski Z (1994b) Effects of biofilm structures on oxygen distribution and mass transport. Biotechnol Bioeng 43(11):1131–1138

de Bentzmann S, Giraud C, Bernard CS, Calderon V, Ewald F, Plesiat P, Nguyen C, Grunwald D, Attree I, Jeannot K, Fauvarque M-O, Bordi C (2012) Unique biofilm signature, drug susceptibility and decreased virulence in Drosophila through the *Pseudomonas aeruginosa* two-component system PprAB. PLoS Pathog 8(11):e1003052

De Kievit TR, Parkins MD, Gillis RJ, Srikumar R, Ceri H, Poole K, Iglewski BH, Storey DG (2001) Multidrug efflux pumps: expression patterns and contribution to antibiotic resistance in *Pseudomonas aeruginosa* biofilms. Antimicrob Agents Chemother 45(6):1761–1770

Diggle SP, Cornelis P, Williams P, Camara M (2006) 4-Quinolone signalling in *Pseudomonas aeruginosa*: old molecules, new perspectives. Int J Med Microbiol 296(2):83–91

Dorel C, Vidal O, Prigent-Combaret C, Vallet I, Lejeune P (1999) Involvement of the Cpx signal transduction pathway of *E. coli* in biofilm formation. FEMS Microbiol Lett 178(1):169–175, Epub 14 Sept 1999

Dorel C, Lejeune P, Rodrigue A (2006) The Cpx system of *Escherichia coli*, a strategic signaling pathway for confronting adverse conditions and for settling biofilm communities? Res Microbiol 157(4):306–314

Dorr T, Lewis K, Vulic M (2009) SOS response induces persistence to fluoroquinolones in *Escherichia coli*. PLoS Genet 5(12):e1000760

Dorr T, Vulic M, Lewis K (2010) Ciprofloxacin causes persister formation by inducing the TisB toxin in *Escherichia coli*. PLoS Biol 8(2):e1000317

Dotsch A, Eckweiler D, Schniederjans M, Zimmermann A, Jensen V, Scharfe M, Geffers R, Haussler S (2012) The *Pseudomonas aeruginosa* transcriptome in planktonic cultures and static biofilms using RNA sequencing. PLoS One 7(2):e31092

Drenkard E, Ausubel FM (2002) Pseudomonas biofilm formation and antibiotic resistance are linked to phenotypic variation. Nature 416(6882):740–743

Driffield K, Miller K, Bostock JM, O'Neill AJ, Chopra I (2008) Increased mutability of *Pseudomonas aeruginosa* in biofilms. J Antimicrob Chemother 61(5):1053–1056

Evans DJ, Allison DG, Brown MRW, Gilbert P (1991) Susceptibility of *Pseudomonas aeruginosa* and *Escherichia coli* biofilms towards ciprofloxacin: effect of specific growth rate. J Antimicrob Chemother 27(2):177–184

Fasani RA, Savageau MA (2013) Molecular mechanisms of multiple toxin-antitoxin systems are coordinated to govern the persister phenotype. Proc Natl Acad Sci U S A 110(27):E2528–E2537

Field TR, White A, Elborn JS, Tunney MM (2005) Effect of oxygen limitation on the in vitro antimicrobial susceptibility of clinical isolates of *Pseudomonas aeruginosa* grown planktonically and as biofilms. Eur J Clin Microbiol Infect Dis 24(10):677–687

Folsom JP, Richards L, Pitts B, Roe F, Ehrlich GD, Parker A, Mazurie AL, Stewart PS (2010) Physiology of *Pseudomonas aeruginosa* in biofilms as revealed by transcriptome analysis. BMC Microbiol 10(1):294

Fraud S, Poole K (2011) Oxidative stress induction of the MexXY multidrug efflux genes and promotion of aminoglycoside resistance development in *Pseudomonas aeruginosa*. Antimicrob Agents Chemother 55(3):1068–1074

Frawley ER, Crouch M-LV, Bingham-Ramos LK, Robbins HF, Wang W, Wright GD, Fang FC (2013) Iron and citrate export by a major facilitator superfamily pump regulates metabolism and stress resistance in *Salmonella typhimurium*. Proc Natl Acad Sci 110(29):12054–12059

Garcia LG, Lemaire S, Kahl BC, Becker K, Proctor RA, Denis O, Tulkens PM, Van Bambeke F (2013) Antibiotic activity against small-colony variants of *Staphylococcus aureus*: review of in vitro, animal and clinical data. J Antimicrob Chemother 68(7):1455–1464, Epub 15 Mar 2013

Gerdes K, Maisonneuve E (2012) Bacterial persistence and toxin-antitoxin loci. Annu Rev Microbiol 66(1):103–123

Gillis RJ, White KG, Choi KH, Wagner VE, Schweizer HP, Iglewski BH (2005) Molecular basis of azithromycin-resistant *Pseudomonas aeruginosa* biofilms. Antimicrob Agents Chemother 49 (9):3858–3867

Gordon CA, Hodges NA, Marriott C (1988) Antibiotic interaction and diffusion through alginate and exopolysaccharide of cystic fibrosis-derived *Pseudomonas aeruginosa*. J Antimicrob Chemother 22(5):667–674

Gotz F (2002) Staphylococcus and biofilms. Mol Microbiol 43(6):1367–1378, Epub 16 Apr 2002

Groisman EA, Kayser J, Soncini FC (1997) Regulation of polymyxin resistance and adaptation to low-Mg^{2+} environments. J Bacteriol 179(22):7040–7045

Hansen S, Lewis K, Vulifá M (2008) Role of global regulators and nucleotide metabolism in antibiotic tolerance in *Escherichia coli*. Antimicrob Agents Chemother 52(8):2718–2726

Harrison JJ, Wade WD, Akierman S, Vacchi-Suzzi C, Stremick CA, Turner RJ, Ceri H (2009) The chromosomal toxin gene yafQ is a determinant of multidrug tolerance for *Escherichia coli* growing in a biofilm. Antimicrob Agents Chemother 53(6):2253–2258

Hausner M, Wuertz S (1999) High rates of conjugation in bacterial biofilms as determined by quantitative in situ analysis. Appl Environ Microbiol 65(8):3710–3713, Epub 31 July 1999

Haussler S, Ziegler I, Lottel A, von Gotz F, Rohde M, Wehmhohner D, Saravanamuthu S, Tummler B, Steinmetz I (2003) Highly adherent small-colony variants of *Pseudomonas aeruginosa* in cystic fibrosis lung infection. J Med Microbiol 52(Pt 4):295–301, Epub 05 Apr 2003

Hill D, Rose B, Pajkos A, Robinson M, Bye P, Bell S, Elkins M, Thompson B, MacLeod C, Aaron SD, Harbour C (2005) Antibiotic susceptibilities of *Pseudomonas aeruginosa* isolates derived from patients with cystic fibrosis under aerobic, anaerobic, and biofilm conditions. J Clin Microbiol 43(10):5085–5090

Hirakawa H, Nishino K, Hirata T, Yamaguchi A (2003) Comprehensive studies of drug resistance mediated by overexpression of response regulators of two-component signal transduction systems in *Escherichia coli*. J Bacteriol 185(6):1851–1856, Epub 06 Mar 2003

Hoyle BD, Alcantara J, Costerton JW (1992) *Pseudomonas aeruginosa* biofilm as a diffusion barrier to piperacillin. Antimicrob Agents Chemother 36(9):2054–2056

Ito A, Taniuchi A, May T, Kawata K, Okabe S (2009) Increased antibiotic resistance of *Escherichia coli* in mature biofilms. Appl Environ Microbiol 75(12):4093–4100

Kaneko Y, Thoendel M, Olakanmi O, Britigan BE, Singh PK (2007) The transition metal gallium disrupts *Pseudomonas aeruginosa* iron metabolism and has antimicrobial and antibiofilm activity. J Clin Invest 117(4):877–888

Kayama S, Murakami K, Ono T, Ushimaru M, Yamamoto A, Hirota K, Miyake Y (2009) The role of rpoS gene and quorum sensing system in ofloxacin tolerance in *Pseudomonas aeruginosa*. FEMS Microbiol Lett 298(2):184–192

Keren I, Kaldalu N, Spoering A, Wang Y, Lewis K (2004) Persister cells and tolerance to antimicrobials. FEMS Microbiol Lett 230(1):13–18, Epub 22 Jan 2004

Khakimova M, Ahlgren H, Harrison JJ, English A, Nguyen D (2013) The stringent response controls catalases in *Pseudomonas aeruginosa*: implications for hydrogen peroxide and antibiotic tolerance. J Bacteriol 195(9):2011–2020

Khan W, Bernier SP, Kuchma SL, Hammond JH, Hasan F, O'Toole GA (2010) Aminoglycoside resistance of *Pseudomonas aeruginosa* biofilms modulated by extracellular polysaccharide. Int Microbiol 13(4):207–212, Epub 16 Mar 2011

Kim YH, Lee Y, Kim S, Yeom J, Yeom S, Seok Kim B, Oh S, Park S, Jeon CO, Park W (2006) The role of periplasmic antioxidant enzymes (superoxide dismutase and thiol peroxidase) of the Shiga toxin-producing *Escherichia coli* O157:H7 in the formation of biofilms. Proteomics 6 (23):6181–6193

Kim J, Hahn J-S, Franklin MJ, Stewart PS, Yoon J (2009) Tolerance of dormant and active cells in *Pseudomonas aeruginosa* PA01 biofilm to antimicrobial agents. J Antimicrob Chemother 63 (1):129–135

Kint CI, Verstraeten N, Fauvart M, Michiels J (2012) New-found fundamentals of bacterial persistence. Trends Microbiol 20(12):577–585

Koh KS, Lam KW, Alhede M, Queck SY, Labbate M, Kjelleberg S, Rice SA (2007) Phenotypic diversification and adaptation of *Serratia marcescens* MG1 biofilm-derived morphotypes. J Bacteriol 189(1):119–130

Kohanski MA, Dwyer DJ, Hayete B, Lawrence CA, Collins JJ (2007) A common mechanism of cellular death induced by bactericidal antibiotics. Cell 130(5):797–810, Epub 07 Sept 2007

Kolenbrander PE (2000) Oral microbial communities: biofilms, interactions, and genetic systems. Annu Rev Microbiol 54(1):413–437

Korch SB, Henderson TA, Hill TM (2003) Characterization of the hipA7 allele of *Escherichia coli* and evidence that high persistence is governed by (p)ppGpp synthesis. Mol Microbiol 50 (4):1199–1213

Król JE, Nguyen HD, Rogers LM, Beyenal H, Krone SM, Top EM (2011) Increased transfer of a multidrug resistance plasmid in *Escherichia coli* biofilms at the air-liquid interface. Appl Environ Microbiol 77(15):5079–5088

Kumon H, Tomochika K-i, Matunaga T, Ogawa M, Ohmori H (1994) A sandwich cup method for the penetration assay of antimicrobial agents through *Pseudomonas* exopolysaccharides. Microbiol Immunol 38(8):615–619

Kvist M, Hancock V, Klemm P (2008) Inactivation of efflux pumps abolishes bacterial biofilm formation. Appl Environ Microbiol 74(23):7376–7382

Laham NA, Rohde H, Sander G, Fischer A, Hussain M, Heilmann C, Mack D, Proctor R, Peters G, Becker K, von Eiff C (2007) Augmented expression of polysaccharide intercellular adhesin in a defined *Staphylococcus epidermidis* mutant with the small-colony-variant phenotype. J Bacteriol 189(12):4494–4501

Lee S, Hinz A, Bauerle E, Angermeyer A, Juhaszova K, Kaneko Y, Singh PK, Manoil C (2009) Targeting a bacterial stress response to enhance antibiotic action. Proc Natl Acad Sci U S A 106 (34):14570–14575, Epub 27 Aug 2009

Lenz AP, Williamson KS, Pitts B, Stewart PS, Franklin MJ (2008) Localized gene expression in *Pseudomonas aeruginosa* biofilms. Appl Environ Microbiol 74(14):4463–4471

Lewis K (2008) Multidrug tolerance of biofilms and persister cells. Curr Top Microbiol Immunol 322:107–131

Lewis K (2010) Persister cells. Annu Rev Microbiol 64(1):357–372

Liao J, Sauer K (2012) The MerR-like transcriptional regulator BrlR contributes to *Pseudomonas aeruginosa* biofilm tolerance. J Bacteriol 194(18):4823–4836

Liao J, Schurr MJ, Sauer K (2013) The MerR-like regulator BrlR confers biofilm tolerance by activating multidrug efflux pumps in *Pseudomonas aeruginosa* biofilms. J Bacteriol 195 (15):3352–3363

Lu X, Roe F, Jesaitis A, Lewandowski Z (1998) Resistance of biofilms to the catalase inhibitor 3-amino-1,2, 4-triazole. Biotechnol Bioeng 59(2):156–162

Luo Y, Helmann JD (2012) Analysis of the role of *Bacillus subtilis* sigma(M) in beta-lactam resistance reveals an essential role for c-di-AMP in peptidoglycan homeostasis. Mol Microbiol 83(3):623–639

Lynch SV, Dixon L, Benoit MR, Brodie EL, Keyhan M, Hu P, Ackerley DF, Andersen GL, Matin A (2007) Role of the rapA gene in controlling antibiotic resistance of *Escherichia coli* biofilms. Antimicrob Agents Chemother 51(10):3650–3658

Macfarlane EL, Kwasnicka A, Ochs MM, Hancock RE (1999) PhoP-PhoQ homologues in *Pseudomonas aeruginosa* regulate expression of the outer-membrane protein OprH and polymyxin B resistance. Mol Microbiol 34(2):305–316, Epub 17 Nov 1999

Mah T-F, Pitts B, Pellock B, Walker GC, Stewart PS, O'Toole GA (2003) A genetic basis for *Pseudomonas aeruginosa* biofilm antibiotic resistance. Nature 426(6964):306–310

Maira-Litran T, Allison DG, Gilbert P (2000) An evaluation of the potential of the multiple antibiotic resistance operon (mar) and the multidrug efflux pump acrAB to moderate resistance towards ciprofloxacin in *Escherichia coli* biofilms. J Antimicrob Chemother 45 (6):789–795

Maisonneuve E, Shakespeare LJ, Jorgensen MG, Gerdes K (2011) Bacterial persistence by RNA endonucleases. Proc Natl Acad Sci 108(32):13206–13211

Maisonneuve E, Castro-Camargo M, Gerdes K (2013) (p)ppGpp controls bacterial persistence by stochastic induction of toxin-antitoxin activity. Cell 154(5):1140–1150

McEllistrem MC, Ransford JV, Khan SA (2007) Characterization of in vitro biofilm-associated pneumococcal phase variants of a clinically relevant serotype 3 clone. J Clin Microbiol 45 (1):97–101

McPhee JB, Lewenza S, Hancock REW (2003) Cationic antimicrobial peptides activate a two-component regulatory system, PmrA-PmrB, that regulates resistance to polymyxin B and cationic antimicrobial peptides in *Pseudomonas aeruginosa*. Mol Microbiol 50(1):205

Meissner A, Wild V, Simm R, Rohde M, Erck C, Bredenbruch F, Morr M, Römling U, Häussler S (2007) *Pseudomonas aeruginosa* cupA-encoded fimbriae expression is regulated by a GGDEF and EAL domain-dependent modulation of the intracellular level of cyclic diguanylate. Environ Microbiol 9(10):2475

Mikkelsen H, Duck Z, Lilley KS, Welch M (2007) Interrelationships between colonies, biofilms, and planktonic cells of *Pseudomonas aeruginosa*. J Bacteriol 189(6):2411–2416

Mikkelsen H, Ball G, Giraud C, Filloux A (2009) Expression of *Pseudomonas aeruginosa* CupD fimbrial genes is antagonistically controlled by RcsB and the EAL-containing PvrR response regulators. PLoS One 4(6):e6018

Miller PF, Sulavik MC (1996) Overlaps and parallels in the regulation of intrinsic multiple-antibiotic resistance in *Escherichia coli*. Mol Microbiol 21(3):441–448

Mills E, Pultz IS, Kulasekara HD, Miller SI (2011) The bacterial second messenger c-di-GMP: mechanisms of signalling. Cell Microbiol 13(8):1122–1129

Molin S, Tolker-Nielsen T (2003) Gene transfer occurs with enhanced efficiency in biofilms and induces enhanced stabilisation of the biofilm structure. Curr Opin Biotechnol 14(3):255–261

Mulcahy H, Charron-Mazenod L, Lewenza S (2008) Extracellular DNA chelates cations and induces antibiotic resistance in *Pseudomonas aeruginosa* biofilms. PLoS Pathog 4(11): e1000213

Nguyen D, Joshi-Datar A, Lepine F, Bauerle E, Olakanmi O, Beer K, McKay G, Siehnel R, Schafhauser J, Wang Y, Britigan BE, Singh PK (2011) Active starvation responses mediate antibiotic tolerance in biofilms and nutrient-limited bacteria. Science 334(6058):982–986

O'Toole G, Kaplan HB, Kolter R (2000) Biofilm formation as microbial development. Annu Rev Microbiol 54(1):49–79

Otto K, Silhavy TJ (2002) Surface sensing and adhesion of *Escherichia coli* controlled by the Cpx-signaling pathway. Proc Natl Acad Sci U S A 99(4):2287–2292, Epub 07 Feb 2002

Pamp SJ, Gjermansen M, Johansen HK, Tolker-Nielsen T (2008) Tolerance to the antimicrobial peptide colistin in *Pseudomonas aeruginosa* biofilms is linked to metabolically active cells, and depends on the pmr and mexAB-oprM genes. Mol Microbiol 68(1):223

Parsek MR, Greenberg EP (2000) Acyl-homoserine lactone quorum sensing in gram-negative bacteria: a signaling mechanism involved in associations with higher organisms. Proc Natl Acad Sci U S A 97(16):8789–8793, Epub 02 Aug 2000

Parsek MR, Singh PK (2003) Bacterial biofilms: an emerging link to disease pathogenesis. Annu Rev Microbiol 57:677–701, Epub 07 Oct 2003

Patell S, Gu M, Davenport P, Givskov M, Waite RD, Welch M (2010) Comparative microarray analysis reveals that the core biofilm-associated transcriptome of *Pseudomonas aeruginosa* comprises relatively few genes. Environ Microbiol Rep 2(3):440–448, Epub 01 June 2010

Patrauchan MA, Sarkisova SA, Franklin MJ (2007) Strain-specific proteome responses of *Pseudomonas aeruginosa* to biofilm-associated growth and to calcium. Microbiology 153 (11):3838–3851

Pérez-Osorio AC, Williamson KS, Franklin MJ (2010) Heterogeneous rpoS and rhlR mRNA levels and 16S rRNA/rDNA (rRNA gene) ratios within *Pseudomonas aeruginosa* biofilms, sampled by laser capture microdissection. J Bacteriol 192(12):2991–3000

Perry RD, Bobrov AG, Kirillina O, Jones HA, Pedersen L, Abney J, Fetherston JD (2004) Temperature regulation of the hemin storage (Hms+) phenotype of *Yersinia pestis* is posttranscriptional. J Bacteriol 186(6):1638–1647

Phillips NJ, Steichen CT, Schilling B, Post DMB, Niles RK, Bair TB, Falsetta ML, Apicella MA, Gibson BW (2012) Proteomic analysis of *Neisseria gonorrhoeae* biofilms shows shift to anaerobic respiration and changes in nutrient transport and outermembrane proteins. PLoS One 7(6):e38303

Poole K (2012) Stress responses as determinants of antimicrobial resistance in Gram-negative bacteria. Trends Microbiol 20(5):227–234

Potera C (1999) Forging a link between biofilms and disease. Science 283(5409):1837–1839

Potrykus K, Cashel M (2008) (p)ppGpp: still magical? Annu Rev Microbiol 62:35–51, Epub 06 May 2008

Potvin E, Sanschagrin F, Levesque RC (2008) Sigma factors in *Pseudomonas aeruginosa*. FEMS Microbiol Rev 32(1):38

Proctor RA, von Eiff C, Kahl BC, Becker K, McNamara P, Herrmann M, Peters G (2006) Small colony variants: a pathogenic form of bacteria that facilitates persistent and recurrent infections. Nat Rev Microbiol 4(4):295–305

Raivio TL, Leblanc SK, Price NL (2013) The *Escherichia coli* Cpx envelope stress response regulates genes of diverse function that impact antibiotic resistance and membrane integrity. J Bacteriol 195(12):2755–2767

Resch A, Rosenstein R, Nerz C, Gotz F (2005) Differential gene expression profiling of *Staphylococcus aureus* cultivated under biofilm and planktonic conditions. Appl Environ Microbiol 71 (5):2663–2676

Romling U (2012) Cyclic di-GMP, an established secondary messenger still speeding up. Environ Microbiol 14(8):1817–1829

Romling U, Galperin MY, Gomelsky M (2013) Cyclic di-GMP: the first 25 years of a universal bacterial second messenger. Microbiol Mol Biol Rev 77(1):1–52

Rotem E, Loinger A, Ronin I, Levin-Reisman I, Gabay C, Shoresh N, Biham O, Balaban NQ (2010) Regulation of phenotypic variability by a threshold-based mechanism underlies bacterial persistence. Proc Natl Acad Sci U S A 107(28):12541–12546

Ryder VJ, Chopra I, O'Neill AJ (2012) Increased mutability of Staphylococci in biofilms as a consequence of oxidative stress. PLoS One 7(10):e47695

Sauer K, Camper AK, Ehrlich GD, Costerton JW, Davies DG (2002) *Pseudomonas aeruginosa* displays multiple phenotypes during development as a biofilm. J Bacteriol 184(4):1140–1154, Epub 25 Jan 2002

Schaible B, Taylor CT, Schaffer K (2012) Hypoxia increases antibiotic resistance in *Pseudomonas aeruginosa* through altering the composition of multidrug efflux pumps. Antimicrob Agents Chemother 56(4):2114–2118

Schramm A, Larsen LH, Revsbech NP, Ramsing NB, Amann R, Schleifer KH (1996) Structure and function of a nitrifying biofilm as determined by in situ hybridization and the use of microelectrodes. Appl Environ Microbiol 62(12):4641–4647, Epub 01 Dec 1996

Seneviratne CJ, Wang Y, Jin L, Wong SSW, Herath TDK, Samaranayake LP (2012) Unraveling the resistance of microbial biofilms: has proteomics been helpful? Proteomics 12(4–5):651–665

Serra DO, Richter AM, Klauck G, Mika F, Hengge R (2013) Microanatomy at cellular resolution and spatial order of physiological differentiation in a bacterial biofilm. MBio 4(2): e00103–e00113

Shah D, Zhang Z, Khodursky A, Kaldalu N, Kurg K, Lewis K (2006) Persisters: a distinct physiological state of *E. coli*. BMC Microbiol 6:53, Epub 14 June 2006

Shigeta M, Tanaka G, Komatsuzawa H, Sugai M, Suginaka H, Usui T (1997) Permeation of antimicrobial agents through *Pseudomonas aeruginosa* biofilms: a simple method. Chemotherapy 43(5):340–345

Shrout JD, Tolker-Nielsen T, Givskov M, Parsek MR (2011) The contribution of cell-cell signaling and motility to bacterial biofilm formation. MRS Bull 36(5):367–373

Singh R, Ray P, Das A, Sharma M (2010) Enhanced production of exopolysaccharide matrix and biofilm by a menadione-auxotrophic *Staphylococcus aureus* small-colony variant. J Med Microbiol 59(5):521–527

Sommerfeldt N, Possling A, Becker G, Pesavento C, Tschowri N, Hengge R (2009) Gene expression patterns and differential input into curli fimbriae regulation of all GGDEF/EAL domain proteins in *Escherichia coli*. Microbiology 155(Pt 4):1318–1331

Southey-Pillig CJ, Davies DG, Sauer K (2005) Characterization of temporal protein production in *Pseudomonas aeruginosa* biofilms. J Bacteriol 187(23):8114–8126

Sriramulu DD, Lunsdorf H, Lam JS, Romling U (2005) Microcolony formation: a novel biofilm model of *Pseudomonas aeruginosa* for the cystic fibrosis lung. J Med Microbiol 54 (Pt 7):667–676, Epub 11 June 2005

Starkey M, Hickman JH, Ma L, Zhang N, De Long S, Hinz A, Palacios S, Manoil C, Kirisits MJ, Starner TD, Wozniak DJ, Harwood CS, Parsek MR (2009) *Pseudomonas aeruginosa* rugose small-colony variants have adaptations that likely promote persistence in the cystic fibrosis lung. J Bacteriol 191(11):3492–3503, Epub 31 Mar 2009

Staudinger BJ, Muller JF, Halldorsson S, Boles B, Angermeyer A, Nguyen D, Rosen H, Baldursson O, Gottfreethsson M, Guethmundsson GH, Singh PK (2014) Conditions associated with the cystic fibrosis defect promote chronic *Pseudomonas aeruginosa* infection. Am J Respir Crit Care Med 189(7):812–824, Epub 29 Jan 2014

Sternberg C, Christensen BB, Johansen T, Nielsen AT, Andersen JB, Givskov M, Molin S (1999) Distribution of bacterial growth activity in flow-chamber biofilms. Appl Environ Microbiol 65 (9):4108–4117

Stewart PS (1996) Theoretical aspects of antibiotic diffusion into microbial biofilms. Antimicrob Agents Chemother 40(11):2517–2522, Epub 01 Nov 1996

Stewart PS, Franklin MJ (2008) Physiological heterogeneity in biofilms. Nat Rev Microbiol 6 (3):199–210, Epub 12 Feb 2008

Stewart PS, Rayner J, Roe F, Rees WM (2001) Biofilm penetration and disinfection efficacy of alkaline hypochlorite and chlorosulfamates. J Appl Microbiol 91(3):525–532, Epub 15 Sept 2001

Tremoulet F, Duche O, Namane A, Martinie B, Labadie JC, European Listeria Genome C (2002) Comparison of protein patterns of *Listeria monocytogenes* grown in biofilm or in planktonic mode by proteomic analysis. FEMS Microbiol Lett 210(1):25–31

Tresse O, Jouenne T, Junter GA (1995) The role of oxygen limitation in the resistance of agar-entrapped, sessile-like *Escherichia coli* to aminoglycoside and β-lactam antibiotics. J Antimicrob Chemother 36(3):521–526

Trunk K, Benkert B, Quack N, Munch R, Scheer M, Garbe J, Jansch L, Trost M, Wehland J, Buer J, Jahn M, Schobert M, Jahn D (2010) Anaerobic adaptation in *Pseudomonas aeruginosa*: definition of the Anr and Dnr regulons. Environ Microbiol 12(6):1719–1733, Epub 18 June 2010

Tuomanen E, Cozens R, Tosch W, Zak O, Tomasz A (1986) The rate of killing of *Escherichia coli* by beta-lactam antibiotics is strictly proportional to the rate of bacterial growth. J Gen Microbiol 132(5):1297–1304

Ude S, Arnold DL, Moon CD, Timms-Wilson T, Spiers AJ (2006) Biofilm formation and cellulose expression among diverse environmental *Pseudomonas* isolates. Environ Microbiol 8 (11):1997–2011

van Alen T, Claus H, Zahedi RP, Groh J, Blazyca H, Lappann M, Sickmann A, Vogel U (2010) Comparative proteomic analysis of biofilm and planktonic cells of *Neisseria meningitidis*. Proteomics 10(24):4512–4521

Vega NM, Allison KR, Khalil AS, Collins JJ (2012) Signaling-mediated bacterial persister formation. Nat Chem Biol 8(5):431–433

Vinella D, Albrecht C, Cashel M, D'Ari R (2005) Iron limitation induces SpoT-dependent accumulation of ppGpp in *Escherichia coli*. Mol Microbiol 56(4):958–970

von Gotz F, Haussler S, Jordan D, Saravanamuthu SS, Wehmhoner D, Strussmann A, Lauber J, Attree I, Buer J, Tummler B, Steinmetz I (2004) Expression analysis of a highly adherent and cytotoxic small colony variant of *Pseudomonas aeruginosa* isolated from a lung of a patient with cystic fibrosis. J Bacteriol 186(12):3837–3847, Epub 04 June 2004

Vrany JD, Stewart PS, Suci PA (1997) Comparison of recalcitrance to ciprofloxacin and levofloxacin exhibited by *Pseudomonas aeruginosa* biofilms displaying rapid-transport characteristics. Antimicrob Agents Chemother 41(6):1352–1358

Waite RD, Papakonstantinopoulou A, Littler E, Curtis MA (2005) Transcriptome analysis of *Pseudomonas aeruginosa* growth: comparison of gene expression in planktonic cultures and developing and mature biofilms. J Bacteriol 187(18):6571–6576

Walters MC 3rd, Roe F, Bugnicourt A, Franklin MJ, Stewart PS (2003) Contributions of antibiotic penetration, oxygen limitation, and low metabolic activity to tolerance of *Pseudomonas aeruginosa* biofilms to ciprofloxacin and tobramycin. Antimicrob Agents Chemother 47 (1):317–323, Epub 25 Dec 2002

Waters CM, Bassler BL (2005) Quorum sensing: cell-to-cell communication in bacteria. Annu Rev Cell Dev Biol 21:319–346, Epub 11 Oct 2005

Werner E, Roe F, Bugnicourt A, Franklin MJ, Heydorn A, Molin S, Pitts B, Stewart PS (2004) Stratified growth in *Pseudomonas aeruginosa* biofilms. Appl Environ Microbiol 70 (10):6188–6196

Whiteley M, Bangera MG, Bumgarner RE, Parsek MR, Teitzel GM, Lory S, Greenberg EP (2001) Gene expression in *Pseudomonas aeruginosa* biofilms. Nature 413(6858):860–864, Epub 26 Oct 2001

Wijman JGE, de Leeuw PPLA, Moezelaar R, Zwietering MH, Abee T (2007) Air-liquid interface biofilms of *Bacillus cereus*: formation, sporulation, and dispersion. Appl Environ Microbiol 73 (5):1481–1488

Wood TK, Knabel SJ, Kwan BW (2013) Bacterial persister cell formation and dormancy. Appl Environ Microbiol 79(23):7116–7121

Wozniak DJ, Wyckoff TJ, Starkey M, Keyser R, Azadi P, O'Toole GA, Parsek MR (2003) Alginate is not a significant component of the extracellular polysaccharide matrix of PA14 and PAO1 *Pseudomonas aeruginosa* biofilms. Proc Natl Acad Sci U S A 100(13):7907–7912, Epub 18 June 2003

Xu KD, Stewart PS, Xia F, Huang C-T, McFeters GA (1998) Spatial physiological heterogeneity in *Pseudomonas aeruginosa* biofilm is determined by oxygen availability. Appl Environ Microbiol 64(10):4035–4039

Xu KD, Franklin MJ, Park CH, McFeters GA, Stewart PS (2001) Gene expression and protein levels of the stationary phase sigma factor, RpoS, in continuously-fed *Pseudomonas aeruginosa* biofilms. FEMS Microbiol Lett 199(1):67–71

Yamaguchi Y, Inouye M (2011) Regulation of growth and death in *Escherichia coli* by toxin, Äiantitoxin systems. Nat Rev Microbiol 9(11):779–790

Yasuda H, Ajiki Y, Koga T, Kawada H, Yokota T (1993) Interaction between biofilms formed by *Pseudomonas aeruginosa* and clarithromycin. Antimicrob Agents Chemother 37 (9):1749–1755, Epub 01 Sept 1993

Yeom J, Imlay JA, Park W (2010) Iron homeostasis affects antibiotic-mediated cell death in *Pseudomonas* species. J Biol Chem 285(29):22689–22695

Yildiz FH, Schoolnik GK (1999) *Vibrio cholerae* O1 El Tor: identification of a gene cluster required for the rugose colony type, exopolysaccharide production, chlorine resistance, and biofilm formation. Proc Natl Acad Sci 96(7):4028–4033

Yu Q, Griffin EF, Moreau-Marquis S, Schwartzman JD, Stanton BA, O'Toole GA (2012) In vitro evaluation of tobramycin and aztreonam versus *Pseudomonas aeruginosa* biofilms on cystic fibrosis-derived human airway epithelial cells. J Antimicrob Chemother 67(11):2673–2681, Epub 31 July 2012

Zegans ME, Wozniak D, Griffin E, Toutain-Kidd CM, Hammond JH, Garfoot A, Lam JS (2012) *Pseudomonas aeruginosa* exopolysaccharide Psl promotes resistance to the biofilm inhibitor polysorbate 80. Antimicrob Agents Chemother 56(8):4112–4122

Zeiler HJ (1985) Evaluation of the in vitro bactericidal action of ciprofloxacin on cells of *Escherichia coli* in the logarithmic and stationary phases of growth. Antimicrob Agents Chemother 28(4):524–527, Epub 01 Oct 1985

Zhang L, Mah T-F (2008) Involvement of a novel efflux system in biofilm-specific resistance to antibiotics. J Bacteriol 190(13):4447–4452

Zhang L, Fritsch M, Hammond L, Landreville R, Slatculescu C, Colavita A, Mah T-F (2013) Identification of genes involved in *Pseudomonas aeruginosa* biofilm-specific resistance to antibiotics. PLoS One 8(4):e61625

Zogaj X, Nimtz M, Rohde M, Bokranz W, Romling U (2001) The multicellular morphotypes of *Salmonella typhimurium* and *Escherichia coli* produce cellulose as the second component of the extracellular matrix. Mol Microbiol 39(6):1452–1463, Epub 22 Mar 2001

Strategies for Circumventing Bacterial Resistance Mechanisms

Jed F. Fisher, Jarrod W. Johnson, and Shahriar Mobashery

Contents

Abstract

The future practices for the control of bacterial infections are uncertain. The intransigent infection is no longer found just among the immune compromised but is now found both in and out the boundaries of the hospital. Preserving the efficacy of the antibacterials we have, in order to secure the time needed to discover and develop new antibacterials, will require abrupt change: in the way antibacterials are dispensed and disposed, in the criteria used to measure clinical safety and efficacy, in the financial incentives for antibacterial development, and in the understanding of the molecular mechanisms governing the relationship between the antibacterial and the bacterium. This review examines this

J.F. Fisher (✉) • J.W. Johnson • S. Mobashery
Department of Chemistry and Biochemistry, University of Notre Dame, Notre Dame, IN, USA
e-mail: jfisher1@nd.edu; jarrod.w.johnson@gmail.com

M. Gotte et al. (eds.), *Handbook of Antimicrobial Resistance*,
DOI 10.1007/978-1-4939-0694-9_12

relationship from the particular perspective of the eventual need to circumvent resistance mechanisms in order to reclaim the lifesaving value of the antibacterial chemical.

Keywords
Antibiotic • Cell Wall • Cytoskeleton • Natural Products • Resistome • Synergy

Introduction

The parlous confluence of expanding bacterial resistance and contracting investment in antibacterial discovery will be well recognized by the readers of this essay (Lewis 2013; Spellberg et al. 2013; Howard et al. 2014; Singh 2014). The reasons underlying this confluence – found at the microbiological, medical, and societal levels – are equally well understood (O'Connell et al. 2013). These reasons include, at the microbiological level, naiveté of the extraordinary breadth (McArthur et al. 2013; Modi et al. 2013) and resilience of the intrinsic resistome (Cox and Wright 2013; Hede 2014) of bacteria and the ease with which this resistome is shared (Carattoli 2013; Otto 2013a; Perry and Wright 2013; Rodriguez-Rojas et al. 2013); at the medical level, failures of antibiotic stewardship (Leuthner and Doern 2013; Munoz-Price and Quinn 2013; Laxminarayan 2014; Livermore 2014); and at the societal level, willful ignorance of the ecological interplay between antibiotics and animals of all species (Allen et al. 2013; Finley et al. 2013; Stanton 2013; Wellington et al. 2013) and of the magnitude of the financial investment required to ameliorate this confluence (Shlaes et al. 2013; Schäberle and Hack 2014). Moreover, sustaining this amelioration will require simultaneous change at *each* of these three levels (Paphitou 2013; Metz and Shlaes 2014). While the resistome is ancient, the profligate exploitation of the antibiotics has accelerated resistance emergence and galvanized its distribution (Galán et al. 2013). While it is uncertain whether an event short of a pandemic will realize this sea change, the scientific and medical objectives for preserving successful antibacterial chemotherapy in the face of a seeming universe of resistance mechanisms are obvious. These objectives include the discovery of new antibacterials (Gammon 2014), the reincarnation of old antibacterials, the optimization of multi-agent chemotherapy by mechanistic correlation of interdependent targets, a better understanding of the control mechanisms for the expression of resistance mechanisms, a better understanding of the bactericidal mechanisms used by clinically successful antibacterials, and improved clinical trial design (Shlaes and Spellberg 2012; Dalhoff et al. 2014). The exploitation of these discoveries, combined with a recognition of the importance of the clinical practices that ensure antibacterial efficacy (Bogan and Marchaim 2013; Ciccolini et al. 2013), can preserve the antibiotic miracle (Bartlett et al. 2013; Davies et al. 2013).

Nonetheless, the magnitude of the challenge of continually intercepting the moving landscape of antibacterial resistance, by correlation of strategy to objectives, cannot be underestimated (Lewis 2013). At the most fundamental biological levels, we simply do not understand the antibacterial substance. The abundance of antibacterial natural products – the antibiotics – gave rise to the belief that their sole purpose was as offensive weapons. This belief is now understood to be a gross oversimplification (Davies 2013, 2014). It is a trivial matter to demonstrate in vitro mechanistic synergy between two antibacterials. Sustaining this synergy in clinical practice, where it is necessary to align both the respective mechanisms and pharmacokinetics of the drugs, is much more difficult (Paul and Leibovici 2013). Yet we must try (Sun et al. 2013). This essay addresses five perspectives on the relationship between antibiotic discovery and the future chemotherapy of resistant bacteria:

- Will the discovery of new antibacterials contribute to overcoming bacterial resistance?
- Will the discovery of new targets contribute to overcoming bacterial resistance?
- Will understanding how bacteria recognize the presence of antibacterials identify new anti-resistance strategies?
- Will understanding the bactericidal mechanisms of antibacterials identify new anti-resistance strategies?
- How will these answers shape the antibiotic future in the face of the inexorable expansion of the resistome?

We discuss here the current strategies that address these questions and illustrate the extraordinary breadth of the current scientific efforts toward antibacterial discovery in the face of the emergence of extensively resistant bacterial pathogens.

Will the Discovery of New Antibacterials Contribute to Overcoming Bacterial Resistance?

In the immediate decades following the discoveries of the sulfonamides, penicillins, and the aminoglycosides, innumerable antibacterial substances were discovered, primarily from Nature (the antibiotics). Although few of these had the requisite pairing of efficacy and safety, the ease with which this universe of antibacterials was found sustained the belief that Nature held a seemingly inexhaustible trove of antibacterial structures. While successive generations of antibacterials have followed based upon these first structures, this optimism has faded in the face of the experimental difficulties of dereplication (is the biological activity the result of an already known structure?) and validation (Berdy 2012). Indeed, while the past decades have yielded new antibacterial classes of synthetic origin (such as the oxazolidinones) and of semisynthetic origin (such as the fluoroquinolones and carbapenems), few new antibiotics (these new antibiotics are exemplified by daptomycin (**1**), pleuromutilin, and fidaxomicin (**2**)) have progressed to the clinic. While the question as to whether new antibiotic structures will be found in Nature and new antibacterials found by synthesis was once provocative, the new structures, the new combinations of structure, and the new targets that have emerged recently provide guarded optimism for the future (Butler et al. 2013; Chopra 2013; Pucci and Bush 2013; Walsh and Wencewicz 2014) (Fig. 1).

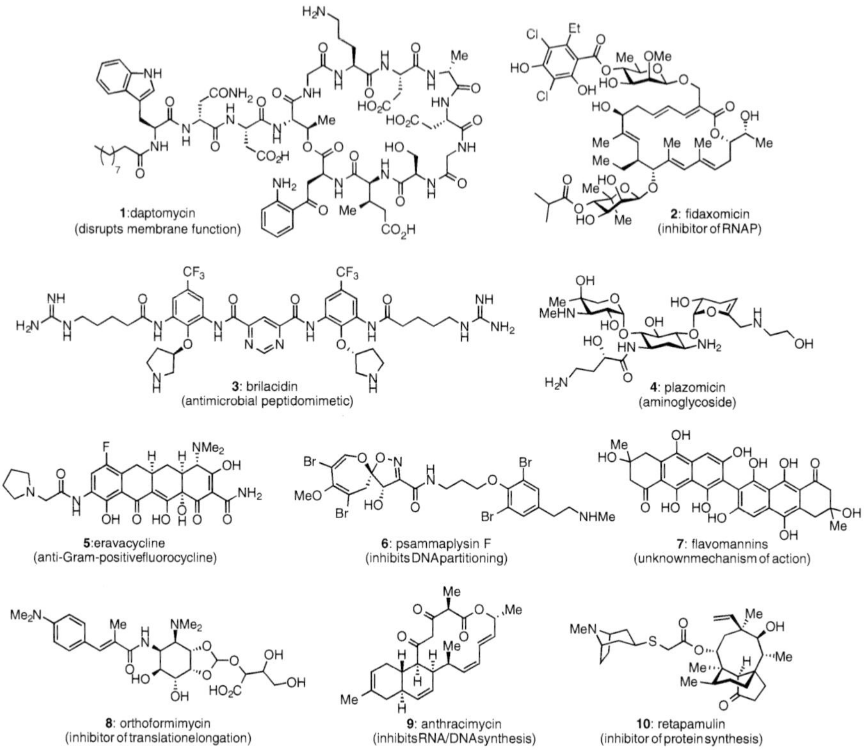

Fig. 1 A selection of recently discovered antibacterials of natural origin

New Natural Products as Antibacterials

The argument that we are entering a new era for the discovery of biologically active natural products is indisputable (Brown et al. 2014). It is not simply that our interrogation now includes both terrestrial and marine organisms (Gerwick and Moore 2012; Gammon 2014) but, additionally, the recognition that our anthropomorphic interest in antibiotics belies the vastly more complex roles these structures have for communication within their ecological niches (Davies 2013). A direct implication from this understanding that the coculture of organisms can profoundly alter secondary metabolite expression is proven (Bertrand et al. 2013; Rateb et al. 2013; Kalghatgi et al. 2013; Hopwood 2013). The vast realm of the so-called "uncultured" bacteria may open for exploration, as we further understand their chemical means of communication (Nikitushkin et al. 2013; Wilson and Piel 2013). Advances in structure analysis (Seger et al. 2013; El-Elimat et al. 2013), including the ability to directly interrogate the presence of secondary metabolites by imaging mass spectrometry (Watrous et al. 2012; Graupner et al. 2012), have diminished dereplication as a barrier to discovery. Finally, numerous advances in the understanding of the genomic organization used for secondary metabolite biosynthesis (Andersen et al. 2013; Wright 2014), coupled to an understanding of the genetic control of biosynthesis by small molecules (Ahmed et al. 2013), by pathway metabolic modeling (Breitling et al. 2013), and by development of new bacterial vectors (Ongley et al. 2013; Komatsu et al. 2013), anticipate a future ability to attain (by manipulation of starting material, enzymes, and vectors) unprecedented antibacterial structure (Baltz 2014; Craney et al. 2013; Walsh et al. 2013; Zakeri and Lu 2013; Thaker et al. 2013; Thaker and Wright 2014).

This opinion implies that disclosures of potentially transformative natural product antibacterials are evident already (Bologa et al. 2013; Kirst 2013). Among the most recently registered antibiotics are daptomycin (**1**) (CUBICIN®, a lipopeptide with a membrane-based mechanism) (Pogliano et al. 2012), retapamulin (**10**) (ALTABAX®/ ALTARGO®, a pleuromutilin that inhibits the 23S rRNA interaction with the 50S subunit of the ribosome with topical Gram-positive activity) (Novak 2011), and fidaxomicin (**2**) (DIFICID®, a macrolide that inhibits the RNA polymerase of Gram-positive bacteria, approved as a narrow-spectrum agent against *C. difficile*) (Sears et al. 2013). The seven parenteral Gram-negative antibacterials (Bush 2012; Boucher et al. 2013) in late-stage clinical evaluation include four β-lactam/β-lactamase inhibitor pairs, plazomicin (**4**) (an aminoglycoside also with Gram-positive activity) (Becker and Cooper 2013), brilacidin (**3**) (an antimicrobial peptidomimetic also having Gram-positive activity), and eravacycline (**5**) (a "fluorocycline" tetracycline derivative and also having Gram-positive activity) (Xiao et al. 2012; Wright et al. 2014). An outstanding characteristic of this list is the explicit role of the evasion of resistance mechanisms in their design (the β-lactam pairs, eravacycline). As was also true of tigecycline (the preceding generation tetracycline), eravacycline was selected on the basis of potency, safety, and the ability to overcome both efflux and ribosomal protection resistance mechanisms (Clark et al. 2012). The other end of the development pipeline – the discovery of structurally unprecedented biological structure – is illustrated with the structures of anthracimycin (**9**), orthoformimycin (**8**), psammaplysin (**6**), and flavomannin (**7**). Anthracimycin is a marine natural product with exceptional potency as an RNA/DNA synthesis inhibitor, especially Gram-positive activity against *Bacillus anthracis*: MIC 0.3 μg mL^{-1} (Jang et al. 2013). Orthoformimycin (Maffioli et al. 2013) is a moderate inhibitor of Gram-positive protein synthesis as a result of binding to the 50S ribosomal subunit, thus blocking elongation. It was identified by the dual screening of microbial fermentation extracts to identify inhibitors of bacterial, but not yeast, protein synthesis. The psammaplysins exemplify a previously known class of marine natural products but now identified as having the remarkable mechanism of inhibiting DNA partitioning into the daughter cell of Gram-positive bacteria (Ramsey et al. 2013). Screening of an extract of *Talaromyces wortmannii* and endophytic fungus of the plant *Aloe vera* identified the flavomannins, atropisomeric dihydroanthracenones with a similar mechanism and equally unknown target (Bara et al. 2013). Antibacterials that are present in small quantities in these extracts but show promising biological activity can be enriched significantly (in the identical fashion as was done decades ago for other antibiotics) by optimization of the fermentation medium. This ability, most recently demonstrated for the platensimycin/platencin class

(Aluotto et al. 2013), enables the further synthetic transformations required to impart clinical potency. While the likelihood that any of these four natural products will progress to the clinic is remote, they illustrate the emerging criteria now used to identify captivating antibiotic structure: evaluation of novel microbial sources and/or the use of sophisticated screening methodologies to discover unprecedented mechanism and target (Thaker et al. 2013).

New Synthetics as Antibacterials

The interrogation of industrial chemicals for compounds with potential biological activity was foundational in the mid-nineteenth century to the creation of the synthetic dye industry, and the interrogation of synthetic dyes was foundational decades later to the discovery of the sulfonamide (sulfa) class of antibacterials. The emergence of an entire breadth of new technologies to address both new antibacterial targets and reassess old targets has led to new horizons for antibacterial discovery. Even with respect to sulfonamide antibacterials, new discoveries have been made with respect to both resistance mutation(s) of the target and to off-target mechanisms. Crystallographic examination of the molecular target of sulfonamides, the enzyme dihydropteroate synthase, allowed cross-correlation of the resistance mutations seen within this enzyme to both the catalytic mechanism and sulfonamide binding (Yun et al. 2012). The probable basis for the CNS side effects of certain antibacterial (and other) sulfonamides was identified as competitive inhibition within the tetrahydrobiopterin biosynthetic pathway (Haruki et al. 2013). Whether access to these protein structures will enable the redesign of a sulfonamide to simultaneously evade resistance mutation and eliminate off-target binding is uncertain. Rather, it is the simple demonstration that it is now possible to conceptualize structural change within a (seemingly aged) antibacterial class based on structure-based design (Agarwal and Fishwick 2010).

Among the most intensively studied targets for the identification of novel antibacterial structure is the bacterial cytoskeleton (Celler et al. 2013; Pilhofer and Jensen 2013; Ojima et al. 2014). The dramatic increase in the understanding of the bacterial cytoskeleton as a control mechanism for coordinating bacterial cell growth has identified new antibacterial opportunity (Ma and Ma 2012; Pinho et al. 2013; Wilson and Gitai 2013). A Gram-negative bacterium cannot merely organize the assembly of its cell-wall polymer, but it must coordinate this assembly with *inter alia* the duplication and translocation of its genome (Sass and Brötz-Oesterhelt 2013), the synthesis of its inner membrane, the export of proteins to the periplasm and outer membrane, the assembly of the inner leaflet of the outer membrane, and the export of the lipopolysaccharide as the outer leaflet of its outer membrane. Among the key contributors to this coordination are the central cell-division mediator (tubulin-like) protein FtsZ (Reimold et al. 2013) and the membrane-adhering (actin-like) protein MreB (Celler et al. 2013). Notwithstanding the challenge of confirming and identifying the precise molecular mechanisms of compounds that bind to these proteins (Anderson et al. 2012; Foss et al. 2013), compounds that disrupt this coordination are antibacterial and/or are synergistic with other antibacterials. The most prominent inhibitors with respect to binding to FtsZ are PC190723 (**15**) and related structures (Anderson et al. 2012; Elsen et al. 2012; Matsui et al. 2012). An *N*-dimethylaminomethyl prodrug derivative of PC190723 (TXY436) shows improved solubility and has oral efficacy in mice infected with MSSA and MRSA (Kaul et al. 2013). One of the best compounds in this series has potent antistaphylococcal activity (MIC 0.12 μg mL^{-1}) in vitro, oral activity in infection models, and an acceptable frequency of FtsZ point mutation resistance selection (4.1×10^{-9}) given the evidence for impaired in vitro fitness accompanying the point mutation (Stokes et al. 2013). PC190723 also acts synergistically with β-lactam antibiotics against *S. aureus*, possibly as a result of mislocalization of FtsZ with concomitant disruption of its binding partner (and target of the β-lactams), the PBP bifunctional enzyme(s) (Tan et al. 2012). A no less significant observation is an even lower resistance frequency (1.6×10^{-9}) for the PC190723–β-lactam pairing. PC190723 and other cytoskeleton-interacting structures are shown in Fig. 2.

The potential of structural biology-enabled screening for the serendipitous discovery of new antibiotic leads is vast. A high-throughput screening of drug-like structures against the MipZ protein identified one compound ("divin," **18**) as a weak inhibitor; subsequent analysis showed neither MipZ nor FtsZ was its true target. The target is unidentified. Divin is bacteriostatic against several Gram-negative bacteria (MIC 1–50 μg mL^{-1}) as a result of its ability to disrupt the assembly of division proteins (including for the cell wall) and to block compartmentalization of the cytoplasm (Eun et al. 2013). A virtual screening effort against the structure of the AgrA response regulator identified an FDA-approved compound, the nonsteroidal anti-inflammatory drug diflunisal, with micromolar anti-virulence (but not antibacterial) activity against MRSA as a result of its inhibition of the production of α-hemolysin and phenol-soluble modulins (Khodaverdian et al. 2013). As a third example, the structure of the *P. aeruginosa* multidrug efflux transporter inhibited by a pyridopyrimidine compound sets the opportunity for successful structure-based design of a "universal" efflux inhibitor (Nakashima et al. 2013). As antibacterial targets are identified, a phalanx of physical and virtual methods is available to interrogate the target.

Will the Discovery of New Targets Contribute to Overcoming Bacterial Resistance?

The correct choice of the therapeutic target is essential (Bugg 2014). Given the smaller genome of the bacteria, an early presumption of the post-genomic era was that the identification of the essential bacterial targets would in turn identify exploratory antibacterials. A reappraisal of the Gram-positive *B. subtilis* genome identified 261 genes (259 proteins, only six without assigned function, and two functional RNAs) as essential (Commichau et al. 2013). Extensive bioinformatic efforts, such as by genome cross-correlation, have further generalized our understanding of the essential bacterial genome (Duffield et al. 2010; McArthur et al. 2013). Nonetheless,

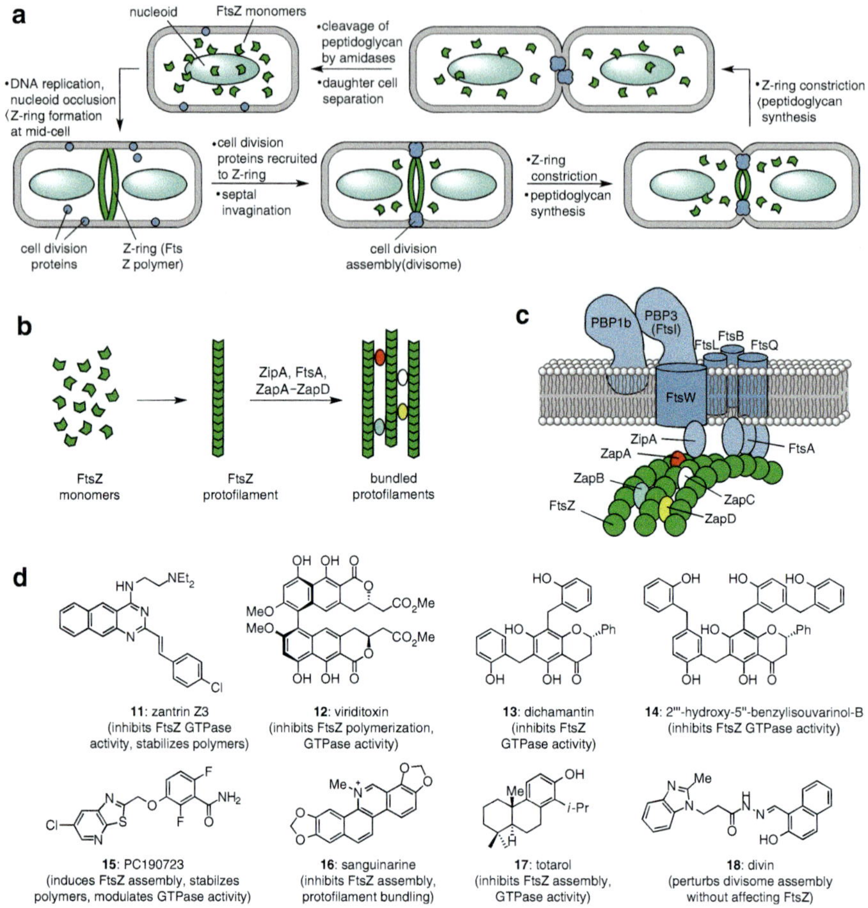

Fig. 2 Bacterial cell division, divisome assembly, and cell-division inhibitors. (**a**) Selected steps in *E. coli* cell division, including nucleoid occlusion, followed by Z-ring formation, recruitment of cell-division assembly proteins, Z-ring contraction, and daughter cell separation. (**b**) Polymerization of FtsZ into protofilaments and bundling of the protofilaments for Z-ring assembly. (**c**) A simplified representation of interactions of Z-ring proteins with selected membrane-bound proteins of *E. coli*. For recent reviews of cell division and divisome assembly, see (Egan and Vollmer 2013; Huang et al. 2013; Pinho et al. 2013). (**d**) Selected cell-division inhibitors. For recent reviews, see Sass and Brötz-Oesterhelt (2013), Schaffner-Barbero et al. (2012)

the limitation of a singular focus on essentiality with respect to successful antibacterial discovery was revealed and candidly discussed by Payne et al. in the context of successive failed high-throughput antibacterial target screens (Payne et al. 2007). The lessons from this collective failure – the surprising genetic diversity of bacteria, the mutational ease of resistance generation, the extraordinary versatility of bacteria to adapt to metabolic challenge, the unusual chemical space for antibacterial structure, and the synthetic challenge in entering that space – have been transformative to current thinking on bacterial targeting (Roemer and Boone

2013). Notwithstanding these transformations in thinking, empirical exploration of chemical structure to identify new targets has not lost value, as exemplified by the most recently approved addition to *Mycobacterium tuberculosis* chemotherapy, bedaquiline (SIRTURO®). The identification of its target as the bacterial ATP synthase was foundational to further exploration of both its structural class and the target with respect to other Gram-positive pathogens (Balemans et al. 2012). Likewise, one of the most promising new exploratory classes of drugs against *M. tuberculosis*, the imidazopyridines, was discovered by the serendipity of classic antibacterial screening (Moraski et al. 2013; Pethe et al. 2013). The imidazopyridines also block ATP synthesis, although at a different target (the cytochrome bc1 complex).

And while structure-based design will indeed contribute to the discovery of new antibacterials – as discussed below and as exemplified by the opportunities implicit in the AEROPATH compilation of *Pseudomonas aeruginosa* target structures (Moynie et al. 2013) – complementary new approaches have emerged to address the central relationship of validating targets with respect to resistance-compromised chemical structure. Proteomic analysis of the resistance response will contribute to an understanding of the overall metabolic adjustment (Lima et al. 2013) and the identification of critical protein interaction networks (Zoraghi and Reiner 2013). Mass spectrometric analysis eventually will demonstrate clinical value for bacterial diagnosis (Mitsuma et al. 2013) and for the detection of resistance mechanisms, as exemplified by the shotgun proteomic identification of a β-barrel outer membrane-located carbapenem-resistance protein (of unknown function) in *Acinetobacter baumannii* (Chang et al. 2013). Underlying many of these efforts is the emerging realization that future chemotherapy of multidrug-resistant bacteria will demand antibacterials either with multi-target activities (East and Silver 2013; Yan et al. 2013) or synergistic mechanisms of action (Lázár et al. 2013; Roemer and Boone 2013; Worthington and Melander 2013a).

The inevitable transition from single-drug treatment of bacterial infection to multidrug treatment – as is already the case for *Mycobacterium tuberculosis* – will not be guided by empirical experimentation. While the enormously successful pairing of β-lactamase inhibitors with β-lactams is the obvious example of the facile selection of synergistic targets (Worthington and Melander 2013b), strategies for the experimental validation of equally promising synergistic pairs are emerging (Roemer et al. 2012; Roemer and Boone 2013; Lázár et al. 2013; Zoraghi and Reiner 2013). We noted the synergistic pairing with β-lactams (targeting the PBP enzymes) with FtsZ antagonists against Gram-positive bacteria. The possibility of synergy with proven antibacterials will certainly be used to prioritize the additional FtsZ antagonists that emerge from screening against both Gram-positive (Foss et al. 2013; Ruiz-Avila et al. 2013) and Gram-negative (Keffer et al. 2013) bacteria.

Small-molecule screening of drug-like structures may now be done using antibacterial synergy as the focus. Using a small (20,000 compounds) library to identify compounds showing synergy with β-lactams (potentiation agents) against methicillin-resistant *S. aureus* (MRSA) identified an inhibitor of MurG (Huber et al. 2009), an enzyme that catalyzes the second glycosyltransferase step in the biosynthesis of the pivotal cell-wall precursor, Lipid II (Mann et al. 2013).

The primary mechanism for this synergy was depletion of Lipid II as a result of MurG inhibition, resulting in the inability of the essential penicillin-binding protein enzyme (and target of the β-lactam) to correctly localize to the division septum. Perhaps not surprisingly, the enzymatic transformations that follow MurG and complete Lipid II biosynthesis also show promise as targets identifying potentiation agents against MRSA (Roemer et al. 2013). An inhibitor specific for one of these *Fem* (*f*actor *e*ssential for *m*ethicillin resistance) enzymes (cyslabdan, **25**) has been already identified and demonstrates β-lactam synergy (Koyama et al. 2012). Moreover, the first crystal structure of a Fem enzyme suggests an unexpected mechanism (Fonvielle et al. 2013) that opens the possibility of both structure- and mechanism-based design. Lastly, glycosylation of the cell-surface teichoic acids of *S. aureus* [is critical for antibacterial resistance, but not for] viability (Bertsche et al. 2013; Brown et al. 2012b; Pasquina et al. 2013) function. The relationship between the integrity of the cell-surface teichoic acids to resistance is substantiated by the identification of a series of inhibitors addressing different events in their biosynthesis, including a synthetic compound (**24**) with in vitro and in vivo antibiotic activity as a result of its inhibition of LtaS (lipoteichoic acid polymerase) (Richter et al. 2013); a registered drug (ticlopidine, **22**) discovered to also act as an inhibitor of TarO (first enzyme of teichoic acid synthesis) and that is synergistic with β-lactams (Farha et al. 2013a); and a synthetic inhibitor (targocil, **20**) of the TarG teichoic acid transporter that also synergizes with β-lactams (Lee et al. 2010; Campbell et al. 2012; Wang et al. 2013). Moreover, blocking the biosynthesis of the wall teichoic acids may suppress horizontal gene transfer in chronic polymicrobial infections (Winstel et al. 2013). Exemplification of the correlation of new structures to classic Gram-positive targets, as well as emerging Gram-positive targets, is given in Fig. 3.

At the same conceptual level as for teichoic acid structure integrity for Gram-positives (Sewell and Brown 2014), there is an identical relationship between integrity and resistance for many antibacterials with respect to the lipopolysaccharide (LPS) leaflet of the outer membrane of Gram-negative bacteria. This relationship is exemplified by the discrete structural alterations that are made to the LPS as a resistance mechanism against polymyxin (Hankins et al. 2012; Fernández et al. 2013; Wanty et al. 2013) and colistin (Pelletier et al. 2013). Given the importance of the integrity of the LPS leaflet, interference with LPS biosynthesis and transport has been identified as a promising strategy to attenuate resistance (Srinivas et al. 2010; Werneburg et al. 2012; Sherman et al. 2013). High-throughput screening identified a lead compound (**32**) as an inhibitor of the ATPase component of the multienzyme complex (IC_{50} 120 μM, compared to 20 μM against the LptB ATPase alone) with antibacterial activity (MIC 12.5 μM) against outer membrane-permeabilized (but not wild type) *E. coli*. This result substantiates the expectation that a more potent compound would potentiate clinically proven antibacterials, as a result of its ability to compromise outer membrane permeability (Sherman et al. 2013).

Clinical validation of in vitro promise is arduous. The seemingly subtle changes that occur with respect to transcription following antibiotic challenge

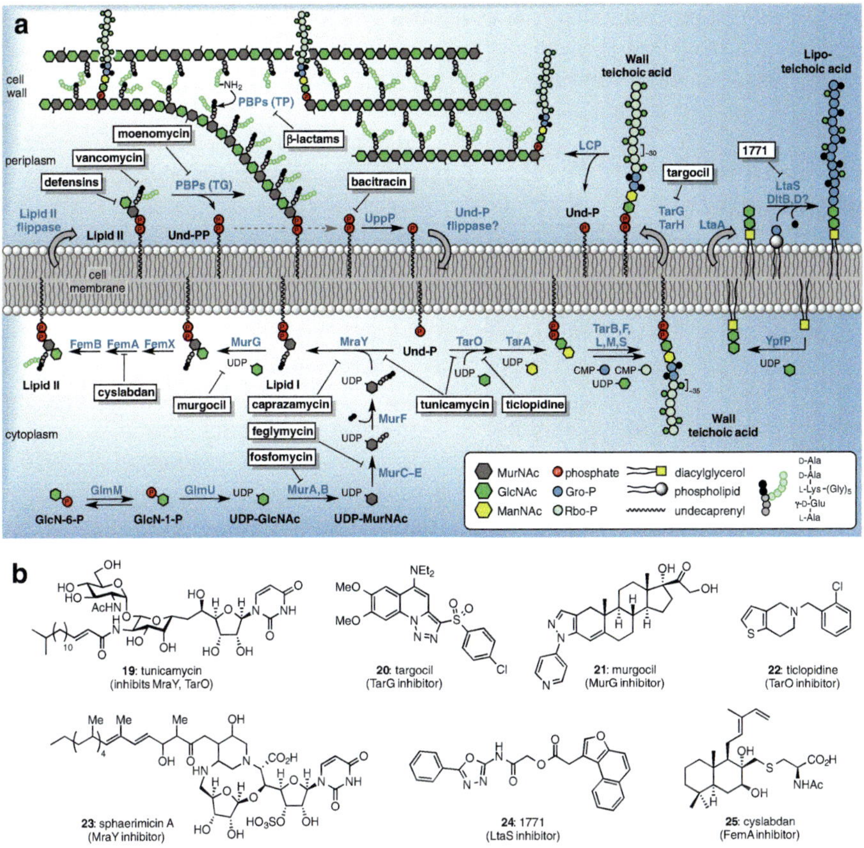

Fig. 3 (**a**) Cell-wall biosynthesis and teichoic acid biosynthesis in *S. aureus*. For recent reviews, see Barreteau et al. (2008), Brown et al. (2013), Pasquina et al. (2013), Sewell and Brown (2014). (**b**) A selection of cell-wall-targeting inhibitors and antibiotics active against Gram-positive bacteria (GlcNAc *N*-acetylglucosamine, MurNAc *N*-acetylmuramic acid, PBP penicillin-binding protein, TG transglycosylase, TP transpeptidase, Und undecaprenyl, Gro glycerol phosphate, Rbo ribitol phosphate)

(Van Oudenhove et al. 2012; Abranches et al. 2013) can be interpreted either as encouraging (even small alterations in activity can reduce fitness) or daunting (numerous compensatory pathways). The remarkable (and not yet understood) “seesaw” effect observed in MRSA – wherein β-lactam susceptibility increases as glycopeptide and lipopeptide susceptibility decreases, suggesting subtle structural interplay between their proximal cell-wall targets (Werth et al. 2013a) – cautions against the expectation that the identification of synergistic target pairs is straightforward. Nonetheless, increasingly sophisticated analytic methodologies have proven that such pairs exist and that the time-proven medicinal chemistry strategies can be expected to deliver on this promise. Indeed, the judicious pairing with vancomycin of a β-lactam with advantageous activity against MRSA (the cephalosporin ceftaroline) shows in vitro synergy (Werth et al. 2013b). A key aspect of future clinical chemotherapy of resistant bacteria will be chemotherapeutic synergy, as identified and confirmed by biochemical, proteomic, and genomic analyses.

Will an Understanding of How Bacteria Recognize the Presence of Antibacterials Identify New Anti-resistance Strategies?

The increasing prevalence of antibiotic-resistant bacteria might be interpreted as evidence that bacterial fitness is not compromised by resistance mechanisms. This interpretation is facile. Rather, it is that bacteria have a remarkable ability to reorganize their metabolic networks so as to accommodate the resistance mechanism(s) at the cost of a reduced ecological range (Händel et al. 2013). While there are numerous examples of the constitutive expression of powerful resistance mechanisms (such as β-lactamase expression by *M. tuberculosis*) (Tremblay et al. 2010), the expression of many resistance mechanisms is regulated. The depth of these mysteries surrounding such regulation is superbly exemplified by vancomycin, an antibiotic with a decades-long history. Although its molecular mechanism – formation of a stable non-covalent complex with the cell-wall peptidoglycan – is long known, in bacteria where vancomycin resistance is induced (such as *S. aureus*) the structural relationship of complex formation to resistance expression is unknown. The study of this relationship in *Streptomyces coelicolor* implicates direct binding of the peptidoglycan–vancomycin complex to the VanS histidine kinase component of the VanRS two-component regulatory system (Koteva et al. 2010; Kwun et al. 2013). This two-component system has no human counterpart, and ensuing structural change to the VanR response regulator is profound (Leonard et al. 2013). A ligand capable of exploiting this difference in structure so as to prevent VraR dimerization would compromise the ability to respond to the presence of vancomycin. This conclusion presumes, however, that regulation of the resistance mechanism is advantageous with respect to fitness. Notwithstanding the complexity of the vancomycin resistance pathway (seven genes organized into two operons), in the enterococci the evolutionary pressure exerted by vancomycin exposure has abolished the fitness cost of maintaining this pathway (Foucault et al. 2010). However, fitness cost is not the only basis used by bacteria to compel regulation of the resistance pathway. Sustaining resistance mechanism against one antibacterial may simultaneously sensitize to another antibacterial. This "seesaw" effect has been observed in vitro between two pairs of cell-wall-targeting antibacterials against resistant staphylococci: daptomycin and β-lactams (Dhand et al. 2011; Vignaroli et al. 2011; Mehta et al. 2012) and vancomycin and β-lactams (Werth et al. 2013a). Should these conclusions be sustained in vivo, the use of such antibacterial pairs may improve efficacy while decreasing the likelihood of transmitting resistance mechanisms.

While the value of β-lactams is increasingly endangered due to resistance (McKenna 2013; Watkins and Bonomo 2013), many Gram-positive and

Gram-negative bacteria use distinct sentinel pathways to initiate a β-lactam resistance response. Neither signal transduction pathway is well understood. The sentinel protein that initiates the β-lactam resistance response in MRSA (Llarrull and Mobashery 2012) detects β-lactams by acylation of a serine residue by the β-lactam, an event with extraordinary identity to the first half-reaction in class D serine β-lactamase turnover (Kumarasiri et al. 2012). Although the penultimate event leading to the β-lactam resistance of MRSA is proteolytic inactivation of a repressor, the intermediate events of signal transduction – between the initial acylation and this proteolysis – are uncertain (Arede et al. 2013). A possible messenger is a co-activator derived from perturbed peptidoglycan recycling (Amoroso et al. 2012). This possibility is especially intriguing as perturbed peptidoglycan recycling (Cavallari et al. 2013; Johnson et al. 2013) – possibly as a result of the selective inactivation of low-molecular-mass penicillin-binding proteins (Moya et al. 2012) – is central to the induction of β-lactamase expression in many Gram-negative bacteria.

The control of β-lactamase expression is instructive. These enzymes exhibit high catalytic efficiency with respect to many β-lactam substrates, and the co-substrate used to detoxify the β-lactam – water – is independent of all other metabolic pathways within the bacterium. Yet for certain β-lactamases there appears to be a permissive correlation with particular bacteria, implying a fitness cost underlying the control of their expression (Fernández et al. 2012). The biochemical basis for the much more complex transition from planktonic bacteria to the biofilm, as regulated by quorum-sensing pathways and correlated to virulence (Beceiro et al. 2013), has revealed strategies – chemical (Morkunas et al. 2012; Stacy et al. 2012, 2013; Imperi et al. 2013b; Melamed Yerushalmi et al. 2013; Saroj and Rather 2013), biochemical (Chatterjee et al. 2013), and microbiological (Gupta et al. 2013) – to interfere with this transition (Blackledge et al. 2013; Hirakawa and Tomita 2013; Zhu and Kaufmann 2013). While the determination of the optimal structure and target for intervention is still uncertain (and is likely different for each bacterium), whole-genome analysis of the bacterial resistome (McArthur et al. 2013) is a credible strategy to identify lineage in outbreaks (Harris et al. 2013; Otto 2013b; Reuter et al. 2013; Holt et al. 2013); to identify resistance–evolution pathways (Abranches et al. 2013; Kamen Ek and Gur-Bertok 2013; Méhi et al. 2013); to correlate biochemical adaptation to resistance (as exemplified for daptomycin (Kelesidis et al. 2013; Peleg et al. 2012; Song et al. 2013; Tran et al. 2013); and to validate targets (Wang et al. 2013). Exemplification of the correlation of new structures to old Gram-negative targets, as well as emerging Gram-negative targets, is given in Fig. 4.

Bacteria recognize and respond to antibiotics and to each other. These responses may be relatively simple (such as lipid remodeling as a resistance mechanism to daptomycin) or complex (such as caused by activation of cell-wall stress stimulons). Within each of these responses are critical nexuses, and disrupting these connections will be future strategies to combat resistance.

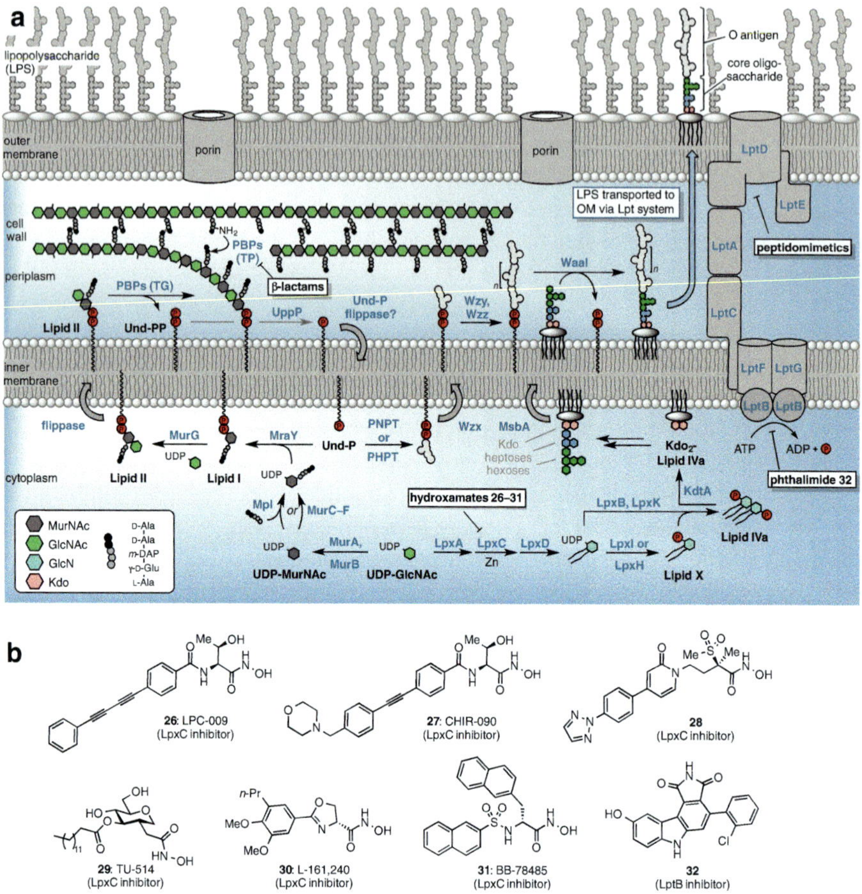

Fig. 4 (**a**) Cell-wall biosynthesis, *O*-antigen biosynthesis, and lipopolysaccharide (*LPS*) biosynthesis and transport in *E. coli*. For recent reviews, see Greenfield and Whitfield (2012), Zhang et al. (2013). (**b**) A selection of LpxC inhibitors (Jackman et al. 2000; Brown et al. 2012a; Montgomery et al. 2012; Warmus et al. 2012) and inhibitors of LptB (Sherman et al. 2013). For peptidomimetic inhibitors of LptD, see Srinivas et al. (2010)

Will Understanding the Bactericidal Mechanisms of Antibacterials Identify New Anti-resistance Strategies?

A parallel opportunity to combat resistance by identifying critical connectivity exists for the bacterial responses subsequent to encounter with the antibacterial. While there is certainly a mechanistic correlation between the engagement of the target by the antibacterial and the ensuing loss of bacterial viability, it is now more than ever evident that the mechanistic relationship between these two events is not linear (Kohanski et al. 2010). Knowledge of the antibacterial activity of silver ions is ancient: but at a molecular level, how should we interpret the ability of silver ions to potentiate (both in vitro and in murine pharmacological assays of infection) a variety of antibiotics against both Gram-negative and Gram-positive bacteria (Morones-Ramirez et al. 2013)? One possible explanation for this synergy is cooperative induction of oxidative stress as the key bactericidal event (Brynildsen et al. 2013; Vatansever et al. 2013). The induction by β-lactams of the RpoS regulon (so as to facilitate mutagenesis) (Gutierrez et al. 2013) and the toxicity of antibacterials to mitochondria are consistent with this hypothesis (Kalghatgi et al. 2013). Other experimental data, however, are inconsistent (Liu and Imlay 2013; Keren et al. 2013; Ezraty et al. 2013) and emphasize the extraordinary challenges both of experimental design and interpretation necessary to decipher tightly integrated response pathways (Mahoney and Silhavy 2013; Manoil 2013).

Oxidative stress is not the only source of connectivity loci directly relevant to resistance. Bacteria control pathways by kinase/phosphatase signaling and the breadth of phosphorylation control – whether histidine or serine/threonine/tyrosine – encompass resistance responses (Worthington et al. 2013; Wilke and Carlson 2013; Hall et al. 2013). The two-component histidine kinases have no eukaryotic counterpart and thus present opportunity as targets for structure-based inhibitor design (Velikova et al. 2013). Conversely, given the diversity of structures already perfected for the control of eukaryotic kinases, the attractiveness of a strategy that re-optimizes these structures as inhibitors of bacterial kinases – as exemplified by the phosphotransferases used to detoxify aminoglycosides (Stogios et al. 2013) – is obvious.

A third connection is recognition of the relationship of the proton-motive force to antibacterial resistance (Farha et al. 2013b; Lázár et al. 2013). This force is, of course, necessary for bacterial vitality: it contributes directly, for example, to the correct localization of an essential high-molecular-mass penicillin-binding protein in *B. subtilis* as shown by the collapse of this force following exposure of the bacterium to the lantibiotic, nisin (Lages et al. 2013). And while the collapse of this force is intimately connected to the cellular damage arising from oxidative stress (Ezraty et al. 2013), the enzymes that sustain the proton-motive force represent independent targets for antibacterial discovery. For example, exposure of bacteria to sub-MIC concentrations of the OAK antimicrobial peptide sufficiently depolarizes its membrane with compromise of antibacterial efflux, thus potentiating the efficacy of erythromycin in a murine infection model of MDR *E. coli* (Zaknoon et al. 2012; Goldberg et al. 2013). A similar potentiation is demonstrated for *S. aureus* (Kaneti et al. 2013). Exploiting the emerging capabilities of high-resolution microscopy for bacterial cytological profiling, Nonejuie et al. identified the mechanism of a Gram-positive active spirotetronate as the collapse of the proton-motive force (Nonejuie et al. 2013). Indeed, this discovery demonstrates the value of emerging technologies for finding solutions to the resistance conundrum: here, a simple and one-step assay that rapidly identifies the antibacterial mechanism.

A final emerging theme for new strategies to combat antibacterial resistance is invigoration of bacterial persisters – slow-growing or hibernating bacterial cells that show tolerance to the presence of antibiotics (Gerdes and Ingmer 2013) – so as to abolish their tolerance. For example, application of a depsipeptide derivative to an in vitro culture of *S. aureus* persisters activates the ClpP protease of these bacteria. When combined with a second antibacterial (rifampicin), the persisters are killed (Conlon et al. 2013). Moreover, this combination eradicates, in a murine infection model, a biofilm infection of *S. aureus* (Conlon et al. 2013). As suggested by these authors, ClpP may not be unique as a target capable of "corruption" by specific agents, with ensuing sensitization of the bacterial persister. A second enzyme target, NAD synthetase, is a target for the eradication of *M. tuberculosis* persisters (Kim et al. 2013). The emerging abilities of whole-genome bacterial analysis to identify resistance mutations (Reuter et al. 2013) and of proteomics to identify resistance responses (Conlon et al. 2013; Chang et al. 2013; Lima et al. 2013) will enable target (s) validation with respect to collateral sensitivity networks for multi-antibiotic therapy (Roemer and Boone 2013) or multi-antibiotic therapeutic cycling (Imamovic and Sommer 2013).

Conclusion: The Antibiotic Future in the Face of an Inexorable Expansion of the Resistome

These examples emphasize the depth of the resources available to discover new structures and to implement new strategies to combat bacterial resistance. The evolution of the resistance pathways, following the clinical introduction of antibiotics, is recognized as the result of the evolutionary refinement by bacteria of *inter alia* their protein structures, their genomes, and their metabolic pathways (Derewacz et al. 2013). These refinements are interdependent, and identifying and exploiting the key nexuses that are the foundation of this interdependence will be critical to the antibacterial future (Roemer et al. 2012; Roemer and Boone 2013; East and Silver 2013; Lewis 2013; Zlitni et al. 2013). The success of β-lactam/β-lactamase therapy – measured both by three decades of clinical practice (Drawz and Bonomo 2010; Hasan et al. 2013) and the current antibacterial pipeline (Butler et al. 2013; Pucci and Bush 2013; Shlaes 2013) – proves the value of this strategy. The failure of efflux inhibitors to attain clinical impact (to date) proves the challenge of the strategy. Adding to this challenge are the increased expectations for the clinically efficacious antibacterial. The antibacterial expectation is no longer measured with respect to a Gram-positive and Gram-negative divide, but with respect to an emerging array of pathogenic species, each with its own unique resistance capabilities (Boucher et al. 2013; Master et al. 2013; Pendleton et al. 2013). Moreover, the new antibacterial may now be expected to retain efficacy against intracellular bacteria (Miskinyte and Gordo 2013) and bacterial persisters (Lewis 2013; Bald and Koul 2013; Cohen et al. 2013; Maisonneuve and Gerdes 2014) and to preferentially target virulent strains (Beceiro et al. 2013) while preserving the nonpathogenic microbiome (Riley et al. 2013). As we transition from populations at particular risk of bacterial infection – such as the transplant recipient (Bodro et al. 2013), the immunocompromised (Bow 2013), and the critically ill (Cohen 2013) – to the entire populations at risk, such may result from the entry of pathogenic bacteria into the food supply (Le Hello et al. 2013), neither new structures nor new technologies may alone suffice to provide the antibacterial future. We will need to aggressively evaluate empirical opportunities, such as pursuing repurposed compounds that act to sensitize (Thorsing et al. 2013) or to attenuate quorum sensing (Imperi et al. 2013b; O'Loughlin et al. 2013), virulence (Imperi et al. 2013a; Long et al. 2013), and efflux (Jiang et al. 2013). Reassessing old discovery strategies as well as implementing new strategies will be required (Shapiro 2013; Tegos and Hamblin 2013). While the scientific paths to move forward against bacterial resistance are largely evident, the resources needed to engage the breadth of these paths are not, nor, as emphasized in the introduction, is the realization that engaging these paths is necessary but not sufficient. The question is not what needs to be done but rather whether a pandemic is the only circumstance that will galvanize an antibiotic future.

References

Abranches J, Tijerina P, Aviles-Reyes A, Gaca AO, Kajfasz JK, Lemos JA (2013) The cell wall-targeting antibiotic stimulon of *Enterococcus faecalis*. PLoS One 8:e64875. doi:10.1371/journal.pone.0064875

Agarwal AK, Fishwick CWG (2010) Structure-based design of anti-infectives. Ann NY Acad Sci 1213:20–45. doi:10.1111/j.1749-6632.2010.05859.x

Ahmed S, Craney A, Pimentel-Elardo SM, Nodwell JR (2013) A synthetic, species-specific activator of secondary metabolism and sporulation in *Streptomyces coelicolor*. ChemBioChem 14:83–91. doi:10.1002/cbic.201200619

Allen HK, Levine UY, Looft T, Bandrick M, Casey TA (2013) Treatment, promotion, commotion: antibiotic alternatives in food-producing animals. Trends Microbiol 21:114–119. doi:10.1016/j.tim.2012.11.001

Aluotto S, Tynan H, Maggio C, Falzone M, Mukherjee A, Gullo V, Demain AL (2013) Development of a semi-defined medium supporting production of platensimycin and platencin by *Streptomyces platensis*. J Antibiot (Tokyo) 66:51–54. doi:10.1038/ja.2012.97

Amoroso A, Boudet J, Berzigotti S, Duval S, Teller N, Mengin-Lecreulx D, Luxen A, Simorre J-P, Joris B (2012) A peptidoglycan fragment triggers β-lactam resistance in *Bacillus licheniformis*. PLoS Pathog 8:e1002571. doi:10.1371/journal.ppat.1002571

Andersen MR, Nielsen JB, Klitgaard A, Petersen LM, Zachariasen M, Hansen TJ, Blicher LH, Gotfredsen CH, Larsen TO, Nielsen KF, Mortensen UH (2013) Accurate prediction of secondary metabolite gene clusters in filamentous fungi. Proc Natl Acad Sci U S A 110:E99–E107. doi:10.1073/pnas.1205532110

Anderson DE, Kim MB, Moore JT, O'Brien TE, Sorto NA, Grove CI, Lackner LL, Ames JB, Shaw JT (2012) Comparison of small molecule inhibitors of the bacterial cell division protein FtsZ and Identification of a reliable cross-species inhibitor. ACS Chem Biol 7:1918–1928. doi:10.1021/cb300340j

Arede P, Ministro J, Oliveira DC (2013) Redefining the role of the β-lactamase locus in methicillin-resistant *Staphylococcus aureus*: β-lactamase regulators disrupt the MecI-mediated strong repression on *mecA* and optimize the phenotypic expression of resistance in strains with constitutive mecA expression. Antimicrob Agents Chemother 57:3037–3045. doi:10.1128/AAC. 02621-12

Bald D, Koul A (2013) Advances and strategies in discovery of new antibacterials for combating metabolically resting bacteria. Drug Discov Today 18:250–255. doi:10.1016/j.drudis.2012.09.007

Balemans W, Vranckx L, Lounis N, Pop O, Guillemont J, Vergauwen K, Mol S, Gilissen R, Motte M, Lancois D, De Bolle M, Bonroy K, Lill H, Andries K, Bald D, Koul A (2012) Novel antibiotics targeting respiratory ATP synthesis in gram-positive pathogenic bacteria. Antimicrob Agents Chemother 56:4131–4139. doi:10.1128/AAC. 00273-12

Baltz RH (2014) Combinatorial biosynthesis of cyclic lipopeptide antibiotics: a model for synthetic biology to accelerate the evolution of secondary metabolite biosynthetic pathways. ACS Synth Biol 3:748–758. doi:10.1021/sb3000673

Bara R, Zerfass I, Aly AH, Goldbach-Gecke H, Raghavan V, Sass P, Mándi A, Wray V, Polavarapu PL, Pretsch A, Lin W, Kurtán T, Debbab A, Brötz-Oesterhelt H, Proksch P (2013) Atropisomeric dihydroanthracenones as inhibitors of multiresistant *Staphylococcus aureus*. J Med Chem 56:3257–3272. doi:10.1021/jm301816a

Barreteau H, Kovac A, Boniface A, Sova M, Gobec S, Blanot D (2008) Cytoplasmic steps of peptidoglycan biosynthesis. FEMS Microbiol Rev 32:168–207. doi:10.1111/j.1574-6976.2008.00104.x

Bartlett JG, Gilbert DN, Spellberg B (2013) Seven ways to preserve the miracle of antibiotics. Clin Infect Dis 56:1445–1450. doi:10.1093/cid/cit070

Beceiro A, Tomás M, Bou G (2013) Antimicrobial resistance and virulence: a successful or deleterious association in the bacterial world? Clin Microbiol Rev 26:185–230. doi:10.1128/CMR. 00059-12

Becker B, Cooper MA (2013) Aminoglycoside antibiotics in the 21st century. ACS Chem Biol 8:105–115. doi:10.1021/cb3005116

Berdy J (2012) Thoughts and facts about antibiotics: where we are now and where we are heading. J Antibiot (Tokyo) 65:385–395. doi:10.1038/ja.2012.27

Bertrand S, Schumpp O, Bohni N, Monod M, Gindro K, Wolfender J-L (2013) De novo production of metabolites by fungal co-culture of *Trichophyton rubrum* and *Bionectria ochroleuca*. J Nat Prod 76:1157–1165. doi:10.1021/np400258f

Bertsche U, Yang SJ, Kuehner D, Wanner S, Mishra NN, Roth T, Nega M, Schneider A, Mayer C, Grau T, Bayer AS, Weidenmaier C (2013) Increased cell wall teichoic acid production and D-alanylation are common phenotypes among daptomycin-resistant MRSA clinical isolates. PLoS One 8:e67398. doi:10.1371/journal.pone.0067398

Blackledge MS, Worthington RJ, Melander C (2013) Biologically inspired strategies for combating bacterial biofilms. Curr Opin Pharmacol 13:699–706. doi:10.1016/j.coph.2013.07.004

Bodro M, Sabe N, Tubau F, Llado L, Baliellas C, Roca J, Cruzado JM, Carratala J (2013) Risk factors and outcomes of bacteremia caused by drug-resistant ESKAPE pathogens in solid-organ transplant recipients. Transplantation 96:843–849. doi:10.1097/TP.0b013e3182a049fd

Bogan C, Marchaim D (2013) The role of antimicrobial stewardship in curbing carbapenem resistance. Future Microbiol 8:979–991. doi:10.2217/fmb.13.73

Bologa CG, Ursu O, Oprea TI, Melançon CE III, Tegos GP (2013) Emerging trends in the discovery of natural product antibacterials. Curr Opin Pharmacol 13:678–687. doi:10.1016/j.coph.2013.07.002

Boucher HW, Talbot GH, Benjamin DK Jr, Bradley J, Guidos RJ, Jones RN, Murray BE, Bonomo RA, Gilbert D (2013) 10 × '20 progress – development of new drugs active against gram-negative bacilli: an update from the infectious Diseases Society of America. Clin Infect Dis 56:1685–1694. doi:10.1093/cid/cit152

Bow EJ (2013) There should be no ESKAPE for febrile neutropenic cancer patients: the dearth of effective antibacterial drugs threatens anticancer efficacy. J Antimicrob Chemother 68:492–495. doi:10.1093/jac/dks512

Breitling R, Achcar F, Takano E (2013) Modeling challenges in the synthetic biology of secondary metabolism. ACS Synth Biol 2:373–378. doi:10.1021/sb4000228

Brown MF, Reilly U, Abramite JA, Arcari JT, Oliver R, Barham RA, Che Y, Chen JM, Collantes EM, Chung SW, Desbonnet C, Doty J, Doroski M, Engtrakul JJ, Harris TM, Huband M, Knafels JD, Leach KL, Liu S, Marfat A, Marra A, McElroy E, Melnick M, Menard CA, Montgomery JI, Mullins L, Noe MC, O'Donnell J, Penzien J, Plummer MS, Price LM,

Shanmugasundaram V, Thoma C, Uccello DP, Warmus JS, Wishka DG (2012a) Potent inhibitors of LpxC for the treatment of gram-negative infections. J Med Chem 55:914–923. doi:10.1021/jm2014748
Brown S, Xia G, Luhachack LG, Campbell J, Meredith TC, Chen C, Winstel V, Gekeler C, Irazoqui JE, Peschel A, Walker S (2012b) Methicillin resistance in *Staphylococcus aureus* requires glycosylated wall teichoic acids. Proc Natl Acad Sci U S A 109:18909–18914. doi:10.1073/pnas.1209126109
Brown S, Santa Maria JPJ, Walker S (2013) Wall teichoic acids of gram-positive bacteria. Annu Rev Microbiol 67:313–336. doi:10.1146/annurev-micro-092412-155620
Brown DG, Lister T, May-Dracka TL (2014) New natural products as new leads for antibacterial drug discovery. Bioorg Med Chem Lett 24:413–418. doi:10.1016/j.bmcl.2013.12.059
Brynildsen MP, Winkler JA, Spina CS, Macdonald IC, Collins JJ (2013) Potentiating antibacterial activity by predictably enhancing endogenous microbial ROS production. Nat Biotechnol 31:160–165. doi:10.1038/nbt.2458
Bugg TDH (2014) Editorial: antibacterial targets for the 21st century. Bioorg Chem 55:1. doi:10.1016/j.bioorg.2014.05.005
Bush K (2012) Improving known classes of antibiotics: an optimistic approach for the future. Curr Opin Pharmacol 12:527–534. doi:10.1016/j.coph.2012.06.003
Butler MS, Blaskovich MA, Cooper MA (2013) Antibiotics in the clinical pipeline in 2013. J Antibiot (Tokyo) 66:571–591. doi:10.1038/ja.2013.86
Campbell J, Singh AK, Swoboda JG, Gilmore MS, Wilkinson BJ, Walker S (2012) An antibiotic that inhibits a late step in wall teichoic acid biosynthesis induces the cell wall stress stimulon in *Staphylococcus aureus*. Antimicrob Agents Chemother 56:1810–1820. doi:10.1128/AAC.05938-11
Carattoli A (2013) Plasmids and the spread of resistance. Int J Med Microbiol 303:298–304. doi:10.1016/j.ijmm.2013.02.001
Cavallari JF, Lamers RP, Scheurwater EM, Matos AL, Burrows LL (2013) Changes to Its peptidoglycan-remodeling enzyme repertoire modulate β-lactam resistance in *Pseudomonas aeruginosa*. Antimicrob Agents Chemother 57:3078–3084. doi:10.1128/AAC. 00268-13
Celler K, Koning RI, Koster AJ, van Wezel GP (2013) Multidimensional view of the bacterial cytoskeleton. J Bacteriol 195:1627–1636. doi:10.1128/JB.02194-12
Chang CJ, Lin JH, Chang KC, Lai MJ, Rohini R, Hu A (2013) Diagnosis of β-lactam resistance in *Acinetobacter baumannii* using shotgun proteomics and LC-nano-ESI ion trap MS. Anal Chem 85:2802–2808. doi:10.1021/ac303326a
Chatterjee A, Cook LCC, Shu C-C, Chen Y, Manias DA, Ramkrishna D, Dunny GM, Hu W-S (2013) Antagonistic self-sensing and mate-sensing signaling controls antibiotic-resistance transfer. Proc Natl Acad Sci U S A 110:7086–7090. doi:10.1073/pnas.1212256110
Chopra I (2013) The 2012 Garrod lecture: discovery of antibacterial drugs in the 21st century. J Antimicrob Chemother 68:496–505. doi:10.1093/jac/dks436
Ciccolini M, Donker T, Köck R, Mielke M, Hendrix R, Jurke A, Rahamat-Langendoen J, Becker K, Niesters HGM, Grundmann H, Friedrich AW (2013) Infection prevention in a connected world: the case for a regional approach. Int J Med Microbiol 303:380–387. doi:10.1016/j.ijmm.2013.02.003
Clark RB, Hunt DK, He M, Achorn C, Chen CL, Deng Y, Fyfe C, Grossman TH, Hogan PC, O'Brien WJ, Plamondon L, Ronn M, Sutcliffe JA, Zhu Z, Xiao XY (2012) Fluorocyclines. 2. Optimization of the C-9 side-chain for antibacterial activity and oral efficacy. J Med Chem 55:606–622. doi:10.1021/jm201467r
Cohen J (2013) Confronting the threat of multidrug-resistant gram-negative bacteria in critically ill patients. J Antimicrob Chemother 68:490–491. doi:10.1093/jac/dks460
Cohen NR, Lobritz MA, Collins JJ (2013) Microbial persistence and the road to drug resistance. Cell Host Microbe 13:632–642. doi:10.1016/j.chom.2013.05.009
Commichau FM, Pietack N, Stulke J (2013) Essential genes in *Bacillus subtilis*: a re-evaluation after ten years. Mol Biosyst 9:1068–1075. doi:10.1039/c3mb25595f

Conlon BP, Nakayasu ES, Fleck LE, LaFleur MD, Isabella VM, Coleman K, Leonard SN, Smith RD, Adkins JN, Lewis K (2013) Activated ClpP kills persisters and eradicates a chronic biofilm infection. Nature 503:365–370. doi:10.1038/nature12790

Cox G, Wright GD (2013) Intrinsic antibiotic resistance: mechanisms, origins, challenges and solutions. Int J Med Microbiol 303:287–292. doi:10.1016/j.ijmm.2013.02.009

Craney A, Ahmed S, Nodwell J (2013) Towards a new science of secondary metabolism. J Antibiot (Tokyo) 66:387–400. doi:10.1038/ja.2013.25

Dalhoff A, Weintraub A, Nord CE (2014) Alternative strategies for proof-of-principle studies of antibacterial agents. Antimicrob Agents Chemother 58:4257–4263. doi:10.1128/AAC. 02473-14

Davies J (2013) Specialized microbial metabolites: functions and origins. J Antibiot (Tokyo) 66:361–364. doi:10.1038/ja.2013.61

Davies J (2014) The origin and evolution of antibiotics. In: Antimicrobials: new and old molecules in the fight against multi-resistant bacteria. Springer, Heidelberg, pp 3–10. doi:10.1007/978-3-642-39968-8_1

Davies SC, Fowler T, Watson J, Livermore DM, Walker D (2013) Annual report of the chief medical officer: Infection and the rise of antimicrobial resistance. Lancet 381:1606–1609. doi:10.1016/S0140-6736(13)60604-2

Derewacz DK, Goodwin CR, McNees CR, McLean JA, Bachmann BO (2013) Antimicrobial drug resistance affects broad changes in metabolomic phenotype in addition to secondary metabolism. Proc Natl Acad Sci U S A 110:2336–2341. doi:10.1073/pnas.1218524110

Dhand A, Bayer AS, Pogliano J, Yang SJ, Bolaris M, Nizet V, Wang G, Sakoulas G (2011) Use of antistaphylococcal β-lactams to increase daptomycin activity in eradicating persistent bacteremia due to methicillin-resistant *Staphylococcus aureus*: role of enhanced daptomycin binding. Clin Infect Dis 53:158–163. doi:10.1093/cid/cir340

Drawz SM, Bonomo RA (2010) Three decades of β-lactamase inhibitors. Clin Microbiol Rev 23:160–201. doi:10.1128/CMR. 00037-09

Duffield M, Cooper I, McAlister E, Bayliss M, Ford D, Oyston P (2010) Predicting conserved essential genes in bacteria: in silico identification of putative drug targets. Mol Biosyst 6:2482–2489. doi:10.1039/c0mb00001a

East SP, Silver LL (2013) Multitarget ligands in antibacterial research: progress and opportunities. Expert Opin Drug Discov 8:143–156. doi:10.1517/17460441.2013.743991

Egan AJ, Vollmer W (2013) The physiology of bacterial cell division. Ann N Y Acad Sci 1277:8–28. doi:10.1111/j.1749-6632.2012.06818.x

El-Elimat T, Figueroa M, Ehrmann BM, Cech NB, Pearce CJ, Oberlies NH (2013) High-resolution MS, MS/MS, and UV database of fungal secondary metabolites as a dereplication protocol for bioactive natural products. J Nat Prod 76:1709–1716. doi:10.1021/np4004307

Elsen NL, Lu J, Parthasarathy G, Reid JC, Sharma S, Soisson SM, Lumb KJ (2012) Mechanism of action of the cell-division inhibitor PC190723: modulation of FtsZ assembly cooperativity. J Am Chem Soc 134:12342–12345. doi:10.1021/ja303564a

Eun YJ, Zhou M, Kiekebusch D, Schlimpert S, Trivedi RR, Bakshi S, Zhong Z, Wahlig TA, Thanbichler M, Weibel DB (2013) Divin: a small molecule inhibitor of bacterial divisome assembly. J Am Chem Soc 135:9768–9776. doi:10.1021/ja404640f

Ezraty B, Vergnes A, Banzhaf M, Duverger Y, Huguenot A, Brochado AR, Su SY, Espinosa L, Loiseau L, Py B, Typas A, Barras F (2013) Fe-S cluster biosynthesis controls uptake of aminoglycosides in a ROS-less death pathway. Science 340:1583–1587. doi:10.1126/science.1238328

Farha MA, Leung A, Sewell EW, D'Elia MA, Allison SE, Ejim L, Pereira PM, Pinho MG, Wright GD, Brown ED (2013a) Inhibition of WTA synthesis blocks the cooperative action of PBPs and sensitizes MRSA to β-lactams. ACS Chem Biol 8:226–233. doi:10.1021/cb300413m

Farha MA, Verschoor CP, Bowdish D, Brown ED (2013b) Collapsing the proton motive force to identify synergistic combinations against *Staphylococcus aureus*. Chem Biol 20:1168–1178. doi:10.1016/j.chembiol.2013.07.006

Fernández A, Pérez A, Ayala JA, Mallo S, Rumbo-Feal S, Tomás M, Poza M, Bou G (2012) Expression of OXA-Type and SFO-1 β-lactamases Induces changes in peptidoglycan composition and affects bacterial fitness. Antimicrob Agents Chemother 56:1877–1884. doi:10.1128/AAC. 05402-11

Fernández L, Álvarez-Ortega C, Wiegand I, Olivares J, Kocíncová D, Lam JS, Martínez JL, Hancock REW (2013) Characterization of the polymyxin B resistome of *Pseudomonas aeruginosa*. Antimicrob Agents Chemother 57:110–119. doi:10.1128/AAC. 01583-12

Finley RL, Collignon P, Larsson DGJ, McEwen SA, Li XZ, Gaze WH, Reid-Smith R, Timinouni M, Graham DW, Topp E (2013) The scourge of antibiotic resistance: the important role of the environment. Clin Infect Dis 57:704–710. doi:10.1093/cid/cit355

Fonvielle M, Li de La Sierra-Gallay I, El-Sagheer AH, Lecerf M, Patin D, Mellal D, Mayer C, Blanot D, Gale N, Brown T, van Tilbeurgh H, Ethève-Quelquejeu M, Arthur M (2013) The structure of FemXWv in complex with a peptidyl-RNA conjugate: mechanism of aminoacyl transfer from Ala-tRNA(Ala) to peptidoglycan precursors. Angew Chem Int Ed 52:7278–7281. doi:10.1002/anie.201301411

Foss MH, Eun Y-J, Grove CI, Pauw DA, Sorto NA, Rensvold JW, Pagliarini DJ, Shaw JT, Weibel DB (2013) Inhibitors of bacterial tubulin target bacterial membranes in vivo. Med Chem Comm 4:112–119. doi:10.1039/c2md20127e

Foucault ML, Depardieu F, Courvalin P, Grillot-Courvalin C (2010) Inducible expression eliminates the fitness cost of vancomycin resistance in enterococci. Proc Natl Acad Sci U S A 107:16964–16969. doi:10.1073/pnas.1006855107

Galán JC, González-Candelas F, Rolain JM, Cantón R (2013) Antibiotics as selectors and accelerators of diversity in the mechanisms of resistance: from the resistome to genetic plasticity in the β-lactamases' world. Front Microbiol 4:9. doi:10.3389/fmicb.2013.00009

Gammon K (2014) Drug discovery: leaving no stone unturned. Nature 509:S10–S12. doi:10.1038/509S10a

Gerdes K, Ingmer H (2013) Antibiotics: killing the survivors. Nature 503:347–349. doi:10.1038/nature12834

Gerwick WH, Moore BS (2012) Lessons from the past and charting the future of marine natural products drug discovery and chemical biology. Chem Biol 19:85–98. doi:10.1016/j.chembiol.2011.12.014

Goldberg K, Sarig H, Zaknoon F, Epand RF, Epand RM, Mor A (2013) Sensitization of gram-negative bacteria by targeting the membrane potential. FASEB J 27:3818–3826. doi:10.1096/fj.13-227942

Graupner K, Scherlach K, Bretschneider T, Lackner G, Roth M, Gross H, Hertweck C (2012) Imaging mass spectrometry and genome mining reveal highly antifungal virulence factor of mushroom soft rot pathogen. Angew Chem Int Ed 51:13173–13177. doi:10.1002/anie.201206658

Greenfield LK, Whitfield C (2012) Synthesis of lipopolysaccharide *O*-antigens by ABC transporter-dependent pathways. Carbohydr Res 356:12–24. doi:10.1016/j.carres.2012.02.027

Gupta S, Bram EE, Weiss R (2013) Genetically programmable pathogen sense and destroy. ACS Synth Biol 2:715–723. doi:10.1021/sb4000417

Gutierrez A, Laureti L, Crussard S, Abida H, Rodriguez-Rojas A, Blazquez J, Baharoglu Z, Mazel D, Darfeuille F, Vogel J, Matic I (2013) β-Lactam antibiotics promote bacterial mutagenesis via an RpoS-mediated reduction in replication fidelity. Nat Commun 4:1610. doi:10.1038/ncomms2607

Hall CL, Tschannen M, Worthey EA, Kristich CJ (2013) IreB, a Ser/Thr kinase substrate, influences antimicrobial resistance in *Enterococcus faecalis*. Antimicrob Agents Chemother 57:6179–6686. doi:10.1128/AAC. 01472-13

Händel N, Schuurmans JM, Brul S, ter Kuile BH (2013) Compensation of the metabolic costs of antibiotic resistance by physiological adaptation in *Escherichia coli*. Antimicrob Agents Chemother 57:3752–3762. doi:10.1128/AAC. 02096-12

Hankins JV, Madsen JA, Giles DK, Brodbelt JS, Trent MS (2012) Amino acid addition to *Vibrio cholerae* LPS establishes a link between surface remodeling in gram-positive and gram-negative bacteria. Proc Natl Acad Sci U S A 109:8722–8727. doi:10.1073/pnas.1201313109

Harris SR, Cartwright EJ, Torok ME, Holden MT, Brown NM, Ogilvy-Stuart AL, Ellington MJ, Quail MA, Bentley SD, Parkhill J, Peacock SJ (2013) Whole-genome sequencing for analysis of an outbreak of meticillin-resistant *Staphylococcus aureus*: a descriptive study. Lancet Infect Dis 13:130–136. doi:10.1016/S1473-3099(12)70268-2

Haruki H, Pedersen MG, Gorska KI, Pojer F, Johnsson K (2013) Tetrahydrobiopterin biosynthesis as an off-target of sulfa drugs. Science 340:987–991. doi:10.1126/science.1232972

Hasan S, Ali SZ, Khan AU (2013) Novel combinations of antibiotics to inhibit extended-spectrum β-lactamase and metallo-β-lactamase producers in vitro: a synergistic approach. Future Microbiol 8:939–944. doi:10.2217/fmb.13.54

Hede K (2014) Antibiotic resistance: an infectious arms race. Nature 509:S2–S3. doi:10.1038/509S2a

Hirakawa H, Tomita H (2013) Interference of bacterial cell-to-cell communication: a new concept of antimicrobial chemotherapy breaks antibiotic resistance. Front Microbiol 4:114. doi:10.3389/fmicb.2013.00114

Holt KE, Thieu Nga TV, Thanh DP, Vinh H, Kim DW, Vu Tra MP, Campbell JI, Hoang NV, Vinh NT, Minh PV, Thuy CT, Nga TT, Thompson C, Dung TT, Nhu NT, Vinh PV, Tuyet PT, Phuc HL, Lien NT, Phu BD, Ai NT, Tien NM, Dong N, Parry CM, Hien TT, Farrar JJ, Parkhill J, Dougan G, Thomson NR, Baker S (2013) Tracking the establishment of local endemic populations of an emergent enteric pathogen. Proc Natl Acad Sci U S A 110:17522–17527. doi:10.1073/pnas.1308632110

Hopwood DA (2013) Imaging mass spectrometry reveals highly specific interactions between actinomycetes to activate specialized metabolic gene clusters. MBio 4:e00612–e00613. doi:10.1128/mBio. 00612-13

Howard SJ, Hopwood S, Davies SC (2014) Antimicrobial resistance: a global challenge. Sci Transl Med 6:236ed10. doi:10.1126/scitranslmed.3009315

Huang KH, Durand-Heredia J, Janakiraman A (2013) FtsZ ring stability: of bundles, tubules, crosslinks, and curves. J Bacteriol 195:1859–1868. doi:10.1128/JB.02157-12

Huber J, Donald RG, Lee SH, Jarantow LW, Salvatore MJ, Meng X, Painter R, Onishi RH, Occi J, Dorso K, Young K, Park YW, Skwish S, Szymonifka MJ, Waddell TS, Miesel L, Phillips JW, Roemer T (2009) Chemical genetic identification of peptidoglycan inhibitors potentiating carbapenem activity against methicillin-resistant *Staphylococcus aureus*. Chem Biol 16:837–848. doi:10.1016/j.chembiol.2009.05.012

Imamovic L, Sommer MOA (2013) Use of collateral sensitivity networks to design drug cycling protocols that avoid resistance development. Sci Transl Med 5:204ra132. doi:10.1126/scitranslmed.3006609

Imperi F, Massai F, Facchini M, Frangipani E, Visaggio D, Leoni L, Bragonzi A, Visca P (2013a) Repurposing the antimycotic drug flucytosine for suppression of *Pseudomonas aeruginosa* pathogenicity. Proc Natl Acad Sci U S A 110:7458–7463. doi:10.1073/pnas.1222706110

Imperi F, Massai F, Pillai CR, Longo F, Zennaro E, Rampioni G, Visca P, Leoni L (2013b) New life for an old drug: the anthelmintic drug niclosamide inhibits *Pseudomonas aeruginosa* quorum sensing. Antimicrob Agents Chemother 57:996–1005. doi:10.1128/AAC. 01952-12

Jackman JE, Fierke CA, Tumey LN, Pirrung M, Uchiyama T, Tahir SH, Hindsgaul O, Raetz CRH (2000) Antibacterial agents that target lipid A biosynthesis in gram-negative bacteria. Inhibition of diverse UDP-3-*O*-(r-3-hydroxymyristoyl)-N-acetylglucosamine deacetylases by substrate analogs containing zinc binding motifs. J Biol Chem 275:11002–11009. doi:10.1074/jbc.275.15.11002

Jang KH, Nam SJ, Locke JB, Kauffman CA, Beatty DS, Paul LA, Fenical W (2013) Anthracimycin, a potent anthrax antibiotic from a marine-derived actinomycete. Angew Chem Int Ed 52:7822–7824. doi:10.1002/anie.201302749

Jiang W, Li B, Zheng X, Liu X, Pan X, Qing R, Cen Y, Zheng J, Zhou H (2013) Artesunate has its enhancement on antibacterial activity of β-lactams via increasing the antibiotic accumulation within methicillin-resistant *Staphylococcus aureus* (MRSA). J Antibiot (Tokyo) 66:339–345. doi:10.1038/ja.2013.22

Johnson JW, Fisher JF, Mobashery S (2013) Bacterial cell-wall recycling. Ann N Y Acad Sci 1277:54–75. doi:10.1111/j.1749-6632.2012.06813.x

Kalghatgi S, Spina CS, Costello JC, Liesa M, Morones-Ramirez JR, Slomovic S, Molina A, Shirihai OS, Collins JJ (2013) Bactericidal antibiotics induce mitochondrial dysfunction and oxidative damage in mammalian cells. Sci Transl Med 5:192ra85. doi:10.1126/scitranslmed.3006055

Kamen Ek S, Gur-Bertok D (2013) Global transcriptional responses to the bacteriocin colicin M in *Escherichia coli*. BMC Microbiol 13:42. doi:10.1186/1471-2180-13-42

Kaneti G, Sarig H, Marjieh I, Fadia Z, Mor A (2013) Simultaneous breakdown of multiple antibiotic resistance mechanisms in *S. aureus*. FASEB J 27:4834–4843. doi:10.1096/fj.13-237610

Kaul M, Mark L, Zhang Y, Parhi AK, LaVoie EJ, Pilch DS (2013) An FtsZ-targeting prodrug with oral antistaphylococcal efficacy in vivo. Antimicrob Agents Chemother 57:5860–5869. doi:10.1128/AAC. 01016-13

Keffer JL, Huecas S, Hammill JT, Wipf P, Andreu JM, Bewley CA (2013) Chrysophaentins are competitive inhibitors of FtsZ and inhibit Z-ring formation in live bacteria. Bioorg Med Chem 21:5673–5678. doi:10.1016/j.bmc.2013.07.033

Kelesidis T, Tewhey R, Humphries RM (2013) Evolution of high-level daptomycin resistance in *Enterococcus faecium* during daptomycin therapy is associated with limited mutations in the bacterial genome. J Antimicrob Chemother 68:1926–1928. doi:10.1093/jac/dkt117

Keren I, Wu Y, Inocencio J, Mulcahy LR, Lewis K (2013) Killing by bactericidal antibiotics does not depend on reactive oxygen species. Science 339:1213–1216. doi:10.1126/science.1232688

Khodaverdian V, Pesho M, Truitt B, Bollinger L, Patel P, Nithianantham S, Yu G, Delaney E, Jankowsky E, Shoham M (2013) Discovery of antivirulence agents against methicillin-resistant *Staphylococcus aureus*. Antimicrob Agents Chemother 57:3645–3652. doi:10.1128/AAC. 00269-13

Kim JH, O'Brien KM, Sharma R, Boshoff HI, Rehren G, Chakraborty S, Wallach JB, Monteleone M, Wilson DJ, Aldrich CC, Barry CE III, Rhee KY, Ehrt S, Schnappinger D (2013) A genetic strategy to identify targets for the development of drugs that prevent bacterial persistence. Proc Natl Acad Sci U S A 110:19095–19100. doi:10.1073/pnas.1315860110

Kirst HA (2013) Developing new antibacterials through natural product research. Expert Opin Drug Discov 8:479–493. doi:10.1517/17460441.2013.779666

Kohanski MA, Dwyer DJ, Collins JJ (2010) How antibiotics kill bacteria: from targets to networks. Nat Rev Microbiol 8:423–435. doi:10.1038/nrmicro2333

Komatsu M, Komatsu K, Koiwai H, Yamada Y, Kozone I, Izumikawa M, Hashimoto J, Takagi M, Omura S, Shin-ya K, Cane DE, Ikeda H (2013) Engineered *Streptomyces avermitilis* host for heterologous expression of biosynthetic gene cluster for secondary metabolites. ACS Synth Biol 2:384–396. doi:10.1021/sb3001003

Koteva K, Hong HJ, Wang XD, Nazi I, Hughes D, Naldrett MJ, Buttner MJ, Wright GD (2010) A vancomycin photoprobe identifies the histidine kinase VanSsc as a vancomycin receptor. Nat Chem Biol 6:327–329. doi:10.1038/nchembio.350

Koyama N, Tokura Y, Munch D, Sahl HG, Schneider T, Shibagaki Y, Ikeda H, Tomoda H (2012) The non-antibiotic small molecule cyslabdan enhances the potency of β-lactams against MRSA by inhibiting pentaglycine interpeptide bridge synthesis. PLoS One 7:e48981. doi:10.1371/journal.pone.0048981

Kumarasiri M, Llarrull LI, Borbulevych O, Fishovitz J, Lastochkin E, Baker BM, Mobashery S (2012) An amino-acid position at the crossroads of evolution of protein function: antibiotic-sensor domain of the BlaR1 protein from *Staphylococcus aureus* vs. class D β-lactamases. J Biol Chem 287:8232–8241. doi:10.1074/jbc.M111.333179

Kwun MJ, Novotna G, Hesketh AR, Hill L, Hong HJ (2013) In vivo studies suggest that induction of VanS-dependent vancomycin resistance requires binding of the drug to D-Ala-D-Ala termini in the peptidoglycan cell wall. Antimicrob Agents Chemother 57:4470–4480. doi:10.1128/AAC. 00523-13

Lages MC, Beilharz K, Morales Angeles D, Veening JW, Scheffers DJ (2013) The localization of key *Bacillus subtilis* penicillin binding proteins during cell growth is determined by substrate availability. Environ Microbiol 15:3272–3281. doi:10.1111/1462-2920.12206

Laxminarayan R (2014) Antibiotic effectiveness: balancing conservation against innovation. Science 345:1299–1301. doi:10.1126/science.1254163

Lázár V, Pal Singh G, Spohn R, Nagy I, Horváth B, Hrtyan M, Busa-Fekete R, Bogos B, Méhi O, Csörgő B, Pósfai G, Fekete G, Szappanos B, Kégl B, Papp B, Pál C (2013) Bacterial evolution of antibiotic hypersensitivity. Mol Syst Biol 9:700. doi:10.1038/msb.2013.57

Le Hello S, Harrois D, Bouchrif B, Sontag L, Elhani D, Guibert V, Zerouali K, Weill FX (2013) Highly drug-resistant *Salmonella enterica* serotype Kentucky ST198-X1: a microbiological study. Lancet Infect Dis 13:672–679. doi:10.1016/S1473-3099(13)70124-5

Lee K, Campbell J, Swoboda JG, Cuny GD, Walker S (2010) Development of improved inhibitors of wall teichoic acid biosynthesis with potent activity against *Staphylococcus aureus*. Bioorg Med Chem Lett 20:1767–1770. doi:10.1016/j.bmcl.2010.01.036

Leonard PG, Golemi-Kotra D, Stock AM (2013) Phosphorylation-dependent conformational changes and domain rearrangements in *Staphylococcus aureus* VraR activation. Proc Natl Acad Sci U S A 110:8525–8530. doi:10.1073/pnas.1302819110

Leuthner KD, Doern GV (2013) Antimicrobial stewardship programs. J Clin Microbiol 51:3916–3920. doi:10.1128/JCM. 01751-13

Lewis K (2013) Platforms for antibiotic discovery. Nat Rev Drug Discov 12:371–387. doi:10.1038/nrd3975

Lima TB, Pinto MFS, Ribeiro SM, Alves de Lima L, Viana JC, Júnior NG, de Souza Candido E, Dias SC, Franco OL (2013) Bacterial resistance mechanism: what proteomics can elucidate. FASEB J 27:1291–1303. doi:10.1096/fj.12-221127

Liu Y, Imlay JA (2013) Cell death from antibiotics without the involvement of reactive oxygen species. Science 339:1210–1213. doi:10.1126/science.1232751

Livermore DM (2014) Of stewardship, motherhood and apple pie. Int J Antimicrob Agents 43:319–322. doi:10.1016/j.ijantimicag.2014.01.011

Llarrull LI, Mobashery S (2012) Dissection of events in the resistance to β-lactam antibiotics mediated by the protein BlaR1 from *Staphylococcus aureus*. Biochemistry 51:4642–4649. doi:10.1021/bi300429p

Long DR, Mead J, Hendricks JM, Hardy ME, Voyich JM (2013) 18β-Glycyrrhetinic acid inhibits methicillin-resistant *Staphylococcus aureus* survival and attenuates virulence gene expression. Antimicrob Agents Chemother 57:241–247. doi:10.1128/AAC. 01023-12

Ma S, Ma S (2012) The development of FtsZ inhibitors as potential antibacterial agents. ChemMedChem 7:1161–1172. doi:10.1002/cmdc.201200156

Maffioli SI, Fabbretti A, Brandi L, Savelsbergh A, Monciardini P, Abbondi M, Rossi R, Donadio S, Gualerzi CO (2013) Orthoformimycin, a selective inhibitor of bacterial translation elongation from *Streptomyces* containing an unusual orthoformate. ACS Chem Biol 8:1939–1946. doi:10.1021/cb4004095

Mahoney TF, Silhavy TJ (2013) The Cpx stress response confers resistance to some, but not all, bactericidal antibiotics. J Bacteriol 195:1869–1874. doi:10.1128/JB.02197-12

Maisonneuve E, Gerdes K (2014) Molecular mechanisms underlying bacterial persisters. Cell 157 (3):539–548. doi:10.1016/j.cell.2014.02.050

Mann PA, Muller A, Xiao L, Pereira PM, Yang C, Lee SH, Wang H, Trzeciak J, Schneeweis J, Dos Santos MM, Murgolo N, She X, Gill C, Balibar CJ, Labroli M, Su J, Flattery A, Sherborne B, Maier R, Tan CM, Black T, Onder K, Kargman S, Monsma FJ, Pinho MG, Schneider T, Roemer T (2013) Murgocil is a highly bioactive staphylococcal-specific Inhibitor of the peptidoglycan glycosyltransferase enzyme MurG. ACS Chem Biol 8:2442–2451. doi:10.1021/cb400487f

Manoil C (2013) Clarifying the role of two-component regulation in antibiotic killing. J Bacteriol 195:1857–1858. doi:10.1128/JB.00190-13
Master RN, Deane J, Opiela C, Sahm DF (2013) Recent trends in resistance to cell envelope-active antibacterial agents among key bacterial pathogens. Ann N Y Acad Sci 1277:1–7. doi:10.1111/nyas.12022
Matsui T, Yamane J, Mogi N, Yamaguchi H, Takemoto H, Yao M, Tanaka I (2012) Structural reorganization of the bacterial cell-division protein FtsZ from *Staphylococcus aureus*. Acta Crystallogr D Biol Crystallogr 68:1175–1188. doi:10.1107/S0907444912022640
McArthur AG, Waglechner N, Nizam F, Yan A, Azad MA, Baylay AJ, Bhullar K, Canova MJ, De Pascale G, Ejim L, Kalan L, King AM, Koteva K, Morar M, Mulvey MR, O'Brien JS, Pawlowski AC, Piddock LJV, Spanogiannopoulos P, Sutherland AD, Tang I, Taylor PL, Thaker M, Wang W, Yan M, Yu T, Wright GD (2013) The comprehensive antibiotic resistance database. Antimicrob Agents Chemother 57:3348–3357. doi:10.1128/AAC. 00419-13
McKenna M (2013) Antibiotic resistance: the last resort. Nature 499:394–396. doi:10.1038/499394a
Méhi O, Bogos B, Csörgo B, Päl C (2013) Genomewide screen for modulators of evolvability under toxic antibiotic exposure. Antimicrob Agents Chemother 57:3453–3456. doi:10.1128/AAC.02454-12
Mehta S, Singh C, Plata KB, Chanda PK, Paul A, Riosa S, Rosato RR, Rosato AE (2012) β-Lactams increase the antibacterial activity of daptomycin against clinical methicillin-resistant *Staphylococcus aureus* strains and prevent selection of daptomycin-resistant derivatives. Antimicrob Agents Chemother 56:6192–6200. doi:10.1128/AAC. 01525-12
Melamed Yerushalmi S, Buck ME, Lynn DM, Lemcoff NG, Meijler MM (2013) Multivalent alteration of quorum sensing in *Staphylococcus aureus*. Chem Commun 49:5177–5179. doi:10.1039/c3cc41645c
Metz M, Shlaes DM (2014) Eight more ways to deal with antibiotic resistance. Antimicrob Agents Chemother 58:4253–4256. doi:10.1128/AAC. 02623-14
Miskinyte M, Gordo I (2013) Increased survival of antibiotic-resistant *Escherichia coli* inside macrophages. Antimicrob Agents Chemother 57:189–195. doi:10.1128/AAC. 01632-12
Mitsuma SF, Mansour MK, Dekker JP, Kim J, Rahman MZ, Tweed-Kent A, Schuetz P (2013) Promising new assays and technologies for the diagnosis and management of infectious diseases. Clin Infect Dis 56:996–1002. doi:10.1093/cid/cis1014
Modi SR, Lee HH, Spina CS, Collins JJ (2013) Antibiotic treatment expands the resistance reservoir and ecological network of the phage metagenome. Nature 499:219–222. doi:10.1038/nature12212
Montgomery JI, Brown MF, Reilly U, Price LM, Abramite JA, Arcari J, Barham R, Che Y, Chen JM, Chung SW, Collantes EM, Desbonnet C, Doroski M, Doty J, Engtrakul JJ, Harris TM, Huband M, Knafels JD, Leach KL, Liu S, Marfat A, McAllister L, McElroy E, Menard CA, Mitton-Fry M, Mullins L, Noe MC, O'Donnell J, Oliver R, Penzien J, Plummer M, Shanmugasundaram V, Thoma C, Tomaras AP, Uccello DP, Vaz A, Wishka DG (2012) Pyridone methylsulfone hydroxamate LpxC inhibitors for the treatment of serious gram-negative infections. J Med Chem 55:1662–1670. doi:10.1021/jm2014875
Moraski GC, Markley LD, Cramer J, Hipskind PA, Boshoff H, Bailey MA, Alling T, Ollinger J, Parish T, Miller MJ (2013) Advancement of imidazo[1,2-*a*]pyridines with improved pharmacokinetics and nM activity vs. *M. tuberculosis*. ACS Med Chem Lett 4:675–679. doi:10.1021/ml400088y
Morkunas B, Galloway WR, Wright M, Ibbeson BM, Hodgkinson JT, O'Connell KM, Bartolucci N, Valle MD, Welch M, Spring DR (2012) Inhibition of the production of the *Pseudomonas aeruginosa* virulence factor pyocyanin in wild-type cells by quorum sensing autoinducer-mimics. Org Biomol Chem 10:8452–8464. doi:10.1039/c2ob26501j
Morones-Ramirez JR, Winkler JA, Spina CS, Collins JJ (2013) Silver enhances antibiotic activity against gram-negative bacteria. Sci Transl Med 5:190ra81. doi:10.1126/scitranslmed.3006276

Moya B, Beceiro A, Cabot G, Juan C, Zamorano L, Alberti S, Oliver A (2012) Pan-β-lactam resistance development in *Pseudomonas aeruginosa* clinical strains: molecular mechanisms, PBP profiles, and binding affinities. Antimicrob Agents Chemother 56:4771–4778. doi:10.1128/AAC. 00680-12

Moynie L, Schnell R, McMahon SA, Sandalova T, Boulkerou WA, Schmidberger JW, Alphey M, Cukier C, Duthie F, Kopec J, Liu H, Jacewicz A, Hunter WN, Naismith JH, Schneider G (2013) The AEROPATH project targeting *Pseudomonas aeruginosa*: crystallographic studies for assessment of potential targets in early-stage drug discovery. Acta Crystallogr Sect F Struct Biol Cryst Commun 69:25–34. doi:10.1107/S1744309112044739

Munoz-Price LS, Quinn JP (2013) Deconstructing the infection control bundles for the containment of carbapenem-resistant Enterobacteriaceae. Curr Opin Infect Dis 26:378–387. doi:10.1097/01.qco.0000431853.71500.77

Nakashima R, Sakurai K, Yamasaki S, Hayashi K, Nagata C, Hoshino K, Onodera Y, Nishino K, Yamaguchi A (2013) Structural basis for the inhibition of bacterial multidrug exporters. Nature 500:102–106. doi:10.1038/nature12300

Nikitushkin VD, Demina GR, Shleeva MO, Kaprelyants AS (2013) Peptidoglycan fragments stimulate resuscitation of "non-culturable" mycobacteria. Antonie Van Leeuwenhoek 103:37–46. doi:10.1007/s10482-012-9784-1

Nonejuie P, Burkart M, Pogliano K, Pogliano J (2013) Bacterial cytological profiling rapidly identifies the cellular pathways targeted by antibacterial molecules. Proc Natl Acad Sci U S A 110:16169–16174. doi:10.1073/pnas.1311066110

Novak R (2011) Are pleuromutilin antibiotics finally fit for human use? Ann NY Acad Sci 1241:71–81. doi:10.1111/j.1749-6632.2011.06219.x

O'Connell KMG, Hodgkinson JT, Sore HF, Welch M, Salmond GPC, Spring DR (2013) Combating multidrug-resistant bacteria: current strategies for the discovery of novel antibacterials. Angew Chem Int Ed 52:10706–10733. doi:10.1002/anie.201209979

O'Loughlin CT, Miller LC, Siryaporn A, Drescher K, Semmelhack MF, Bassler BL (2013) A quorum-sensing inhibitor blocks *Pseudomonas aeruginosa* virulence and biofilm formation. Proc Natl Acad Sci U S A 110:17981–17986. doi:10.1073/pnas.1316981110

Ojima I, Kumar K, Awasthi D, Vineberg JG (2014) Drug discovery targeting cell division proteins, microtubules and FtsZ. Bioorg Med Chem 22(18):5060–5077. doi:10.1016/j.bmc.2014.02.036

Ongley SE, Bian X, Zhang Y, Chau R, Gerwick WH, Müller R, Neilan BA (2013) High-titer heterologous production in *E. coli* of lyngbyatoxin, a PKC activator from an uncultured marine cyanobacterium. ACS Chem Biol 8:1888–1893. doi:10.1021/cb400189j

Otto M (2013a) Blocking the spread of resistance. Sci Transl Med 5:184fs17. doi:10.1126/scitranslmed.3006128.

Otto M (2013b) Community-associated MRSA: what makes them special? Int J Med Microbiol 303:324–330. doi:10.1016/j.ijmm.2013.02.007

Paphitou NI (2013) Antimicrobial resistance: action to combat the rising microbial challenges. Int J Antimicrob Agents 42(Suppl 1):S25–S28. doi:10.1016/j.ijantimicag.2013.04.007

Pasquina LW, Santa Maria JP, Walker S (2013) Teichoic acid biosynthesis as an antibiotic target. Curr Opin Microbiol 16:531–537. doi:10.1016/j.mib.2013.06.014

Paul M, Leibovici L (2013) Combination therapy for *Pseudomonas aeruginosa* bacteremia: where do we stand? Clin Infect Dis 57:217–220. doi:10.1093/cid/cit220

Payne DJ, Gwynn MN, Holmes DJ, Pompliano DL (2007) Drugs for bad bugs: confronting the challenges of antibacterial discovery. Nat Rev Drug Discov 6:29–40. doi:10.1038/nrd2201

Peleg AY, Miyakis S, Ward DV, Earl AM, Rubio A, Cameron DR, Pillai S, Moellering RC Jr, Eliopoulos GM (2012) Whole genome characterization of the mechanisms of daptomycin resistance in clinical and laboratory derived isolates of *Staphylococcus aureus*. PLoS One 7: e28316. doi:10.1371/journal.pone.0028316

Pelletier MR, Casella LG, Jones JW, Adams MD, Zurawski DV, Hazlett KR, Doi Y, Ernst RK (2013) Unique structural modifications are present in the lipopolysaccharide from colistin-resistant strains of *Acinetobacter baumannii*. Antimicrob Agents Chemother 57:4831–4840. doi:10.1128/AAC. 00865-13

Pendleton JN, Gorman SP, Gilmore BF (2013) Clinical relevance of the ESKAPE pathogens. Expert Rev Anti-Infect Ther 11:297–308. doi:10.1586/eri.13.12

Perry JA, Wright GD (2013) The antibiotic resistance "mobilome": searching for the link between environment and clinic. Front Microbiol 4:138. doi:10.3389/fmicb.2013.00138

Pethe K, Bifani P, Jang J, Kang S, Park S, Ahn S, Jiricek J, Jung J, Jeon HK, Cechetto J, Christophe T, Lee H, Kempf M, Jackson M, Lenaerts AJ, Pham H, Jones V, Seo MJ, Kim YM, Seo M, Seo JJ, Park D, Ko Y, Choi I, Kim R, Kim SY, Lim S, Yim SA, Nam J, Kang H, Kwon H, Oh CT, Cho Y, Jang Y, Kim J, Chua A, Tan BH, Nanjundappa MB, Rao SP, Barnes WS, Wintjens R, Walker JR, Alonso S, Lee S, Kim J, Oh S, Oh T, Nehrbass U, Han SJ, No Z, Lee J, Brodin P, Cho SN, Nam K, Kim J (2013) Discovery of Q203, a potent clinical candidate for the treatment of tuberculosis. Nat Med 19:1157–1160. doi:10.1038/nm.3262

Pilhofer M, Jensen GJ (2013) The bacterial cytoskeleton: more than twisted filaments. Curr Opin Cell Biol 25:125–133. doi:10.1016/j.ceb.2012.10.019

Pinho MG, Kjos M, Veening JW (2013) How to get (a)round: mechanisms controlling growth and division of coccoid bacteria. Nat Rev Microbiol 11:601–614. doi:10.1038/nrmicro3088

Pogliano J, Pogliano N, Silverman JA (2012) Daptomycin-mediated reorganization of membrane architecture causes mislocalization of essential cell division proteins. J Bacteriol 194:4494–4504. doi:10.1128/JB.00011-12

Pucci MJ, Bush K (2013) Investigational antimicrobial agents of 2013. Clin Microbiol Rev 26:792–821. doi:10.1128/CMR. 00033-13

Ramsey DM, Amirul Islam M, Turnbull L, Davis RA, Whitchurch CB, McAlpine SR (2013) Psammaplysin F: a unique inhibitor of bacterial chromosomal partitioning. Bioorg Med Chem Lett 23:4862–4866. doi:10.1016/j.bmcl.2013.06.082

Rateb ME, Hallyburton I, Houssen WE, Bull AT, Goodfellow M, Santhanam R, Jaspars M, Ebel R (2013) Induction of diverse secondary metabolites in *Aspergillus fumigatus* by microbial co-culture. RSC Adv 3:14444–14450. doi:10.1039/C3RA42378F

Reimold C, Defeu Soufo HJ, Dempwolff F, Graumann PL (2013) Motion of variable-length MreB filaments at the bacterial cell membrane influences cell morphology. Mol Biol Cell 24:2340–2349. doi:10.1091/mbc.E12-10-0728

Reuter S, Ellington MJ, Cartwright EJ, Koser CU, Torok ME, Gouliouris T, Harris SR, Brown NM, Holden MT, Quail M, Parkhill J, Smith GP, Bentley SD, Peacock SJ (2013) Rapid bacterial whole-genome sequencing to enhance diagnostic and public health microbiology. JAMA Intern Med 173:1397–1404. doi:10.1001/jamainternmed.2013.7734

Richter SG, Elli D, Kim HK, Hendrickx APA, Sorg JA, Schneewind O, Missiakas D (2013) Small molecule inhibitor of lipoteichoic acid synthesis is an antibiotic for gram-positive bacteria. Proc Natl Acad Sci U S A 110:3531–3536. doi:10.1073/pnas.1217337110

Riley MA, Robinson SM, Roy CM, Dorit RL (2013) Rethinking the composition of a rational antibiotic arsenal for the 21st century. Future Med Chem 5:1231–1242. doi:10.4155/fmc.13.79

Rodriguez-Rojas A, Rodriguez-Beltran J, Couce A, Blazquez J (2013) Antibiotics and antibiotic resistance: a bitter fight against evolution. Int J Med Microbiol 303:293–297. doi:10.1016/j.ijmm.2013.02.004

Roemer T, Boone C (2013) Systems-level antimicrobial drug and drug synergy discovery. Nat Chem Biol 9:222–231. doi:10.1038/nchembio.1205

Roemer T, Davies J, Giaever G, Nislow C (2012) Bugs, drugs and chemical genomics. Nat Chem Biol 8:46–56. doi:10.1038/nchembio.744

Roemer T, Schneider T, Pinho MG (2013) Auxiliary factors: a chink in the armor of MRSA resistance to beta-lactam antibiotics. Curr Opin Microbiol 16:538–548. doi:10.1016/j.mib.2013.06.012

Ruiz-Avila LB, Huecas S, Artola M, Vergoñós A, Ramírez-Aportela E, Cercenado E, Barasoain I, Vázquez-Villa H, Martín-Fontecha M, Chacón P, López-Rodríguez ML, Andreu JM (2013)

Synthetic inhibitors of bacterial cell division targeting the GTP binding site of FtsZ. ACS Chem Biol 8:2072–2083. doi:10.1021/cb400208z
Saroj SD, Rather PN (2013) Streptomycin inhibits quorum sensing in *Acinetobacter baumannii*. Antimicrob Agents Chemother 57:1926–1929. doi:10.1128/AAC. 02161-12
Sass P, Brötz-Oesterhelt H (2013) Bacterial cell division as a target for new antibiotics. Curr Opin Microbiol 16:522–530. doi:10.1016/j.mib.2013.07.006
Schäberle TF, Hack IM (2014) Overcoming the current deadlock in antibiotic research. Trends Microbiol 22:165–167. doi:10.1016/j.tim.2013.12.007
Schaffner-Barbero C, Martin-Fontecha M, Chacon P, Andreu JM (2012) Targeting the assembly of bacterial cell division protein FtsZ with small molecules. ACS Chem Biol 7:269–277. doi:10.1021/cb2003626
Sears P, Ichikawa Y, Ruiz N, Gorbach S (2013) Advances in the treatment of *Clostridium difficile* with fidaxomicin: a narrow spectrum antibiotic. Ann NY Acad Sci 1291:33–41. doi:10.1111/nyas.12135
Seger C, Sturm S, Stuppner H (2013) Mass spectrometry and NMR spectroscopy: modern high-end detectors for high resolution separation techniques–state of the art in natural product HPLC-MS, HPLC-NMR, and CE-MS hyphenations. Nat Prod Rep 30:970–987. doi:10.1039/c3np70015a
Sewell EW, Brown ED (2014) Taking aim at wall teichoic acid synthesis: new biology and new leads for antibiotics. J Antibiot (Tokyo) 67:43–51. doi:10.1038/ja.2013.100
Shapiro S (2013) Speculative strategies for new antibacterials: all roads should not lead to Rome. J Antibiot (Tokyo) 66:371–386. doi:10.1038/ja.2013.27
Sherman DJ, Okuda S, Denny WA, Kahne D (2013) Validation of inhibitors of an ABC transporter required to transport lipopolysaccharide to the cell surface in *Escherichia coli*. Bioorg Med Chem 21:4846–4851. doi:10.1016/j.bmc.2013.04.020
Shlaes DM (2013) New β-lactam–β-lactamase inhibitor combinations in clinical development. Ann N Y Acad Sci 1277:105–114. doi:10.1111/nyas.12010
Shlaes DM, Spellberg B (2012) Overcoming the challenges to developing new antibiotics. Curr Opin Pharmacol 12:522–526. doi:10.1016/j.coph.2012.06.010
Shlaes DM, Sahm D, Opiela C, Spellberg B (2013) The FDA reboot of antibiotic development. Antimicrob Agents Chemother 57:4605–4607. doi:10.1128/AAC. 01277-13
Singh SB (2014) Confronting the challenges of discovery of novel antibacterial agents. Bioorg Med Chem Lett 24(16):3683–3689. doi:10.1016/j.bmcl.2014.06.053
Song Y, Rubio A, Jayaswal RK, Silverman JA, Wilkinson BJ (2013) Additional routes to *Staphylococcus aureus* daptomycin resistance as revealed by comparative genome sequencing, transcriptional profiling, and phenotypic studies. PLoS One 8:e58469. doi:10.1371/journal.pone.0058469
Spellberg B, Bartlett JG, Gilbert DN (2013) The future of antibiotics and resistance. N Engl J Med 368:299–302. doi:10.1056/NEJMp1215093
Srinivas N, Jetter P, Ueberbacher BJ, Werneburg M, Zerbe K, Steinmann J, Van der Meijden B, Bernardini F, Lederer A, Dias RL, Misson PE, Henze H, Zumbrunn J, Gombert FO, Obrecht D, Hunziker P, Schauer S, Ziegler U, Kach A, Eberl L, Riedel K, DeMarco SJ, Robinson JA (2010) Peptidomimetic antibiotics target outer-membrane biogenesis in *Pseudomonas aeruginosa*. Science 327:1010–1013. doi:10.1126/science.1182749
Stacy DM, Welsh MA, Rather PN, Blackwell HE (2012) Attenuation of quorum sensing in the pathogen *Acinetobacter baumannii* using non-native *N*-acyl homoserine lactones. ACS Chem Biol 7:1719–1728. doi:10.1021/cb300351x
Stacy DM, Le Quement ST, Hansen CL, Clausen JW, Tolker-Nielsen T, Brummond JW, Givskov M, Nielsen TE, Blackwell HE (2013) Synthesis and biological evaluation of triazole-containing *N*-acyl homoserine lactones as quorum sensing modulators. Org Biomol Chem 11:938–954. doi:10.1039/c2ob27155a
Stanton TB (2013) A call for antibiotic alternatives research. Trends Microbiol 21:111–113. doi:10.1016/j.tim.2012.11.002

Stogios PJ, Spanogiannopoulos P, Evdokimova E, Egorova O, Shakya T, Todorovic N, Capretta A, Wright GD, Savchenko A (2013) Structure-guided optimization of protein kinase inhibitors reverses aminoglycoside antibiotic resistance. Biochem J 454:191–200. doi:10.1042/BJ20130317

Stokes NR, Baker N, Bennett JM, Berry J, Collins I, Czaplewski LG, Logan A, Macdonald R, MacLeod L, Peasley H, Mitchell JP, Nayal N, Yadav A, Srivastava A, Haydon DJ (2013) An improved small-molecule inhibitor of FtsZ with superior in vitro potency, drug-like properties, and in vivo efficacy. Antimicrob Agents Chemother 57:317–325. doi:10.1128/AAC. 01580-12

Sun X, Vilar S, Tatonetti NP (2013) High-throughput methods for combinatorial drug discovery. Sci Transl Med 5:205rv1. doi:10.1126/scitranslmed.3006667.

Tan CM, Therien AG, Lu J, Lee SH, Caron A, Gill CJ, Lebeau-Jacob C, Benton-Perdomo L, Monteiro JM, Pereira PM, Elsen NL, Wu J, Deschamps K, Petcu M, Wong S, Daigneault E, Kramer S, Liang L, Maxwell E, Claveau D, Vaillancourt J, Skorey K, Tam J, Wang H, Meredith TC, Sillaots S, Wang-Jarantow L, Ramtohul Y, Langlois E, Landry F, Reid JC, Parthasarathy G, Sharma S, Baryshnikova A, Lumb KJ, Pinho MG, Soisson SM, Roemer T (2012) Restoring methicillin-resistant *Staphylococcus aureus* susceptibility to β-lactam antibiotics. Sci Transl Med 4:126ra35. doi:10.1126/scitranslmed.3003592.

Tegos GP, Hamblin MR (2013) Disruptive innovations: new anti-infectives in the age of resistance. Curr Opin Pharmacol 13:673–677. doi:10.1016/j.coph.2013.08.012

Thaker MN, Wright GD (2014) Opportunities for synthetic biology in antibiotics: expanding glycopeptide chemical diversity. ACS Synth Biol. doi:10.1021/sb300092n

Thaker MN, Wang W, Spanogiannopoulos P, Waglechner N, King AM, Medina R, Wright GD (2013) Identifying producers of antibacterial compounds by screening for antibiotic resistance. Nat Biotechnol 31:922–927. doi:10.1038/nbt.2685

Thorsing M, Klitgaard JK, Atilano ML, Skov MN, Kolmos HJ, Filipe SR, Kallipolitis BH (2013) Thioridazine induces major changes in global gene expression and cell wall composition in methicillin-resistant *Staphylococcus aureus* USA300. PLoS One 8:e64518. doi:10.1371/journal.pone.0064518

Tran TT, Panesso D, Gao H, Roh JH, Munita JM, Reyes J, Diaz L, Lobos EA, Shamoo Y, Mishra NN, Bayer AS, Murray BE, Weinstock GM, Arias CA (2013) Whole-genome analysis of a daptomycin-susceptible *Enterococcus faecium* strain and its daptomycin-resistant variant arising during therapy. Antimicrob Agents Chemother 57:261–268. doi:10.1128/AAC. 01454-12

Tremblay LW, Xu H, Blanchard JS (2010) Structures of the Michaelis complex (1.2 Å) and the covalent acyl intermediate (2.0 Å) of cefamandole bound in the active sites of the *M. tuberculosis* β-lactamase K73A and E166A mutants. Biochemistry 49:9685–9687. doi:10.1021/bi1015088

Van Oudenhove L, De Vriendt K, Van Beeumen J, Mercuri PS, Devreese B (2012) Differential proteomic analysis of the response of *Stenotrophomonas maltophilia* to imipenem. Appl Microbiol Biotechnol 95:717–733. doi:10.1007/s00253-012-4167-0

Vatansever F, de Melo WC, Avci P, Vecchio D, Sadasivam M, Gupta A, Chandran R, Karimi M, Parizotto NA, Yin R, Tegos GP, Hamblin MR (2013) Antimicrobial strategies centered around reactive oxygen species – bactericidal antibiotics, photodynamic therapy, and beyond. FEMS Microbiol Rev 37:955–989. doi:10.1111/1574-6976.12026

Velikova N, Bem AE, van Baarlen P, Wells JM, Marina A (2013) WalK, the path towards new antibacterials with low potential for resistance development. ACS Med Chem Lett 4:891–894. doi:10.1021/ml400320s

Vignaroli C, Rinaldi C, Varaldo PE, Lee CH, Chen FJ, Lauderdale TL (2011) Striking "seesaw effect" between daptomycin nonsusceptibility and β-lactam susceptibility in *Staphylococcus haemolyticus*. Antimicrob Agents Chemother 55:2495–2497. doi:10.1128/AAC. 00224-11

Walsh CT, Wencewicz TA (2014) Prospects for new antibiotics: a molecule-centered perspective. J Antibiot (Tokyo) 67:7–22. doi:10.1038/ja.2013.49

Walsh CT, O'Brien RV, Khosla C (2013) Nonproteinogenic amino acid building blocks for nonribosomal peptide and hybrid polyketide scaffolds. Angew Chem Int Ed 52:7098–7124. doi:10.1002/anie.201208344

Wang H, Gill CJ, Lee SH, Mann P, Zuck P, Meredith TC, Murgolo N, She X, Kales S, Liang L, Liu J, Wu J, Santa Maria J, Su J, Pan J, Hailey J, Mcguinness D, Tan CM, Flattery A, Walker S, Black T, Roemer T (2013) Discovery of wall teichoic acid inhibitors as potential anti-MRSA β-lactam combination agents. Chem Biol 20:272–284. doi:10.1016/j.chembiol.2012.11.013

Wanty C, Anandan A, Piek S, Walshe J, Ganguly J, Carlson RW, Stubbs KA, Kahler CM, Vrielink A (2013) The structure of the neisserial lipooligosaccharide phosphoethanolamine transferase A (LptA) required for resistance to polymyxin. J Mol Biol 425:3389–3402. doi:10.1016/j.jmb.2013.06.029

Warmus JS, Quinn CL, Taylor C, Murphy ST, Johnson TA, Limberakis C, Ortwine D, Bronstein J, Pagano P, Knafels JD, Lightle S, Mochalkin I, Brideau R, Podoll T (2012) Structure based design of an in vivo active hydroxamic acid inhibitor of *P. aeruginosa* LpxC. Bioorg Med Chem Lett 22:2536–2543. doi:10.1016/j.bmcl.2012.01.140

Watkins RR, Bonomo RA (2013) Increasing prevalence of carbapenem-resistant *Enterobacteriaceae* and strategies to avert a looming crisis. Expert Rev Anti-Infect Ther 11:543–545. doi:10.1586/eri.13.46

Watrous J, Roach P, Alexandrov T, Heath BS, Yang JY, Kersten RD, van der Voort M, Pogliano K, Gross H, Raaijmakers JM, Moore BS, Laskin J, Bandeira N, Dorrestein PC (2012) Mass spectral molecular networking of living microbial colonies. Proc Natl Acad Sci U S A 109: E1743–E1752. doi:10.1073/pnas.1203689109

Wellington EMH, Boxall ABA, Cross P, Feil EJ, Gaze WH, Hawkey PM, Johnson-Rollings AS, Jones DL, Lee NM, Otten W, Thomas CM, Williams AP (2013) The role of the natural environment in the emergence of antibiotic resistance in gram-negative bacteria. Lancet Infect Dis 13:155–165. doi:10.1016/S1473-3099(12)70317-1

Werneburg M, Zerbe K, Juhas M, Bigler L, Stalder U, Kaech A, Ziegler U, Obrecht D, Eberl L, Robinson JA (2012) Inhibition of lipopolysaccharide transport to the outer membrane in *Pseudomonas aeruginosa* by peptidomimetic antibiotics. ChemBioChem 13:1767–1775. doi:10.1002/cbic.201200276

Werth BJ, Steed ME, Kaatz GW, Rybak MJ (2013a) Evaluation of ceftaroline activity against heteroresistant vancomycin-intermediate *Staphylococcus aureus* and vancomycin-intermediate methicillin-resistant *S. aureus* strains in an in vitro pharmacokinetic/pharmacodynamic model: exploring the 'Seesaw Effect'. Antimicrob Agents Chemother 57:2664–2668. doi:10.1128/AAC. 02308-12

Werth BJ, Vidaillac C, Murray KP, Newton KL, Sakoulas G, Nonejuie P, Pogliano J, Rybak MJ (2013b) Novel combinations of vancomycin plus ceftaroline or oxacillin against methicillin-resistant vancomycin-intermediate *Staphylococcus aureus* (VISA) and heterogeneous VISA. Antimicrob Agents Chemother 57:2376–2379. doi:10.1128/AAC. 02354-12

Wilke KE, Carlson EE (2013) All signals lost. Sci Transl Med 5:203ps12. doi:10.1126/scitranslmed.3006670.

Wilson MZ, Gitai Z (2013) Beyond the cytoskeleton: mesoscale assemblies and their function in spatial organization. Curr Opin Microbiol 16:177–183. doi:10.1016/j.mib.2013.03.008

Wilson MC, Piel J (2013) Metagenomic approaches for exploiting uncultivated bacteria as a resource for novel biosynthetic enzymology. Chem Biol 20:636–647. doi:10.1016/j.chembiol.2013.04.011

Winstel V, Liang C, Sanchez-Carballo P, Steglich M, Munar M, Bröker BM, Penadés JR, Nübel U, Holst O, Dandekar T, Peschel A, Xia G (2013) Wall teichoic acid structure governs horizontal gene transfer between major bacterial pathogens. Nat Commun 4:2345. doi:10.1038/ncomms3345

Worthington RJ, Melander C (2013a) Combination approaches to combat multidrug-resistant bacteria. Trends Biotechnol 31:177–184. doi:10.1016/j.tibtech.2012.12.006

Worthington RJ, Melander C (2013b) Overcoming resistance to β-lactam antibiotics. J Org Chem 78:4207–4213. doi:10.1021/jo400236f

Worthington RJ, Blackledge MS, Melander C (2013) Small-molecule inhibition of bacterial two-component systems to combat antibiotic resistance and virulence. Future Med Chem 5:1265–1284. doi:10.4155/fmc.13.58

Wright G (2014) Perspective: synthetic biology revives antibiotics. Nature 509:S13. doi:10.1038/509S13a

Wright PM, Seiple IB, Myers AG (2014) The evolving role of chemical synthesis in antibacterial drug discovery. Angew Chem Int Ed 53:8840–8869. doi:10.1002/anie.201310843

Xiao XY, Hunt DK, Zhou J, Clark RB, Dunwoody N, Fyfe C, Grossman TH, O'Brien WJ, Plamondon L, Ronn M, Sun C, Zhang WY, Sutcliffe JA (2012) Fluorocyclines. 1. 7-fluoro-9-pyrrolidinoacetamido-6-demethyl-6-deoxytetracycline: a potent, broad spectrum antibacterial agent. J Med Chem 55:597–605. doi:10.1021/jm201465w

Yan J, Wang K, Dang W, Chen R, Xie J, Zhang B, Song J, Wang R (2013) Two hits are better than one: Membrane-active and DNA binding-related double-action mechanism of NK-18, a novel antimicrobial peptide derived from mammalian NK-Lysin. Antimicrob Agents Chemother 57:220–228. doi:10.1128/AAC. 01619-12

Yun M-K, Wu Y, Li Z, Zhao Y, Waddell MB, Ferreira AM, Lee RE, Bashford D, White SW (2012) Catalysis and sulfa drug resistance in dihydropteroate synthase. Science 335:1110–1114. doi:10.1126/science.1214641

Zakeri B, Lu TK (2013) Synthetic biology of antimicrobial discovery. ACS Synth Biol 2:358–372. doi:10.1021/sb300101g

Zaknoon F, Goldberg K, Sarig H, Epand RF, Epand RM, Mor A (2012) Antibacterial properties of an oligo-acyl-lysyl hexamer targeting gram-negative species. Antimicrob Agents Chemother 56:4827–4832. doi:10.1128/AAC.00511-12

Zhang G, Meredith TC, Kahne D (2013) On the essentiality of lipopolysaccharide to gram-negative bacteria. Curr Opin Microbiol 16:779–785. doi:10.1016/j.mib.2013.09.007

Zhu J, Kaufmann GF (2013) Quo vadis quorum quenching? Curr Opin Pharmacol 13:688–698. doi:10.1016/j.coph.2013.07.003

Zlitni S, Ferruccio LF, Brown ED (2013) Metabolic suppression identifies new antibacterial inhibitors under nutrient limitation. Nat Chem Biol 9:796–804. doi:10.1038/nchembio.1361

Zoraghi R, Reiner NE (2013) Protein interaction networks as starting points to identify novel antimicrobial drug targets. Curr Opin Microbiol 16:566–572. doi:10.1016/j.mib.2013.07.010

Drug-Resistant Tuberculosis

Faiz Ahmad Khan, Greg Fox, and Dick Menzies

Contents

Dr. Ahmad Khan and Dr. Fox contributed equally to this work and are co-first authors.

F. Ahmad Khan (✉)
Montreal Chest Institute, Montreal, QC, Canada
e-mail: faizresp@gmail.com

G. Fox (✉)
Woolcock Institute of Medical Research, The University of Sydney, Sydney, Australia
e-mail: foxsimile@gmail.com

D. Menzies
Respiratory Division, McGill University, Montreal, QC, Canada
e-mail: dick.menzies@mcgill.ca

M. Gotte et al. (eds.), *Handbook of Antimicrobial Resistance*,
DOI 10.1007/978-1-4939-0694-9_13

Abstract
Tuberculosis, an airborne infectious disease caused by the organism *Mycobacterium tuberculosis*, has been a leading cause of death for centuries and remains a major cause of morbidity and mortality in many parts of the world. In 2012, 8.6 million people became sick with tuberculosis, and 1.3 million died from this curable disease (World Health Organization 2013a). While the majority of cases are caused by strains susceptible to all antituberculosis antibiotics, drug resistance is a major concern that carries the potential to reverse decades of progress in tuberculosis control. This chapter examines the global epidemiology of drug-resistant tuberculosis and the drivers for development of drug resistance and its spread within populations. We explore the reasons for the complex nexus between drug resistance and access to health care, including case studies of countries whose epidemics have taken different trajectories. We examine the important implications of drug-resistant tuberculosis for health systems in both the developed world and low- and middle-income countries. Finally, we discuss the elements needed to control the spread of drug-resistant tuberculosis.

Keywords
Tuberculosis • MDR-TB • XDR-TB • nosocomial tuberculosis • health systems

Introduction

Tuberculosis, an airborne infectious disease caused by the bacterium *Mycobacterium tuberculosis*, has been a leading cause of death for centuries and remains a major cause of morbidity and mortality in many parts of the world. In 2012, 8.6 million people became sick with tuberculosis, and 1.3 million died from this curable disease (World Health Organization 2013a). While the majority of cases are caused by strains susceptible to all antituberculosis antibiotics, drug resistance is a major concern that carries the potential to reverse decades of progress in tuberculosis control. This chapter examines the global epidemiology of drug-resistant tuberculosis and the drivers for the development of drug resistance and its spread within populations. We explore the reasons for the complex nexus between drug resistance and access to health care, including case studies of countries whose epidemics have taken different trajectories. We examine the important implications of drug-resistant tuberculosis for health systems in both high-income and low/middle-income countries. Finally, we discuss the elements needed to control the spread of drug-resistant tuberculosis.

Background and Global Epidemiology of Drug-Resistant Tuberculosis

A Brief History of Tuberculosis Treatment and Drug Resistance

Prior to the era of antibiotic treatment for tuberculosis, patients remained contagious for years, few were cured, and case fatality approached 100 % (Rieder and International Union Against Tuberculosis and Lung Disease 1999). The advent of medications capable of curing the disease was a major breakthrough and hastened the fall in tuberculosis incidence and mortality in many industrialized nations (Armstrong et al. 1999; Murray 2004).

In the initial clinical trials of tuberculosis treatment, it became evident that *Mycobacterium tuberculosis* rapidly acquires resistance in patients treated with a single antibiotic (Crofton and Mitchison 1948; Medical Research Council Streptomycin in Tuberculosis Trials Committee 1948; Daniels and Hill 1952; Knox et al. 1952). Studies from this era also suggested that poor adherence to treatment increased the risk of drug-resistant tuberculosis (Crofton 1959; Simpson 1959) and that treatment outcomes were worse among patients infected with resistant organisms (Daniels and Hill 1952). In 1960, the International Union Against Tuberculosis published results from the first global survey of tuberculosis drug resistance. The survey, which pooled data from patients admitted to sanitoria or hospitals in Europe, North America, Brazil, and India, found 42 % of previously treated patients, and 6.5 % of previously untreated patients, had strains resistant to at least one of the three antituberculosis drugs in use at the time (Crofton 1960).

The rising prevalence of drug-resistant tuberculosis among previously untreated cases prompted the use of regimens utilizing three drugs. This ensured that patients with undiagnosed resistance to one drug would receive treatment with at least two medications to which the strain remained susceptible (Bell and Brown 1960).

Standard treatment of drug-susceptible tuberculosis lasted 1–2 years until the 1970s, when several clinical trials led to the establishment of "short-course chemotherapy" (SCC) regimens, which were able to cure the disease in 6–8 months with low rates of relapse (East African/British Medical Research Council 1973a, b; Fox et al. 1999). Despite the advent of effective, shorter treatment regimens, tuberculosis continued to afflict millions and remained the leading cause of death due to a single infectious agent (Kochi 1999; Snider and La Montagne 1994). The emergence of the HIV epidemic in the 1980s further strained tuberculosis control programs in many parts of the world. To improve tuberculosis control and increase the number of affected persons being treated, a new global strategy was developed and advocated by the World Health Organization (WHO) – "DOTS," an acronym for Directly Observed Treatment Short-course (Kochi 1999; Snider and La Montagne 1994). DOTS was intended to build the capacity to diagnose and treat drug-susceptible tuberculosis, while using direct observation of pill ingestion to ensure adequate adherence and prevent the emergence of resistance.

In the early 1990s, a series of deadly outbreaks of highly drug-resistant tuberculosis occurred in the United States. As data became available, it was soon clear that resistance posed a threat to tuberculosis control in many parts of the world (Centers for Disease Control and Prevention 1999; Coninx et al. 1999; Farmer et al. 1998; Kim et al. 1997; Kimerling et al. 1999a; Pablos-Mendez et al. 1998). Today, drug-resistant tuberculosis is found in every country and is recognized as a global problem that needs to be addressed urgently.

Definitions and Clinical Implications of Drug-Resistant Tuberculosis

Antituberculosis antibiotics are often broadly grouped into two categories: first-line drugs and second-line drugs. Orally administered first-line drugs are isoniazid, rifampin, pyrazinamide, and ethambutol. Streptomycin is an injectable first-line drug. All other antituberculosis drugs are considered second line, although, as shown in Box 1, these second-line drugs are further categorized into four categories. This categorization is useful when creating regimens to treat drug-resistant tuberculosis (World Health Organization 2011a; World Health Organization and Stop TB Department 2008).

All cases of tuberculosis, regardless of resistance or susceptibility, can be categorized as either "new" or "previously treated." New cases have never been treated for tuberculosis in the past (or have been treated for less than 1 month), whereas previously treated cases are those that have previously received more than 1 month of treatment (World Health Organization 2013b).

Antibiotic resistance is broadly divided into two forms, according to the host in which the resistance-conferring mutations arose. *Primary drug resistance* occurs when the bacilli were already resistant to antibiotics at the time they were transmitted from another patient. This is seen in new cases. *Acquired drug resistance* (also called "secondary drug resistance") occurs when new drug resistance arises in an individual during the course of their infection (Dye 2009). This is seen in previously treated cases. Further, it is possible for a strain resistant to some drugs to be transmitted to an individual who then acquires resistance to additional antibiotics during treatment.

Categorization of drug-resistant tuberculosis is also based upon the number and type of medications to which the organism is resistant, as these characteristics impact treatment and outcomes (Box 2).

Among the different types of drug-resistant tuberculosis, the categories of multidrug-resistant (MDR-TB) and extensively drug-resistant tuberculosis (XDR-TB) have the greatest impact on treatment and outcomes. MDR- and XDR-TB are resistant to the most potent categories of antituberculosis medications, and their treatment requires more drugs (at least 5) and lasts much longer (at least 20 months for MDR-TB, at least 2 years for XDR-TB). Their treatment is also more challenging because it necessitates utilization of injectable antibiotics as well as second-line oral agents which are more expensive, more commonly associated with adverse events, and less effective than first-line drugs. The average cure rate for MDR-TB in the published literature has been approximately 60 % and mortality during treatment 15 % (Ahuja et al. 2012), although, with adequate resources and timely diagnosis, it is possible to achieve cure rates of >80 % (Mitnick et al. 2003). Cure rates for XDR-TB are 25–30 % – similar to spontaneous cure rates seen in the pre-antibiotic era (Falzon et al. 2012).

Because MDR- and XDR-TB have the greatest impact on treatment and outcomes, we focus on these forms when describing the global epidemiology of drug-resistant tuberculosis.

Further reading on the diagnosis and treatment of tuberculosis and drug-resistant tuberculosis can be found at:

http://www.who.int/tb/publications/tb_treatmentguidelines/en/

http://www.who.int/tb/challenges/mdr/programmatic_guidelines_for_mdrtb/en/

Box 1: Groups of Antituberculosis Medications†

First-line agents	
Group 1. First-line oral agents	Isoniazid, rifampin, ethambutol, pyrazinamide
Second-line agents	
Group 2. Injectable antituberculosis drugs[a]	Kanamycin, amikacin, capreomycin
Group 3. Fluoroquinolones	Levofloxacin, moxifloxacin, gatifloxacin
Group 4. Second-line oral agents	Ethionamide, prothionamide, cycloserine, PAS
Group 5. Agents of unclear efficacy against drug-resistant tuberculosis	Clofazimine, linezolid, amoxicillin-clavulanate, thioacetazone, imipenem-cilastatin, clarithromycin, high-dose isoniazid

†Two new second-line antituberculosis medications, bedaquiline and delamanid, have yet to be classified and are not included in this table.

[a]Streptomycin, an injectable, is not a second-line medication as it is not used to treat multidrug-resistant tuberculosis (see Box 2)

Box 2: Categorization of Tuberculosis Drug Resistance

Resistance pattern	***Definition***
Pan-susceptible	Susceptibility to all antituberculosis medications
Mono-resistant	Resistance to one antituberculosis medication
	For example, "isoniazid mono-resistant" organisms are resistant to isoniazid and susceptible to other antituberculosis medications
Polydrug-resistant (PDR)	Resistance to at least two tuberculosis medications, excluding organisms resistant to both isoniazid *and* rifampin
Multidrug-resistant (MDR)	Resistance to at least isoniazid *and* rifampin
Extensively drug-resistant (XDR)	MDR strains that are also resistant to fluoroquinolones *and* at least one second-line injectable agent

Global Epidemiology of Drug-Resistant Tuberculosis

Isoniazid mono-resistance is of epidemiologic importance as it is common in many parts of the world and increases the risk of relapse and of developing MDR-TB (Menzies et al. 2009). A recent study described the global prevalence, distribution, and trends in isoniazid-resistant tuberculosis between 1994 and 2007 (Jenkins et al. 2011). The global average prevalence of isoniazid-resistant tuberculosis among new and previously treated cases was estimated to be 13.9 % and 29.0 %, respectively. These estimates were calculated excluding data from Eastern Europe, where prevalence was much higher (33.5 % among new and 61.4 % among previously treated cases). The highest rates among new cases were reported in some countries of the former Soviet Union, China, Vietnam, the Dominican Republic, and parts of India.

In 2012, MDR-TB represented 3.6 % of new and 20.2 % of previously treated tuberculosis cases (World Health Organization 2013a). Thus, among tuberculosis notified to the WHO, it is estimated that 170,000 new and 140,000 previously treated cases had MDR-TB. While MDR-TB caused 5 % of the world's incident tuberculosis cases in 2012, it was responsible for 13 % of tuberculosis deaths (World Health Organization 2013a). XDR-TB accounts for 9.6 % of all MDR-TB and has been reported in 92 countries (World Health Organization 2013a).

Worldwide summary statistics do not adequately describe the epidemiology of drug-resistant tuberculosis, a disease whose global burden is unequally distributed (Fig. 1). "High-burden countries" are those that have reported at least 4,000 cases of

Percentage of new TB cases with MDR-TB[a]

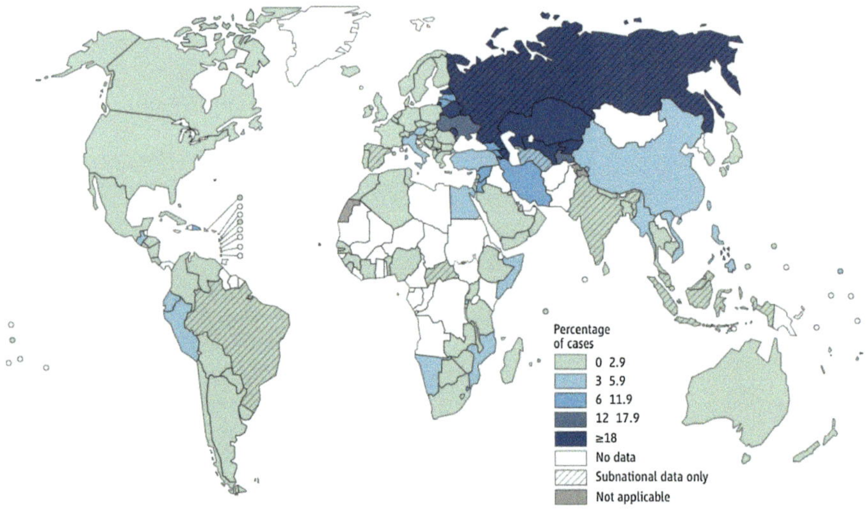

[a] Figures are based on the most recent year for which data have been reported, which varies among countries.

Fig. 1 Proportion of new tuberculosis cases with MDR-TB. With permission from the World Health Organization (http://www.who.int/tb/publications/global_report/en/) (World Health Organization 2013a)

MDR-TB or where at least 10 % of new cases have MDR-TB (World Health Organization 2010a). Over 50 % of the world's MDR cases are found in three countries: China, India, and Russia (Zignol et al. 2012a). In China, 10 % of tuberculosis patients have MDR-TB, and over half of these are cases of primary drug resistance, caused by transmission of resistant strains (World Health Organization 2010a; Zhao et al. 2009; Zhao et al. 2012). In India, where only subnational data on the prevalence of drug resistance have been gathered, the WHO estimates that 100,000 cases of MDR-TB emerge annually (World Health Organization 2010b). In Russia, 23 % of new and 49 % of previously treated cases have MDR-TB; however, certain regions have a higher prevalence than others. For example, the highest proportion of MDR-TB among new cases in the world – 41.9 % – has been found in the Russian Federation's Yamalo-Nenets Autonomous Area (World Health Organization 2013b), and in the Ulyanovsk oblast, over 70 % of all tuberculosis cases have MDR-TB (World Health Organization 2013b). The elevated prevalence of MDR-TB in Russia is part of a larger epidemic involving several Eastern European and Central Asian countries.

Unfortunately, drug resistance surveillance data are lacking for most of Africa, a region that accounts for over one-fifth of the world's tuberculosis cases and 80 % of those occurring among people living with HIV (World Health Organization 2013b). Available data suggest MDR-TB accounts for a smaller proportion of tuberculosis in Africa than other parts of the world (World Health Organization 2013b); however, because tuberculosis is highly prevalent in this region, the absolute number of MDR-TB cases could be high enough to strain resources (Zignol et al. 2012b). In South Africa, the prevalence of drug-resistant tuberculosis has risen rapidly – MDR-TB accounted for 3.1 % of all tuberculosis cases in 2002 and for 9.6 % in 2008 (Streicher et al. 2012). The majority of MDR-TB in South Africa is seen in new cases of tuberculosis, and it has been estimated that 80 % of MDR-TB in this country is caused by transmission of resistant organisms (Streicher et al. 2012).

The Pathogenesis of Drug-Resistant Tuberculosis

The Biological Basis of Drug Resistance

Antibiotic resistance arises when the mutation of mycobacterial genes confers bacilli with a survival advantage that enables them to withstand antituberculosis antibiotics. If mycobacteria are exposed to inadequate concentrations of an antibiotic, those that are resistant to that medication become dominant (David 1970). These bacteria then replicate and can be transmitted to others. Many different genetic changes can confer resistance to any given drug. For example, studies using whole genomic sequencing have demonstrated that resistance to the drug isoniazid may be caused by hundreds of possible genetic changes (Hazbon et al. 2006; Almeida Da Silva and Palomino 2011).

In some cases, genetic changes that confer resistance may be associated with a fitness cost to the bacteria that renders them potentially less pathogenic or transmissible. However, it has been suggested that over time the increased survival and transmission of fittest isolates will lead them to become dominant (Sun et al. 2012). Relative strain fitness is considered one of the most important factors in mathematical modeling of the dissemination of drug resistance in populations, as it is thought to influence the transmissibility of the strain and hence its epidemiological impact (Almeida Da Silva and Palomino 2011; Borrell and Gagneux 2011).

Another important mycobacterial factor in the development of drug resistance is the very slow replication rate of *M. tuberculosis*. In contrast to most bacterial pathogens, which replicate in minutes to hours, the doubling time of *M. tuberculosis* is about 24 h. As a result, effective therapeutic drug levels must be maintained for long periods in order to eradicate all viable mycobacteria (David 1970).

The rate at which bacilli develop drug-resistant mutations may also be related to the mycobacterial strain. There is some evidence from clinical (Cox et al. 2007) and in vitro (Ford et al. 2013) studies showing that the prevalent Beijing strains of *M. tuberculosis* may acquire drug resistance more rapidly than others, although this has been disputed. All *Mycobacterium tuberculosis* strains originated from an original ancestor, in the distant past. Over time, selective pressures have caused genetic differences to emerge, creating strain diversity. The "Beijing" family of strains (also known as the W family of strains) comprises one dominant branch of the phylogenetic tree (Borrell and Gagneux 2011). This particular strain represents about 50 % of strains in Asia and more than 13 % of all strains worldwide (Parwati et al. 2010).

At a population level, the incidence of drug-resistant disease is determined by the complex interplay between (a) the rate at which resistant isolates are generated, (b) the effect these resistance-conferring genetic changes have upon infectiousness and transmissibility of the pathogen, (c) the susceptibility of the exposed population to tuberculosis, and (d) the selective pressures generated by antibiotic use (Dye 2009). Consequently, there has been considerable clinical and research interest in developing strategies to address each aspect.

In the following section, we examine the epidemiological factors affecting acquired and primary drug resistance and present several case studies to illustrate their impact.

Epidemiological Factors Associated with Acquired Drug Resistance

Nonadherence with Therapy

Standard treatment for drug-susceptible tuberculosis involves taking multiple antibiotics at least 3 times per week for a minimum of 6 months (World Health Organization and Stop TB Department 2010). These patients are generally prescribed four antibiotics during the initial 2-month "intensive phase," followed by two drugs in the 4-month "continuation phase." The duration and complexity of this therapy is a substantial barrier to adherence. Furthermore, common side effects of tuberculosis medications such as nausea, anorexia, and rash often deter patients from continuing treatment. Interrupted or inadequate drug therapy can lead to subtherapeutic drug levels and give rise to drug resistance.

Past tuberculosis treatment is a strong predictor of drug resistance (Dalton et al. 2012). A frequently cited mechanism by which treatment leads to drug resistance is noncompliance with medications, with irregular treatment leading to subtherapeutic levels and the selection of resistant isolates (David 1970). However, the data to support this theory is limited and largely confined to retrospective studies (Pablos-Mendez et al. 1997; Gelmanova et al. 2007). A study in San Francisco found that noncompliance was 20 times (95 % CI 1.7–234) more likely to be associated with acquired drug resistance (Bradford et al. 1996). The study showed that side effects of therapy may have contributed to the nonadherence, with gastrointestinal symptoms of therapy increasing the odds of acquired resistance by 11.5 times (95 % CI 1.2–107). A widely reported epidemic of drug-resistant tuberculosis in New York City in the early 1990s found nonadherent cases took almost four times as long to achieve sputum culture conversion (254 vs. 64 days, $p < 0.00001$) – suggesting that interrupted treatment was also considerably less effective. However, there was no overall association between acquired resistance and noncompliance with therapy (Pablos-Mendez et al. 1997).

Inappropriate Drug Regimens

The selection of drug regimens containing an inadequate number of antituberculosis medications to which the bacteria are susceptible substantially increases the likelihood of acquired drug resistance. The success of standard therapy may be reduced markedly if tuberculosis is caused by a mycobacterial strain that is already resistant to one or more antibiotics. A review of two studies that characterized drug resistance before treatment of non-MDR-TB showed that the relative risk of developing MDR-TB was 29 (3.8–226.7) times increased among individuals who were given inappropriate treatment, as defined by drug susceptibility (van der Werf et al. 2012). Another review of the effect of standardized treatments found the odds of acquiring drug resistance were between five- and tenfold higher if disease was caused by a resistant strain compared to a pan-sensitive strain (Menzies et al. 2009). This study also found that the number of drugs to which strains were susceptible was inversely related to the likelihood of acquired drug resistance.

Despite the availability of evidence-based guidelines for managing drug resistance, the reality "on the ground" is often very different. In many countries with limited access to diagnostics or optimal tuberculosis treatment, the haphazard prescription of drugs to patients failing treatment creates the preconditions for acquired drug resistance. The use of substandard drug regimens was an important factor driving the high rates of drug resistance that emerged in the former Soviet Union in the 1990s (Drobniewski et al. 1996a).

Case Study: Drug Resistance in the Former Soviet Union
The rapid rise in MDR-TB incidence after the collapse of the former Soviet Union illustrates how the disease can become prevalent in a population. In the two decades until 1990, Russia had achieved a 3.7 % annual decline in tuberculosis notifications. After a sudden economic downturn with the end of the Soviet Union, tuberculosis notifications rose by 7.5 % per year (Shilova and Dye 2001). As early as 1996, the incidence of MDR-TB among new cases in prisons had risen to 20 % (Kimerling et al. 1999b). The emergence of drug resistance was largely driven by the widespread use of suboptimal regimens. A study among prisoners in the mid-1990s found that 79 % of patients with tuberculosis had experienced treatment interruption (Kimerling et al. 1999b). Inappropriate first-line treatment for patients with past tuberculosis histories and inadequate re-treatment regimens that added a single additional drug to failing regimens (the WHO "Category 2" regimens) also contributed to the rise of MDR-TB. There was also evidence that prisons became reservoirs of MDR-TB and XDR-TB, and drug-resistant tuberculosis spread from there to the general population (Drobniewski et al. 1996b). As a result, in 2012, MDR-TB comprised 23 % of all newly diagnosed tuberculosis cases in Russia (World Health Organization 2013a). An interesting contrast with the Russian experience was Latvia and Estonia, which maintained their functioning tuberculosis control programs and saw a decline in the incidence of MDR-TB during the same time period (Dye 2009). The contrast between the settings emphasizes the importance of the public health response to tuberculosis in the control of drug-resistant tuberculosis.

Suboptimal Drug Levels and Poor Drug Quality

Even when appropriate antibiotics are prescribed and patients are compliant, treatment still may be ineffective. Poor drug quality is a major problem for tuberculosis control in many countries. Problems with manufacturing standards, storage of medications, or expiry of drugs may all contribute to suboptimal drug levels. One study of drug quality in hospitals and pharmacies in six low- and middle-income countries found that 10 % of all samples contained inadequate quantities of the active tuberculosis drugs (Laserson et al. 2001). Interestingly, fixed dose combinations were 1.7 times more likely to be associated with low drug quantities than individually administered tablets.

Physiological differences between individuals may also contribute to diminished drug effectiveness. There is some evidence that HIV may reduce drug absorption, leading to higher treatment failure rates and acquired drug resistance (Andrews et al. 2007). This finding was supported by a study of tuberculosis pharmacokinetics, which also found a substantial proportion of individuals without other comorbidities had subtherapeutic drug levels despite being compliant with therapy (Babalik et al. 2011).

Case Study of Factors Contributing to Drug Resistance: India

India, which is home to over 20 % of all MDR-TB cases (World Health Organization 2013a), illustrates how weakness in tuberculosis control creates the environment where drug-resistant tuberculosis can readily emerge. There are several factors that may explain why drug resistance has become an important problem in India. Firstly, weaknesses in drug prescribing may create a setting where drug resistance can emerge. The diagnosis and treatment of tuberculosis in India is highly decentralized, with more than half of all tuberculosis patients receiving care through poorly regulated private providers (Prasad 2010). One study from Mumbai illustrated the problems with treatment practices in the private sector. Among 106 health-care workers, 63 different regimens were recommended, of which only six were considered adequate (Udwadia et al. 2010). Surprisingly, the survey showed no improvement in prescribing practices compared to a similar one 20 years earlier. Such variable prescription practices are likely to give rise to ineffective treatment, treatment failure, and acquired drug resistance. Poor-quality drugs may contribute to substandard regimens, with reports of low quality of medications, poor drug storage, and drug supply chain problems (Prasad 2010; Bhaumik 2013). Thirdly, diagnostic delay may also contribute to prolonged periods of transmission of disease, with one study finding that patients saw 6–9 doctors before receiving standardized therapy (Prasad 2010). Finally, access to appropriate second-line treatment in India remains low – with less than 25 % of patients with MDR-TB receiving appropriate treatment (World Health Organization 2013a). In summary, recognized weaknesses in the Indian health-care system, particularly in the private sector, have created many of the preconditions for the development of drug-resistant tuberculosis. However, limitations in routine disease reporting have made it difficult to quantify the epidemiological impact of these trends.

Epidemiological Drivers of Primary Drug Resistance

Delays in Diagnosis and Effective Treatment

In many high-tuberculosis-burden settings, the most widely used diagnostic test for tuberculosis is "smear microscopy" wherein sputum, after special staining, is examined under a microscope for the presence of tuberculosis bacilli. While it is inexpensive, smear microscopy is unable to determine whether drug resistance is present. Traditional methods for determining drug resistance can take several months, involving sputum culture and then culture-based (phenotypic) drug susceptibility testing (DST). There can be long delays in the diagnosis of MDR-TB, particularly if sputum culture is initiated only after a patient fails first-line therapy. Newer, more rapid methods of DST use PCR-based technologies to identify the presence of *M. tuberculosis* and resistance-conferring DNA sequences with a turnaround time of hours to days, substantially decreasing time to diagnosis (Boehme et al. 2010). However, it is unclear whether availability of these tests translates to meaningful reductions in the time to treatment initiation.

The risk of transmission of tuberculosis to exposed contacts is influenced by the duration and closeness of exposure to the index patient and environmental factors such as ventilation (Kenyon et al. 1996; Lienhardt et al. 2003; Escombe et al. 2007). Transmission of drug-resistant tuberculosis is most pronounced in settings where there are lengthy delays in the diagnosis and appropriate treatment of patients with disease. Diagnostic delay is common for patients with drug-resistant disease, in light of the patient and health system factors described above.

Diagnosis of drug resistance – the necessary precursor to effective therapy – is particularly challenging in settings where access to confirmatory testing is limited. In many countries where there is limited access to laboratory-based diagnostics, a diagnosis of "clinical" MDR-TB is routinely made after a patient fails empirical therapy with first-line drugs, which can take 5 months (World Health Organization and Stop TB Department 2010), and often only when patients fail empiric therapy with a re-treatment regimen (which also utilize first-line medications). Even in settings where DST is routinely available, there may be delays of 12 weeks or more until drug susceptibility results are available. Even after diagnosis and commencement of appropriate second-line drug therapy, patients may remain infectious for weeks to months, until they no longer secrete viable bacilli (Ahuja et al. 2012). During this time, whether patients are managed at home or in hospital, they can transmit drug-resistant disease to many others before they are cured.

During the prolonged infectious period, strategies to reduce transmission for which there is some evidence include standard infection control procedures such as isolation, ventilation, and other environmental controls and use of personal protective devices (Jensen et al. 2005). Administrative controls also play a critical role in avoiding unnecessary exposure. However, some infection control strategies may be practically difficult or expensive to implement routinely in the overstretched health-care systems of resource-limited settings. Therefore, transmission of MDR-TB and XDR-TB is likely to be substantial in settings where health systems are weak or overstretched (Gandhi et al. 2006).

Unfortunately, the vast majority of patients with drug-resistant tuberculosis are never diagnosed nor treated, because diagnostic capacity is very limited in most countries where this disease is common. Although the WHO recommends DST for all tuberculosis patients at increased risk of drug resistance, in 2012, only 9 % of previously treated cases underwent DST (World Health Organization 2013a). In 2012, in India and China – home to over half of the world's MDR-TB cases – only 26 % and 5 % of MDR-TB patients were detected and reported (World Health

Organization 2013a). Left undiagnosed and untreated, most people with drug-resistant tuberculosis are likely to transmit the disease to others and die.

Environmental Risk Factors for Transmission

The environment in which an infectious patient resides affects the likelihood of transmission and the populations who are likely to have been exposed. Household contacts in particular are a high-risk group, owing to the duration and proximity of their exposure to the patient (Becerra et al. 2011; Fox et al. 2013). The risk of transmission is also high in health-care settings, prisons, and other congregate settings (Nodieva et al. 2010). A widely reported outbreak of XDR-TB in Tugela Ferry, Kwazulu-Natal Province, in South Africa tragically illustrated the problem of nosocomial transmission (transmission of infection within health-care settings). The authors found that 39 % of all tuberculosis patients had MDR-TB and 6.3 % were infected with XDR-TB. Subsequent epidemiological investigation showed that 67 % of the XDR-TB patients had been admitted to hospital within the preceding 2 years before diagnosis, and none had other history of close contact with tuberculosis (Gandhi et al. 2006). Further support for the hypothesis of transmission of resistant strains was given by genotypic testing, which found that 85 % of isolates were genetically similar. This suggested that a dominant strain of XDR-TB had spread throughout the province (Moodley et al. 2011). Importantly, 80 % of patients in the Tugela Ferry outbreak were infected with HIV. Not only did HIV coinfection contribute to the high mortality rates, but HIV also has the effect of "telescoping" outbreaks, by reducing the time for infected individuals to develop the disease and hence the time to further propagation of the infection.

Challenges in Measuring the Impact of Drug-Resistant Tuberculosis

An accurate assessment of the global impact of drug-resistant tuberculosis is extremely challenging. Estimates of disease incidence in many high-burden countries are extrapolated from very limited data and rely upon numerous assumptions such as the representativeness of the population sampling and the correct classification of cases. Given this, the estimates of the global annual incidence of MDR-TB are imprecise, with the 95 % confidence limits ranging from 300,000 to 600,000 new cases (World Health Organization 2013a). In its 2013 report, the WHO was unable to obtain any data on drug resistance from 30 % of its member states (Fig. 1). Even among the 136 countries for which data is available, many estimates rely upon subnational surveys that may not accurately reflect the national situation (Cohen 2013).

There is also a considerable gap between the predicted number of incident cases and the number that are actually reported, making it difficult to verify the estimates.

The settings with the greatest case-detection gaps are the Western Pacific and Southeast Asian regions of the WHO, where only 6 % and 21 % of incident cases of MDR-TB, respectively, were diagnosed in 2012 (World Health Organization 2013a).

Furthermore, only 48 % of patients that were reported to WHO as diagnosed in 2010 had successfully completed treatment 2 years later (World Health Organization 2013a). In summary, there remain significant limitations in the data available about the incidence of MDR-TB, particularly in many of the highest-burden settings.

The Health System Impacts of Drug-Resistant Tuberculosis

Treatment of MDR-TB and XDR-TB is both complex and costly, necessitating at least 20 months of expensive multidrug therapy to achieve optimal outcomes (World Health Organization 2011a). While the cost of sputum smear to diagnose new tuberculosis is less than $2, the costs to diagnose MDR-TB are considerably greater. Culture and phenotypic DST to make the diagnosis of MDR-TB cost at least $20, and rapid PCR-based tests cost at least $10. Treatment regimens for MDR-TB typically cost at least $2,000, compared to a $20 course of standard therapy for drug-susceptible disease (Oxlade et al. 2012). Given these high costs, the WHO estimates that treating MDR-TB consumes over 20 % of the eight billion dollars that low- and middle-income countries require for treating tuberculosis, despite representing less than 6 % of disease (World Health Organization 2013a). Expensive second-line medications can comprise 20–50 % of all treatment costs despite being off-patent. Clearly, this has major financial implications for both patients and tuberculosis control programs.

A major determinant of costs relates to the manner in which tuberculosis care is provided. In one study, participants in MDR-TB treatment studies in Russia and Estonia were found to have lengthy inpatient hospital stays. This hospital-based approach more than doubled the cost compared to similar programs in Peru and the Philippines (Fitzpatrick and Floyd 2012). To address this issue, WHO guidelines recommend an ambulatory model of care for MDR-TB where possible (World Health Organization 2011a; Falzon et al. 2011).

The timing of diagnostic testing also affects the cost of MDR-TB treatment. A modeling study showed that in a country with a moderate incidence of MDR-TB (2.1 % of incident cases), a strategy of rapid DST (such as GeneXpert) at the beginning of active tuberculosis treatment was more cost-effective than a strategy of waiting until treatment failure before diagnosing MDR-TB and starting MDR-TB therapy (Oxlade et al. 2012). While parameters may vary between epidemiological contexts, the study illustrates the importance of MDR-TB management policies that match the local epidemiological and socioeconomic circumstances.

Case Study: The Cost of MDR-TB Control in the United States

The high cost of controlling drug-resistant tuberculosis is demonstrated by the experience in the early 1990s in New York City. Between 1979 and 1991, the number of incident cases of tuberculosis rose from 1,530 to 3,673 (Landesman 1993). During the same period, there was a 130 % increase in drug-resistant disease, with the proportion of MDR-TB in previously untreated cases rising from 3 % to 7 % (Frieden et al. 1993). The MDR outbreak predominantly affected the homeless, people of low socioeconomic status, people living with HIV, and intravenous drug users (Frieden et al. 1993). Prior treatment was the strongest predictor of MDR disease, with only 54 % of patients with all forms of tuberculosis completing treatment (Landesman 1993).

The rise of MDR-TB coincided with a period of sustained funding cuts to New York's public health infrastructure, characterized by a lack of coordination between tuberculosis services and poor infection control (Sterling 2006). At its nadir, owing to chronic underinvestment by government, only six nurses were responsible for community-based supervised treatment, despite there being over 3,000 incident cases of tuberculosis each year (Brudney and Dobkin 1991). By the time the problem was finally addressed in the early 1990s, the number of patients in New York had tripled in the previous 15 years, and the incidence of MDR-TB among previously untreated patients had increased from 10 % in 1983 to 23 % in 1991 (Frieden et al. 1995). Further, the mortality among MDR-TB patients approached 80 %. As the scale of the problem became apparent and funding was restored, the epidemic was rapidly contained. However, by the end of the decade, the overall cost of reestablishing tuberculosis control was estimated to be over one billion dollars (Coker 1998).

This outbreak in New York demonstrates the substantial financial and human costs of neglecting tuberculosis control and the importance of maintaining a sustained and effective public health response in order to prevent drug-resistant tuberculosis.

Addressing Drug-Resistant Tuberculosis: What Will It Take?

Scaling Up the Response

Very few patients who develop drug-resistant tuberculosis are able to access timely and appropriate therapy. A major scale-up of the existing repertoire of tuberculosis diagnostics, therapies, and public health strategies could substantially reduce MDR-TB. For example, modeling analyses suggest the WHO's "Consolidated

Action Plan to Prevent and Combat MDR and XDR Tuberculosis in the European Region" – which is based on the utilization of existing diagnostics and therapies – would place 127,000 MDR-TB patients on treatment, save 120,000 lives, and could prevent the emergence of 250,000 MDR and 13,000 XDR cases (World Health Organization and Regional Office for Europe 2011). Another modeling study suggested that scaling up diagnostic capacity in South Africa, in order to perform DST in 37 % of new and 85 % of previously treated cases, could prevent the emergence of 7,759 cases of MDR-TB and lower MDR-TB mortality by 50 % over a 10-year period (Dowdy et al. 2008).

Inadequate funding for MDR-TB control is an important obstacle to scale up. In 2010, funding for MDR-TB control in high-burden countries was only 3 % of what was needed (World Health Organization 2010b). While funding has since increased, the gaps remain substantial: in 2013, funding for MDR-TB management in low- and middle-income countries fell $84 million short of the required amount (World Health Organization 2012).

The high cost of medications to treat MDR-TB is another obstacle to scale up. A major global initiative, the Global Drug Facility, was developed to lower costs and facilitate procurement and distribution of second-line medications to WHO-approved MDR-TB treatment programs (Kim et al. 2003). While the program has successfully driven down prices of second-line drugs, MDR-TB treatment regimens continue to be costly (at least $1500 for a full course) (Global Drug Facility Stop TB Partnership). Drug costs for XDR-TB treatment may exceed tens of thousands of dollars (Pooran et al. 2013).

While scaling up of existing approaches for the diagnosis and treatment of MDR-TB could have a major effect, the impact of greater investment could be improved by innovations in MDR-TB diagnosis or treatment.

Advances in Diagnostics for MDR-TB

The advent of nucleic acid amplification tests (NAATs) has marked a major leap forward in our ability to diagnose MDR-TB (Boehme et al. 2010; Steingart et al. 2013). With these assays, drug-resistant tuberculosis can be diagnosed in a few hours, rather than weeks. Cartridge-based NAATs, such as the GeneXpert MTB/RIF assay, have the added advantage of not requiring the stringent biosafety levels needed for other DST methods (including non-cartridge PCR-based assays), which means they can be used in district- and sub-district-level facilities. A cost and affordability analysis suggests that widespread use of the Xpert assay could *lower* the cost of diagnosing MDR-TB in high-burden countries, compared to scale-up of conventional DST (Pantoja et al. 2013). The rapid result time may also reduce time to initiation of MDR-TB treatment, although this has not yet been demonstrated in the published literature. By June 2012, the Xpert MTB/RIF assay had been implemented in 67 low- and middle-income countries (Weyer et al. 2013). While this progress is promising, advances in diagnostics need to be paralleled with advances in the availability of effective treatment.

Advances in the Treatment of MDR-TB

At the time of writing, two new antituberculosis drugs have been approved by regulatory agencies: bedaquiline and delamanid. As noted in a review by Brigden and colleagues, while the development of new drugs is important, it is also essential to develop new drug combinations (i.e., treatment regimens) for MDR- and XDR-TB that are shorter in duration, less toxic, and yet more effective (Brigden et al. 2014). In a cohort of 206 MDR-TB patients in Bangladesh, a 9-month regimen using seven drugs in the intensive phase cured 88 % of patients, with a default rate of only 5.8 % (recall, the WHO recommendation is at least 20 months of treatment with a minimum of five intensive phase medications) (Van Deun et al. 2010). While these results are promising, this was an observational study rather than a randomized controlled trial; hence, it is unclear whether the high rates of good outcomes were truly attributable to the treatment regimen utilized and not due to characteristics of the patients, *M. tuberculosis* strain, or study setting. The STREAM study, a multicenter, randomized trial taking place in South Africa, Vietnam, and Ethiopia, is under way to determine whether these results are attributable to the treatment regimen and can be achieved in other settings.

Strengthening Infection Control

Innovation is also needed to curb nosocomial transmission of drug-resistant tuberculosis. In certain high-burden settings, such transmission is thought to be contributing to MDR-TB in new cases (Nardell and Dharmadhikari 2010; Basu et al. 2011) and also among patients hospitalized while being treated for drug-susceptible tuberculosis (Zhao et al. 2012; Gelmanova et al. 2007). With MDR-TB, it can be challenging to implement measures needed to prevent nosocomial transmission (World Health Organization 2009). In many parts of the world, tuberculosis patients share living quarters while they are hospitalized. If patients with drug-resistant tuberculosis are not separated from those with drug-susceptible strains, the latter will be at risk of infection by resistant strains. The risk of transmission will be particularly elevated if patients with drug-resistant tuberculosis are not being treated with effective second-line regimens, a situation that could arise when resistance is undiagnosed and a patient only receives first-line medications. Box 3 describes an innovative protocol that incorporates the use of rapid molecular diagnostics to reduce the likelihood of nosocomial transmission of MDR-TB.

Box 3: The FAST Strategy

Molecular-based diagnostics that rapidly diagnose resistance could play an important role in curbing nosocomial transmission of drug-resistant tuberculosis. One infection control strategy that incorporates these tests is called FAST, which stands for **F**inding MDR tuberculosis **A**ctively, **S**eparating safely, **T**reating effectively. In this strategy, a molecular-based test is used to screen all tuberculosis suspects presenting to hospital, and all hospitalized tuberculosis patients, for drug-resistant tuberculosis. The strategy should lower nosocomial MDR-TB transmission because patients with resistant strains will be rapidly identified, separated, and started on the second-line regimens needed to render them noncontagious. The strategy is being implemented in Bangladesh and in parts of the Russian Federation (http://tbcare2.org/resources/infection-control).

Expanding the MDR-TB Research Agenda

The development of new diagnostics to reduce time to diagnosis, and new medications and treatment regimens to reduce the length and complexity of therapy, will facilitate the scale-up of global drug-resistant tuberculosis control (World Health Organization 2011b). However, tuberculosis research and development has been chronically underfunded, in part because the disease is uncommon in most high-income countries (Addington et al. 1977; Bloom and Murray 1992; O'Brien and Nunn 2001). As a result, drug development has been slow: after rifampin was approved in 1971, it took 41 years for another new class of drug designed for tuberculosis treatment to be developed and approved for use (while fluoroquinolone antibiotics are also highly effective drugs for tuberculosis, they were developed for other indications) (Cohen 2013). Because so few drugs have been developed, the treatment of drug-resistant tuberculosis now relies mostly on old and less effective medications, most of which were discovered prior to the 1960s and whose use in drug-susceptible disease was largely abandoned due to poor tolerability and efficacy. Additional new antibiotics to treat tuberculosis are now in the drug development pipeline, and investment in research for tuberculosis has improved since the early 2000s. However, progress remains precarious, with funding declining by $30.4 million (USD) between 2011 and 2012 (Frick and Jiminez-Levi 2013).

Conclusion

The hurdles to effectively prevent, diagnose, and treat MDR- and XDR-TB are daunting. Yet the global response to the HIV epidemic, which has seen millions of people placed on lifelong HIV therapy in some of the world's most poverty-stricken areas, suggests that complex public health problems can be addressed with sustained political will and resource allocation. The Stop TB Partnership has outlined an ambitious goal of tuberculosis elimination by the year 2050 (World Health Organization and Stop TB Partnership 2010) and has highlighted MDR-TB as an urgent priority. Greater resources have been committed to tuberculosis control from international donors, new rapid diagnostic tests are now available, and new drugs have recently been developed. These gains have been underpinned by a growing political commitment at a national and international level. There is cause for cautious optimism. Lessons learned in the MDR outbreaks of New York City in the 1990s, and a successful national program for treatment of MDR-TB in Peru, show that treatment success is attainable in a variety of settings. Despite the development of new diagnostic technologies and promising treatment regimens, these alone will not control the drug resistance epidemic without strategies to improve access to health care by the poorest communities, among whom tuberculosis is most prevalent.

Get Involved: The MSF Access Campaign

Grassroots campaigns can help convince governments, pharmaceutical companies, and international donor agencies to enact policies and provide funding needed to increase health-care access in poor parts of the world. Médecins Sans Frontières (MSF) is an international humanitarian organization that won the Nobel Peace Prize in 1999 for providing medical relief to populations living in poverty-stricken and war-torn areas. In 1999, MSF started the "Access Campaign" whose purpose is "to push for access to, and the development of life-saving and life prolonging medicines, diagnostic tests and vaccines for patients in MSF programmes and beyond." Ensuring access to effective diagnostics and treatment for drug-resistant tuberculosis is one of the issues the Access Campaign has been tackling. To get involved in the campaign for drug-resistant tuberculosis, visit http://msfaccess.org/TBmanifesto/

To learn more about the Access Campaign in general, visit http://msfaccess.org/

References

Addington WW, Agarwal MK, Banner AS (1977) Toward shorter-course antituberculosis chemotherapy. Chest 71(5):565

Ahuja SD, Ashkin D, Avendano M et al (2012) Multidrug resistant pulmonary tuberculosis treatment regimens and patient outcomes: an individual patient data meta-analysis of 9,153 patients. PLoS Med 9(8):e1001300

Almeida Da Silva PE, Palomino JC (2011) Molecular basis and mechanisms of drug resistance in *Mycobacterium tuberculosis*: classical and new drugs. J Antimicrob Chemother 66 (7):1417–1430

Andrews JR, Shah NS, Gandhi N et al (2007) Multidrug-resistant and extensively drug-resistant tuberculosis: implications for the HIV epidemic and antiretroviral therapy rollout in South Africa. J Infect Dis 196(Suppl 3):S482–S490

Armstrong GL, Conn LA, Pinner RW (1999) Trends in infectious disease mortality in the United States during the 20th century. JAMA 281(1):61–66

Babalik A, Babalik A, Mannix S, Francis D, Menzies D (2011) Therapeutic drug monitoring in the treatment of active tuberculosis. Can Respir J 18(4):225–229

Basu S, Stuckler D, McKee M (2011) Addressing institutional amplifiers in the dynamics and control of tuberculosis epidemics. Am J Trop Med Hyg 84(1):30

Becerra M, Appleton S, Franke M et al (2011) Tuberculosis burden in households of patients with multidrug-resistant and extensively drug-resistant tuberculosis: a retrospective cohort study. Lancet 377:147–152

Bell WJ, Brown PP (1960) Bacterial resistance to streptomycin, pas and isoniazid in untreated patients with symptomatic pulmonary tuberculosis in Ashanti. Tubercle 41:247–252

Bhaumik S (2013) India's human rights commission seeks answers over shortage of TB drugs. Br Med J 347:f4301

Bloom BR, Murray CJ (1992) Tuberculosis: commentary on a reemergent killer. Science 257 (5073):1055–1064

Boehme CC, Nabeta P, Hillemann D et al (2010) Rapid molecular detection of tuberculosis and rifampin resistance. N Engl J Med 363(11):1005–1015

Borrell S, Gagneux S (2011) Strain diversity, epistasis and the evolution of drug resistance in *Mycobacterium tuberculosis*. Clin Microbiol Infect 17(6):815–820

Bradford WZ, Martin JN, Reingold AL, Schecter GF, Hopewell PC, Small PM (1996) The changing epidemiology of acquired drug-resistant tuberculosis in San Francisco, USA. Lancet 348(9032):928–931

Brigden G, Nyang'wa BT, du Cros P et al (2014) Principles for designing future regimens for multidrug-resistant tuberculosis. Bull World Health Organ 92(1):68–74

Brudney K, Dobkin J (1991) Resurgent tuberculosis in New York City. Human immunodeficiency virus, homelessness, and the decline of tuberculosis control programs. Am Rev Respir Dis 144 (4):745–749

Centers for Disease Control and Prevention (1999) Primary multidrug-resistant tuberculosis–Ivanovo Oblast, Russia, 1999. MMWR Morb Mortal Wkly Rep 48(30):661–664

Cohen J (2013) Infectious disease. Approval of novel TB drug celebrated–with restraint. Science 339(6116):130

Coker R (1998) Lessons from New York's tuberculosis epidemic. Tuberculosis is a political as much as a medical problem-and so are the solutions. Br Med J 317(7159):616

Coninx R, Mathieu C, Debacker M et al (1999) First-line tuberculosis therapy and drug-resistant *Mycobacterium tuberculosis* in prisons. Lancet 353(9157):969–973

Cox HS, Niemann S, Ismailov G et al (2007) Risk of acquired drug resistance during short-course directly observed treatment of tuberculosis in an area with high levels of drug resistance. Clin Infect Dis 44(11):1421–1427

Crofton J (1959) Chemotherapy of pulmonary tuberculosis. Br Med J 1(5138):1610–1614

Crofton J (1960) Tuberculosis undefeated. Br Med J 2(5200):679–687

Crofton J, Mitchison DA (1948) Streptomycin resistance in pulmonary tuberculosis. Br Med J 2 (4588):1009–1015

Dalton T, Cegielski P, Akksilp S et al (2012) Prevalence of and risk factors for resistance to second-line drugs in people with multidrug-resistant tuberculosis in eight countries: a prospective cohort study. Lancet 380(9851):1406–1417

Daniels M, Hill AB (1952) Chemotherapy of pulmonary tuberculosis in young adults; an analysis of the combined results of three medical research council trials. Br Med J 1 (4769):1162–1168

David HL (1970) Probability distribution of drug-resistant mutants in unselected populations of *Mycobacterium tuberculosis*. Appl Microbiol 20(5):810–814

Dowdy DW, Chaisson RE, Maartens G, Corbett EL, Dorman SE (2008) Impact of enhanced tuberculosis diagnosis in South Africa: a mathematical model of expanded culture and drug susceptibility testing. Proc Natl Acad Sci U S A 105(32):11293–11298

Drobniewski F, Tayler E, Ignatenko N et al (1996a) Tuberculosis in Siberia: 2. Diagnosis, chemoprophylaxis and treatment. Tuberc Lung Dis 77(4):297–301

Drobniewski F, Tayler E, Ignatenko N et al (1996b) Tuberculosis in Siberia: 1. An epidemiological and microbiological assessment. Tuberc Lung Dis 77(3):199–206

Dye C (2009) Doomsday postponed? Preventing and reversing epidemics of drug-resistant tuberculosis. Nat Rev Microbiol 7(1):81–87

East African/British Medical Research Council (1973a) Controlled clinical trial of four short-course (6-month) regimens of chemotherapy for treatment of pulmonary tuberculosis: second report. The Lancet 301(7816):1331–1339

East African/British Medical Research Council (1973b) Controlled clinical trial of four short-course (6-month) regimens of chemotherapy for treatment of pulmonary tuberculosis: third report. The Lancet 304(7875):237–240

Escombe AR, Oeser CC, Gilman RH et al (2007) Natural ventilation for the prevention of airborne contagion. PLoS Med 4(2):e68

Falzon D, Jaramillo E, Schunemann HJ et al (2011) WHO guidelines for the programmatic management of drug-resistant tuberculosis: 2011 update. Eur Respir J 38(3):516–528

Falzon D, Gandhi N, Migliori G et al (2013) Resistance to fluoroquinolones and second-line injectable drugs: impact on multidrug-resistant TB outcomes. Eur Respir J 42(1):156–168

Farmer P, Bayona J, Becerra M et al (1998) The dilemma of MDR-TB in the global era. Int J Tuberc Lung Dis 2(11):869

Fitzpatrick C, Floyd K (2012) A systematic review of the cost and cost effectiveness of treatment for multidrug-resistant tuberculosis. Pharmacoeconomics 30(1):63–80

Ford CB, Shah RR, Maeda MK et al (2013) *Mycobacterium tuberculosis* mutation rate estimates from different lineages predict substantial differences in the emergence of drug-resistant tuberculosis. Nat Genet 45(7):784–790

Fox W, Ellard GA, Mitchison DA (1999) Studies on the treatment of tuberculosis undertaken by the British Medical Research Council tuberculosis units, 1946–1986, with relevant subsequent publications. Int J Tuberc Lung Dis 3(10 Suppl 2):S231–S279

Fox GJ, Barry SE, Britton WJ, Marks GB (2013) Contact investigation for tuberculosis: a systematic review and meta-analysis. Eur Respir J 41(1):140–156

Frick M, Jiminez-Levi E (2013) Report on tuberculosis research funding trends, 2005–2012. In: Harrington M (ed) New York: Treatment Action Group http://www.treatmentactiongroup.org/sites/tagone.drupalgardens.com/files/201310/TAG_TB_2013_8.5.pdf

Frieden TR, Sterling T, Pablos-Mendez A, Kilburn JO, Cauthen GM, Dooley SW (1993) The emergence of drug-resistant tuberculosis in New York City. N Engl J Med 328(8):521–526

Frieden TR, Fujiwara PI, Washko RM, Hamburg MA (1995) Tuberculosis in New York City–turning the tide. N Engl J Med 333(4):229–233

Gandhi NR, Moll A, Sturm AW et al (2006) Extensively drug-resistant tuberculosis as a cause of death in patients co-infected with tuberculosis and HIV in a rural area of South Africa. Lancet 368(9547):1575–1580

Gelmanova IY, Keshavjee S, Golubchikova VT et al (2007) Barriers to successful tuberculosis treatment in Tomsk, Russian federation: non-adherence, default and the acquisition of multidrug resistance. Bull World Health Organ 85(9):703–711

Global Drug Facility Stop TB Partnership GDF impact on SLD dynamics. Available at: http://www.stoptb.org/assets/documents/gdf/whatis/SecondLineDrugs.pdf. Accessed Jan 2014

Hazbon MH, Brimacombe M, Bobadilla del Valle M et al (2006) Population genetics study of isoniazid resistance mutations and evolution of multidrug-resistant *Mycobacterium tuberculosis*. Antimicrob Agents Chemother 50(8):2640–2649

Jenkins HE, Zignol M, Cohen T (2011) Quantifying the burden and trends of isoniazid resistant tuberculosis, 1994–2009. PLoS One 6(7):e22927

Jensen PA, Lambert LA, Iademarco MF, Ridzon R (2005) Guidelines for preventing the transmission of *Mycobacterium tuberculosis* in health-care settings. MMWR Morb Mortal Wkly Rep 54:1–141

Kenyon TA, Valway SE, Walter WI, Onorato IM, Castro KG (1996) Transmission of multidrug-resistant *Mycobacterium tuberculosis* during a long airplane flight. N Engl J Med 334 (15):933–938

Kim S, Bai G, Hong Y (1997) Drug-resistant tuberculosis in Korea, 1994. Int J Tuberc Lung Dis 1 (4):302–308

Kim JY, Mukherjee JS, Rich ML, Mate K, Bayona J, Becerra MC (2003) From multidrug-resistant tuberculosis to dots expansion and beyond: making the most of a paradigm shift. Tuberculosis 83(1–3):59–65

Kimerling ME, Kluge H, Vezhnina N et al (1999a) Inadequacy of the current WHO re-treatment regimen in a Central Siberian prison: treatment failure and MDR-TB. Int J Tuberc Lung Dis 3 (5):451–453

Kimerling ME, Kluge H, Vezhnina N et al (1999b) Inadequacy of the current WHO re-treatment regimen in a Central Siberian prison: treatment failure and MDR-TB. Int J Tuberc Lung Dis 3 (5):451–453

Knox R, MacLean KS, Robson JM (1952) New results with isonicotinic acid hydrazide. Br Med J 1 (4767):1081

Kochi A (1999) Directly observed treatment for tuberculosis. Lancet 353(9147):147–148

Landesman SH (1993) Commentary: tuberculosis in New York City–the consequences and lessons of failure. Am J Public Health 83(5):766–768

Laserson KF, Kenyon AS, Kenyon TA, Layloff T, Binkin NJ (2001) Substandard tuberculosis drugs on the global market and their simple detection. Int J Tuberc Lung Dis 5(5):448–454

Lienhardt C, Sillah J, Fielding K et al (2003) Risk factors for tuberculosis infection in children in contact with infectious tuberculosis cases in the Gambia, West Africa. Pediatrics 111(5 Pt 1):e608–e614

Medical Research Council Streptomycin in Tuberculosis Trials Committee (1948) Streptomycin treatment of pulmonary tuberculosis. Br Med J 2(4582):769–782

Menzies D, Benedetti A, Paydar A et al (2009) Standardized treatment of active tuberculosis in patients with previous treatment and/or with mono-resistance to isoniazid: a systematic review and meta-analysis. PLoS Med 6(9):e1000150

Mitnick C, Bayona J, Palacios E et al (2003) Community-based therapy for multidrug-resistant tuberculosis in Lima, Peru. N Engl J Med 348(2):119–128

Moodley P, Shah NS, Tayob N et al (2011) Spread of extensively drug-resistant tuberculosis in Kwazulu-Natal Province, South Africa. PLoS One 6(5):e17513

Murray JF (2004) A century of tuberculosis. Am J Respir Crit Care Med 169(11):1181–1186

Nardell E, Dharmadhikari A (2010) Turning off the spigot: reducing drug-resistant tuberculosis transmission in resource-limited settings. Int J Tuberc Lung Dis 14(10):1233–1243

Nodieva A, Jansone I, Broka L, Pole I, Skenders G, Baumanis V (2010) Recent nosocomial transmission and genotypes of multidrug-resistant *Mycobacterium tuberculosis*. Int J Tuberc Lung Dis 14(4):427–433

O'Brien RJ, Nunn PP (2001) The need for new drugs against tuberculosis. Obstacles, opportunities, and next steps. Am J Respir Crit Care Med 163(5):1055–1058

Oxlade O, Falzon D, Menzies D (2012) The impact and cost-effectiveness of strategies to detect drug-resistant tuberculosis. Eur Respir J 39(3):626–634. doi:10.1183/09031936.0065311. Epub 2011 Aug 4

Pablos-Mendez A, Knirsch CA, Barr RG, Lerner BH, Frieden TR (1997) Nonadherence in tuberculosis treatment: predictors and consequences in New York City. Am J Med 102 (2):164–170

Pablos-Mendez A, Raviglione MC, Laszlo A et al (1998) Global surveillance for antituberculosis-drug resistance, 1994–1997. World Health Organization-International Union against Tuberculosis and Lung Disease Working Group on Anti-Tuberculosis Drug Resistance Surveillance. N Engl J Med 338(23):1641–1649

Pantoja A, Fitzpatrick C, Vassall A, Weyer K, Floyd K (2013) Xpert Mtb/Rif for diagnosis of tuberculosis and drug-resistant tuberculosis: a cost and affordability analysis. Eur Respir J 42 (3):708–720

Parwati I, van Crevel R, van Soolingen D (2010) Possible underlying mechanisms for successful emergence of the *Mycobacterium tuberculosis* beijing genotype strains. Lancet Infect Dis 10 (2):103–111

Pooran A, Pieterson E, Davids M, Theron G, Dheda K (2013) What is the cost of diagnosis and management of drug resistant tuberculosis in South Africa? PLoS One 8(1):e54587

Prasad R (2010) Multidrug and extensively drug-resistant TB (M/XDR-TB): problems and solutions. Indian J Tuberc 57(4):180–191

Rieder HL, International Union Against Tuberculosis and Lung Disease (1999) Epidemiologic basis of tuberculosis control. International Union Against Tuberculosis and Lung Disease, Paris

Shilova MV, Dye C (2001) The resurgence of tuberculosis in Russia. Philos Trans R Soc Lond B Biol Sci 356(1411):1069–1075

Simpson JM (1959) Drug resistance in out-patients treated with sodium pas and isoniazid cachets. Tubercle 40:453–456

Snider DE Jr, La Montagne JR (1994) The neglected global tuberculosis problem: a report of the 1992 world congress on tuberculosis. J Infect Dis 169(6):1189–1196

Steingart KR, Sohn H, Schiller I et al (2013) Xpert(R) Mtb/Rif assay for pulmonary tuberculosis and rifampicin resistance in adults. Cochrane Database Syst Rev 1, CD009593

Sterling TR (2006) Drug-resistant tuberculosis in New York City: lessons to remember. Clin Infect Dis 42(12):1711–1712

Streicher EM, Muller B, Chihota V et al (2012) Emergence and treatment of multidrug resistant (MDR) and extensively drug-resistant (XDR) tuberculosis in South Africa. Infect Genet Evol 12 (4):686–694

Sun G, Luo T, Yang C et al (2012) Dynamic population changes in *Mycobacterium tuberculosis* during acquisition and fixation of drug resistance in patients. J Infect Dis 206 (11):1724–1733

Udwadia ZF, Pinto LM, Uplekar MW (2010) Tuberculosis management by private practitioners in Mumbai, India: has anything changed in two decades? PLoS One 5(8):e12023

van der Werf MJ, Langendam MW, Huitric E, Manissero D (2012) Multidrug resistance after inappropriate tuberculosis treatment: a meta-analysis. Eur Respir J 39(6):1511–1519

Van Deun A, Maug AK, Salim MA et al (2010) Short, highly effective, and inexpensive standardized treatment of multidrug-resistant tuberculosis. Am J Respir Crit Care Med 182 (5):684–692

Weyer K, Mirzayev F, Migliori GB et al (2013) Rapid molecular TB diagnosis: evidence, policy making and global implementation of Xpert Mtb/Rif. Eur Respir J 42(1):252–271

World Health Organization (2009) WHO policy on TB infection control in health-care facilities, congregate settings and households. World Health Organization, Geneva

World Health Organization (2010a) Multidrug and extensively drug-resistant TB (M/XDR-TB): 2010 global report on surveillance and response. World Health Organization, Geneva

World Health Organization (2010b) Multidrug and extensively drug-resistant TB (M/XDR-TB): 2010 global report on surveillance and response. WHO, Geneva

World Health Organization (2011a) Guidelines for the programmatic management of drug-resistant tuberculosis – 2011 update. WHO, Geneva

World Health Organization (2011b) Towards universal access to diagnosis and treatment of multidrug-resistant and extensively drug-resistant tuberculosis by 2015: WHO progress report 2011. World Health Organization, Geneva

World Health Organization (2012) Global tuberculosis report 2012. WHO, Geneva

World Health Organization (2013a) Global tuberculosis report 2013. WHO, Geneva

World Health Organization (2013b) Definitions and reporting framework for tuberculosis – 2013 revision. World Health Organization, Geneva

World Health Organization, Regional Office for Europe (2011) Roadmap to prevent and combat drug-resistant tuberculosis : the consolidated action plan to prevent and combat multidrug- and extensively drug-resistant tuberculosis in the WHO European Region 2011–2015. WHO/Regional Office for Europe, Copenhagen

World Health Organization, Stop TB Department (2008) Guidelines for the programmatic management of drug-resistant tuberculosis. World Health Organization, Geneva
World Health Organization, Stop TB Department (2010) Treatment of tuberculosis: guidelines, 4th edn. World Health Organization, Geneva
World Health Organization, Stop TB Partnership (2010) The Global Plan to Stop TB 2011–2015: transforming the fight towards elimination of tuberculosis. World Health Organization, Geneva
Zhao M, Li X, Xu P et al (2009) Transmission of MDR and XDR tuberculosis in Shanghai, China. PLoS One 4(2):e4370
Zhao Y, Xu S, Wang L et al (2012) National survey of drug-resistant tuberculosis in China. N Engl J Med 366(23):2161–2170
Zignol M, Gemert WV, Falzon D et al (2012a) Surveillance of anti-tuberculosis drug resistance in the world: an updated analysis, 2007–2010. Bull World Health Organ 90(2):111–119
Zignol M, van Gemert W, Falzon D et al (2012b) Surveillance of anti-tuberculosis drug resistance in the world: an updated analysis, 2007–2010. Bull World Health Organ 90(2):111–119D

Part III

Parasitology

The Biochemistry of Quinoline Antimalarial Drug Resistance

Paul S. Callaghan and Paul D. Roepe

Contents

Abstract

Mutations in the *Plasmodium falciparum* chloroquine-resistance transporter (PfCRT) have been shown to be central to the molecular mechanism of quinoline antimalarial drug resistance. However, additional facets to resistance biochemistry are emerging, and it is now clear that multiple quinoline drug resistance phenotypes exist in different regions of the globe. Different public health policies and drug use histories across the globe, along with natural genetic drift, have created this diversity, such that there are now dozens of distinct chloroquine-resistant (CQR) strains of *P. falciparum*. Some of these can be described in detail, but information is incomplete. This leads to some degree of continued uncertainty on how best to proceed in controlling malaria in some regions. This issue is even

P.S. Callaghan • P.D. Roepe (✉)
Department of Chemistry, Department of Biochemistry, Cellular and Molecular Biology, and Center for Infectious Disease, Georgetown University, Washington, DC, USA
e-mail: callaghan.psamuel@gmail.com; roepep@georgetown.edu

M. Gotte et al. (eds.), *Handbook of Antimicrobial Resistance*,
DOI 10.1007/978-1-4939-0694-9_16

more critical for controlling chloroquine-resistant *P. vivax*, about which even less is known. This review summarizes key features of quinoline antimalarial drug resistance in *P. falciparum* malaria and suggests concepts relevant for "staying ahead of the resistance curve."

Keywords

Malaria • *Plasmodium falciparum* • PfCRT • Chloroquine resistance • Quinoline multidrug resistance

List of Abbreviations

ABC	ATP-binding cassette
ACT	Artemisinin combination therapy
ATP	Adenosine triphosphate
CQ	Chloroquine
CQR	CQ resistant (resistance)
CQS	CQ sensitive
DV	Digestive vacuole
FPIX	Ferriprotoporphyrin IX
Hb	Hemoglobin
HF	Halofantrine
Hz	Hemozoin
iRBC	Red blood cell infected with *P. falciparum*
ISOV	Inside–out yeast plasma membrane vesicle
MDR	Multidrug resistant (resistance)
MQ	Mefloquine
pfcrt/PfCRT	*Plasmodium falciparum* chloroquine-resistance transporter (*gene*/PROTEIN)
PfMDR1	*P. falciparum* multidrug resistance protein 1
PfNHE	*P. falciparum* Na^+/H^+ exchanger
pvs	Parasitophorous vacuolar space
QD	Quinidine
QN	Quinine
QNR	Quinine resistance
QTL	Quantitative trait loci
RBC	Red blood cell
VPL	Verapamil

Introduction

Five *Plasmodia* spp. infect humans, and these cause distinct malarias that are distinguished by different pathophysiology and rates of mortality. These unicellular eukaryotic parasites belonging to the phylum Apicomplexa exist in the body as multiple highly differentiated forms. Mixed infections with multiple strains and multiple species can occur, and the pathophysiology of malaria in pre-immune versus naïve children, adults, and pregnant women differs. The overall point is that malaria is actually a spectrum of diseases with a variety of effects on different human populations, which presents many unique challenges in controlling the disease. The emergence and spread of drug-resistant strains of *P. falciparum* and *P. vivax* have further complicated treatment and threaten the lives of millions annually.

The life cycle of malarial parasites is complex, involving two hosts (*Anopheles* mosquitoes and humans) or, for *P. knowlesi*, three (transmission of this species is zoonotic via macaques). *P. falciparum* and *P. vivax* infections are the most common, with the former causing most mortality. *P. falciparum* sporozoites injected into the skin during an *Anopheles* blood meal quickly migrate to the liver, invade hepatocytes, and are then released back into the blood stream approximately 2 weeks later as large clusters of merozoites called merosomes. The individual merozoites then rapidly invade red blood cells (RBC). Once in the erythrocyte, the parasite proceeds through ring, trophozoite, and schizont stages of development before lysing the RBC within 48 h and emerging as ≥ 8 new merozoites. These then reinvade fresh RBC. Most clinical symptoms of malaria are a consequence of the RBC cycle, and most antimalarial drugs act against the RBC stages. See Bogitsch et al. (2005) for a detailed discussion of the parasite life cycle.

Quinoline Drugs, Emergence of Resistance, and Drug–Heme Interactions

Multiple effective classes of antimalarial drugs exist including the quinolines (4-amino-quinoline, 8-amino-quinoline, and quinoline methanols), the reactive endoperoxides (artemisinins), and antifolates such as pyrimethamine (typically administered in combination with sulfadoxine) that poison pyrimidine biosynthesis or utilization. Quinoline-based drugs (Fig. 1) have long been used in the battle against malaria, beginning with quinine [QN], originally extracted from the leaves of the cinchona tree. Upon the synthesis of chloroquine (CQ) and other 4-aminoquinolines during World War II (see Kauer et al. (2010) for a recent review), efficacious, cost-effective antimalarial drug therapy became readily available worldwide. Resulting widespread use of CQ led to the emergence of CQ-resistant (CQR) *P. falciparum* parasites, which was aided by prophylactic use and population-based dosing directed towards global eradication (Foley and Tilley 1998). Today, the majority of *P. falciparum* infections in S.E. Asia are CQR, and >50 % are CQR in many African countries, but pockets of CQ-sensitive (CQS) *P. falciparum* malaria still exist in South America and elsewhere. Importantly, quinoline antimalarials (QN), amodiaquine (AQ) (first synthesized at Parke-Davis in the late 1940s Burckhalter et al. 1948), and mefloquine (MQ), despite prolonged use, are still effective against most CQR parasites, and AQ and MQ are also important partners in approved artemisinin-based combination therapies (ACTs) (Schlagenhauf et al. 2010). Quinoline-quinoline and quinoline-non-quinoline combinations (Bell 2005), as well as quinoline-resistance reversal strategies (Peyton 2012), are additional components of ongoing development of new therapy.

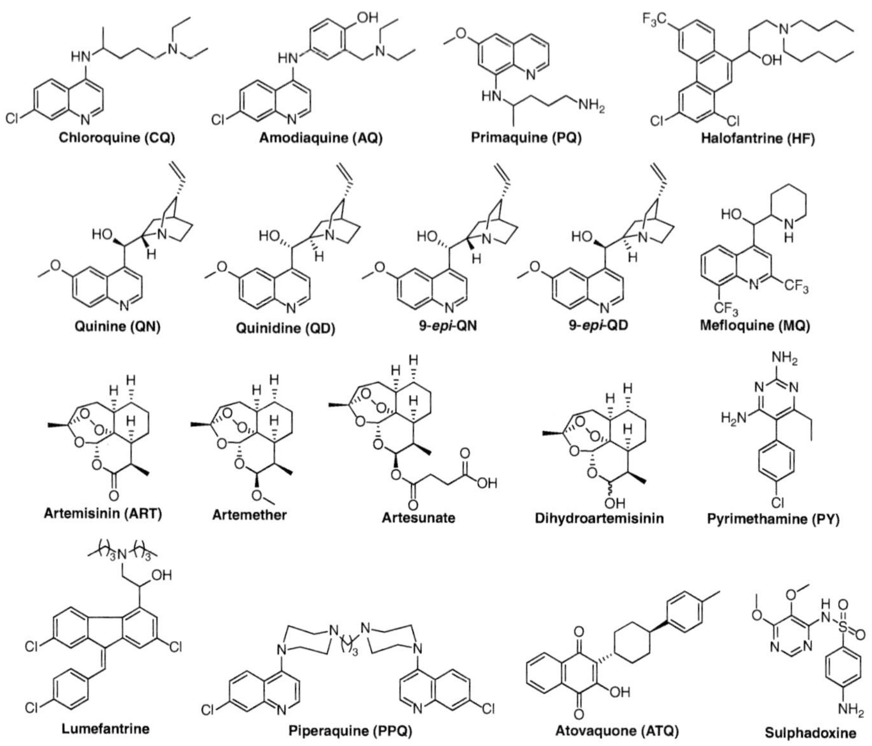

Fig. 1 Common antimalarial drugs

In recent decades, as CQR strains have both spread around the globe and continued to evolve, new geographically distinct CQR strains with unique genotypes and phenotypes have appeared. Resistance to the antifolate drugs is also now widespread, and delayed clearance of parasites is now seen in some patients treated with artemisinin-based drugs (Cheeseman et al. 2012; Takala-Harrison et al. 2013) which may be an early sign of emerging resistance to this class of compounds as well. To use current drugs more effectively, and to develop new therapies, molecular details of antimalarial drug resistance phenomena must be elucidated.

Detailed biochemical and molecular analyses of drug resistance is complicated, but conceptually, drug resistance phenomena are quite simple. A drug must interact with one or more molecular targets to exert its effect, and so resistance to that drug is due to either (or both) disruption of that interaction or to altered signal transduction propagated from the drug–target interaction that would normally promote growth arrest or cell death. Disruption of drug–target interactions seen in drug resistance phenomena typically fall into one of three categories: increased enzymatic degradation of the drug, mutation or altered expression of the drug target, or altered cellular transport of the drug. In some cases, particularly in examples of "multidrug" resistance, more than one mechanism may be relevant. There are many examples of altered signal transduction related to drug resistance, with the best understood being disrupted apoptotic signal transduction (disrupted induction of programmed cell death) in multidrug-resistant tumor cells.

In the case of *P. falciparum* resistance to CQ and related quinoline antimalarial drugs, there is no known enzymatic degradation of drug that reduces drug–target interactions. As described in more detail below, the principal target for quinoline drugs is believed to be ferriprotoporphyrin IX (FPIX) heme released upon the host red blood cell hemoglobin (Hb) catabolism. Thus, the drug target cannot be mutated by the drug-resistant parasite because it is synthesized by the host. This leaves altered cellular transport of quinoline drugs as the likely pathway to disrupting drug–target interactions. However, as more has been learned about how free FPIX is processed by the parasite, it may also be possible that target accessibility is reduced in interesting novel ways, as briefly described below, which would then also disrupt drug–target interactions.

Regarding signal transduction related to parasite growth or death, very little is currently known about how quinoline drugs might affect that signaling, or how that signaling might be altered in drug-resistant parasites. Being a single-celled microorganism without clear caspases and other key apoptosis effectors encoded within its genome, *P. falciparum* does not appear to express a typical apoptosis pathway (Sinai and Roepe 2012), and our understanding of cell cycle regulation for the parasite is limited (Doerig et al. 2002; Halbert et al. 2010). Thus, changes in the signal transduction relevant for cell cycle regulation or cell death have not yet been inspected in any detail for drug-resistant *P. falciparum* malaria, although one very recent paper suggests that autophagy signaling may be related to parasite cell death (Gaviria et al. 2013). Progress in understanding signal transduction and other biology relevant for drug resistance in the related pathogen *P. vivax* is even more limited, but just as crucial (Shanks 2012; Douglas et al. 2012).

To analyze how drug–target interactions might be perturbed in drug resistance, the drug target must be understood in molecular terms. Quinoline antimalarials have long been thought to target FPIX heme within the digestive vacuole (DV) of the parasite, which is released upon Hb digestion during the trophozoite stage of the intraerythrocytic cycle (Banerjee et al. 2002; Gamboa de Domínguez and Rosenthal 1996; Elliot et al. 2008). The parasite must digest most Hb found in the RBC cytosol, both to provide room for very rapid trophozoite growth and to obtain necessary amino acids. FPIX is toxic in its free state (Fitch et al. 1983), and due to the lack of a heme oxygenase pathway, the malarial parasite must sequester FPIX as nontoxic crystalline hemozoin (Hz). At cytostatic dosages, quinoline drugs slow the production of Hz, presumably by interacting with uncrystallized Hz precursors, growing Hz crystal faces, or both. This inhibition of Hz presumably leads to the buildup of free heme which is then believed to inhibit Hb-degrading proteases (Vander Jagt et al. 1987) leading to growth arrest. Precisely how quinoline drugs target heme to inhibit Hz formation in vivo is not fully known nor is it understood whether different quinoline antimalarials inhibit Hz via similar or different pathways. Different pathways are likely since some CQR parasites remain sensitive to related quinoline drugs such as QN, AQ, and MQ (Fig. 1), whereas others do not.

Hz is a crystal of heme dimers, and the unit cell is a unique heme structure, with the ferric iron of each FPIX coordinated to a carboxyl side chain of an adjacent moiety. These "head-to-tail" dimers are stabilized in the crystal lattice via hydrogen bonding (Pagola et al. 2000; Bohle et al. 2012). Current evidence strongly supports catalysis of Hz formation by lipid in vivo (Jackson et al. 2004; Pisciotta et al. 2007; Gorka et al. 2013b), and certain lipids are known to efficiently catalyze Hz crystal growth in vitro (Jackson et al. 2004; Pisciotta et al. 2007; Egan et al. 2006). Structures for a number of quinoline drug-FPIX heme structures have recently been solved, and these are reviewed elsewhere (Gorka et al. 2013a).

As a diprotic weak base with pK_a of 8.4 and 10.2, CQ exists as neutral, singly, or doubly charged compound under biological conditions, and these different drug species have different reactivity towards multiple chemical forms of free heme (i.e., monomers vs dimers in either aqueous or lipid phase, see Gorka et al. 2013a). In vitro, some drug–heme species aggregate and fall out of solution, generating amorphous drug–heme aggregates that then reestablish aqueous equilibria between heme species not complexed with drug. Others prefer to partition into lipid as 1:1 drug–heme complexes (Alumasa et al. 2010; Casabianca et al. 2008). This drug–heme chemistry likely competes with heme-to-hemozoin conversion; however, quantification of drug–heme aggregation or lipid partitioning phenomena within the parasite has not yet been done. Factors that reduce efficiency of quinoline drug–FPIX heme binding will alter DV retention of drug as well as the rate of Hz formation and could therefore contribute to resistance in multiple ways.

Genetic Basis of CQR

CQR is both spreading and continuing to genetically evolve via ongoing selective pressure. As briefly summarized in the next section, it was initially thought that ATP-binding cassette (ABC) protein drug pumps for CQ and other antimalarials must exist in drug-resistant *P. falciparum* and that these would be similar to the drug pump proposed for tumor cells (HsMDR1, or Pgp) believed by many investigators to directly translocate vinblastine, doxorubicin, and other antitumor drugs out of drug-resistant tumor cells. However, subsequent work showed that genotypes of some drug-resistant *P. falciparum* do not necessarily include mutation or increased expression of *pfmdr* genes (Wellems et al. 1990; Barnes et al. 1992) and that other genetic events must therefore be important. Similar to *P. falciparum* multidrug resistance (PfMDR) protein versus malarial MDR, the precise role of HsMDR1 protein in tumor MDR has been questioned (e.g., Roepe et al. 1996) as clinical pathology data have not correlated HsMDR1 overexpression with clinically relevant drug resistance as strongly as initially suspected.

Initial Genetic Studies of CQR: CG2 Versus Na^+/H^+ Exchange

More detailed genetic definition of CQR begins with cloning of *pfcg2*, which was suggested to be a resistance determinant based on quantitative trait loci (QTL) analysis of the progeny of a CQS × CQR parasite cross (Su et al. 1997). Subsequently, Lanzer and coworkers concluded that mutated PfCG2 protein was a dysregulated Na^+/H^+ exchanger that also pumped CQ out of parasites (Sanchez et al. 1998; Wünsch et al. 1998). Wellems and colleagues questioned this (Wellems et al. 1998). Subcellular localization of PfCG2 reveals it resides in vesicle-like structures near the parasitophorous vacuolar space (pvs) and the DV (Cooper et al. 2005) but is not localized within the plasma or pv membranes of the parasite as originally envisioned (Sanchez et al. 1998). A follow-up study (Bray et al. 1999) questioned Na^+ dependency for CQR phenomena, arguing against a strong role for Na^+/H^+ exchange in CQ transport or CQR. More recently, QTL analysis, availability of the *P. falciparum* genome, and novel single-cell imaging of Na^+/H^+ exchange in a series of drug resistant progeny suggested that altered Na^+/H^+ might be related to QN resistance (QNR), but not to CQR, and that the relevant exchanger is not PfCG2, but *Plasmodium falciparum* Na^+/H^+ exchanger (PfNHE) (Ferdig et al. 2004; Bennett et al. 2007).

Wellems and colleagues found that mutant PfCG2 did not confer CQR in and of itself (Fidock et al. 2000a). Attention thus focused on another gene found within the same 36 kbp fragment that harbored *pfcg2*, namely, *pfcrt* (Fidock et al. 2000b). Results described in this and additional papers (Sidhu et al. 2002; Cooper et al. 2002) show that mutations in the PfCRT protein are the ultimate determinant of CQR (and of some degree of resistance to other drugs) in *P. falciparum* malaria (see "PfCRT," below). While PfCRT mutations play a dominant role, importantly, PfMDR1 protein appears to modulate cross-resistance patterns in interesting ways.

The Elusive Role of PfMDR1

Early studies of CQR showed that drug resistance was associated with decreased drug accumulation (Krogstad et al. 1987) that was reversed by the ion channel blocker verapamil (VPL). Similar phenomena had been seen in drug-resistant tumor cells; thus, early on Wirth and colleagues screened *P. falciparum* for *Hsmdr1* homologues and identified *Pfmdr1* and *Pfmdr2* (Wilson et al. 1989). Another group found *Pfmdr1* to be upregulated in some CQR *P. falciparum* (Foote et al. 1989). But subsequent experiments (Barnes et al. 1992) showed that *Pfmdr1* overexpression did not correlate with CQR. This was not entirely surprising since Wellems et al. had earlier shown that CQR did not segregate with the *Pfmdr1* chr 5 locus in progeny from a CQS × CQR genetic cross (Wellems et al. 1990).

On the other hand, polymorphisms in *pfmdr1* were also associated with CQR early on (Foote et al. 1990). While CQS isolates had identical *pfmdr1* sequences, there were five changes in CQR isolates. In strains K1 and ITG2, N86Y was the only change. CQR strain 7G8 had four mutations: Y184F, S1034C, N1042D, and

D1246Y. The 184F mutation was postulated as not likely involved in CQR since it was also found in CQS strains. Thus, the *pfmdr1* overexpression hypothesis was revised to suggest that CQR strains expressed mutant *pfmdr1* but did not necessarily overexpress wild-type *pfmdr* (Foote et al. 1990).

Subsequently, when MQR *P. falciparum* were selected to higher levels of MQR, *pfmdr1* was found to be amplified (Cowman et al. 1994), and a very interesting inverse relationship between resistance to MQ and CQ was observed in the series of strains. Also, halofantrine (HF) and QN resistance increased with increasing *pfmdr1*, whereas AQ resistance did not (Cowman et al. 1994). However, when CQR strain K1 was selected versus HF, it did not result in MQR or amplification of *pfmdr1* (Ritchie et al. 1996). In another study, which used allelic exchange of *pfmdr* to probe these questions, incorporation of *pfmdr1* 7G8 polymorphisms into a CQS strain not previously exposed to drug had no effect on CQR, but incorporating wild-type *pfmdr1* into a CQR strain expressing mutant *pfmdr1* did decrease the level of resistance by half (Reed et al. 2000). Also, the CQS strains expressing mutant *pfmdr1* alleles showed some mild QNR and altered sensitivity to MQ and HF. Variations on this theme have also been described by Fidock and colleagues (Sidhu et al. 2005). Essentially, these data suggest that the *pfmdr1* effects measured by Reed et al. may be strain specific, and they bring us to our current understanding (Roepe 2009). It seems unlikely that mutations in *pfmdr1* confer CQR in and of themselves, but they can provide an important modulatory effect in some strains and isolates (Price et al. 2004; Dorsey et al. 2001; Patel et al. 2010). Interestingly, a recent report shows that PfMDR1 binds a high-affinity CQ photoaffinity analogue, suggesting that the protein does indeed react with quinoline drugs in some fashion (Pleeter et al. 2010), but the significance of this binding remains to be elucidated.

PfCRT

As mentioned, work by Wellems and colleagues showed that *pfmdr1* was unlikely to cause CQR since the relevant region of chr 5 harboring *pfmdr1* did not segregate with the CQR phenotype in a genetic cross (Wellems et al. 1990). Another key paper suggested that the CQR locus resided within the *cg2* gene on chr 7 (Su et al. 1997), but this paper also showed that one CQS strain (Sudan 106/1) carried CQR-associated *cg2* yet was nonetheless CQS. The 36 kbp chr 7 locus that segregated with CQR was thus reexamined, and a previously unrecognized gene, now known as *pfcrt,* was found (Fidock et al. 2000b). Mutations in *pfcrt* are the central determinant for *P. falciparum* CQR. The 13 exons of *pfcrt* span 3.1 kbp and encode a 424 amino acid, 48.6 kDa protein. Mutant-*crt* alleles found in CQR parasites contain a number of point mutations that confer multiple amino acid substitutions, with the pattern of mutations depending on the region of the globe from which the CQR parasite originates (Table 1). CQR arose (and continues to evolve) independently in at least five locations – S.E. Asia (which then spread to Africa), Papua New Guinea,

Peru, Colombia, and the Philippines (Wooton et al. 2002; Chen et al. 2003). CQR parasites from S.E. Asia and Africa carry 7–8 point mutations, whereas South American CQR strains carry 5. Novel patterns continue to be discovered, including new alleles recently identified in the Philippines (Chen et al. 2003), Cambodia (Durrand et al. 2004), Columbia (Echeverry et al. 2007) China (Yang et al. 2007), and Thailand (Chaijarkoenkul et al. 2011). Based on these mutations, it appears that at least four amino acid substitutions are required for conversion to CQR, with a change at codon 76 always required. It is not completely understood why South American CQR strains segregate into two groups with distinct mutations, but a likely explanation is variable AQ selective pressure (Sá et al. 2009). The pattern of PfCRT mutations thus provides identification of the likely geographic origin of a CQR isolate. The number of mutations apparently required for conversion to CQR explains two riddles, namely, why CQR took so long to appear on a large scale and why it had historically been impossible to create CQR strains from CQS in the laboratory via drug selection pressure.

Thus, over the past 10 years, it has become clear that a number of distinct *pfcrt* alleles encoding unique PfCRT isoforms exist (see Table 1). These have presumably arisen for two reasons: (1) different antimalarial drug use in various regions of the globe has provided different selective pressure for the persistence of PfCRT mutations in these regions and (2) the patterns of mutations may provide different "fitness" advantages, some of which could be more specific to one region versus another. Ongoing efforts to sequence entire genomes of multiple *P. falciparum* strains and isolates will help further explain this ongoing parasite evolution (e.g., Wooton et al. 2002; Volkman et al. 2007). *To date, a full molecular understanding of the relative resistance-conferring function of the different PfCRT isoforms known to exist is yet to be elucidated.*

Similar to PfMDR1, PfCRT protein is localized to the DV membrane (Cooper et al. 2002) and is a polytopic integral membrane protein that performs some type of transport function (see Roepe 2011; Ecker et al. 2012 for recent reviews). Most functional hypotheses for PfCRT involve either ion or drug transport or both, since CQR parasites accumulate less antimalarial drug versus time relative to CQS (see below) and quinoline antimalarial drugs are hydrophobic weak bases. In fact, CQ and related drugs are dibasic, and the DV is known to be quite acidic. So, passive concentration of CQ within the DV (where FPIX heme CQ target is found) is dependent upon the square of the net pH gradient and will be 10^5–10^6-fold by the predictions of weak-base partitioning theory. A repercussion is that very subtle changes in DV pH will have quite significant consequences for drug sequestration. Regulation of DV pH is not fully understood, but it includes a V type H^+ ATPase that hydrolyzes cytosolic ATP to pump H^+ into the DV. Interestingly, small changes in DV pH and volume caused by mutation of PfCRT have been measured in some studies (Roepe 2011; Gligorijevic et al. 2006). These can affect drug partitioning, FPIX heme to Hz biomineralization, and the chemistry of Hz inhibition by drug (see Gorka et al. (2013a) for a more extensive discussion).

Table 1 All known PfCRT isoforms. Amino acid substitutions relative to wild type are shown in *green*. Where literature shows more than one measured IC50 for a strain harboring the PfCRT isoform, the high and low values are reported

	*Pf*CRT Amino Acid Positions																												
Origin	Clone/Isolate	39	72	74	75	76	77	97	123	144	148	152	160	163	194	198	205	220	251	271	275	277	326	3270	333	334	350	352	356	371	IC_{50} (Low, High)
Honduras	HB3	S	C	M	N	K	I	H	H	A	L	T	L	S	I	E	T	A	F	Q	P	N	N	I	T	S	C	Q	I	R	12.3, 33.9
Netherlands	3D7	S	C	M	N	K	I	H	H	A	L	T	L	S	I	E	T	A	F	Q	P	N	N	I	T	S	C	Q	I	R	5.8, 30.4
PNG	D10	S	C	M	N	K	I	H	H	A	L	T	L	S	I	E	T	A	F	Q	P	N	N	I	T	S	C	Q	I	R	6.0, 40.7
Kenya	K39	S	C	M	N	K	I	H	H	A	L	T	L	S	I	E	T	A	F	Q	P	N	N	I	T	S	C	Q	I	R	3.9, 43.2
Thailand	T2/C6	S	C	M	N	K	I	H	H	A	L	T	L	S	I	E	T	A	F	Q	P	N	N	I	T	S	C	Q	I	R	9.7, 29.5
S. Africa	Fab9	S	C	M	N	K	I	H	H	A	L	T	L	S	I	E	T	A	F	Q	P	N	N	I	T	S	C	Q	I	R	9.7, 27.5
Sierra Leone	SL/D6	S	C	M	N	K	I	H	H	A	L	T	L	S	I	E	T	A	F	Q	P	N	N	I	T	S	C	Q	I	R	7.8, 25.9
Kenya	M24	S	C	M	N	K	I	H	H	A	L	T	L	S	I	E	T	A	F	Q	P	N	N	I	T	S	C	Q	I	R	5.8, 23.4
Sudan	REN	S	C	M	N	K	I	H	H	A	L	T	L	S	I	E	T	A	F	Q	P	N	N	I	T	S	C	Q	I	R	5.8, 16.2
Liberia	LF4/1	S	C	M	N	K	I	H	H	A	L	T	L	S	I	E	T	A	F	Q	P	N	N	I	T	S	C	Q	I	R	7.8, 15.0
Malaysia	Camp/A1	S	C	M	N	K	I	H	H	A	L	T	L	S	I	E	T	A	F	Q	P	N	N	I	T	S	C	Q	I	R	7.8, 12.5
Mali	BC5	S	C	M	N	K	I	H	H	A	L	T	L	S	I	E	T	A	F	Q	P	N	N	I	T	S	C	Q	I	R	11.6
Mali	M5	S	C	M	N	K	I	H	H	A	L	T	L	S	I	E	T	A	F	Q	P	N	N	I	T	S	C	Q	I	R	21.0
Haiti	Haiti	S	C	M	N	K	I	H	H	A	L	T	L	S	I	E	T	A	F	Q	P	N	N	I	T	S	C	Q	I	R	5.8, 16.2
Sudan	106/I	S	C	I	E	K	I	H	H	A	L	T	L	S	I	E	T	S	F	E	P	N	S	I	T	S	C	Q	I	I	37.8, 15
Thailand	Dd2	S	C	I	E	T	I	H	H	A	L	T	L	S	I	E	T	S	F	E	P	N	S	I	T	S	C	Q	T	I	404.1, 48
Thailand	Thai16	S	C	I	E	T	I	H	H	A	L	T	L	S	I	E	T	S	F	E	P	N	S	I	T	S	C	Q	T	I	436.0
Thailand	Thai19	S	C	I	E	T	I	H	H	A	L	T	L	S	I	E	T	S	F	E	P	N	S	I	T	S	C	Q	T	I	874.1
Thailand	TM284	S	C	I	E	T	I	H	H	A	L	T	L	S	I	E	T	S	F	E	P	N	S	I	T	S	C	Q	T	I	155.1, 363.3
Thailand	C2A	S	C	I	E	T	I	H	H	A	L	T	L	S	I	E	T	S	F	E	P	N	S	I	T	S	C	Q	T	I	301.5
Vietnam	V1/S	S	C	I	E	T	I	H	H	A	L	T	L	S	I	E	T	S	F	E	P	N	S	I	T	S	C	Q	T	I	186.1, 659.1
Cambodia	JCK	S	C	I	E	T	I	H	H	A	L	T	L	S	I	E	T	S	F	E	P	N	S	I	T	S	C	Q	T	I	521.3
Sudan	102/1	S	C	I	E	T	I	H	H	A	L	T	L	S	I	E	T	S	F	E	P	N	S	I	T	S	C	Q	T	I	164.8, 431.6
SEA	D5	S	C	I	E	T	I	H	H	A	L	T	L	S	I	E	T	S	F	E	P	N	S	I	T	S	C	Q	T	I	353.6
Thailand	TM93-C1088	S	C	I	E	T	I	L		A	L	T	L	S	I	E	T	S	F	E	P	N	S	I	T	S	C	Q	T	I	1200.2
Thailand	FCB	S	C	I	E	T	I	H	H	A	L	T	L	S	I	E	T	S	F	E	P	N	S	I	T	S	C	Q	I	I	135.7, 492.2
Thailand	K1	S	C	I	E	T	I	H	H	A	L	T	L	S	I	E	T	S	F	E	P	N	S	I	T	S	C	Q	I	I	75.22, 320.0
Uganda	PAR	S	C	I	E	T	I	H	H	A	L	T	L	S	I	E	T	S	F	E	P	N	S	I	T	S	C	Q	I	I	124.1
Gambia	FCR-3	S	C	I	E	T	I	H	H	A	L	T	L	S	I	E	T	S	F	E	P	N	S	I	T	S	C	Q	I	I	200.0
Kenya	KMWII	S	C	I	E	T	I	H	H	A	L	T	L	S	I	E	T	S	F	E	P	N	S	I	T	S	C	Q	I	I	77.5
South Africa	RB8	S	C	I	E	T	I	H	H	A	L	T	L	S	I	E	T	S	F	E	P	N	S	I	T	S	C	Q	I	I	116.3, 152.5
South Africa	RB20	S	C	I	E	T	I	H	H	A	L	T	L	S	I	E	T	S	F	E	P	N	S	I	T	S	C	Q	I	I	232.6
Ghana	9020	S	C	I	E	T	I	H	H	A	L	T	L	S	I	E	T	S	F	E	P	N	S	I	T	S	C	Q	I	I	468.4
Ghana	9013	S	C	I	E	T	I	H	H	A	L	T	L	S	I	E	T	S	F	E	P	N	S	I	T	S	C	Q	I	I	305.5
SEA	P31	S	C	I	E	T	I	H	H	A	L	T	L	S	I	E	T	S	F	E	P	N	S	I	T	S	C	Q	I	I	454.6
Sudan	124/8	S	C	I	E	T	I	H	H	A	L	T	L	S	I	E	T	S	F	E	P	N	S	I	T	S	C	Q	I	I	439.3
Sudan	128/4	S	C	I	E	T	I	H	H	A	L	T	L	S	I	E	T	S	F	E	P	N	S	I	T	S	C	Q	I	I	87.2, 379.4
Mali	M2	S	C	I	E	T	I	H	H	A	L	T	L	S	I	E	T	S	F	E	P	N	S	I	T	S	C	Q	I	I	116.3, 320.0
SEA	ItG2F6	S	C	I	E	T	I	H	H	A	L	T	L	S	I	E	T	S	F	E	P	N	S	I	T	S	C	Q	I	I	124.1, 128.0
Gambia	M97	S	C	I	E	T	I	H	H	A	L	T	L	S	I	E	T	S	F	E	P	N	S	I	T	S	C	Q	I	I	517.7
Sao Tome	Cai	S	C	I	E	T	I	H	H	A	L	T	L	S	I	E	T	S	F	E	P	N	S	I	T	S	C	Q	I	I	96.9
Thailand	TM6	S	C	I	E	T	I	H	R	A	L	T	L	S	I	E	A	S	F	E	P	N	S	I	T	S	C	Q	I	I	111, 167.0
Thailand	BC7	S	C	I	E	T	I	H	H	A	L	T	L	S	I	E	T	S	F	E	P	N	S	-	T	S	C	Q	T	I	54.0
Thailand	J9	P	C	I	E	A	I	H	H	A	L	T	L	S	I	E	T	S	F	E	P	D	S	I	T	S	C	Q	T	I	123.0
Thailand	KS28	S	C	I	E	T	I	H	H	A	L	T	L	S	I	E	T	S	-	E	P	N	S	I	T	S	C	Q	T	I	74.0
Thailand	BC22	S	C	I	E	T	I	H	H	A	L	T	L	S	I	K	T	S	F	E	P	N	S	I	T	S	C	Q	T	I	42.0

Brazil	7G8	S	S	M	N	T	I	H	H	A	L	T	L	S	I	E	T	S	F	Q	P	N	D	I	T	S	C	Q	L	R	34, 220
Peru	PC26	S	S	M	N	T	I	H	H	A	L	T	L	S	I	E	T	S	F	Q	P	N	D	I	T	S	C	Q	L	R	689.4
Brazil	DIV17	S	S	M	N	T	I	H	H	A	L	T	L	S	I	E	T	S	F	Q	P	N	D	I	T	S	C	Q	L	R	441.3
Brazil	DIV14	S	S	M	N	T	I	H	H	A	L	T	L	S	I	E	T	S	F	Q	P	N	D	I	T	S	C	Q	L	R	430.0
Brazil	ECP	S	S	M	N	T	I	H	H	A	L	T	L	S	I	E	T	S	F	Q	P	N	D	I	T	S	C	Q	L	R	287.7
Brazil	PAD	S	S	M	N	T	I	H	H	A	L	T	L	S	I	E	T	S	F	Q	P	N	D	I	T	S	C	Q	L	R	269.1
Brazil	ICS	S	S	M	N	T	I	H	H	A	L	T	L	S	I	E	T	S	F	Q	P	N	D	I	T	S	C	Q	L	R	347.1
PNG	PNG3	S	S	M	N	T	I	H	H	A	L	T	L	S	I	E	T	S	F	Q	P	N	D	I	T	S	C	Q	L	R	242.9
PNG	PNG2	S	S	M	N	T	I	H	H	A	L	T	L	S	I	E	T	S	F	Q	P	N	D	I	T	S	C	Q	L	R	225.9
Brazil	DIV30	S	S	M	N	T	I	H	H	A	L	T	L	S	I	E	T	S	F	Q	P	N	D	I	T	S	C	Q	L	R	217.4
PNG	PNG13	S	S	M	N	T	I	H	H	A	L	T	L	S	I	E	T	S	F	Q	P	N	D	I	T	S	C	Q	L	R	198.4
Solomon	PNG4	S	S	M	N	T	I	H	H	A	L	T	L	S	I	E	T	A	F	Q	P	N	D	I	T	S	C	Q	L	R	250.5
Ghana	GB4	S	C	I	E	T	I	H	H	A	L	T	L	S	I	E	T	S	F	E	P	N	N	I	T	S	C	Q	I	I	89.8, 144.8
Mali	S35CQ	S	C	I	E	T	I	H	H	A	L	T	L	S	I	E	T	S	F	E	P	N	N	I	T	S	C	Q	I	I	229.5
Cambodia	742		C	I	E	T	I	H	H	A	L	T	L	S	I	E	T	S	F	E	P	N	N	I	T	S	C	Q	I	I	466.7
Cambodia	766		C	I	E	T	I	H	H	A	L	T	L	S	I	E	T	S	F	E	P	N	N	I	T	S	C	Q	I	I	53.9
Cambodia	783		C	I	E	T	I	H	H	A	L	T	L	S	I	E	T	S	F	E	P	N	N	I	T	S	C	Q	T	I	133.7
Cambodia	738		C	I	D	T	I	H	H	A	I	T	L	S	T	E	T	S	F	E	P	N	N	I	S	S	C	Q	I	R	156.8
Cambodia	734		C	I	D	T	I	H	H	F	I	T	L	S	T	E	T	S	F	E	P	N	N	I	S	S	C	Q	I	R	169.4
Cambodia	613		C	I	D	T	I	H	H	F	I	T	L	S	T	E	T	S	F	E	P	N	N	I	S	S	C	Q	I	R	33.6
Phillipines	PH1	S	C	M	N	T	I	H	H	T	L	T	Y	S	I	E	T	A	F	Q	P	N	D	I	T	S	C	Q	I	R	95.0
Phillipines	PH2		S	M	N	T	I	H		T	L	T	Y	S	I	E	T	A	F	Q	P	N	D	I	T	S	C	Q	I	R	N.D.
Ecuador	Ecu1110	S	C	M	N	T	I	H	H	A	L	T	L	S	I	E	T	S	F	Q	P	N	D	I	T	S	C	Q	L	R	90.0, 156.4
Peru	PC17	S	C	M	N	T	I	H	H	A	L	T	L	S	I	E	T	S	F	Q	P	N	D	I	T	S	C	Q	L	R	373.8
Colombia	Jav	S	C	M	E	T	I	Q	H	A	L	T	L	S	I	E	T	S	F	Q	P	N	N	I	T	S	C	Q	I	T	137.3, 305.9
Colombia	TU741	S	C	M	N	T	I	H	H	A	L	T	L	S	I	E	T	S	F	Q	P	N	D	I	T	N	C	Q	L	R	N.D.
Colombia	TA7519	S	C	M	E	T	I	Q	H	A	L	T	L	S	I	E	T	S	F	Q	P	N	N	I	T	S	C	Q	I	T	N.D.
Colombia	TA6182	S	C	M	E	T	I	Q	H	A	L	T	L	S	I	E	T	S	F	Q	P	N	S	I	T	S	C	Q	I	I	N.D.
China	Isolate B	S	C	I	D	T	I	H		Y	L	T	L	S	I	E	T	A	F	E	P	N	N	I	T	S	C	Q	I	R	N.D.
China	Isolate C	S	C	I	D	T	I	H		Y	L	T	L	S	I	E	T	A	F	E	P	N	N	I	T	S	C	Q	I	I	N.D.
China	Isolate D	S	C	I	E	T	I	H		Y	L	T	L	S	I	E	T	A	F	E	P	N	N	I	T	S	C	Q	I	R	N.D.
China	Isolate E	S	C	I	E	T	I	H		A	L	T	L	S	I	E	T	S	F	E	P	N	N	I	T	S	C	Q	I	R	N.D.
Indo. Papau	2300	S	C	I	K	T	I	H	H	A	L	T	L	S	I	E	T	S	F	E	P	N	S	I	I	S	C	Q	I	I	N.D.
French Guiana	H209	S	S	M	N	T	I	H	H	A	L	T	L	S	I	E	T	S	F	Q	P	N	D	I	T	S	R	Q	L	R	35

Altered Drug Transport Observed in CQR *P. falciparum*

Coy Fitch first observed reduced accumulation of CQ into iRBC infected with drug-resistant parasites (Fitch 1969), and decreased retention of CQ for CQR parasites was subsequently reported in zero-trans efflux experiments (Krogstad et al. 1987). This was termed "increased efflux" and quantified as the percent preloaded ^{3}H-CQ remaining versus time after dilution into a drug-free medium. Efflux was hypothesized to be 40–50 times faster for CQR parasites (Krogstad et al. 1987); however, no molar quantification of transport (moles-free CQ per parasite per unit time) was possible. Soon thereafter, as described above several papers suggested that CQR was due to outward pumping of CQ by a *P. falciparum* homologue of human P-glycoprotein (HsMDR1 or Pgp), named PfMDR1, and encoded by the *pfmdr1* gene on Pf chr 5 (Wilson et al. 1989; Foote et al. 1990). However, at about the same time, Wellems and colleagues reported that the determinant for CQR identified in a Mendelian cross resided on Pf chr 7, not chr 5 (Wellems et al. 1990), which led to the search for other genes involved in CQR and the subsequent identification of *pfcrt* 10 years later (Fidock et al. 2000b) (see "Genetic Basis of CQR" above).

Many cell-based drug influx and/or efflux studies have been reported for CQS versus CQR parasites (e.g., Geary et al. 1986; Bray et al. 1992; Roepe 2011). These were performed using iRBC populations or detergent-extracted parasites and various filtration or oil layer centrifugation approaches. Non-saturable drug accumulation was often calculated (e.g., see Hawley et al. 1998), and the different protocols quickly generated a variety of data. Consensus was nonetheless eventually reached, namely, at low external [CQ] (1–50 nM) CQR parasites typically accumulate 2–10-fold less CQ in similar time relative to CQS. Depending on calculated non-saturable accumulation subtracted from these data, some studies (Bray et al. 1992) hypothesize that saturable uptake differs by as much as 100–1,000 fold for CQR versus CQS parasites; however, this conclusion rests on mathematical modeling assumptions. Measured differences in net CQ accumulation are typically 2–10 fold (see Roepe 2011 for more detailed review).

A proposed faster rate of drug efflux back out of the iRBC was one popular explanation for reduced iRBC drug accumulation early on (Krogstad et al. 1987; Martin et al. 1987), and initially the PfMDR1 protein (see section "The Elusive Role of PfMDR1") was thought to mediate the hypothesized increased efflux. After identification of PfCRT (see section "The Elusive Role of PfMDR1"), it was proposed that PfCRT, not PfMDR1, was responsible for the putative increased cellular drug efflux. Several interpretations were offered: (1) PfCRT-mediated outward pumping of drug from CQR parasites, (2) PfCRT-mediated drug counterflow (exchange) in the presence of appropriate drug gradients, (3) altered binding to intracellular targets caused by PfCRT mutations promoted decreased drug retention (increased efflux) in zero-trans efflux experiments.

However, both PfCRT and PfMDR1 proteins reside in a subcellular organellar membrane (the DV membrane), with three additional membranes between it and the outside of the iRBC. How one transporter at the DV membrane (via whatever thermodynamic mechanism one chooses to invoke) could kinetically compete with the fast passive influx of drug across these other membranes to result in net movement of drug out of the entire iRBC remains unclear. This leads to the proposal that PfCRT facilitates downhill leak of charged CQ from the DV to the cytosol (Zhang et al. 2004). Thus, PfCRT would not "pump" CQ from the iRBC per se but would promote decreased accumulation over time by lowering time-dependent CQ binding to intra-DV targets (e.g., FPIX heme, discussed above).

Interestingly, with one noted exception (Geary et al. 1986), all cell-based transport during this period was assayed at 1–10 nM levels of CQ. However, these concentrations are approximately 100–1,000 times below peak plasma [CQ] in malaria patients. In situ autoradiography of trophozoites showed that accumulated ^{3}H-CQ localized nearly exclusively to the DV of the mid-stage trophozoite (Sullivan et al. 1996), but these experiments were done at even lower external levels of drug (pM). Nonetheless, when abundant PfCRT was found expressed in the DV membrane, nearly all evidence seemed to point in favor of a straightforward interpretation of the Fitch hypothesis (Fitch 1969) and a DV membrane drug pump or drug channel explanation for CQR. Only recently have resistance phenomena related to higher (cytocidal) levels of CQ been investigated and evaluated versus drug transport phenomena (see below "New Insights: Cytostatic Versus Cytocidal Resistance").

An additional caveat for interpreting altered drug accumulation in iRBC is that some studies have reported altered DV pH and volume for CQR parasites (reviewed in Roepe 2011). It seems likely that traffic of endogenous DV osmolytes (ions and/or small molecule metabolites) is perturbed upon mutation of wild-type PfCRT to CQR isoforms found in CQR parasites (Roepe 2011). Altered osmolyte traffic perturbs regulation of important biochemical characteristics of the DV (e.g., pH, volume, ionic composition) that have direct effects on the efficiency of quinoline drug–FPIX heme interactions, and hence on net drug accumulation versus time (see Gorka et al. 2013a).

Vesicle Studies

From studies with whole cells, it was not entirely clear whether reduced accumulation of drug versus time for iRBC harboring CQR parasites was due to transporter-mediated efflux from the DV, altered binding of drug to FPIX heme targets caused by perturbations in DV physiology, or some combination. In most cases, analysis of drug transport with vesicles or proteoliposomes reduces complexity in interpretation. Initial vesicle-based studies of hypothesized PfCRT drug transport function used plasma membranes from yeast and first tested for direct binding of ^{3}H-CQ to PfCRT (Zhang et al. 2004). Scatchard analysis indicated a single-drug binding site in PfCRT, and, surprisingly, that CQS and CQR isoforms of PfCRT have similar affinity for CQ (K_d = 435 and 385 nM, respectively). A recent follow-up study of CQ binding used covalent attachment of a perfluoroazido-tagged CQ probe to quantify CQ probe binding versus other quinoline antimalarials and to further define the drug binding site in PfCRT, which is predicted to be disposed towards the DV side of the DV membrane (Lekostaj et al. 2008). Satisfyingly, this binding site can also easily place the quinoline ring of CQ near mutations in PfCRT isoforms that are known to modulate response to drugs (Fidock et al. 2000b; Cooper et al. 2002). It is clear at this point that both wild-type (CQS) and mutant (CQR) isoforms of PfCRT bind CQ at a single-drug binding site, that related quinoline drugs such as MQ and QN compete with CQ for binding to this site, and that chemoreversal agents such as VPL inhibit CQ binding only for some PfCRT isoforms (Lekostaj et al. 2008).

The paper showing direct binding of ^{3}H-CQ (Zhang et al. 2004) also examined ^{3}H-CQ efflux from inside–out plasma membrane vesicles (ISOV) via flow dialysis techniques and concluded that one CQR isoform of PfCRT mediated downhill passive efflux of ^{3}H-CQ faster than that observed for control ISOV or ISOV harboring CQS PfCRT. This was the first direct biochemical evidence in support of CQ transport by PfCRT. Subsequently, another paper applying a similar approach with vesicles made from *D. discoideum* reached similar conclusions after observing that vesicles harboring mutant PfCRT accumulated less CQ than those harboring wild-type PfCRT (Naude et al. 2005). In this study as well as an earlier yeast vesicle study (Zhang et al. 2002), additional evidence for ion or osmolyte transport via PfCRT was also obtained. A more recent *D. discoideum* vesicle study supports the notion that CQ transport is likely driven by electrochemical potential (Papakrivos et al. 2012).

Analysis of CQ Transport Using Proteoliposomes and Oocytes

Injection of oocytes with modified *pfcrt* mRNA followed by measuring ^{3}H-CQ accumulation into individual eggs (Martin et al. 2009) and purification of recombinant PfCRT from yeast followed by reconstitution into proteoliposomes (PLs) and analysis of fluorescently tagged CQ efflux from these PLs (Paguio et al. 2009) have both recently been pursued to test conclusions regarding PfCRT-mediated drug transport (see Roepe 2011 for more detailed review). Both the PL and oocyte approaches provide the best evidence for direct CQ transport by PfCRT; however, there are important differences in interpretation between the two studies. One is quantification of apparent turnover (mole drug/mol transporter(s)), and the other is whether both CQS and CQR isoforms are capable of drug transport. The paper reporting CQ transport in oocytes (Martin et al. 2009) does not calculate explicit turnover, presumably because the transport measured in this study is quite slow and does not plateau. However, initial rates are calculated and expressed as pmol CQ/oocyte/h. Assuming site density of PfCRT is within the range reported for many other transporters and channels expressed in oocytes (68), then these data convert to 0.002–0.02 CQ molecules/PfCRT(s) (CQS isoform) and 0.009–0.09 CQ molecules/PfCRT(s) (CQR isoform) at 300 nM external ^{3}H-CQ. This estimated turnover is 1–2 orders of magnitude lower than that measured with fluorescent drug probe and purified protein reconstituted into PLs (Paguio et al. 2009) and does not appear sufficient to account for reduced CQ accumulation in the parasite DV for CQR parasites (Cabrera et al. 2009; Roepe 2011).

The PL experiments are done with preparations wherein efflux of free CQ probe from an acidified PL interior can be measured instead of influx into the oocyte from a neutral egg perfusate. Experiments with these PLs and the fluorescent CQ analogue yield turnovers that are much higher than those computed from the oocyte data and that are also found to be highly dependent on the magnitude of ΔpH and ΔΨ (Paguio et al. 2009). This is expected for a DV transporter since high electrochemical driving forces exist across the DV membrane. At 5 μM NBD-CQ, turnover numbers were determined to be 0.8 NBD-CQ molecules/PfCRT(s) in the presence of a 1 unit ΔpH and 0 mV ΔΨ, 1.6 NBD-CQ molecules/PfCRT(s) in the presence of a 2 unit ΔpH and 0 mV ΔΨ, and 3.4 NBD-CQ molecules/PfCRT(s) in the presence of a 2 unit ΔpH and ~120 mV $\Delta\Psi^{+}$ (Paguio et al. 2009).

Data from the two approaches probably differs for several reasons. First, oocyte plasma membranes have low electrochemical driving force that cannot be conveniently manipulated, whereas driving force can be both increased significantly and conveniently manipulated for the PLs. Also in the PL experiments, the only modification to the amino acid sequence of PfCRT is a hexa-His tag added at the C-terminus, but in oocytes, four putative lysosomal-/endosomal-targeting motifs were removed in PfCRT by replacing 15 residues (a.a. # 17, 20, 22, 23, 26, 27, 47, 48, 50, 51, 409, 412, 414, 421, 422) with alanine (Martin et al. 2009). It is possible that, along with very different electrochemical driving force, these extensive modifications to the PfCRT primary sequence affect catalytic efficiency of CQ transport.

A second key difference in comparing these studies is the relative transport measured for CQS versus CQR isoforms of PfCRT. In the PL study, small differences in CQ transport by the two isoforms are noted when transport is measured at the same ΔpH and ΔΨ. In contrast, the oocyte system does not show statistically significant CQ transport above background for the CQS isoform of PfCRT. Levels of transporter are difficult to quantify for the oocyte system, and western blot data that directly compares CQS to CQR PfCRT isoform expression in the oocytes is not shown in this study (Martin et al. 2009). Also, as mentioned, the extensive N-terminal modifications that are necessary for effective oocyte expression of PfCRT could be compromising activity, as could different lipid composition in the different membrane systems.

Most recently, Baro et al. (2011) engineered galactose-inducible expression of PfCRT in metabolically active growing yeast. Since the majority of PfCRT protein in this system is expressed at the plasma membrane and since the topology of the protein (cytosolic domains remain cytosolic, intra-DV domains are disposed outside the cell) as well as DV membrane bioenergetics (high delta pH acid outside) are preserved relative to DV-disposed PfCRT, function of PfCRT can be analyzed by plating or growing the live yeast versus various external [CQ]. In these experiments, both CQS and CQR isoforms of PfCRT are found to transport CQ, but the CQR isoforms transport at higher efficiency and with a stronger dependence on membrane potential (Baro et al. 2011), consistent with observations made with purified PfCRT reconstituted into proteoliposomes (Paguio et al. 2009). A recent review (Roepe 2011) discusses other factors that could explain the disagreements between oocyte versus yeast and proteoliposome data; regardless, the important point is that considerable evidence now exists in support of direct transport of CQ by PfCRT driven by membrane potential. There is not yet complete agreement on whether this transport is more "channel-like" versus "carrier-like" (see also Papakrivos et al. 2012), thus additional studies with purified protein will be needed to refine the remaining hypotheses.

Most recently, (Baro et al. 2013) the inducible yeast expression system has been used to quantify differences in CQ transport by multiple CQR-associated PfCRT isoforms. Surprisingly, plots of CQ transport efficiency versus CQ IC_{50} for the strains in which the PfCRT isoforms are found reveal very poor correlation. A simple interpretation is that mutant PfCRT alone does not explain the degree of CQR.

New Insights: Cytostatic Versus Cytocidal Resistance

The above summary presents a satisfying model for PfCRT-mediated CQR further modulated by PfMDR1 and perhaps other factors. However, this assessment of CQR phenomena is based upon an incomplete definition of CQ pharmacology. With one exception (Paguio et al. 2011), for decades, all quantification of CQR has been via computing a ratio in CQ IC_{50} for CQR versus CQS strains or isolates. IC_{50} are determined from long-term growth inhibition assays wherein live parasites are grown for 1–3 iRBC cycles in the constant presence of CQ. These IC_{50} are in the 10^1–10^2 nM range (depending on the strain) and are relatively easy to obtain, including in high-throughput fashion with live cells (Smilkstein et al. 2004; Bennett et al. 2004a). Growth inhibition of parasites is highly relevant to the development of antimalarial therapy, because a good antimalarial drug should prevent increases in parasitemia and recrudescence. But it is also true that when CQ is administered to a malaria patient, the plasma concentration of the drug is typically >1 μM (not 10–100 nM), for at least the first 6–12 h. The most important initial effect of CQ therapy is significant reduction of parasitemia from 10^{12} to 10^{11} parasites to $\leq 10^9$, within hours. Meaning, successful clinical administration of CQ kills many parasites, it does not merely prevent their growth. A patient infected with CQR *P. falciparum* does not show this dramatic drop in parasitemia due to parasite death from micromolar CQ dose. Meaning, clinically relevant CQR can also be defined via an elevated LD_{50} ("**L**ethal **D**ose"). LD_{50} (defined as survival after bolus dose of CQ, see Paguio et al. 2011; Cabrera et al. 2009) have only been reported for two laboratory strains of *P. falciparum*. Many more such studies obviously need to be done. In one recent study, when drug accumulation is analyzed for intact iRBC using LD_{50} levels of drug (not IC_{50} levels), reduction in DV accumulation is not found for the CQR parasites relative to CQS (Cabrera et al. 2009). In fact, this study reports that CQR parasites can accumulate **more** toxic CQ relative to CQS and still exhibit resistance to drug-induced cell death. It is of course not uncommon for antimicrobial or anticancer drugs to show both growth inhibitory (cytostatic) and cell killing (cytocidal) effects. When they do, cytocidal activity often (but not always) requires higher levels of drug or longer exposure to drug. It is also not uncommon for targets that are relevant for cytostatic functions of a drug to differ from those that are relevant for cytocidal. It is critical then to point out that, with two exceptions (Geary et al. 1986; Cabrera et al. 2009), nearly all detailed CQ transport analyses for CQR versus CQS parasites, vesicles, or oocytes that have been used to develop models for CQR and PfCRT function have been done at sub IC_{50} levels of drug (typically, 1–50 nM). This has led to logical explanations for CQR that are relevant for resistance to the cytostatic functions of CQ ("CQR^{CS}") but that, at least initially, do not appear to be completely relevant for resistance to the cytocidal functions of CQ ("CQR^{CC}," Cabrera et al. 2009). To fully elucidate CQR, and in the design of additional antimalarial chemotherapy, both facets are critical, and more work is required to understand the latter.

At LD_{50} doses of the drug, [CQ] in the DV will be very far above K_d for PfCRT, suggesting any direct PfCRT-mediated CQ transport would be overwhelmed by increased passive diffusion of the drug. Assuming therefore that targets for CQ static versus cidal effects differ (see also Gorka et al. 2013b), then those relevant for the latter might exist outside the DV, in the cytosol, in the nucleus, or in some other organelle. A search for these possible targets, better definition of LD_{50} versus IC_{50} for a number of drugs, and continued analysis of the differences between strains harboring various PfCRT and PfMDR1 isoforms are important topics for future research. These points are likely also relevant for defining what is apparently a non-mutated CRT mechanism for CQR in *P. vivax* malaria (Nomura et al. 2001; Baro et al. 2011).

Most recently, at least some of the additional biochemistry relevant for CQR^{CC} has been revealed (Gaviria et al. 2013). By performing LD_{50}-directed QTL for progeny of the HB3 (CQS) × Dd2 (CQR) cross (instead of IC_{50}-directed; Fidock et al. 2000b), it was found that CQS^{CS} and CQR^{CC} are genetically distinct, and additional chromosomal loci were found to be inherited in an LD_{50}-dependent fashion. Analysis of these loci suggests biological processes that could be altered in the development of resistance to the cytocidal effects of CQ. One process in particular, similar to autophagy, was found to be dysregulated in CQR parasites via analysis of PfATG8 protein distribution upon exposure to LD_{50} levels of CQ (Gaviria et al. 2013).

Conclusion

Resistance to CQ and other common antimalarials has historically been quantified by ratioing IC_{50} that quantify drug cytostatic activity. Drug transport experiments at IC_{50} dosages, genetics, and molecular pharmacology of drug–heme interactions have generated a molecular model for cytostatic CQR wherein mutations in PfCRT cause increased, electrochemically downhill, leak of CQ (and possibly other quinoline drugs) from the DV. This model is strongly supported by recent experiments with purified PfCRT protein that both define a single CQ-binding site and that show membrane potential-driven transport by PfCRT. Some conflicting interpretations regarding the efficiency of drug transport by different PfCRT isoforms exist based on other recent experiments with oocytes, but overall these experiments also support PfCRT-mediated CQ transport. Questions that remain to be elucidated include defining relative affinities of related quinoline drugs for PfCRT isoforms and determining the efficiency with which they might be transported. Also, resistance to the cytocidal action of CQ does not appear to require decreased cellular accumulation of CQ. The precise role that PfCRT and other transport proteins (PfMDR1, PfNHE) play in this phenomenon remains to be explored.

The Fitch/Macomber/Sprinz hypothesis (Fitch 1969; Macomber and Spintz 1967) states that the DV is the principal site of CQ accumulation because heme released from Hb catabolism within the DV is its principal molecular target. Simply moving CQ from the DV faster than it passively diffuses back inward from the cytosol would then decrease binding to heme target that is continuously delivered as Hb is digested, and thereby cause CQR. In addition, the dynamics of CQ^{2+} versus CQ^{+} versus CQ binding to different chemical forms of heme (monomer vs μ-oxo dimer vs head-to-tail dimer) might be different in CQS versus CQR parasites, further contributing to decreased retention of CQ. In support of both models, several studies have defined both covalent and non-covalent heme–drug complexes for CQ and related drugs that are influenced by CQ protonation (Gorka et al. 2013a). Decreased pH and volume-dependent CQ-heme adduct accumulation within the DV of CQR parasites may be part of the explanation for elevated IC_{50} in these CQR parasites. However, the early observations of Geary and Ginsburg (Geary et al. 1986), along with recent distinction between IC_{50} versus LD_{50} phenomena (Paguio et al. 2011; Gaviria et al. 2013), continue to hint that the mechanism of clinically relevant cytocidal CQR is likely multifaceted. Perhaps related to this, interestingly, mutations in the *P. vivax* orthologue PvCRT apparently do not cause CQR in *P. vivax* malaria (Nomura et al. 2001). We suggest the additional layers to CQR in *P. falciparum*, which likely represent biochemistry relevant to raising CQ LD_{50} (but not necessarily IC_{50}), will provide important clues for the mechanism of CQR in *P. vivax* malaria.

Lastly, for both *P. falciparum* and *P. vivax* malaria, parasite CQR can be overcome with new chemotherapy that can be perfected by screening versus CQR strains (e.g., Peyton 2012). It has been hoped that detailed knowledge of CQR would expedite second-tier drug development versus malaria, and this hope is now beginning to be realized. A key component to new antimalarial chemotherapy is (and will continue to be) the additive or synergistic effects of two or more drugs given in combination. We suggest more detailed quantification of IC_{50} versus LD_{50} synergies is an important new avenue to explore in antimalarial drug discovery (Gorka et al. 2013c).

Acknowledgments Many outstanding laboratory colleagues have contributed to the studies from the Roepe laboratory mentioned in this chapter. We thank in particular Drs. L. Ursos, S. Dzekunov, E. Howard, T. Bennett, B. Gligorejevic, A. Kosar, L. Amoah, J. Lekostaj, M. Paguio, M. Cabrera, C. Xie, J. Alumasa, N. Baro, A. Gorka, and D. Gaviria. We also thank A. Siriwardana, Y. Liu, K. Sherlach, L. Jacobs, L. Turnbull, Drs. A. Sinai and M. Ferdig for additional helpful discussions, and Dr. A. Gorka for helping with Fig. 1. The work done in the Roepe laboratory since the cloning of *pfcrt* has been supported by the Burroughs Wellcome Foundation, the Luce Foundation, the US Department of Defense, and the NIH (RO1 AI045957, AI056312, AI052312, AI060792, and AI071121).

References

Alumasa JA, Gorka A, Casabianca L, Comstock E, Wolf C, deDios A, Roepe PD (2010) The hydroxyl functionality is vital to quinine antimalarial activity. J Inorg Biochem 105:467–475

Banerjee R, Liu J, Beatty W, Pelosof L, Klemba M, Goldberg DE (2002) Four plasmepsins are active in the *Plasmodium falciparum* food vacuole, including a protease with an active-site histidine. Proc Natl Acad Sci U S A 99:990–995

Barnes DA, Foote SJ, Galatis D, Kemp DJ, Cowman AF (1992) Selection for high-level chloroquine resistance results in deamplification of the pfmdr1 gene and increased sensitivity to mefloquine in *Plasmodium falciparum*. EMBO J 11:3067–3075

Baro NK, Pooput C, Roepe PD (2011) Analysis of chloroquine resistance transporter (CRT) isoforms and orthologues in *S. cerevisiae* yeast. Biochemistry 50:6701–6710

Baro NK, Callaghan PS, Roepe PD (2013) Function of resistance conferring *Plasmodium falciparum* chloroquine resistance transporter isoforms. Biochemistry 52:4242–4249

Bell A (2005) Antimalarial drug synergism and antagonism: mechanistic and clinical significance. FEMS Microbiol Lett 253:171–184

Bennett TN, Paguio M, Gligorijevic B, Seudieu C, Kosar AD, Davidson E, Roepe PD (2004a) Novel, rapid, and inexpensive cell-based quantification of antimalarial drug efficacy. Antimicrob Agents Chemother 48:1807–1810

Bennett TN, Kosar AD, Ursos LMB, Dzekunov S, Sidhu ABS, Fidock DA, Roepe PD (2004b) Drug resistance-associated pfCRT mutations confer decreased *Plasmodium falciparum* digestive vacuolar pH. Mol Biochem Parasitol 133:99–114

Bennett TN, Patel J, Ferdig MT, Roepe PD (2007) Altered *Plasmodium falciparum* Na^+/H^+ exchange activity is correlated with quinine resistance. Mol Biochem Parasitol 153:48–58

Bogitsch BJ, Carter CE, Oeltmann TN (2005) Human parasitology. Elsevier Press, London

Bohle DS, Dodd EL, Stephens PW (2012) Structure of malaria pigment and related propanoate-linked metalloporphyrin dimers. Chem Biodivers 9:1891–1902

Bray PG, Howells RE, Ritchie GY, Ward SA (1992) Rapid chloroquine efflux phenotype in both chloroquine-sensitive and chloroquine-resistant *Plasmodium falciparum*. A correlation of chloroquine sensitivity with energy-dependent drug accumulation. Biochem Pharmacol 44:1317–1324

Bray PG, Janneh O, Raynes KJ, Mungthin M, Ginsburg H, Ward SA (1999) Cellular uptake of chloroquine is dependent on binding to FPIX and is independent of NHE activity in *Plasmodium falciparum*. J Cell Biol 145:363–376

Burckhalter JH, Tendick FH, Jones EM, Jones PA, Holcomb WF, Rawlins AL (1948) Aminoalkylphenols as antimalarials. II. (Heterocyclic-amino)-α-amino-*o*-cresols. The synthesis of camoquin. J Am Chem Soc 70:1363–1373

Cabrera M, Paguio MF, Xie C, Roepe PD (2009) Reduced digestive vacuolar accumulation of chloroquine is not linked to resistance to chloroquine toxicity. Biochemistry 48:11152–11154

Casabianca LB, An D, Natarajan JK, Alumasa JN, Roepe PD, Wolf C, de Dios AC (2008) Quinine and chloroquine differentially perturb heme monomer-dimer equilibrium. Inorg Chem 47:6077–6081

Chaijarkoenkul W, Ward SA, Mungthin M, Owen A, Bray PG, Na-Bangchang K (2011) Sequence and gene expression of chloroquine resistance transporter (pfcrt) in the association of in vitro drugs resistance of *Plasmodium falciparum*. Malar J 10:42–51

Cheeseman IH, Miller BA, Nair S, Nkhoma S, Tan A, Tan JC, Al Saai S, Phyo AP, Moo CL, Lwin KM, McGready R, Ashley E, Imwong M, Stepniewska K, Yi P, Dondorp AM, Mayxay M, Newton PN, White NJ, Nosten F, Ferdig MT, Anderson TJ (2012) A major genome region underlying artemisinin resistance in malaria. Science 336:79–82

Chen N, Kyle DE, Pasay C, Fowler EV, Baker J, Peters JM, Cheng Q (2003) Pfcrt Allelic types with two novel amino – acid mutations in chloroquine- resistant *Plasmodium falciparum* isolates from the Philippines. Antimicrob Agents Chemother 47:3500–3505

Cooper RA, Ferdig MT, X-z S, Ursos LMB, Mu J, Nomura T, Fujioka H, Fidock DA, Roepe PD, Wellems TE (2002) Alternative mutations at position 76 of the vacuolar transmembrane protein

PfCRT produce chloroquine resistance and unique stereospecific quinine and quinidine responses in *Plasmodium falciparum*. Mol Pharmacol 61:1–8

Cooper RA, Papakrivos J, Lane KD, Fujioka H, Lingelbach K, Wellems TE (2005) PfCG2, A *Plasmodium falciparum* protein peripherally associated with the parasitophorous vacuolar membrane, is expressed in the period of maximum hemoglobin uptake and digestion by trophozoites. Mol Biochem Parasitol 144:167–176

Cowman AF, Galatis D, Thompson JK (1994) Selection for mefloquine resistance in *Plasmodium falciparum* is linked to amplification of the pfmdr1 gene and cross-resistance to halofantrine and quinine. Proc Natl Acad Sci U S A 91:1143–1147

Doerig C, Endicott J, Chakrabarti D (2002) Cyclin-dependent kinase homologues of *Plasmodium falciparum*. Int J Parasitol 32:1575–1585

Dorsey G, Kamya MR, Singh A, Rosenthal PJ (2001) Polymorphisms in the *Plasmodium falciparum* pfcrt and pfmdr-1 genes and clinical response to Chloroquine in Kampala, Uganda. J Infect Dis 183:1417–1420

Douglas NM, John GK, von Seidlein L, Anstey NM, Price RN (2012) Chemotherapeutic strategies for reducing transmission of *Plasmodium vivax* malaria. Adv Parasitol 80:271–300

Durrand V, Berry A, Sem R, Glaziou P, Beaudou J, Fandeur, T (2004) Variations in the sequence and expression of the plasmodium falciparum chloroquine resistance transporter (PfCRT) and their relationship to chloroquine resistance in vitro. Mol Biochem Parasitol 136:273–285

Echeverry D, Holmgren G, Murillo C, Higuita J, Bjorkman A, Gil J, Osorio L (2007) Short report: Polymorphisms in the PfCRT and pfmdrl genes of *Plasmodium falciparum* and in vitro susceptibility to amodiaquine and desethylamodiaquine. Am J Trop Med Hyg 77:1034–1038

Ecker A, Lehane AM, Clain J, Fidock DA (2012) PfCRT and its role in antimalarial drug resistance. Trends Parasitol 28:504–514

Egan TJ, Chen JY, de Villiers KA, Mabotha TE, Naidoo KJ, Ncokazi KK, Langford SJ, McNaughton D, Pandiancherii S, Wood BR (2006) Hemozoin (β-hematin) biomineralization occurs by self-assembly near the lipid/water interface. FEBS Lett 580:5105–5110

Elliot DA, McIntosh MT, Hosgood HD III, Chen S, Zhang G, Baevova P, Joiner KA (2008) Four distinct pathways of hemoglobin uptake in the malaria parasite *Plasmodium falciparum*. Proc Natl Acad Sci U S A 105:2463–2468

Ferdig MT, Cooper RA, Mu J, Deng B, Joy DA, Su XZ, Wellems TE (2004) Dissecting the loci of Low-level quinine resistance in malaria parasites. Mol Microbiol 52:985–997

Fidock DA, Nomura T, Talley AK, Cooper RA, Dzekunov SA, Ferdig MT, Ursos LM, Sidhu AB, Naude B, Deitsch KW, Su XZ, Wootton JC, Roepe PD, Wellems TE (2000a) Mutations in the *P. falciparum* digestive vacuole transmembrane protein PfCRT and evidence for their role in chloroquine resistance. Mol Cell 6:861–871

Fidock DA, Nomura T, Cooper RA, Su X, Talley AK, Wellems TE (2000b) Allelic modifications of the cg2 and cgl genes do not alter the chloroquine response of drug-resistant *Plasmodium falciparum*. Mol Biochem Parasitol 110:1–10

Fitch CD (1969) Chloroquine resistance in malaria: a deficiency of chloroquine binding. Proc Natl Acad Sci U S A 64:1181–1187

Fitch CD, Chevli R, Kanjananggulpan P, Dutta P, Chevli K, Chou AC (1983) Intracellular ferriprotoporphyrin IX is a lytic agent. Blood 62:1165–1168

Foley M, Tilley L (1998) Quinoline antimalarials: mechanisms of action and resistance and prospects for new agents. Pharmacol Therapeutics 79:55–87

Foote SJ, Thompson JK, Cowman AF, Kemp DJ (1989) Amplification of the multidrug resistance gene in some chloroquine – resistant isolates of *P. falciparum*. Cell 57:921–930

Foote SJ, Kyle DE, Martin RK, Oduola AMJ, Forsyth K, Kemp DJ, Cowman AF (1990) Several alleles of the multidrug-resistance gene are closely linked to chloroquine resistance in *Plasmodium falciparum*. Nature 345:255–258

Gamboa de Domínguez ND, Rosenthal PJ (1996) Cysteine proteinase inhibitors block early steps in hemoglobin degradation by cultured malaria parasites. Blood 87:4448–4454

Gaviria D, Paguio M, Turnbull LB, Siriwardana A, Ferdig MT, Sinai AP, Roepe PD (2013) A process similar to autophagy is associated with cytocidal chloroquine resistance in *Plasmodium falciparum*. PLoS One 8(11):e79059

Geary TG, Jensen JB, Ginsburg H (1986) Uptake of [^{3}H]chloroquine by drug-sensitive and -resistant strains of the human malaria parasite *Plasmodium falciparum*. Biochem Pharmacol 35:3805–3812

Gligorijevic B, Bennett T, McAllister R, Urbach JS, Roepe PD (2006) Spinning disk confocal microscopy of live, intraerythrocytic malarial parasites. 2. Altered vacuolar volume regulation in drug resistant malaria. Biochemistry 45:12411–12423

Gorka A, deDios AC, Roepe PD (2013a) Quinoline drug-heme interactions and implications for antimalarial cytostatic versus cytocidal activities. J Med Chem 56:5231–5246

Gorka AP, Alumasa JN, Sherlach KS, Jacobs LM, Nickley KB, Brower JP, de Dios AC, Roepe PD (2013b) Cytostatic versus cytocidal activities of chloroquine analogues and inhibition of hemozoin crystal growth. Antimicrob Agents Chemother 57:356–564

Gorka AP, Jacobs LM, Roepe PD (2013c) Cytostatic versus cytocidal profiling of quinoline drug combinations via modified fixed-ratio isobologram analysis. Malar J 12(1):332–339

Halbert J, Ayong L, Equinet L, Le Roch K, Hardy M, Goldring D, Reininger L, Waters N, Chakrabarti D, Doerig C (2010) A *Plasmodium falciparum* transcriptional cyclin-dependent kinase-related kinase with a crucial role in parasite proliferation associates with histone deacetylase activity. Eukaryot Cell 9:952–959. doi:10.1128/EC.00005-10

Hawley SR, Bray PG, Mungthin M, Atkinson JD, O'Neill PM, Ward SA (1998) Relationship between antimalarial drug activity, accumulation, and inhibition of heme polymerization in *Plasmodium falciparum* in vitro. Antimicrob Agents Chemother 42:682–686

Jackson KE, Klonis N, Ferguson DJ, Adisa A, Dogovski C, Tilley L (2004) Food vacuole-associated lipid bodies and heterogeneous lipid environments in the malaria parasite, *Plasmodium falciparum*. Mol Microbiol 54:109–122

Kauer K, Jain M, Reddy RP, Jain R (2010) Quinolines and structurally related heterocycles as antimalarials. Eur J Med Chem 45:3245–3264

Krogstad DJ, Gluzman IY, Kyle DE, Oduola AM, Martin SK, Milhous WK, Schlesinger PH (1987) Efflux of chloroquine from *Plasmodium falciparum:* mechanism of chloroquine resistance. Science 238:1283–1285

Lekostaj JK, Natarajan JK, Paguio MF, Wolf C, Roepe PD (2008) Photoaffinity labeling of the *Plasmodium falciparum* chloroquine resistance transporter with a novel perfluorophenylazido chloroquine. Biochemistry 47:10394–10406

Macomber PB, Spintz H (1967) Morphological effects of chloroquine on *Plasmodium berghei* in Mice. Nature 214:937–939

Martin SK, Oduola AM, Milhous WK (1987) Reversal of chloroquine resistance in *Plasmodium falciparum* by verapamil. Science 235:899–901

Martin RE, Marchetti RV, Cowan AI, Howitt SM, Bröer S, Kirk K (2009) Chloroquine transport via the malaria parasite's chloroquine resistance transporter. Science 325:1680–1682

Naude B, Brzostowski JA, Kimmel AR, Wellems TE (2005) *Dictyostelium discoideum* expresses a malaria chloroquine resistance mechanism upon transfection with mutant, but not wild-type, *Plasmodium falciparum* transporter PfCRT. J Biol Chem 280:25596–25603

Nomura T, Carlton JM, Baird JK, del Portillo HA, Fryauff DJ, Rathore D, Fidock DA, Su X, Collins WE, McCutchan TF, Wootton JC, Wellems TE (2001) Evidence for different mechanisms of chloroquine resistance in 2 *Plasmodium* species that cause human malaria. J Infect Dis 183:1653–1661

Pagola S, Stephens PW, Bohle DS, Kosar AD, Madsen SK (2000) The structure of malaria pigment β-haematin. Nature 404:307–310

Paguio MF, Cabrera M, Roepe PD (2009) Chloroquine transport in *P. falciparum*. 2. Analysis of PfCRT-mediated drug transport using proteoliposomes and a fluorescent chloroquine probe. Biochemistry 48:9482–9491

Paguio MF, Bogle KL, Roepe PD (2011) *Plasmodium falciparum* resistance to cytocidal versus cytostatic effects of chloroquine. Mol Biochem Parasitol 178:1–6

Papakrivos J, Sá JM, Wellems TE (2012) Functional characterization of the *Plasmodium falciparum* chloroquine-resistance transporter (PfCRT) in transformed *Dictyostelium discoideum vesicles*. PLoS One 7:e39569

Patel JJ, Thacker D, Tan JC, Pleeter P, Checkley L, Gonzales JM, Deng B, Roepe PD, Cooper RA, Ferdig MT (2010) Chloroquine susceptibility and reversibility in a *Plasmodium falciparum* genetic cross. Mol Microbiol 78:770–787

Peyton DH (2012) Reversed chloroquine molecules as a strategy to overcome resistance in malaria. Curr Top Med Chem 12:400–407

Pisciotta JM, Coppens I, Tripathi AK, Scholl PF, Shuman J, Bajad S, Shulaev V, Sullivan DJ Jr (2007) The role of neutral lipid nanospheres in *Plasmodium falciparum* haem crystallization. Biochem J 402:197–204

Pleeter P, Lekostaj JK, Roepe PD (2010) Purified *Plasmodium falciparum* multi-drug resistance protein (PfMDR 1) binds a high affinity chloroquine analogue. Mol Biochem Parasitol 173:158–161

Price RN, Uhlemann AC, Brockman A, McGready R, Ashley E, Phaipun L, Patel R, Laing K, Looareesuwan S, White NJ, Nosten F, Krishna S (2004) Mefloquine resistance in *Plasmodium falciparum* and increased pfmdr1 gene copy number. Lancet 364:438–447

Reed MB, Saliba KJ, Caruana SR, Kirk K, Cowman AF (2000) Pgh1 modulates sensitivity and resistance to multiple antimalarials in *Plasmodium falciparum*. Nature 403:906–909

Ritchie GY, Mungthin M, Green JE, Bray PG, Hawley SR, Ward SA (1996) In vitro selection of halofantrine resistance in *Plasmodium falciparum* is not associated with increased expression of Pgh1. Mol Biochem Parasitol 83:35–46

Roepe PD (2009) Molecular and physiologic basis of quinoline drug resistance in *Plasmodium falciparum* malaria. Future Microbiol 4:441–455

Roepe PD (2011) PfCRT-mediated drug transport in malarial parasites. Biochemistry 50:163–171

Roepe PD, Wei LY, Hoffman MM, Fritz F (1996) Altered drug translocation mediated by the MDR protein: direct, indirect, or both? J Bioenerg Biomembr 28:541–555

Sá JM, Twu O, Hayton K, Reyes S, Fay MP, Ringwald P, Wellems TE (2009) Geographic patterns of *Plasmodium falciparum* drug resistance distinguished by differential responses to amodiaquine and chloroquine. Proc Natl Acad Sci U S A 106:18883–18889

Sanchez CP, Horrocks P, Lanzer M (1998) Is the putative chloroquine resistance mediator CG2 the Na^+/H^+ exchanger of *Plasmodium falciparum*? Cell 92:601–602

Schlagenhauf P, Adamcova M, Regep L, Schaerer MT, Rhein HG (2010) The position of mefloquine as a 21st century malaria chemoprophylaxis. Malar J 9:357

Shanks GD (2012) Control and elimination of *Plasmodium vivax*. Adv Parasitol 80:301–341

Sidhu AB, Verdier-Pinard D, Fidock DA (2002) Chloroquine resistance in *Plasmodium falciparum* malaria parasites conferred by PfCRT mutations. Science 298:210–213

Sidhu AB, Valderramos SG, Fidock DA (2005) pfmdr1 mutations contribute to quinine resistance and enhance mefloquine and artemisinin sensitivity in *Plasmodium falciparum*. Mol Microbiol 57:913–926

Sinai AP, Roepe PD (2012) Autophagy in Apicomplexa: a life sustaining death mechanism? Trends Parasitol 28:358–364. doi:10.1016/j.pt.2012.06.006

Smilkstein M, Sriwilaijaroen N, Kelly JX, Wilairat P, Riscoe M (2004) Simple and inexpensive fluorescence-based technique for high-throughput antimalarial drug screening. Antimicrob Agent Chemotherap 48:1803–1806

Su X-z, Kirkman LA, Fujioka H, Wellems TE (1997) Complex polymorphisms in an 330 kDa protein are linked to chloroquine – resistant *P. falciparum* in Southeast Asia and Africa. Cell 91:593–603

Sullivan DJ Jr, Gluzman IY, Russell DG, Goldberg DE (1996) On the molecular mechanism of chloroquine's antimalarial action. Proc Natl Acad Sci U S A 93:11865–11870

Takala-Harrison S, Clark TG, Jacob CG, Cummings MP, Miotto O, Dondorp AM, Fukuda MM, Nosten F, Noedl H, Imwong M, Bethell D, Se Y, Lon C, Tyner SD, Saunders DL, Socheat D,

Ariey F, Phyo AP, Starzengruber P, Fuehrer HP, Swoboda P, Stepniewska K, Flegg J, Arze C, Cerqueira GC, Silva JC, Ricklefs SM, Porcella SF, Stephens RM, Adams M, Kenfic LJ, Campino S, Auburn S, Macinnis B, Kwiatkowski DP, Su X-z, White NJ, Ringwald P, Plowe CV (2013) Genetic loci associated with delayed clearance of *Plasmodium falciparum* following artemisinin treatment in Southeast Asia. Proc Natl Acad Sci U S A 110:240–245

Vander Jagt DL, Hunsaker LA, Campos NM (1987) Comparison of proteases from chloroquine-sensitive and chloroquine-resistant strains of *Plasmodium falciparum*. Biochem Pharmacol 36:3285–3291

Volkman SK, Sabeti PC, DeCaprio D, Neafesy DE, Schaffner SF, Milner DA, Daily JP, Sarr O, Ndiaye D, Ndir O, Mboup S, Duraisingh MT, Lukens A, Derr A, Stange-Thomann N, Waggoner S, Onofrio R, Ziaugra L, Mauceli E, Gnerre S, Jaffe DB, Zainoun J, Wiegand RC, Birren BW, Hartl DL, Galagan JE, Lander ES, Wirth DF (2007) A genome-wide map of diversity in *Plasmodium falciparum*. Nat Genet 39:113–119

Wellems TE, Panton LJ, Gluzman IY, do Rosario VE, Gwadz RW, Walker-Jonah A, Krogstad DJ (1990) Chloroquine resistance not linked to mdr – like genes in a *Plasmodium falciparum* cross. Nature 345:253–255

Wellems TE, Wootton JC, Fujioka H, X-z S, Cooper R, Baruch D, Fidock DA (1998) *P. falciparum* CG2, linked to chloroquine resistance, does not resemble Na^+/H^+ exchangers. Cell 94:285–286

Wilson CM, Serrano AE, Wasley A, Bogenschutz MP, Shankar AH, Wirth DF (1989) Amplification of a gene related to mammalian mdr genes in drug-resistant *Plasmodium falciparum*. Science 244:1184–1186

Wooton J, Feng X, Ferdig M, Cooper R, Mu J, Baruch D, Magill A, X-z S (2002) Genetic diversity and chloroquine selective sweeps in *Plasmodium falciparum*. Nature 418:320–323

Wünsch S, Sanchez CP, Gekle M, Große-Wortmann L, Wiesner J, Lanzer M (1998) Differential stimulation of the Na^+/H^+ exchanger determines chloroquine uptake in *Plasmodium falciparum*. J Cell Biol 140:335–345

Yang Z, Zhang Z, Sun X, Wan W, Cui L, Zhang X, Zhong D, Yan G, Cui L (2007) Molecular analysis of chloroquine resistance in *Plasmodium falciparum* in Yunnan Province, China. Trop Med Int Health 12:1051–1060

Zhang H, Howard EM, Roepe PD (2002) Analysis of the antimalarial drug resistance protein PfCRT expressed in yeast. J Biol Chem 277:49767–49775

Zhang H, Paguio M, Roepe PD (2004) The antimalarial drug resistance protein *Plasmodium falciparum* chloroquine resistance transporter binds chloroquine. Biochemistry 43:8290–8296

Drug Resistance in *Leishmania*

Danielle Légaré and Marc Ouellette

Contents

Abstract

Protozoan parasites of the genus *Leishmania* cause a wide range of diseases affecting 12 million people worldwide with 1.5–2 million new cases each year. With no vaccine available yet, the control of these parasites relies solely on chemotherapy. Low-cost antimony-derived compounds remain the primary antileishmanial treatment in most developing countries. Increasing drug resistance towards these molecules has forced the use of alternative therapies in highly endemic areas including amphotericin B, paromomycin, and miltefosine. This chapter is presenting our current understanding of the mode of action and underlying resistance mechanisms of the few therapeutic drugs used against *Leishmania*.

D. Légaré • M. Ouellette (✉)
Centre de Recherche en Infectiologie du Centre de Recherche du CHU de Québec, Pavillon CHUL and Département de Microbiologie-Infectiologie et Immunologie, Faculté de Médecine, Université Laval, QC, Canada
e-mail: danielle.legare@crchul.ulaval.ca; marc.ouellette@crchul.ulaval.ca

M. Gotte et al. (eds.), *Handbook of Antimicrobial Resistance*,
DOI 10.1007/978-1-4939-0694-9_17

Keywords
Leishmania • Drug resistance • Pentavalent antimonials • Amphotericin B • Miltefosine • Paromomycin

Abbreviations

AMB	Amphotericin B
CL	Cutaneous leishmaniasis
DCL	Diffuse cutaneous leishmaniasis
GSH	Glutathione
MCL	Mucocutaneous leishmaniasis
MIL	Miltefosine
PKDL	Post-kala-azar dermal leishmaniasis
PM	Paromomycin
SAG	Sodium antimony gluconate
Sb^{III}	Trivalent antimonials
Sb^{V}	Pentavalent antimonials
SILAC	Stable isotope labeling by amino acids in cell culture
TSH	Trypanothione
VL	Visceral leishmaniasis

Introduction

With 12 million people infected in 98 countries on 5 continents and close to 350 million people at risk of infection globally, human leishmaniasis is considered by the World Health Organization as one of the top ten threatening infective conditions worldwide (WHO 2010). In fact, it corresponds to the second-biggest parasitic killer after malaria with an annual death rate of up to 50,000 people and an estimated 2 million disability-adjusted life years (DALYs) lost (Alvar et al. 2012; King and Bertino 2008). Each year, ~1.5–2 million new cases are estimated to occur, although this is probably an underestimate because the disease is reportable only in approximately half of the countries in which it is known to occur. Furthermore, many *Leishmania* infections are asymptomatic, subclinical, or misdiagnosed. Leishmaniasis affects the poorest of the poor, particularly in Africa, South and Central America, Asia, the Mediterranean basin, and the Middle East. Protozoa of the genus *Leishmania* are passed on to humans and animals (mainly small rodents and dogs which act as reservoirs) by female *Phlebotomus* spp. or *Lutzomyia* sand flies that need blood for their eggs. Other forms of transmission such as via intravenous needles shared by drug users (Cruz et al. 2002), transfusion, transplant, or placental contaminations have been reported (Antinori et al. 2008; Grogl et al. 1993). Once injected, promastigote parasites are engulfed by macrophages in the dermis and throughout the reticuloendothelial system (mainly macrophages) where they transform into obligatory intracellular amastigotes within acidified phagosomes. In this sanctuary, after a short period of latency of weeks to few months that may extend to many years, the parasite starts to proliferate. This multiplication will cause a systemic infection of neighboring macrophages that will propagate the disease and result in a large diversity of pathologies. To date, 21 *Leishmania* species pathogenic for humans have been recognized, traditionally divided between Old World (Africa, Asia, Europe) and New World (Americas) parasites, although the taxonomy of the *Leishmania* species is still in debate (Boite et al. 2012). Depending of the species and the host immune status, the clinical manifestations of leishmaniasis range from limited cutaneous (CL) lesions to disseminating visceral disease (VL) also called "kala-azar" which translates to "black disease" because of the skin pigmentation (Alvar et al. 2012; Kaye and Scott 2011). In more than 90 % of patients, CL undergoes self-cure within 3 to 18 months, even though it may develop into a more serious and complex clinical disease such as mucocutaneous (MCL, also known as espundia) or diffuse cutaneous leishmaniasis (DCL). In contrast to CL, VL is uniformly fatal within 2 years if untreated. Even with treatment, VL may result in case-fatality rates of 10–20 % (Alvar et al. 2012). After recovery from a VL, some patients experience dermal leishmaniasis referred to as "post-kala-azar" (PKDL) characterized by indurated nodules or depigmented papules frequently scattered on exposed parts of the body, mainly the face and neck. PKDL patients are extremely difficult to treat, and because these skin lesions are highly infectious to sand flies (e.g., lesions contain many parasites), this particular clinical manifestation is considered as a significant contributor to the spread of VL, particularly in Sudan and India where, respectively, 50 % and 1 to 3 % of the VL patients will develop this insidious cutaneous form (Zijlstra et al. 1995, 2000, 2003). Interestingly, host genetics may have a role in susceptibility to VL and PKDL since studies have reported that some tribes are more vulnerable to VL and PKDL than others (Bucheton et al. 2003; Farouk et al. 2010; Mohamed et al. 2003, 2004; Saha et al. 2007; Salih et al. 2007).

Another rising concern and major threat to the control of VL is its intersection with HIV-1 infection. To date, HIV-*Leishmania* coinfections are reported from more than 35 countries with Ethiopia having by far the highest prevalence of HIV/VL worldwide (e.g., 15–30 % of VL cases) (Orsini et al. 2012). HIV-infected people are particularly vulnerable to VL; the HIV condition increases the risk of developing an active VL by between 100 and 2,320 times, while VL accelerates HIV replication and progression to AIDS (Alvar et al. 2008; Bentwich 2003; Bernier et al. 1995; Mock et al. 2012; Wolday et al. 1999). Polyinfection also exists with *Mycobacterium tuberculosis* which represents an even greater public health challenge (Delobel et al. 2003; Mohamed et al. (2004) Rathnayake et al. 2010; Wang et al. 1999; el-Safi et al. 2004). There is as yet no effective vaccine for prevention of any form of leishmaniasis, although significant effort is being invested (Costa et al. 2011; Kobets et al. 2012; Palatnik-de-Sousa 2008). Leishmanization, e.g., inoculating people with live virulent parasites to cause a local limited lesion and provide protection, has been traditionally used for CL but is not recommended as a control measure. Current limited treatment options are based on chemotherapy but remain unsatisfactory for reasons such as toxic side effects, high cost, route of administration and duration of treatment, need for monitoring and hospitalization, and the increasing incidence of drug-resistant parasite strains.

Current Therapies for Leishmaniasis

Chemotherapy has always been a critical issue in the management of leishmaniasis. Excellent up-to-date reviews have been published recently on the current pharmacotherapy deployed against the parasite *Leishmania*, and readers are referred to them for a more exhaustive description on this topic (Kobets et al. 2012; Singh et al. 2012; Sundar and Chakravarty 2013; Zucca et al. 2013). Only a brief overview of the main therapeutic options available will be presented. The reality is that access to antileishmanial medicines is not always easy in every endemic country, that all forms are difficult to treat, and that current therapies for leishmaniasis are far from ideal. The VL, MCL, DCL, and PKDL forms are principally treated by intravenous drugs, whereas CL is generally treated with local drug injections or topical ointments according to country-specific drug regimens (Table 1). The injectable pentavalent antimonials (Sb^V) have been the cornerstone of antileishmanial chemotherapy for more than 70 years and still remain the first pharmacotherapeutic choice for all clinical forms worldwide, except in Bihar state, India, where resistance has reached such high proportions (~65 % refractory cases) that the use of these compounds is now limited. Two branded antimonials are available, the sodium stibogluconate (SSG, Pentostam®) and meglumine antimoniate (Glucantime®). Second-line drugs include the polyene antibiotic amphotericin B and its various deoxycholate (Fungizone®) or liposomal (AmBisome®) formulations, the hexadecylphosphocholine miltefosine (Impavido®) which is the first orally administrated antileishmanial drug, the diamidine or pentamidine isethionate (Lomidine®, Pentacarinat®), and the aminosidine antibiotic paromomycin sulfate. Also, the primaquine analogue sitamaquine would potentially represent the second promising antileishmanial oral drug if late-stage clinical trials are successful. Preliminary results suggest however that sitamaquine will need to be given in combined therapies because of resistance issues as well as adverse effects observed in clinical trials (Loiseau et al. 2011). Few other drugs are currently in development.

A number of alternative treatments for CL have been developed in the hope to decrease the toxic effects of chemotherapeutic injectable drugs and the difficulty to administer them. Since *Leishmania* amastigotes are heat sensitive (39 °C or higher), thermotherapy has revealed to be a good option for CL treatment. This treatment implies local applications of the device (e.g., ThermoMed® or other radiofrequency heat devices), maintained at 50 °C, to the infected skin sores. The equipment however is very expensive and thus remains difficult to access in endemic countries. Other alternative CL treatments include cryotherapy using liquid nitrogen, CO_2 laser, photodynamic therapy, curettage, and surgical excision either alone or in combination with intralesional antimony (Table 1). These treatment options are however labor intensive and not suitable for multiple or complicated lesions.

Table 1 Leishmaniasis treatments[a]

Antileishmanial compound	Syndrome	Adult regimen	Comments
Current standard chemotherapeutics			
Pentavalent antimony (Pentostam®)	CL VL and MCL PKDL	IL injections at 20 mg/kg/day for 20 days or up to healing IV or IM at 20 mg/kg/day for 28–30 days IM at 20 mg/kg/day for 4–5 months	Antimonial compounds were used against *Leishmania* as early as 1912 and are still active against all species. For pregnant woman, Sb^V should not be used. Increasing resistance in India, Sudan, France, and parts of South America. About 90 % efficacy in US patients. GlaxoSmithKline has never applied for FDA approval so Pentostam® is not licensed for US commercial use and has to be obtained from CDC drug services. Toxicities include myalgias, arthralgias, abdominal symptoms, liver enzyme elevation, pancreatic and cardiac toxicity, and sudden death. Mortality during treatment is high (up to 20 %) in HIV-*Leishmania*-coinfected patients
Pentamidine isethionate (Pentacarinat®)	All	Intravenous or intramuscular 2–4 mg/kg/day for up to 15 days	A diamidine drug active mainly against CL and VL, when other drugs are not available. It may require up to 4 months of treatment. Pentamidine is now mostly used against African trypanosomiasis and patients with HIV and *Leishmania* coinfections
Pentamidine mesylate (Lomidine®)			Pentamidine mesylate is no longer available in certain countries including France. It may cause hypotension and later insulin-dependent diabetes mellitus
Amphotericin B deoxycholate	All	Intravenous 1–5 mg/kg/day, alternate days for 3–4 weeks	In the early 2000s, amphotericin B became the first-line treatment of VL in Bihar, India, because of antimony resistance. Amphotericin B causes secondary effects such as renal disturbances, anemia, fever,

(*continued*)

Table 1 (continued)

Antileishmanial compound	Syndrome	Adult regimen	Comments
			malaise, hypokalemia, and renal failure. These can be reduced by adequate hydration and infusion over several hours
Liposomal amphotericin B (Amphomul®, AmBisome®, Amphotec®, Abelcet®)	All	Intravenous 5–20 mg/kg/day for 3–4 weeks	The most active antileishmanial agent in use and the only US FDA-approved agent against VL. AmBisome® is however very expensive, being almost 3,000 times higher than the sodium stibogluconate price and ~900 times more than that of paromomycin in India. A preferentially low price has been secured however by the MSF and WHO. Toxicities include nephrotoxicity, electrolyte disturbances, fever, and rigors. AmBisome® seems less toxic than other amphotericin B lipid formulations. AmBisome® is a complex of amphotericin B and distearoylphosphatidylgycerol bound to a liposome of cholesterol and phosphatidylcholine. Abelcet® is a lipid complex and Amphocil® is a colloidal dispersion
Miltefosine (Impavido®)	VL and CL	Oral 100–150 mg daily for 28 days	Miltefosine, also called hexadecylphosphocholine, is a phospholipid analogue originally developed as an anticancer drug. Its effectiveness is species and local dependent. Does not work well against *L. braziliensis*, *L. guyanensis*, and *L. mexicana*. Contraindicated in pregnancy and requires effective contraception during and for 3 months after therapy. May cause vomiting, gastrointestinal disturbance, and diarrhea

(continued)

Table 1 (continued)

Antileishmanial compound	Syndrome	Adult regimen	Comments
Paromomycin sulfate	CL and VL	Intravenous or intramuscular 11–15 mg/kg daily for 21 days	Also known as aminosidine. Aminoglycoside antibiotic produced by *Streptomyces rimosus*. Often used in combination with miltefosine. Highest activity was against *L. major* and *L. tropica* while of the New World species *L. panamensis* was most, and *L. mexicana* was least sensitive. *L. donovani* species showed variable sensitivity
Paromomycin sulfate (15 %) ointment	CL	Apply twice daily for 20–30 days	Combined therapy with intralesional Sb^V (weekly or alternate-day injections at multiple doses). Commercially available in Israel. Randomized trials are showing only modest efficiency against *L. major*
Allopurinol	CL	Oral 300–600 mg/day for 4–6 weeks	Allopurinol is phosphorylated by the purine salvage enzyme hypoxanthine-guanine phosphoribosyltransferase (HGPRT) and incorporated into nucleic acid, thus leading to selective death of *Leishmania* parasites (Fish et al. 1985). Parasites of the Old World seem more susceptible, especially *L. major*. Works better in combination with an azole (e.g., itraconazole). Adverse effects include rash, itching, fever, eosinophilia, hepatic granulomas, nephritis, vasculitis, and exfoliative dermatitis
Rifampicin	CL	Oral 200 mg/day for 6 weeks	
Fluconazole (Triflucan® or generic)	CL	Oral 200 mg daily for 6 weeks	Imidazole compound with high skin concentration. Seems effective against *L. major* but remains untested for most species of *Leishmania*. Fluconazole, itraconazole, and ketoconazole inhibit a key enzyme of the ergosterol

(*continued*)

Table 1 (continued)

Antileishmanial compound	Syndrome	Adult regimen	Comments
			biosynthesis pathway, the 14-α-demethylase
Itraconazole	CL	Oral 200 mg twice daily for 28 days	Imidazole compound. Better tolerated than ketoconazole but may be less effective than ketoconazole, at least against the *vianna* subgenus. Works well for *L. major*
Ketoconazole (Nizoral®)	CL	Oral 600 mg/day for 28 days	Imidazole compound. Ketoconazole has modest activity against *L. mexicana* and *L. (V.) panamensis* infections. Its usefulness against *L. major* is still unclear. Does not work for *L. tropica*, *L. aethiopica*, and *L. braziliensis*. Fluconazole seems less toxic and better than ketoconazole
Azithromycin			Macrolide antibiotic that concentrates in macrophages. Seems active against *L. major* in mice model
Dapsone	CL	Oral 2 x 100 mg/day for 6 weeks	
Recombinant interferon gamma (*Imukin*®, Torental®, other immunomodulators)		Subcutaneous or intramuscular	Adjunct therapy, often in combination with miltefosine and paromomycin. Pentoxifylline under the brand name Torental® is an inhibitor of tumor necrosis factor-α
Immunotherapy	CL	Intramuscular. Three doses of killed *L. amazonensis* preparation plus BCG	In South America, particularly in Venezuela, immunostimulation by injections of heat-killed promastigotes plus BCG is used in the treatment of CL due to *L (v.) braziliensis*. This approach promotes healing. BCG vaccination may cause adverse reactions
Preclinical stages leads or compounds tested in academia (only few example are given)			
Fexinidazole	VL	Oral formulation	Fexinidazole is already in phase 1 clinical trials for African sleeping sickness, but it seems also active against *Leishmania* (Wyllie

(*continued*)

Table 1 (continued)

Antileishmanial compound	Syndrome	Adult regimen	Comments
			et al. 2012) with cure rate of 98 % in mice model
Lipid-based amphotericin B (iCo's formulation)	VL	Oral formulation	Developed by Dr. Kishor M. Wasan at the University of British Columbia, Canada, with collaborators. This formulation is stable at the temperatures of WHO Climatic Zones 3 and 4 (30–43 °C) and seems effective against systemic fungal infections and drug-resistant VL. In 2010, iCo's formulation for treating VL received "orphan drug" designation by the FDA, an important recognition of its promise
Imiquimod	CL	Topical formulation	Immunomodulatory agent initially developed as an antiviral drug recommended for facial CL lesions. Seems effective in combination with antimony compounds (Khalili et al. 2011). Imiquimod induces the production of cytokines and nitric oxide in macrophages at the site of application
ER-119884 and E5700			Two quinuclidine derivatives active against the leishmanial squalene synthase enzyme (SQS) in the sterol biosynthetic pathway. These compounds have been tested against *L. amazonensis* (Fernandes Rodrigues et al. 2008)
Bisphosphonates			Bisphosphates inhibit the isoprenoid pathway in *Leishmania* that is catalyzed by the enzyme farnesyl diphosphate synthase (FPPS)
Sitamaquine (WR 6026)	VL	Oral 1–3 mg/kg/day for 28 days	8-Aminoquinoline in development in combination with miltefosine. Abdominal complaints of discomfort, pain, vomiting, diarrhea, and headache are the commonest side effects. Nephrotoxicity

(*continued*)

Table 1 (continued)

Antileishmanial compound	Syndrome	Adult regimen	Comments
			may occur. Tafenoquine is another 8-aminoquinoline in advanced stage of development that will also be administrated orally. Tafenoquine is active against both Sb^V-resistant and Sb^V-sensitive *L. donovani* strains (Yardley et al. 2010)
Nelfinavir			Highly active against strains of *L. braziliensis*, *L. donovani*, and *L. chagasi* with inhibition rates over 90 % (Santos et al. 2013)
Several adenosine analogues			Specific inhibitors for the glycolytic enzyme glyceraldehyde-3-phosphate dehydrogenase (GAPDH) (Aronov et al. 1999)
Trypanothione reductase (TR) inhibitors			Several compounds that inhibit TR have been identified including polyamine derivatives, tricyclics, and aminodiphenyl sulfides (Venkatesan and Dubey 2012). One of these is auranofin, a gold-containing drug already in clinical use as an antiarthritic agent (Ilari et al. 2012)
Inhibitors of topoisomerases			
PTR1 and DHFR-TS inhibitors			PTR1 and DHFR-TS are key in folate metabolism in *Leishmania*. Specific inhibitors are being developed against these proteins (Corona et al. 2012; Rajasekaran and Chen 2012)
Other treatments			
Phototherapy (Omnilux PDT®, Photo Therapeutics Inc)	CL	~100 J/cm^2/treatment at 635 nm in the presence of photosensitizing agents for several weeks	The production of highly reactive oxygen species (ROS) will inhibit and even kill by photolysis the amastigote parasite
Cryotherapy	CL	Freeze/thaw cycles of 15–20 s each using	In combination with Sb^V (intralesional). Effective against *L. tropica* and *L. major*

(*continued*)

Table 1 (continued)

Antileishmanial compound	Syndrome	Adult regimen	Comments
		liquid nitrogen, treatment of 1–2 weeks	CL uncomplicated lesions, e. g., dryer and smaller (<1 cm) lesions
Thermotherapy (ThermoMed®)	CL	Radiofrequency waves with 50 °C for 30 s intralesional	Parasites are mostly killed by heat

[a]Only the main leishmaniasis treatments and some promising compounds are presented in this table. *Leishmania* species are known to present intrinsic variation in drug sensitivity to almost all antileishmanial agents. *IV* intravenous, *IM* intramuscular, *IL* intralesional, *CL* cutaneous leishmaniasis, *MCL* mucocutaneous leishmaniasis, *DCL* diffuse cutaneous leishmaniasis, *PKDL* post-kala-azar dermal leishmaniasis, *VL* visceral leishmaniasis, *MSF* Médecins Sans Frontières, *WHO* World Health Organization

Mechanisms of Drug Resistance

Leishmaniasis is treatable by chemotherapy, but resistance can be developed experimentally for all drugs, suggesting that clinical resistance is just a question of time. The next section will describe the ingenious mechanism(s) of resistance evolved by *Leishmania* parasites to survive the toxic effects of drugs. Emphasis will be put on the main therapeutic options currently used in endemic countries. The mode of action and the underlying resistance mechanisms either demonstrated in vitro, in vivo, or in clinical isolates will be presented when available.

Pentavalent Antimonials

Pentavalent antimonials (Sb^{V}) are the classical first-line treatment against leishmaniasis and the only drugs that are barely affordable in most endemic countries. These drugs are toxic and poorly tolerated with the consequence that a significant proportion of the patients do not complete their full course regimen. This situation appears to be the principal reason behind the selection and emergence of antimony-resistant parasite strains. Apart low compliance, the use of counterfeit medicines with none optimal curative efficacy was also incriminated recently in further promoting the emergence of antimonial resistance in endemic countries (Cockburn et al. 2005; Mackey and Liang 2011). Another interesting hypothesis is that arsenic contamination (arsenic is a metal related to antimony) in drinking water in Bihar has also contributed to the selection of resistant mutants (Ait-Oudhia et al. 2011; Perry et al. 2011).

Antimonials mediate part of their antileishmanial activity via the generation of oxidative stress which leads to the disruption of the synthesis of macromolecules in the parasite cell. To survive, the parasite therefore must control this oxidative assault and this is achieved by a complex molecular response. After nearly 20 years of in vitro studies punctuated with few reports describing work in clinical isolates, a global model for antimonial resistance in *Leishmania* has been proposed (Fig. 1). It is generally accepted that all pentavalent antimonials are prodrugs that require biological reduction to their trivalent form (Sb^{III}) in order to acquire antileishmanial activity (Shaked-Mishan et al. 2001). Antimony reduction apparently may occur in both the host cell and in parasites. The reduced trivalent form in macrophages enters the parasite cell through the aquaglyceroporin AQP1 localized at the parasite surface (Gourbal et al. 2004). It has been shown that a lower activity of AQP1 by gene deletion of reduced expression resulted in Sb^{III} increased resistance (Gourbal et al. 2004; Marquis et al. 2005). Recently, a deletion of the AQP1 gene was observed in in vitro antimony-resistant parasites through a telomeric gene deletion (Mukherjee et al. 2013a). Sb^{V} enters into the parasite via a protein that is different than AQP1. It has been hypothesized that this transporter may either recognize phosphate or a sugar moiety shared with gluconate (Brochu et al. 2003). Increased intracellular levels of the antioxidant molecule trypanothione (TSH, the most abundant thiol in trypanosomatids) have been observed in antimony-resistant parasites, an event usually related to the overexpression of rate-limiting enzymes involved in the synthesis of glutathione (gamma-glutamylcysteine synthetase, γ-GCS) and polyamines (ornithine decarboxylase, ODC) (Fig. 1). Another resistance protein implicates the ABC transporter MRPA (ABCC3 alias PgpA) which confers resistance by sequestering drug-trypanothione conjugates within an intracellular organelle near the flagellar pocket, where the antimonial target(s) is probably absent (Legare et al. 2001). It is thought that the sequestered drugs are then expelled from the parasite through exocytosis occurring at the flagellar pocket (Fig. 1). Finally, a protein localized at the parasite cell surface was reported to be responsible for the active efflux of TSH conjugated-antimonial compounds outside the parasite (Dey et al. 1996) (Fig. 1). One possible candidate would be the recently characterized ABCI4 protein (Manzano et al. 2013). Part of the in vitro antimonial resistance model presented in Fig. 1 was recently confirmed in natural antimony-resistant *Leishmania* clinical isolates recovered from patients unresponsive to sodium antimony gluconate (SAG). Indeed, an active role for MRPA, γ-GCS, and ODC in resistance was confirmed (Mukherjee et al. 2007; Singh et al. 2010), which tends to corroborate the resistance model proposed for in vitro-resistant strains. Nonetheless, since different paths lead to resistance in *Leishmania*, alternative mechanisms other than those described here may also operate in field isolates (Downing et al. 2011; Singh 2006; Vanaerschot et al. 2012). Recently, it has been discovered that *Leishmania* influences cell functions of its host cell via glycans deployed at its cell surface (Mukherjee et al. 2013b). Indeed, particular glycans at the parasite cell surface outwit the immune system of the host and permit to resist to the toxic effect of antimonial drugs by making the human host cell expelling antimony drugs through the ATP-binding cassette (ABC) transporter MDR1 localized at the macrophage cell surface (Fig. 1, left insert). Thus, antimony resistance in *Leishmania* is multifactorial with contributions of several independent events, leading to parasite resistance.

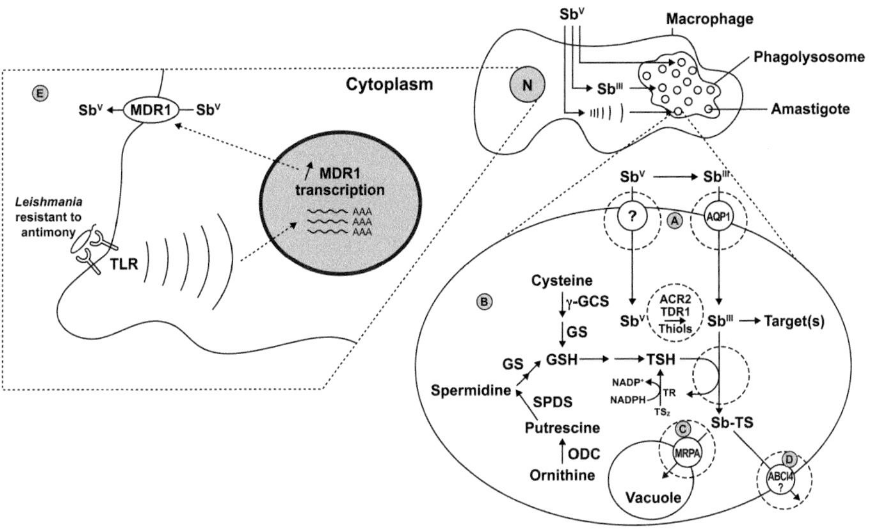

Fig. 1 Resistance mechanisms to antimonials in *Leishmania*. Resistance to antimonials involves modulation of influx in the parasite cell **(a)**, thiol and antimony metabolisms **(b)**, drug sequestration through MRPA **(c)**, drug efflux potentially by the ABC transporter ABCI4 **(d)** at the parasite cell surface, and overproduction of host MDR1 at the macrophage cell surface **(e)**. The drug Sb^V is converted to its reduced form (Sb^{III}, the toxic form of the metal) in the macrophage and/or in the parasite cell. Sb^V and Sb^{III} enter *Leishmania* through two different transporters, a still uncharacterized transporter (depicted by a question mark at the parasite cell surface) and AQP1, respectively. The intracellular Sb^V is potentially converted to Sb^{III} by two parasite enzymes (ACR2 and TDR1) or by reduced thiols. Once reduced, Sb^{III} is detoxified by its conjugation with trypanothione (TSH). Trypanothione is maintained in its reduced form by the enzyme trypanothione reductase (TR) which uses NADPH. In antimony-resistant parasites, the trypanothione biosynthesis pathway is activated which leads to an increase in the concentration of intracellular THS. The Sb^{III}-TS conjugate is either effluxed out of the cell through an efflux pump (potentially ABCI4) or is sequestered in a vacuole by the activity of the ABC transporter MRPA. It is thought that these vacuoles are then exocytosed at the flagellar pocket. Particular glycans at the parasite cell surface are responsible of the MDR1 modulation at the macrophage plasma membrane. The interaction of a unique terminal sugar at the surface of Sb^V-resistant parasites with host TLR2 will result in the activation of a series of transcriptional factors and IL10 production by the macrophage that will ultimately drive the overexpression of MDR1 transcripts in the macrophage nucleus. Translation of MDR1 transcripts will lead to an overproduction of MDR1 proteins at the host plasma membrane, resulting in an increased efflux of antimony outside the macrophage, leading to resistance. *AQP1* aquaglyceroporin 1 transporter, *GSH* glutathione, *TSH* reduced trypanothione, TS_2 oxidized trypanothione, Sb^V pentavalent antimony, Sb^{II}, trivalent antimony, *Sb-TS* trypanothione-antimony conjugate, *MRPA* multidrug resistance protein A alias PgpA. *?* still uncharacterized transporter for Sb^V, *ACR2* antimony reductase, *TDR1* thiol-dependent reductase, *ABCI4* an ABC transporter that may act as an efflux pump, *N* nucleus, *MDR1* multidrug resistance protein 1, *γ-GCS* gamma-glutamylcysteine synthase, *ODC* ornithine decarboxylase, *SPDS* spermidine synthase, *GS* glutathione synthetase, *TR* trypanothione reductase, *TLR* Toll-like receptor

Amphotericin B

Amphotericin B (AMB) is a polyene antibiotic originally extracted from the filamentous bacterium *Streptomyces nodosus* (Lemke et al. 2005; Trejo and Bennett 1963) and first developed as an antifungal drug. AMB is the current secondary treatment of choice against leishmaniasis and the best treatment against antimonial refractive leishmaniasis in highly endemic regions such as Bihar state in India. It is currently available as a plain AMB solution, as cholesteryl sulfate or lipid complexes, and as liposomal formulations (Table 1). AMB is a highly effective antileishmanial drug, but major drawbacks and side effects limit however its widespread use. Indeed, AMB is nephrotoxic and is only available in injectable formulations requiring several hours' administration schedules by infusion and close monitoring. A study aiming at testing the efficacy and safety of one single infusion of AMB over only a 2 h infusion is currently in trials (Sundar and Chakravarty 2013). Similarly, AMB-lipid formulations have been developed to improve tolerability for patients and to increase plasma concentration for a better efficacy, but the cost of these formulations is highly prohibitive. Oral and safer formulations of AMB for the treatment of leishmaniasis are being developed. Positive preclinical data are suggesting an absence of kidney toxicity and a dramatic knockdown of parasitic VL infections with greater than 99 % eradication of parasitic infection at the tested dosages (Wasan et al. 2009, 2010).

The mechanism of action of AMB is based on the binding of the AmB molecule to ergosterol, the predominant sterol in the membranes of *Leishmania* parasites. It produces an aggregate that creates a transmembrane channel (e.g., aqueous pores in the lipid bilayers), allowing the cytoplasmic contents to leak out (especially K^+), probably accelerating cell death (Brajtburg et al. 1990; Ramos et al. 1996; Urbina et al. 1987). Another mechanism by which AMB could affect the parasite is its autooxidation and subsequent formation of free radicals which are highly toxic to *Leishmania*. Thus, both ion movement and oxidative effects induced by AMB may lead to parasite cell death, and any molecular change that interferes with these processes may lead to resistance. The level of sensitivity to AMB is species dependent and depends on the variation in the ergosterol content in membranes (Escobar et al. 2002). Resistance in in vitro-generated *Leishmania* promastigotes was shown to be caused by a significant change in plasma membrane sterols, with ergosterol being replaced by a precursor, cholesta-5,7,24-trien-3β-ol (Mbongo et al. 1998) (Fig. 2a). This change is apparently due to a loss of function of the s-adenosyl-L-methionine-C24-Δ-sterol methyltransferase (SCMT) that impaired C24 transmethylation (Fig. 2a). In addition, AMB uptake was decreased in an in vitro-generated *L. donovani* AMB-resistant cell line, and efflux, most likely due to the overexpression/deregulation of an ABC transporter (MDR1?), was increased (Fig. 2b) (Mbongo et al. 1998). Deep understanding of the putative role of ABC proteins in AMB resistance in *Leishmania* needs to be formally addressed however since it remains possible that the decrease in uptake and/or increase in efflux in this in vitro-generated AMB-resistant mutant may also be due to a weak affinity of AMB for such modified membranes in resistant parasites.

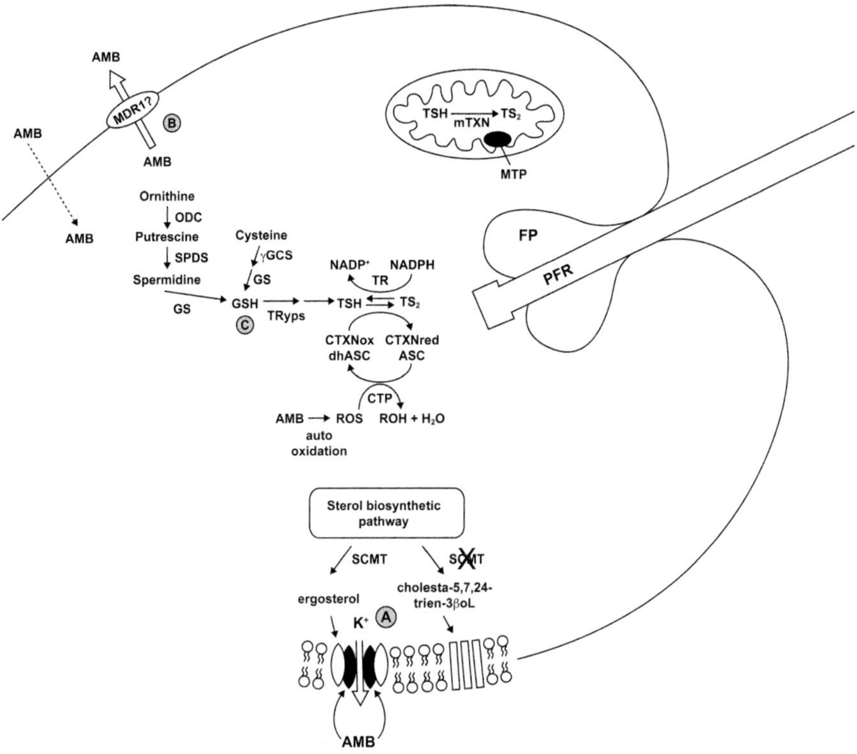

Fig. 2 **Resistance mechanisms to amphotericin B in *Leishmania*.** Multiple mechanisms conferring AMB resistance have been reported in in vitro-generated mutants, with some recently detected in field isolates. These include an altered membrane sterol profile **(a)**; efflux, possibly by the parasite ABC transporter MDR1 (Mbongo et al. 1998; Purkait et al. 2012), although this remains to be formally addressed **(b)**; and detoxification of the AMB-mediated reactive oxygen species (ROS) through the trypanothione/tryparedoxin cascade **(c)**. AMB binds to ergosterol of sensitive *Leishmania* parasites, causing membrane depolarization and leakage of ion K^+, leading to cell death. In AMB-resistant parasites, AMB binding to membrane ergosterol is impaired due to an altered membrane sterol profile caused by a loss of function of the enzyme *S*-adenosyl-L-methionine: C24-D-sterol methyltransferase (SCMT) **(a)**. Although the plasma membrane composition is altered in resistant parasites, it still remains possible that a low amount of AMB manages to enter the parasite cells (schematized by a *dotted line* in figure crossing the parasite plasma membrane). Part of the small amount of AMB that manages to be taken up into the resistant parasites is thought to be rapidly effluxed out by a plasma membrane ABC transporter (possibly MDR1), although this assumption remains to be formally addressed **(b)**. The remaining intracellular AMB auto-oxidizes and will lead to the production of ROS. The toxic effects of ROS may be nullified by the parasite trypanothione/tryparedoxin cascade **(c)**. Two enzymes, the cytoplasmic tryparedoxin peroxidase (CTP) and the mitochondrial tryparedoxin peroxidase (MTP), involved in the terminal steps of the trypanothione/tryparedoxin cascade may cleave the ROS, producing water and alcohols (ROH) **(c)**. *GSH* glutathione, *TSH* reduced trypanothione, *TS_2* oxidized trypanothione, *MDR1* multidrug resistance protein 1, *γ-GCS* gamma-glutamylcysteine synthase, *ODC* ornithine decarboxylase, *SPDS* spermidine synthase, *GS* glutathione synthetase, *Tryps* trypanothione synthase, *TR* trypanothione reductase, $cTXN_{ox}$ oxidized cytosolic tryparedoxin, $cTXN_{red}$ reduced cytosolic tryparedoxin, *mTXN* mitochondrial tryparedoxin, *dhASC* dehydroascorbate, *ASC* ascorbate, *FP* flagellar pocket, *PFR* paraflagellar rod. This schematic is adapted from Purkait et al. (2012)

To date, only few cases of AMB clinical resistance were reported (Purkait et al. 2012; Srivastava et al. 2011). The analysis of one clinical isolate of *L. donovani* has shown that similar resistance mechanisms previously observed in in vitro AMB-resistant mutants are also operating in clinical isolates (Purkait et al. 2012). Indeed, the resistant clinical strain had an altered membrane composition (with the cholesta-5,7,24-trien-3β-ol substitution, Fig. 2a), resulting in a higher fluidity of the plasma membrane compared to sensitive clinical strains. A decrease in AMB uptake as well as an increase in the expression level of MDR1 (Fig. 2b) at the parasite cell surface was also found in the resistant clinical strain, suggesting an increase in efflux of AMB. The tryparedoxin cascade was also upregulated in resistant parasites as well as a more reduced intracellular thiol level (Fig. 2c). It was suggested that this increase in reduced thiol in resistant isolates may help in better scavenging of reactive oxygen species (ROS) produced by AMB (Purkait et al. 2012), although this assumption needs further investigation. It must be stressed however that resistance to AMB must be rare. A study has shown that HIV patients with several relapses with the same strains were treated with several courses of AMB and the parasites never became resistant (Lachaud et al. 2009).

Paromomycin

The aminoglycoside *paromomycin* (PM) has been available in India since 2006. It seems highly effective in this endemic country, but its efficacy in Africa seems however lower. Since there is a concern on the development of clinical resistance, the longevity of PM would be better preserved in combination regimens than as a single agent therapy. Recently, a quantitative SILAC-based proteomic analysis of an in vitro-generated PM-resistant strain has brought some light on the mode of action of PM and the underlying resistance mechanisms (Chawla et al. 2011). The uptake of PM is thought to proceed by endocytosis, a process facilitated by the binding of PM to a number of parasite surface proteins (Fig. 3a). Two of them were the paraflagellar rod (PFR) proteins 1D and 2C that are only found at the flagellum of the parasite. Another protein interacting with PM is prohibitin that is also found at the surface of the flagellar and the aflagellar poles. Apparently, these PM-interacting proteins may help the drug to be taken up by the parasite through endocytosis (Fig. 3a). Another protein that interacts with PM is the putative P-type H^+ ATPase (Fig. 3b). Its localization in *Leishmania* is unclear, but in the parasite *Trypanosoma cruzi*, the orthologous protein is localized in vacuolar compartments and is probably involved in the acidification of these intracellular vacuoles (Vieira et al. 2005). It is thus suspected that this protein plays a similar role in *Leishmania* parasites and that the potential interaction of PM with this putative vacuolar pump promotes its endocytosis/sequestration process or helps to keep the drug inside vacuoles. Interestingly, the resistant strain had a higher number of vesicular vacuoles and an increase in a number of proteins involved in vesicular trafficking compared to the parental sensitive strain. This suggests that PM could affect vesicle-mediated trafficking. The quantitative proteomic analysis also revealed an upregulation of ribosomal

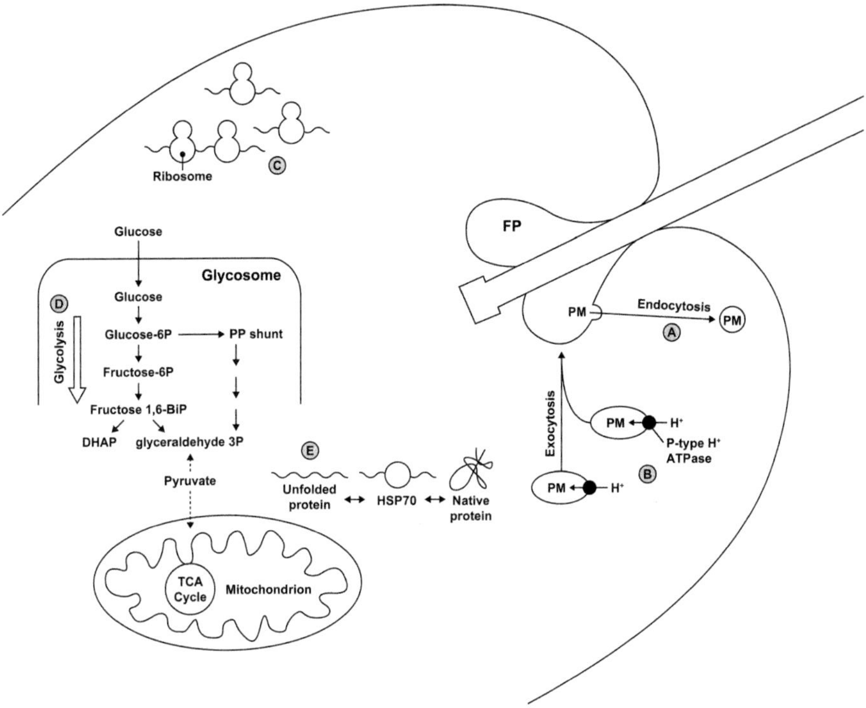

Fig. 3 Proposed resistance mechanisms to paromomycin in *Leishmania*. (a) The drug paromomycin (PM) is probably taken up by the parasite by endocytosis **(a)**. PM is then sequestered into vacuoles. The pump vacuole ATPase is upregulated and the number of vacuoles is increased in resistant parasites **(b)**. A number of ribosomal protein subunits are upregulated in PM-resistant parasites increasing the overall protein synthesis **(c)**. The glycolytic pathway is also upregulated in resistant parasites **(d)**. The chaperone proteins are found upregulated in resistant cells as a result of the stress caused by PM, and these proteins are also involved in protein turnover **(e)**. FP, flagellar pocket. This schematic was inspired from Chawla et al. (2011)

proteins, suggesting that PM also affects translation by targeting these ribosomal proteins (Chawla et al. 2011) (Fig. 3c), although the exact molecular mechanistic remains to be elucidated (Fernandez et al. 2011). Elevated levels of glycolytic enzymes were also detected in the PM-resistant strain, indicating that the resistant strain heavily relies on glycolysis (either aerobic or anaerobic) for its energy requirement (Fig. 3d). An increase in the basal levels of a number of stress protein parts of the HSP70 family was also observed in resistant parasites when compared to the parental sensitive strain (Fig. 3e). All together these results are suggesting that once PM is internalized by endocytosis, a process facilitated by a number of parasite cell surface proteins, it is probably sequestered in vacuole compartments that are most likely exocytosed at the flagellar pocket, thus conferring resistance. The sequestering hypothesis remains however to be formally addressed. Thus, modulation of translation rate, interaction with vesicle-mediated trafficking, an increase in energetic metabolism through glycolysis, and an effective protection of important key players in resistance and survival by chaperone/stress-related proteins are all important features of PM resistance in *Leishmania*.

Miltefosine

Miltefosine (MIL, under the brand name Impavido®) is an alkylphosphocholine initially developed as an anticancer drug. It is the latest antileishmanial agent to reach the market and currently the only oral treatment commercially available, although oral formulations of AMB (as described above) and sitamaquine (a primaquine analogue) are currently under development. MIL is a well-tolerated and effective oral treatment of VL with only minor side effects. It is also highly effective in antimony-resistant cases but cannot be given to women of childbearing age due to a substantial risk of birth defects or fetal malformation. This antileishmanial agent has been licensed in India and Nepal for at least 5 years now, but its use is not under strict control. In addition, since MIL has a long half-life (between 150 and 200 h) (Bryceson 2001), the emergence of resistance remains a concern for public health authorities in these countries. Consequently, after only 5 years, the failure rate for MIL has increased in certain endemic regions (Rijal et al. 2013; Sundar et al. 2012). Recent data would suggest that treatment failure is not associated with resistant parasites, however (Rijal et al. 2013).

Drug uptake is a prerequisite for MIL activity against *Leishmania* which is reputed to act principally by perturbing the metabolism of lipids and especially phospholipids (Imbert et al. 2012). Inhibition of cytochrome c oxidase activity and mitochondrial depolarization resulting to an apoptosis/PCD-like death have also been reported (Luque-Ortega and Rivas 2007). Since experimental resistance to MIL is very easily achieved (Perez-Victoria et al. 2006b) and only cross-resistance (and not primary resistance) to MIL has been observed in clinical isolates from VL patients resistant to Sb^V (Kumar et al. 2009; Vergnes et al. 2007), MIL resistance mechanisms have been only studied in in vitro-generated resistant strains to date. A common feature in all MIL-resistant lines is a decreased drug accumulation. This is achieved by a decrease in uptake (Fig. 4a) and/or an increase in efflux (Fig. 4b). The MIL uptake machinery is composed of 2 proteins, the miltefosine transporter MT (a member of the P4-ATPase subfamily) and its specific beta subunit ROS3 (reviewed in Perez-Victoria et al. 2006b). Both are essential for MIL uptake at the parasite cell surface, and any mutations inactivating or decreasing the expression of any of these 2 components render the parasite cells highly resistant to MIL (Perez-Victoria et al. 2003, 2006a). Interestingly, the resistance phenotype seems stable in in vitro macrophages infected with MT-null mutant and MT-mutated parasites (Seifert et al. 2007), suggesting that what is observed in MIL-resistant promastigotes might be applied to intracellular amastigotes. Moreover, several mutations in MT can lead to resistance, and within a resistant population, they may be several different MT genotypes, leading to resistance (Coelho et al. 2012).

Decreasing MIL uptake (Fig. 4a) seems to be the easiest way for *Leishmania* to develop high levels of MIL resistance, but if a certain amount of MIL manages to

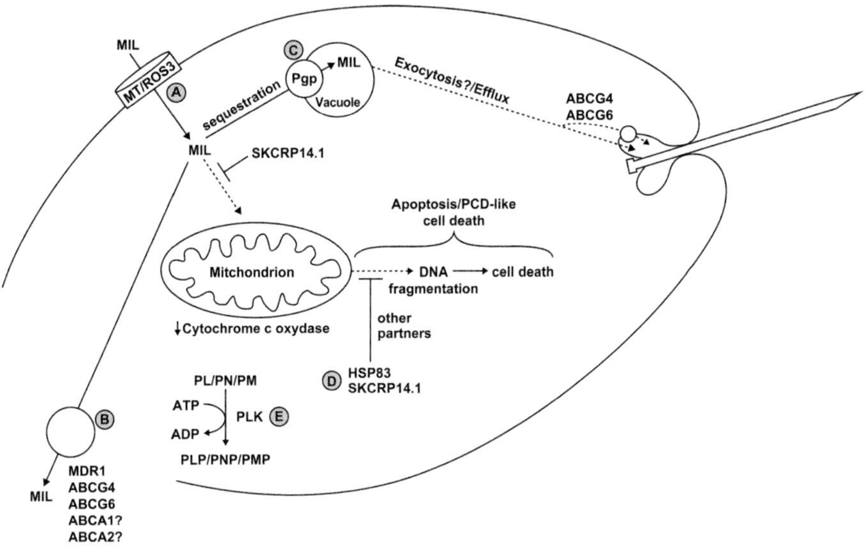

Fig. 4 Resistance mechanisms to miltefosine in *Leishmania*. Miltefosine interacts either directly or indirectly with the mitochondrion, eventually leading to its depolarization. Point mutations in the miltefosine translocation machinery MT/ROS3 have been detected in resistant mutants **(a)**. Changes in the expression level of a number of ABC transporters involved either in the sequestration or efflux (MDR1/PGP, ABCG4, ABCG6) of miltefosine out of the parasite cells have been incriminated in the resistance phenotype **(b** and **c)**. Other factors such as the HSP83 and the calpain-like protein SKCRP14.1 may help to confer miltefosine resistance by interfering with the parasite apoptosis/programmed cell-like death pathway (PCD) **(d)**. The SKCRP14.1 protein also protects against miltefosine-induced PCD by preventing depolarization of the mitochondrion. The enzyme pyridoxal kinase (PLK) catalyzes the addition of phosphate from ATP to the 5′ alcohol group of pyridoxal (PL), pyridoxine (PN), and pyridoxamine (PM) to form, respectively, pyridoxal-5-phosphate (PLP), pyridoxine-5-phosphate (PNP), and pyridoxamine-5-phosphate (PMP) **(e)**. Mutations in PLK were discovered in a number of miltefosine-resistant mutants selected in vitro, and transfection of the WT PLK version in mutants has shown that this enzyme plays a role in miltefosine resistance

enter the parasite cells, an increase in efflux (Fig. 4b) or in sequestration (Fig. 4c) may also lead to in vitro MIL resistance. The parasite protein MDR1, a P-glycoprotein-like transporter part of the *Leishmania* ABC family, was the first molecule shown to be involved in in vitro MIL resistance (Perez-Victoria et al. 2001). This plasma membrane transporter pumps xenobiotic drugs including MIL out of the parasite, thereby decreasing their intracellular concentration. Two members of the ABCG subfamily were also reported to be involved in MIL resistance in *Leishmania*, namely, ABCG4 and ABCG6, whose localization is mainly to the parasite plasma membrane and flagellar pocket (BoseDasgupta et al. 2008; Castanys-Munoz et al. 2007, 2008) (Fig. 4). Interestingly, both genes were also shown to be involved in sitamaquine resistance (Castanys-Munoz et al. 2007, 2008) due to rapid efflux at the plasma membrane. The physiological roles of ABCG4 and ABCG6 remain to be established, but these two half-transporters were reported to be involved in phospholipid trafficking at the plasma membrane (trans-bilayer lipid movement) as they were shown to reduce the accumulation of short-chain phospholipid analogues when overexpressed (Castanys-Munoz et al. 2008). Since ABCG4 and ABCG6 show similar spectra of activity (i.e., similar substrates) and both proteins are half ABC transporters co-localizing mainly at the plasma membrane, it was speculated that these two ABC proteins may not only homodimerize but may heterodimerize together to confer MIL resistance or to extend the substrate specificity of each individual homodimer (Castanys-Munoz et al. 2008). Along with MDR1, ABCG4, and ABCG6, it is not excluded that other ABC proteins (ABCA1, ABCA2) might also contribute to MIL resistance (Fig. 4b). Finally, other proteins involved in experimental MIL resistance in *Leishmania* include the heat shock protein HSP83 and a calpain-like protein (SKCRP14.1) that both could protect against programmed cell death (PCD) induced by MIL (Vergnes et al. 2007) (Fig. 4d). Finally, the sequencing of the genome of miltefosine-resistant mutants pinpointed a mutation in the pyridoxal kinase (*PLK*) gene (Fig. 4e), and the role of this gene in MIL resistance was confirmed by gene transfection experiments (Coelho et al. 2012).

Resistance Reversal Agents

The concept of using a compound able to reverse resistance in refractory cases of leishmaniasis due to parasite-acquired resistance was inspired from what has been achieved in tumor cells. Multidrug resistance (MDR) is a main impediment to successful anticancer chemotherapy and is mediated, for instance, by the P-glycoprotein (MDR1/ABCB1/Pgp) and/or the multidrug resistance protein 1 (MRP1/ABCC1), two ATP-binding cassette (ABC) transporters, that either efflux or sequester drugs. Classical MDR was later associated with other ABC proteins including MDR2/ABCB4, cMOAT/MRP2/ABCC2, BCRP/ABCG2, and more recently MRP7/ABCC10 (Sun et al. 2013). In an attempt to overcome MDR in tumor cells, specific Pgp/MRP inhibitors have been developed with the rationale that blocking the action of these pumps will result in an increased net accumulation of drugs and thus a greater clinical efficacy of chemotherapeutic agents in tumors overexpressing these pumps. Unfortunately, after more than four decades of intensive efforts, there is no MDR reversal drug that has yet been approved by the US Food and Drug Administration (FDA). Nonetheless, third-generation lead compounds with less toxic effects and better pharmacokinetic interactions are currently being tested in advanced clinical studies (Kelly et al. 2012; Robey et al. 2008). Similar to tumor cells, reversal agents were assayed in *Leishmania* cell lines resistant to various therapeutic agents (reviewed in Pradines 2013). It has been shown that sitamaquine reversed miltefosine resistance in an MDR *L. tropica* line that overexpressed MDR1 (Perez-Victoria et al. 2011). The same study demonstrated that sitamaquine was also able to modulate antimony resistance mediated by MRPA/ABCC3, another key player in experimental and clinical antimony resistance in this parasite. If sitamaquine pass clinical trials with success, combination therapy with miltefosine or antimony may represent a promising strategy to avoid the appearance of resistance mediated by ABC proteins in *Leishmania*. Recently, new natural or synthetic sesquiterpenes, flavonoids, acridone carboxamide derivatives (zosuquidar and elacridar), or phenothiazines were shown to revert the resistance phenotype in *Leishmania* to sodium stibogluconate and miltefosine by modulating intracellular drug concentrations (reviewed in Pradines 2013). These compounds may also represent promising modulators of Pgp-/MRP-mediated resistance in *Leishmania*.

Innovative Strategies to Combat Drug Resistance

The WHO has enlisted leishmaniasis to be eliminated in the Indian continent by 2015, which is in less than two years (Gupta et al. 2013). As stated before, the unavailability of a vaccine in clinical use and the widespread emergence of resistance in India to the most effective and affordable drugs against leishmaniasis, pentavalent antimonials, constitute major obstacles in achieving this goal. A number of therapeutic options are in the pipeline however (Table 1), but the large pharmas are not necessarily prioritizing research in neglected diseases including leishmaniasis. Innovative ways coming from academia-industry partnerships are thus more than needed to tackle this deadly parasite and to control the emergence of resistance to the limited number of drugs still active against the parasite.

Studies of in vitro resistance mechanisms in the 1980s and 1990s have shown that one frequent road to achieve resistance in *Leishmania* is gene amplification (e.g., amplification of target or efflux pump genes). These studies demonstrated that amplified DNAs can be either circular or linear with their formation mediated through homologous recombination between direct or inverted repeats of ~400–1000 bp in length. Homologous recombination (HR) between directly repeated homologous sequences leads to circular amplicons, whereas the annealing of inverted homologous repeats leads to either circular or linear amplicons. No further mechanistic insights related to gene amplification in *Leishmania* have emerged in the last decade except for the important observation that gene amplification was also detected in several clinical isolates resistant to chemotherapeutic drugs (Mittal et al. 2007; Singh et al. 2003). Resistance through point mutations (e.g., in drug importer genes such as in the miltefosine transporter MT/ROS3) has also been described but seems rare in the field. Recently, loss of function associated with drug resistance was found to be mediated by gene deletions that also occurred by HR between directly repeated sequences (Mukherjee et al. 2013a). Since *Leishmania* lacks transcriptional control at initiation, there is apparently no easy way for this pathogen to increase (or decrease) the expression of one specific gene except by gene amplification (or deletion). Thus, one can speculate that any molecules or compounds interfering with gene amplification events or HR in *Leishmania* may represent a valuable and innovative strategy to limit the development of resistance in this parasite. We are pursuing this exciting working hypothesis in the hope to develop more effective medicines against *Leishmania*. This type of molecules might be used in combination with current drugs to circumvent or prevent the emergence of drug resistance.

Apart targeting amplification and/or deletion molecular events for limiting the development of resistance in the parasite *Leishmania*, we are also evaluating the peculiar mode of gene expression in *Leishmania* as a valuable therapeutic target and innovative strategy to limit the development of drug resistance in this parasite. More precisely, we are looking at genome signatures or nucleic acid 3D structures encoding signals potentially involved in replication or translation control in the parasite. It is well known that *Leishmania* displays unique features regarding genome organization (no cluster of functional genes) and control of gene expression. Indeed, its ~8,300 genes (of which only ~40 % have a putative assigned function) are organized into unidirectional gene clusters comprising up to 100 functionally unrelated genes that are co-transcribed in the absence of typical polII promoters into long polycistronic primary transcripts. Individual mRNAs are produced from polycistronic molecules by two posttranscriptional RNA-processing reactions, namely, *trans*-splicing and 3′-cleavage/polyadenylation, to generate mature monocistronic mRNAs. Thus, the regulation of gene expression in *Leishmania* occurs almost exclusively at the posttranscriptional level, and sequences within 3′-untranslated regions have been shown to play a key role in controlling either the stability of mRNAs or the efficiency of their translation (reviewed in Requena 2011). In our quest of understanding the regulation of gene/protein expression in *Leishmania*, we have recently discovered numerous G-DNA structures (G4) spread between genes and in telomeres of the parasite's genome (unpublished results). In mammals, there is now compelling evidence for functions of some G4 motifs in essential processes including initiation of DNA replication, telomere maintenance, regulated recombination events, control of gene expression, and genetic and epigenetic instability (Maizels and Gray 2013). Since the control of gene expression in *Leishmania* appears to be posttranscriptional, our hypothesis is that G-structures present in mature monocistronic mRNAs will, upon binding or release of specific factors/proteins, respectively block or allow the translation of mRNAs by ribosomes. This hypothesis may be tested with the newly established "ribosome profiling" methodology (Ingolia et al. 2012) which correlates ribosome occupancy on mRNAs with relative mRNA translation efficiencies. The design of small-molecule compounds able to interact with specific G4-structures and block the translation of mRNA encoding essential proteins or proteins involved in resistance pathways may lead to new alternatives in the treatment and control of leishmaniasis.

Conclusion

Antimicrobial resistance is one of the key health challenges of the twenty-first century. Globally, the threats of resistance are increasing at an alarming rate. Resistance in *Leishmania* parasites has been slow to emerge but is now encountered more frequently in endemic areas including northeastern India where the incidence of kala-azar is highest. With the limited armamentarium of drugs in clinical use, we need to preserve the efficacy of the ones still active against this deadly parasite. Combination therapy, better compliance of patients, good practices in drug supply, and hopefully the development of effective reversal agents should expand the lifespan of existing medicines and slow the spread of drug resistance, but the development of novel antileishmanial medicines remains a priority. The plant kingdom and anticancer drugs are providing an impressive series of medicinal compounds with antileishmanial activities that still need to be tested in clinical trials. The licensing of an effective vaccine for human usage along with more effective strategies for point-of-care diagnostic will be also important milestones that will impact the control and management of leishmaniasis. Concerted efforts are thus required from the whole scientific community in partnership with the pharmaceutical industry.

Acknowledgments The authors are grateful to the members of the laboratory at the Centre de Recherche en Infectiologie du CHU de Québec for their dedication, professionalism, and critical reading of the manuscript. The authors owe an apology to their colleagues in the field of leishmaniasis and even wider area of drug resistance whose work could not be properly acknowledged due to space limitations. This work was funded by a CIHR grant to M.O. M.O. holds the Canada Research Chair in Antimicrobial Resistance.

References

Ait-Oudhia K, Gazanion E, Vergnes B, Oury B, Sereno D (2011) Leishmania antimony resistance: what we know what we can learn from the field. Parasitol Res 109:1225–1232

Alvar J, Aparicio P, Aseffa A, Den Boer M, Canavate C, Dedet JP, Gradoni L, Ter Horst R, Lopez-Velez R, Moreno J (2008) The relationship between leishmaniasis and AIDS: the second 10 years. Clin Microbiol Rev 21:334–359, table of contents

Alvar J, Velez ID, Bern C, Herrero M, Desjeux P, Cano J, Jannin J, den Boer M (2012) Leishmaniasis worldwide and global estimates of its incidence. PLoS One 7:e35671

Antinori S, Cascio A, Parravicini C, Bianchi R, Corbellino M (2008) Leishmaniasis among organ transplant recipients. Lancet Infect Dis 8:191–199

Aronov AM, Suresh S, Buckner FS, Van Voorhis WC, Verlinde CL, Opperdoes FR, Hol WG, Gelb MH (1999) Structure-based design of submicromolar, biologically active inhibitors of trypanosomatid glyceraldehyde-3-phosphate dehydrogenase. Proc Natl Acad Sci U S A 96:4273–4278

Bentwich Z (2003) Concurrent infections that rise the HIV viral load. J HIV Ther 8:72–75

Bernier R, Turco SJ, Olivier M, Tremblay M (1995) Activation of human immunodeficiency virus type 1 in monocytoid cells by the protozoan parasite *Leishmania donovani*. J Virol 69:7282–7285

Boite MC, Mauricio IL, Miles MA, Cupolillo E (2012) New insights on taxonomy, phylogeny and population genetics of Leishmania (Viannia) parasites based on multilocus sequence analysis. PLoS Negl Trop Dis 6:e1888

Bose Dasgupta S, Ganguly A, Roy A, Mukherjee T, Majumder HK (2008) A novel ATP-binding cassette transporter, ABCG6 is involved in chemoresistance of Leishmania. Mol Biochem Parasitol 158:176–188

Brajtburg J, Powderly WG, Kobayashi GS, Medoff G (1990) Amphotericin B: current understanding of mechanisms of action. Antimicrob Agents Chemother 34:183–188

Brochu C, Wang J, Roy G, Messier N, Wang XY, Saravia NG, Ouellette M (2003) Antimony uptake systems in the protozoan parasite Leishmania and accumulation differences in antimony-resistant parasites. Antimicrob Agents Chemother 47:3073–3079

Bryceson A (2001) A policy for leishmaniasis with respect to the prevention and control of drug resistance. Trop Med Int Health 6:928–934

Bucheton B, Abel L, El-Safi S, Kheir MM, Pavek S, Lemainque A, Dessein AJ (2003) A major susceptibility locus on chromosome 22q12 plays a critical role in the control of kala-azar. Am J Hum Genet 73:1052–1060

Castanys-Munoz E, Alder-Baerens N, Pomorski T, Gamarro F, Castanys S (2007) A novel ATP-binding cassette transporter from Leishmania is involved in transport of phosphatidylcholine analogues and resistance to alkyl-phospholipids. Mol Microbiol 64:1141–1153

Castanys-Munoz E, Perez-Victoria JM, Gamarro F, Castanys S (2008) Characterization of an ABCG-like transporter from the protozoan parasite Leishmania with a role in drug resistance and transbilayer lipid movement. Antimicrob Agents Chemother 52:3573–3579

Chawla B, Jhingran A, Panigrahi A, Stuart KD, Madhubala R (2011) Paromomycin affects translation and vesicle-mediated trafficking as revealed by proteomics of paromomycin -susceptible -resistant *Leishmania donovani*. PLoS One 6:e26660

Cockburn R, Newton PN, Agyarko EK, Akunyili D, White NJ (2005) The global threat of counterfeit drugs: why industry and governments must communicate the dangers. PLoS Med 2:e100

Coelho AC, Boisvert S, Mukherjee A, Leprohon P, Corbeil J, Ouellette M (2012) Multiple mutations in heterogeneous miltefosine-resistant Leishmania major population as determined by whole genome sequencing. PLoS Negl Trop Dis 6:e1512

Corona P, Gibellini F, Cavalli A, Saxena P, Carta A, Loriga M, Luciani R, Paglietti G, Guerrieri D, Nerini E, Gupta S, Hannaert V, Michels PA, Ferrari S, Costi PM (2012) Structure-based selectivity optimization of piperidine-pteridine derivatives as potent Leishmania pteridine reductase inhibitors. J Med Chem 55:8318–8329

Costa CH, Peters NC, Maruyama SR, de Brito EC, Santos IK (2011) Vaccines for the leishmaniases: proposals for a research agenda. PLoS Negl Trop Dis 5:e943

Cruz I, Morales MA, Noguer I, Rodriguez A, Alvar J (2002) Leishmania in discarded syringes from intravenous drug users. Lancet 359:1124–1125

Delobel P, Launois P, Djossou F, Sainte-Marie D, Pradinaud R (2003) American cutaneous leishmaniasis, lepromatous leprosy, and pulmonary tuberculosis coinfection with downregulation of the T-helper 1 cell response. Clin Infect Dis 37:628–633

Dey S, Ouellette M, Lightbody J, Papadopoulou B, Rosen BP (1996) An ATP-dependent as(III)-glutathione transport system in membrane vesicles of Leishmania tarentolae. Proc Natl Acad Sci U S A 93:2192–2197

Downing T, Imamura H, Decuypere S, Clark TG, Coombs GH, Cotton JA, Hilley JD, de Doncker S, Maes I, Mottram JC, Quail MA, Rijal S, Sanders M, Schonian G, Stark O, Sundar S, Vanaerschot M, Hertz-Fowler C, Dujardin JC, Berriman M (2011) Whole genome sequencing of multiple *Leishmania donovani* clinical isolates provides insights into population structure and mechanisms of drug resistance. Genome Res 21:2143–2156

Escobar P, Matu S, Marques C, Croft SL (2002) Sensitivities of Leishmania species to hexadecylphosphocholine (miltefosine), ET-18-OCH(3) (edelfosine) and amphotericin B. Acta Trop 81:151–157

Farouk S, Salih MA, Musa AM, Blackwell JM, Miller EN, Khalil EA, Elhassan AM, Ibrahim ME, Mohamed HS (2010) Interleukin 10 gene polymorphisms and development of post kala-azar dermal leishmaniasis in a selected Sudanese population. Public Health Genomics 13:362–367

Fernandes Rodrigues JC, Concepcion JL, Rodrigues C, Caldera A, Urbina JA, de Souza W (2008) In vitro activities of ER-119884 and E5700, two potent squalene synthase inhibitors, against

Leishmania amazonensis: antiproliferative, biochemical, and ultrastructural effects. Antimicrob Agents Chemother 52:4098–4114

Fernandez MM, Malchiodi EL, Algranati ID (2011) Differential effects of paromomycin on ribosomes of *Leishmania mexicana* and mammalian cells. Antimicrob Agents Chemother 55:86–93

Fish WR, Marr JJ, Berens RL, Looker DL, Nelson DJ, LaFon SW, Balber AE (1985) Inosine analogs as chemotherapeutic agents for African trypanosomes: metabolism in trypanosomes and efficacy in tissue culture. Antimicrob Agents Chemother 27:33–36

Gourbal B, Sonuc N, Bhattacharjee H, Legare D, Sundar S, Ouellette M, Rosen BP, Mukhopadhyay R (2004) Drug uptake and modulation of drug resistance in Leishmania by an aquaglyceroporin. J Biol Chem 279:31010–31017

Grogl M, Daugirda JL, Hoover DL, Magill AJ, Berman JD (1993) Survivability and infectivity of viscerotropic Leishmania tropica from operation desert storm participants in human blood products maintained under blood bank conditions. Am J Trop Med Hyg 49:308–315

Gupta A, Nagar M, Mishra SS, Lahariya C (2013) Visceral leishmaniasis (Kala Azar) elimination from Indian Sub-continent by 2015. Int J Trop Dis Health 3:73–81

Ilari A, Baiocco P, Messori L, Fiorillo A, Boffi A, Gramiccia M, Di Muccio T, Colotti G (2012) A gold-containing drug against parasitic polyamine metabolism: the X-ray structure of trypanothione reductase from Leishmania infantum in complex with auranofin reveals a dual mechanism of enzyme inhibition. Amino Acids 42:803–811

Imbert L, Ramos RG, Libong D, Abreu S, Loiseau PM, Chaminade P (2012) Identification of phospholipid species affected by miltefosine action in *Leishmania donovani* cultures using LC-ELSD, LC-ESI/MS, and multivariate data analysis. Anal Bioanal Chem 402:1169–1182

Ingolia NT, Brar GA, Rouskin S, McGeachy AM, Weissman JS (2012) The ribosome profiling strategy for monitoring translation in vivo by deep sequencing of ribosome-protected mRNA fragments. Nat Protoc 7:1534–1550

Kaye P, Scott P (2011) Leishmaniasis: complexity at the host-pathogen interface. Nat Rev Microbiol 9:604–615

Kelly RJ, Robey RW, Chen CC, Draper D, Luchenko V, Barnett D, Oldham RK, Caluag Z, Frye AR, Steinberg SM, Fojo T, Bates SE (2012) A pharmacodynamic study of the P-glycoprotein antagonist CBT-1(R) in combination with paclitaxel in solid tumors. Oncologist 17:512

Khalili G, Dobakhti F, Mahmoudzadeh-Niknam H, Khaze V, Partovi F (2011) Immunotherapy with imiquimod increases the efficacy of glucantime therapy of Leishmania major infection. Iran J Immunol 8:45–51

King CH, Bertino AM (2008) Asymmetries of poverty: why global burden of disease valuations underestimate the burden of neglected tropical diseases. PLoS Negl Trop Dis 2:e209

Kobets T, Grekov I, Lipoldova M (2012) Leishmaniasis: prevention, parasite detection and treatment. Curr Med Chem 19:1443–1474

Kumar D, Kulshrestha A, Singh R, Salotra P (2009) In vitro susceptibility of field isolates of *Leishmania donovani* to Miltefosine and amphotericin B: correlation with sodium antimony gluconate susceptibility and implications for treatment in areas of endemicity. Antimicrob Agents Chemother 53:835–838

Lachaud L, Bourgeois N, Plourde M, Leprohon P, Bastien P, Ouellette M (2009) Parasite susceptibility to amphotericin B in failures of treatment for visceral leishmaniasis in patients coinfected with HIV type 1 and leishmania infantum. Clin Infect Dis 48:e16–e22

Legare D, Richard D, Mukhopadhyay R, Stierhof YD, Rosen BP, Haimeur A, Papadopoulou B, Ouellette M (2001) The Leishmania ATP-binding cassette protein PGPA is an intracellular metal-thiol transporter ATPase. J Biol Chem 276:26301–26307

Lemke A, Kiderlen AF, Kayser O (2005) Amphotericin B. Appl Microbiol Biotechnol 68:151–162

Loiseau PM, Cojean S, Schrevel J (2011) Sitamaquine as a putative antileishmanial drug candidate: from the mechanism of action to the risk of drug resistance. Parasite 18:115–119

Luque-Ortega JR, Rivas L (2007) Miltefosine (hexadecylphosphocholine) inhibits cytochrome c oxidase in *Leishmania donovani* promastigotes. Antimicrob Agents Chemother 51:1327–1332

Mackey TK, Liang BA (2011) The global counterfeit drug trade: patient safety and public health risks. J Pharm Sci 100:4571–4579

Maizels N, Gray LT (2013) The G4 genome. PLoS Genet 9:e1003468

Manzano JI, Garcia-Hernandez R, Castanys S, Gamarro F (2013) A new ABC half-transporter in Leishmania major is involved in resistance to antimony. Antimicrob Agents Chemother 57:3719–3730

Marquis N, Gourbal B, Rosen BP, Mukhopadhyay R, Ouellette M (2005) Modulation in aquaglyceroporin AQP1 gene transcript levels in drug-resistant Leishmania. Mol Microbiol 57:1690–1699

Mbongo N, Loiseau PM, Billion MA, Robert-Gero M (1998) Mechanism of amphotericin B resistance in *Leishmania donovani* promastigotes. Antimicrob Agents Chemother 42:352–357

Mittal MK, Rai S, Ashutosh R, Gupta S, Sundar S, Goyal N (2007) Characterization of natural antimony resistance in *Leishmania donovani* isolates. Am J Trop Med Hyg 76:681–688

Mock DJ, Hollenbaugh JA, Daddacha W, Overstreet MG, Lazarski CA, Fowell DJ, Kim B (2012) Leishmania induces survival, proliferation and elevated cellular dNTP levels in human monocytes promoting acceleration of HIV co-infection. PLoS Pathog 8:e1002635

Mohamed HS, Ibrahim ME, Miller EN, Peacock CS, Khalil EA, Cordell HJ, Howson JM, El Hassan AM, Bereir RE, Blackwell JM (2003) Genetic susceptibility to visceral leishmaniasis in the Sudan: linkage and association with IL4 and IFNGR1. Genes Immun 4:351–355

Mohamed HS, Ibrahim ME, Miller EN, White JK, Cordell HJ, Howson JM, Peacock CS, Khalil EA, El Hassan AM, Blackwell JM (2004) SLC11A1 (formerly NRAMP1) and susceptibility to visceral leishmaniasis in the Sudan. Eur J Hum Genet 12:66–74

Mukherjee A, Padmanabhan PK, Singh S, Roy G, Girard I, Chatterjee M, Ouellette M, Madhubala R (2007) Role of ABC transporter MRPA, gamma-glutamylcysteine synthetase and ornithine decarboxylase in natural antimony-resistant isolates of *Leishmania donovani*. J Antimicrob Chemother 59:204–211

Mukherjee A, Boisvert S, Monte-Neto RL, Coelho AC, Raymond F, Mukhopadhyay R, Corbeil J, Ouellette M (2013a) Telomeric gene deletion and intrachromosomal amplification in antimony-resistant Leishmania. Mol Microbiol 88:189–202

Mukherjee B, Mukhopadhyay R, Bannerjee B, Chowdhury S, Mukherjee S, Naskar K, Allam US, Chakravortty D, Sundar S, Dujardin JC, Roy S (2013b) Antimony-resistant but not antimony-sensitive *Leishmania donovani* up-regulates host IL-10 to overexpress multidrug-resistant protein 1. Proc Natl Acad Sci U S A 110:E575–E582

Orsini M, Canela JR, Disch J, Maciel F, Greco D, Toledo A Jr, Rabello A (2012) High frequency of asymptomatic Leishmania spp. Infection among HIV-infected patients living in endemic areas for visceral leishmaniasis in Brazil. Trans R Soc Trop Med Hyg 106:283–288

Palatnik-de-Sousa CB (2008) Vaccines for leishmaniasis in the fore coming 25 years. Vaccine 26:1709–1724

Perez-Victoria JM, Perez-Victoria FJ, Parodi-Talice A, Jimenez IA, Ravelo AG, Castanys S, Gamarro F (2001) Alkyl-lysophospholipid resistance in multidrug-resistant Leishmania tropica and chemosensitization by a novel P-glycoprotein-like transporter modulator. Antimicrob Agents Chemother 45:2468–2474

Perez-Victoria FJ, Castanys S, Gamarro F (2003) Leishmania donovani resistance to miltefosine involves a defective inward translocation of the drug. Antimicrob Agents Chemother 47:2397–2403

Perez-Victoria FJ, Sanchez-Canete MP, Castanys S, Gamarro F (2006a) Phospholipid translocation and miltefosine potency require both *L. donovani* miltefosine transporter and the new protein LdRos3 in Leishmania parasites. J Biol Chem 281:23766–23775

Perez-Victoria FJ, Sanchez-Canete MP, Seifert K, Croft SL, Sundar S, Castanys S, Gamarro F (2006b) Mechanisms of experimental resistance of Leishmania to miltefosine: implications for clinical use. Drug Resist Updat 9:26–39

Perez-Victoria JM, Bavchvarov BI, Torrecillas IR, Martinez-Garcia M, Lopez-Martin C, Campillo M, Castanys S, Gamarro F (2011) Sitamaquine overcomes ABC-mediated

resistance to miltefosine and antimony in Leishmania. Antimicrob Agents Chemother 55:3838–3844
Perry MR, Wyllie S, Prajapati VK, Feldmann J, Sundar S, Boelaert M, Fairlamb AH (2011) Visceral leishmaniasis and arsenic: an ancient poison contributing to antimonial treatment failure in the Indian subcontinent? PLoS Negl Trop Dis 5:e1227
Pradines B (2013) P-glycoprotein-like transporters in Leishmania: a search for reversal agents. In: Ponte-Sucre A, Diaz E, Padròn-Nieves M. Ponte-Sucre A (ed) Drug resistance in Leishmania parasites. Springer, Vienna
Purkait B, Kumar A, Nandi N, Sardar AH, Das S, Kumar S, Pandey K, Ravidas V, Kumar M, De T, Singh D, Das P (2012) Mechanism of amphotericin B resistance in clinical isolates of *Leishmania donovani*. Antimicrob Agents Chemother 56:1031–1041
Rajasekaran R, Chen YP (2012) Probing the structure of Leishmania major DHFR TS and structure based virtual screening of peptide library for the identification of anti-leishmanial leads. J Mol Model 18:4089–4100
Ramos H, Valdivieso E, Gamargo M, Dagger F, Cohen BE (1996) Amphotericin B kills unicellular leishmanias by forming aqueous pores permeable to small cations and anions. J Membr Biol 152:65–75
Rathnayake D, Ranawake RR, Sirimanna G, Siriwardhane Y, Karunaweera N, De Silva R (2010) Co-infection of mucosal leishmaniasis and extra pulmonary tuberculosis in a patient with inherent immune deficiency. Int J Dermatol 49:549–551
Requena JM (2011) Lights and shadows on gene organization and regulation of gene expression in Leishmania. Front Biosci 16:2069–2085
Rijal S, Ostyn B, Uranw S, Rai K, Bhattarai NR, Dorlo TP, Beijnen JH, Vanaerschot M, Decuypere S, Dhakal SS, Das ML, Karki P, Singh R, Boelaert M, Dujardin JC (2013) Increasing failure of miltefosine in the treatment of kala-azar in Nepal and the potential role of parasite drug resistance, reinfection, or noncompliance. Clin Infect Dis 56:1530–1538
Robey RW, Shukla S, Finley EM, Oldham RK, Barnett D, Ambudkar SV, Fojo T, Bates SE (2008) Inhibition of P-glycoprotein (ABCB1)- and multidrug resistance-associated protein 1 (ABCC1)-mediated transport by the orally administered inhibitor, CBT-1((R)). Biochem Pharmacol 75:1302–1312
el-Safi SH, Hamid N, Omer A, Abdel-Haleem A, Hammad A, Kareem HG, Boelaert M (2004) Infection rates with *Leishmania donovani* and *Mycobacterium tuberculosis* in a village in eastern Sudan. Trop Med Int Health 9:1305–1311
Saha S, Mondal S, Ravindran R, Bhowmick S, Modak D, Mallick S, Rahman M, Kar S, Goswami R, Guha SK, Pramanik N, Saha B, Ali N (2007) IL-10- and TGF-beta-mediated susceptibility in kala-azar and post-kala-azar dermal leishmaniasis: the significance of amphotericin B in the control of *Leishmania donovani* infection in India. J Immunol 179:5592–5603
Salih MA, Ibrahim ME, Blackwell JM, Miller EN, Khalil EA, ElHassan AM, Musa AM, Mohamed HS (2007) IFNG and IFNGR1 gene polymorphisms and susceptibility to post-kala-azar dermal leishmaniasis in Sudan. Genes Immun 8:75–78
Santos LO, Vitorio BS, Branquinha MH, Pedroso e Silva CM, Santos AL, d'Avila-Levy CM (2013) Nelfinavir is effective in inhibiting the multiplication and aspartic peptidase activity of Leishmania species, including strains obtained from HIV-positive patients. J Antimicrob Chemother 68:348–353
Seifert K, Perez-Victoria FJ, Stettler M, Sanchez-Canete MP, Castanys S, Gamarro F, Croft SL (2007) Inactivation of the miltefosine transporter, LdMT, causes miltefosine resistance that is conferred to the amastigote stage of *Leishmania donovani* and persists in vivo. Int J Antimicrob Agents 30:229–235
Shaked-Mishan P, Ulrich N, Ephros M, Zilberstein D (2001) Novel intracellular SbV reducing activity correlates with antimony susceptibility in *Leishmania donovani*. J Biol Chem 276:3971–3976

Singh N (2006) Drug resistance mechanisms in clinical isolates of *Leishmania donovani*. Indian J Med Res 123:411–422

Singh N, Singh RT, Sundar S (2003) Novel mechanism of drug resistance in kala azar field isolates. J Infect Dis 188:600–607

Singh R, Kumar D, Duncan RC, Nakhasi HL, Salotra P (2010) Overexpression of histone H2A modulates drug susceptibility in Leishmania parasites. Int J Antimicrob Agents 36:50–57

Singh N, Kumar M, Singh RK (2012) Leishmaniasis: current status of available drugs and new potential drug targets. Asian Pac J Trop Med 5:485–497

Srivastava P, Prajapati VK, Rai M, Sundar S (2011) Unusual case of resistance to amphotericin B in visceral leishmaniasis in a region in India where leishmaniasis is not endemic. J Clin Microbiol 49:3088–3091

Sun YL, Chen JJ, Kumar P, Chen K, Sodani K, Patel A, Chen YL, Chen SD, Jiang WQ, Chen ZS (2013) Reversal of MRP7 (ABCC10)-mediated multidrug resistance by tariquidar. PLoS One 8: e55576

Sundar S, Chakravarty J (2013) Leishmaniasis: an update of current pharmacotherapy. Expert Opin Pharmacother 14:53–63

Sundar S, Singh A, Rai M, Prajapati VK, Singh AK, Ostyn B, Boelaert M, Dujardin JC, Chakravarty J (2012) Efficacy of miltefosine in the treatment of visceral leishmaniasis in India after a decade of use. Clin Infect Dis 55:543–550

Trejo WH, Bennett RE (1963) Streptomyces nodosus sp. n., the amphotericin-producing organism. J Bacteriol 85:436–439

Urbina JA, Cohen BE, Perozo E, Cornivelli L (1987) Spin-labeled amphotericin B: synthesis, characterization, biological and spectroscopic properties. Biochim Biophys Acta 897:467–473

Vanaerschot M, Decuypere S, Downing T, Imamura H, Stark O, De Doncker S, Roy S, Ostyn B, Maes L, Khanal B, Boelaert M, Schonian G, Berriman M, Chappuis F, Dujardin JC, Sundar S, Rijal S (2012) Genetic markers for SSG resistance in *Leishmania donovani* and SSG treatment failure in visceral leishmaniasis patients of the Indian subcontinent. J Infect Dis 206:752–755

Venkatesan SK, Dubey VK (2012) Footprinting of inhibitor interactions of in silico identified inhibitors of trypanothione reductase of Leishmania parasite. Sci World J 2012:963658

Vergnes B, Gourbal B, Girard I, Sundar S, Drummelsmith J, Ouellette M (2007) A proteomics screen implicates HSP83 and a small kinetoplastid calpain-related protein in drug resistance in *Leishmania donovani* clinical field isolates by modulating drug-induced programmed cell death. Mol Cell Proteomics 6:88–101

Vieira M, Rohloff P, Luo S, Cunha-e-Silva NL, de Souza W, Docampo R (2005) Role for a P-type H + –ATPase in the acidification of the endocytic pathway of *Trypanosoma cruzi*. Biochem J 392:467–474

Wang J, Vanley C, Miyamoto E, Turner JA, Peng SK (1999) Coinfection of visceral leishmaniasis and Mycobacterium in a patient with acquired immunodeficiency syndrome. Arch Pathol Lab Med 123:835–837

Wasan KM, Wasan EK, Gershkovich P, Zhu X, Tidwell RR, Werbovetz KA, Clement JG, Thornton SJ (2009) Highly effective oral amphotericin B formulation against murine visceral leishmaniasis. J Infect Dis 200:357–360

Wasan EK, Gershkovich P, Zhao J, Zhu X, Werbovetz K, Tidwell RR, Clement JG, Thornton SJ, Wasan KM (2010) A novel tropically stable oral amphotericin B formulation (iCo-010) exhibits efficacy against visceral Leishmaniasis in a murine model. PLoS Negl Trop Dis 4:e913

WHO (2010) Control of the leishmaniases. World Health Organ Tech Rep Ser: xii–xiii, pp 1–186

Wolday D, Akuffo H, Demissie A, Britton S (1999) Role of *Leishmania donovani* and its lipophosphoglycan in CD4+ T-cell activation-induced human immunodeficiency virus replication. Infect Immun 67:5258–5264

Wyllie S, Patterson S, Stojanovski L, Simeons FR, Norval S, Kime R, Read KD, Fairlamb AH (2012) The anti-trypanosome drug fexinidazole shows potential for treating visceral leishmaniasis. Sci Transl Med 4(119):119re111

Yardley V, Gamarro F, Croft SL (2010) Antileishmanial and antitrypanosomal activities of the 8-aminoquinoline tafenoquine. Antimicrob Agents Chemother 54:5356–5358
Zijlstra EE, el-Hassan AM, Ismael A (1995) Endemic kala-azar in eastern Sudan: post-kala-azar dermal leishmaniasis. Am J Trop Med Hyg 52:299–305
Zijlstra EE, Khalil EA, Kager PA, El-Hassan AM (2000) Post-kala-azar dermal leishmaniasis in the Sudan: clinical presentation and differential diagnosis. Br J Dermatol 143:136–143
Zijlstra EE, Musa AM, Khalil EA, el-Hassan IM, el-Hassan AM (2003) Post-kala-azar dermal leishmaniasis. Lancet Infect Dis 3:87–98
Zucca M, Scutera S, Savoia D (2013) New chemotherapeutic strategies against malaria, leishmaniasis and trypanosomiases. Curr Med Chem 20:502–526

Part IV

Mycology

Microevolution of Antifungal Drug Resistance

Leah E. Cowen

Contents

Abstract

The evolution of drug resistance in fungal pathogens threatens the utility of the limited number of antifungal drugs available to treat life-threatening invasive fungal infections. Fungal infections are on the rise with the increasing populations of individuals with impaired immune function who are most vulnerable to the opportunistic pathogens. Most antifungal drugs target the distinct composition of

L.E. Cowen (✉)
Department of Molecular Genetics, University of Toronto, Toronto, ON, Canada
e-mail: leah.cowen@utoronto.ca

M. Gotte et al. (eds.), *Handbook of Antimicrobial Resistance*,
DOI 10.1007/978-1-4939-0694-9_19

the fungal cell membrane (azoles and polyenes) or the fungal cell wall (echinocandins). Mortality rates associated with invasive fungal infections often exceed 50 % even with current treatment options, demanding new strategies to minimize the evolution of resistance and reverse it once it has evolved. This chapter focuses on the evolution of drug resistance in the leading human fungal pathogens, including species of *Candida, Aspergillus*, and *Cryptococcus*. The emphasis is on the microevolution of drug resistance that occurs on timescales relevant to experimental populations and human hosts receiving treatment. The relevant agents of selection are introduced, followed by a discussion of the diversity in drug resistance phenotypes, the scope of adaptive mechanisms, the fitness consequences of drug resistance, and strategies to thwart the evolution of drug resistance.

Keywords
Antifungal drug resistance • Fungal pathogen • Azole • Echinocandin • Stress response • Hsp-90 • Fitness • Experimental evolution • Microevolution • *Candida* • *Cryptococcus* • *Aspergillus*

Introduction

The emergence of drug resistance provides one of the most poignant examples of microevolution with a severe impact on human health. It is a ubiquitous process in nature, as microbes produce a dazzling array of small molecules that exert selection for resistance in neighboring microbial communities (Allen et al. 2010; Wright 2007, 2012). The rate at which resistance evolves has been accelerated by the widespread use of antimicrobial agents in medicine and agriculture, which selects for organisms capable of survival and reproduction despite drug exposure (Anderson 2005; Davies and Davies 2010). As a consequence, the rapid emergence of drug resistance in diverse pathogen populations now threatens the utility of many of the drugs that we critically depend on. The annual economic cost of the evolution of drug resistance is staggering, and in the United States alone, it is in excess of $33 billion to cover treatment of patients with drug-resistant infections, to manage resistant plant pathogens, and to compensate for crop loss to resistant pests (Palumbi 2001).

The evolution of drug resistance is an acute problem in the context of fungal pathogens. Fungal pathogens are eukaryotes and closely related to their human hosts, which limits the number of drug targets that can be selectively inhibited in the pathogen (Cowen 2008). Consequently, there are a limited number of clinically useful antifungal drugs to treat the increasing incidence of fungal infections worldwide. The global impact of fungal pathogens on human health remains largely unappreciated. They can cause life-threatening invasive infections in immunocompromised individuals, as well as in healthy hosts (Pfaller and Diekema 2004, 2010). The incidence of fungal bloodstream infections has increased by 207 % in recent decades, along with the growing population of individuals with impaired immune function, such as those undergoing immunosuppressive therapy for transplants or chemotherapy for cancer, as well as those infected with HIV (Martin et al. 2003;

Pfaller and Diekema 2007). Despite the latest therapeutic options, invasive fungal infections are associated with mortality rates in excess of 50 %, and fungal pathogens kill as many people as tuberculosis or malaria worldwide (Brown et al. 2012a, b). The majority of all deaths due to fungal infection are due to species of *Candida*, *Aspergillus*, and *Cryptococcus*.

Here, we focus on the evolution of drug resistance in the leading fungal pathogens of humans. We explore the microevolution of drug resistance as it operates on timescales that can be observed in experimental populations or in human hosts undergoing treatment. We introduce the relevant agents of selection, diversity in drug resistance phenotypes, adaptive mechanisms, fitness consequences, and strategies to thwart the evolution of drug resistance.

Agents of Selection

Antifungal drug targets must be sufficiently divergent between fungal pathogens and their human hosts to enable selective inhibition in the pathogen, thereby minimizing host toxicity. The majority of clinically relevant antifungal drugs exploit the distinct plasma membrane composition of fungi and target ergosterol or its biosynthesis (Fig. 1). Ergosterol is analogous to cholesterol in mammals, and serves to modulate membrane integrity and fluidity, and the function of enzymes; anchored in the membrane (Ostrosky-Zeichner et al. 2010; Shapiro et al. 2011). The fungal cell wall provides other attractive antifungal drug targets (Fig. 1), as it is not conserved in mammals. Fungal cell walls are rigid structures composed of covalent linkages of (1,3)-β-D-glucans with (1,6)-β-D-glucans and chitin (Netea et al. 2008; Tada et al. 2013). Here, we focus on the antifungal drugs currently employed to treat the most prevalent fungal infections.

Azoles

The azoles have been the most broadly and extensively used class of antifungal drug in recent decades. They include both imidazoles and triazoles and are five-membered, nitrogen-containing, heterocyclic compounds that inhibit ergosterol biosynthesis (Cowen and Steinbach 2008; Odds et al. 2003). Imidazoles are restricted to topical formulations due to toxicity and bioavailability issues, while there are currently four triazoles available in oral or injection formats: fluconazole, itraconazole, voriconazole, and posaconazole, each with distinct pharmacokinetic properties. Isavuconazole is an additional triazole in clinical development. The azoles enter the fungal cell by facilitated diffusion (Mansfield et al. 2010) and inhibit the ergosterol biosynthetic enzyme lanosterol demethylase (a cytochrome P450), encoded by *ERG11* in *Candida* and *Cryptococcus* and by *cyp51A* and *cyp51B* in *Aspergillus*. In addition to blocking ergosterol biosynthesis, azoles cause accumulation of 14 α-methyl-3,6-diol, a toxic sterol produced by the Δ-5,6-desaturase encoded by *ERG3* (Shapiro et al. 2011). Azoles are effective against diverse fungi, including *Candida*, *Cryptococcus*, and

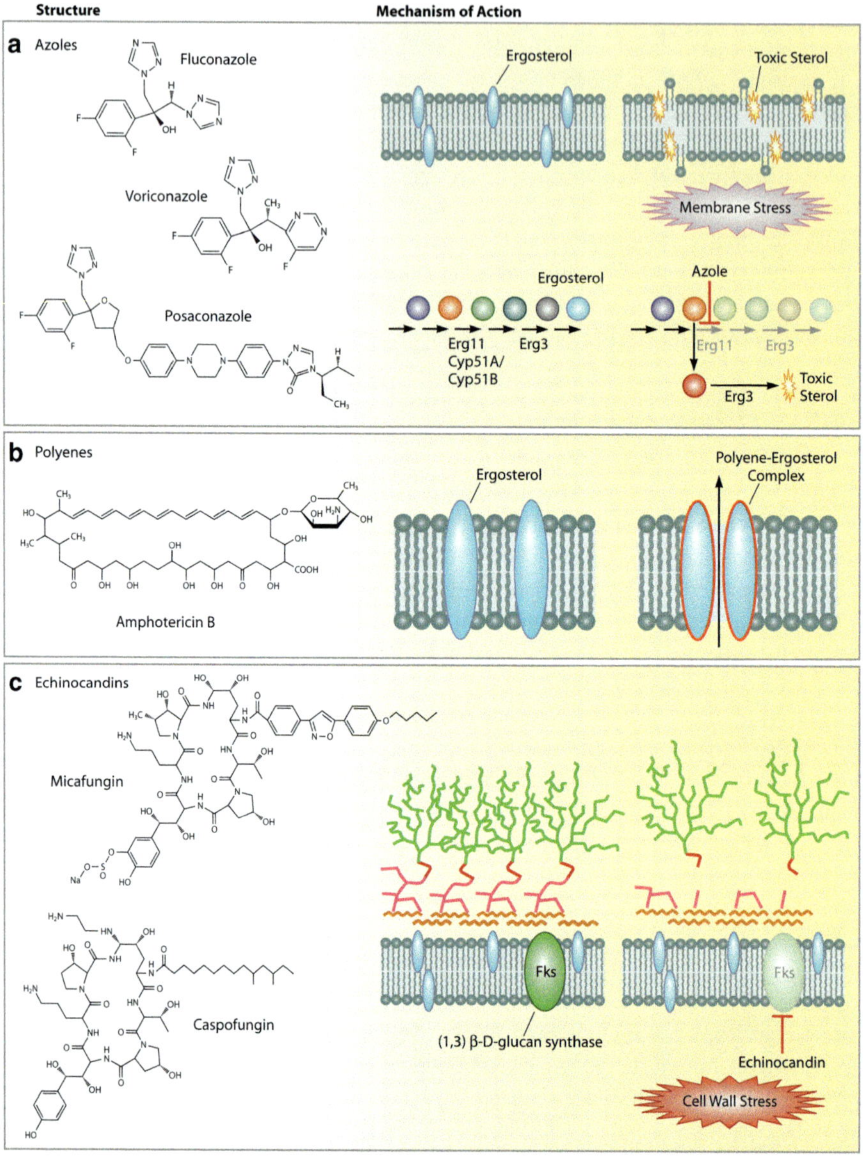

Fig. 1 Antifungal drugs and their targets. (**a**) The azoles inhibit the ergosterol biosynthesis enzyme lanosterol demethylase, which is encoded by *ERG11* in *Candida albicans* and *Cryptococcus neoformans* or by *cyp51A* and *cyp51B* in *Aspergillus fumigatus*, thereby blocking ergosterol production and leading to the accumulation of a toxic sterol produced by Erg3. (**b**) The polyenes bind to ergosterol creating drug-lipid complexes that intercalate into fungal cell membranes to form a membrane-spanning channel that causes leakage of cellular ions, destruction of the proton gradient, and ultimately osmotic cellular lysis. (**c**) The echinocandins inhibit (1,3)-β-D-glucan synthase, which is encoded by *FKS1* in *C. albicans*, *C. neoformans*, and *A. fumigatus* and by *FKS1* and *FKS2* in *Candida glabrata* and *Saccharomyces cerevisiae* (Reproduced by permission from Copyright © American Society for Microbiology [Microbiology and Molecular Biology Reviews, 75, 2011, 213–67 and ▶ 10.1128/MMBR.00045-10] (Shapiro et al. 2011))

Aspergillus species, as well as dimorphic fungi and dermatophytes. Posaconazole also has efficacy against zygomycetes (Alastruey-Izquierdo et al. 2009). The azoles typically exert fungistatic activity against yeasts, such as *Candida* species, and fungicidal activity against molds, such as *Aspergillus*. The fungistatic activity against yeasts generates strong selection on the surviving population that facilitates the evolution of azole resistance in the laboratory and in the clinic.

Polyenes

The polyenes have been in clinical use for over 50 years. These amphipathic drugs have both hydrophobic and hydrophilic moieties and exert fungicidal activity by binding to ergosterol to form drug-lipid complexes that intercalate into the cell membrane (Shapiro et al. 2011; Odds et al. 2003; Gruszecki et al. 2003). The resulting pores that span the membrane cause leakage of ions and destruction of the proton gradient. Nystatin is a commonly used polyene for superficial infections, and amphotericin B is a polyene that is effective against systemic fungal infections caused by species of *Candida*, *Cryptococcus*, and *Aspergillus*. The major limitation of polyenes is host toxicity, including renal dysfunction, which is likely a consequence of structural similarities between ergosterol and cholesterol (Fanos and Cataldi 2000). Toxicity can be mitigated by lipid-complexed formulations that can enhance fungal selectivity (Cifani et al. 2012). Polyene resistance has emerged in clinical cases, although it is not widespread, perhaps due to fitness costs of resistance mutations (Vincent et al. 2013).

Echinocandins

The echinocandins are the only new class of antifungal drug to enter clinical use in recent decades. There are currently three echinocandins on the market: caspofungin, micafungin, and anidulafungin. These large lipopeptide molecules are noncompetitive inhibitors of the fungal cell wall biosynthetic enzyme (1,3)-β-D-glucan synthase, leading to loss of cell wall integrity (Denning 2003; Turner et al. 2006). The echinocandins typically exert fungicidal activity against yeasts such as *Candida* species and fungistatic activity against molds such as *Aspergillus* species. Notably, echinocandins are not effective against *Cryptococcus neoformans* (Denning 2003). The echinocandins have little host toxicity and are the drug of choice for treatment of azole-resistant invasive fungal infections. Despite their relatively short history of clinical use, resistance has already begun to emerge in the clinic.

Other Antifungal Drugs

There are several additional antifungal drugs currently in clinical use or in development (Ostrosky-Zeichner et al. 2010; Pitman et al. 2011). The long-standing antifungal drug 5-flucytosine inhibits fungal nucleic acid biosynthesis; its efficacy is restricted by fungistatic activity and by the rapid emergence of resistance, and thus it is typically only prescribed in combinations with other antifungal drugs. Antifungals in development include sordarins and nikkomycin Z. Sordarins are semisynthetic natural products that inhibit protein biosynthesis by targeting fungal elongation factor 2. Nikkomycin Z impairs cell wall biosynthesis by competitively inhibiting chitin synthases.

Diversity in Drug Resistance

The emergence of antifungal drug resistance can manifest in a multitude of different forms. Antifungal drug resistance itself can be defined in distinct ways in clinical and laboratory contexts. In the clinical context, drug resistance is the persistence or progression of infection despite appropriate antifungal treatment (White et al. 1998). In the laboratory context, drug resistance is a continuous trait that is quantified using susceptibility assays, in which fungal growth is measured across a series of drug concentrations (Shapiro et al. 2011). The minimum inhibitory concentration (MIC) is the drug concentration that inhibits fungal growth by a defined amount, most often either 50 % or 90 %. There is extensive variation in response to antifungal drugs between fungal species, as well as between strains of the same species and even between cells of a single strain (Hill et al. 2012). Fungi can differ in their inherent capacity to survive antifungal drug exposure, referred to as basal tolerance when the drug has activity against the relevant fungal species (Shapiro et al. 2011). Tolerance can facilitate the evolution of drug resistance by enabling surviving cells to respond to selection and acquire resistance mutations. Here we focus on variation in antifungal drug resistance.

Perhaps most fascinating from the perspective of microevolution of antifungal drug resistance is variation within a population. In contrast to the largely stable diversity in resistance phenotypes observed between strains and species, variation within a population of cells is often more transient in nature. One intriguing example of variation in azole resistance in *Cryptococcus* is heteroresistance, which is the emergence of both azole-resistant and azole-susceptible cells from a susceptible progenitor (Sionov et al. 2009). In this case, resistance increases incrementally and is lost with passage in the absence of drug. The resistant cells tend to be disomic for chromosome 1, which harbors genes important for resistance such as those encoding the target of the azoles, *ERG11*, and an azole efflux transporter, *AFR1* (Sionov et al. 2010). The phenomenon of heteroresistance has also been reported for *Candida albicans* (Marr et al. 2001).

Another source of diversity in drug resistance within a population is heterogeneous resistance, which is a broad term for a phenomenon in fungi and bacteria that involves a susceptible population giving rise to resistant cells at a frequency of $\sim 10^{-1} - 10^{-4}$; the distinguishing feature is that the resistant cells reproducibly generate the same distribution of resistance phenotypes among their progeny as the original susceptible parent (White and Oliver 2004). Such heterogeneous resistance has been observed in *Candida*, as has the related phenomenon of high-frequency azole resistance in which some strains give rise to azole-resistant progeny at a frequency that is higher than the mutation rate (White and Oliver 2004). High-frequency azole resistance is associated with stable resistance phenotypes, which may be a result of altered mitochondrial function.

Diversity in drug resistance among genotypically identical cells is also prevalent in the clinic and in nature in the context of biofilms. Fungal biofilms are surface-associated communities that initiate upon adherence to specific surfaces such as plastics, catheters, and other medical devices (Blankenship and Mitchell 2006). Biofilms are surrounded by an extracellular matrix and are characterized by a level of antifungal drug resistance that vastly exceeds what is observed in their planktonic counterparts. Species of *Candida*, *Cryptococcus*, and *Aspergillus* all form drug-resistant biofilms that present a major clinical challenge (Ramage et al. 2009). There are numerous resistance mechanisms that operate in biofilms (d'Enfert 2006), but one of the most striking is the emergence of persister cells. Persister cells are phenotypic variants that can tolerate high drug concentrations (LaFleur et al. 2006). They arise from biofilms, which offer protection from the full impact of antifungal drugs and host immune response. While bacterial persisters are quiescent, the state of metabolic activity of fungal persisters remains unknown.

Adaptive Mechanisms

Antifungal drug resistance can evolve by numerous mechanisms including mutation or overexpression of the drug target, increased drug efflux, and activation of cellular stress responses (Fig. 2). High-level drug resistance observed in clinical isolates is often a consequence of the stepwise acquisition of multiple mechanisms, such as those discussed below.

Alteration of the Drug Target

A prevalent mechanism of resistance to diverse drugs is mutation of the drug target that impairs drug binding. In the context of azoles, numerous mutations in genes encoding the drug target (*ERG11* in *Candida* and *Cryptococcus* and *cyp51A* and *cyp51B* in *Aspergillus*) have been identified in mutational "hot spots" that cause amino acid substitutions in or adjacent to the active site (Alcazar-Fuoli et al. 2011; MacCallum et al. 2010; Pfaller 2012; Sionov et al. 2012; Lamb et al. 1997). These mutations are thought to reduce the azole binding affinity of the target lanosterol demethylase, thereby causing increased azole resistance. Increased dosage of the mutant allele is associated with elevated resistance, as is observed with loss of heterozygosity (White 1997a). In the context of echinocandins, the best characterized mechanism of resistance is mutations in hot spots of the genes *FKS1* and *FKS2*, which encode the catalytic subunit of the target glucan synthase (Perlin 2007). These mutations reduce sensitivity of the enzyme to inhibition by echinocandins

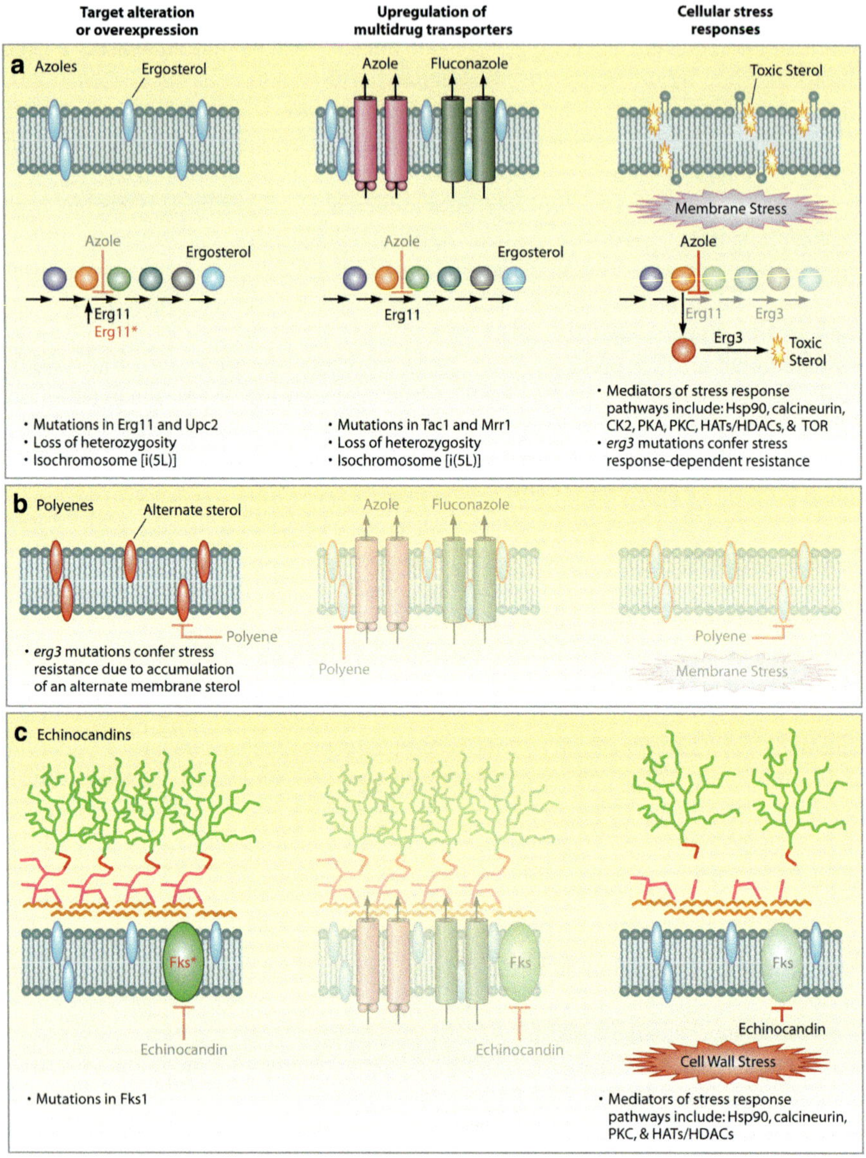

Fig. 2 Drug resistance mechanisms of *C. albicans*. (**a**) Resistance to azoles can arise by multiple mechanisms including overexpression or alteration of the drug target Erg11 and overexpression of the multidrug efflux transporters Cdr1, Cdr2, or Mdr1 or by modulation of cellular stress responses. (**b**) Resistance to polyenes can be caused by loss of function of Erg3, which blocks the production of ergosterol, thereby inhibiting the formation of the drug-lipid complex that causes osmotic cellular lysis. Drug transporters do not have a major impact on polyene resistance, and stress responses have not been identified as key resistance determinants. (**c**) Resistance to echinocandins is most often due to mutations in two hot-spot regions of *FKS1*. Drug transporters do have a major impact on resistance, although cellular stress responses do. Bright images indicate important mechanisms of

(Garcia-Effron et al. 2009), and their phenotypic effect is amplified with increased dosage of the resistance alleles (Niimi et al. 2010).

Overexpression of the Drug Target

Elevated resistance can also result from increased drug target expression. This has been studied extensively in *C. albicans*, where overexpression of *ERG11* can be attributed to gain-of-function mutations in the transcription factor encoded by *UPC2*, which controls expression of ergosterol biosynthesis genes (Dunkel et al. 2008a; Hoot et al. 2011). Mutations in the C-terminal region *UPC2* are associated with azole resistance, which is amplified with increased dosage of the mutant allele (Dunkel et al. 2008a; Hoot et al. 2011; Heilmann et al. 2010). In *Candida glabrata* there are two *UPC2* homologs, which influence azole susceptibility (Nagi et al. 2011). In many other Ascomycetes and in Basidiomycetes such as *C. neoformans*, transcriptional control of ergosterol biosynthesis genes is regulated by an SREBP-like transcription factor Sre1 (Bien and Espenshade 2010), which has functional homology to the mammalian cholesterol regulatory transcription factor SREBP. In *Aspergillus fumigatus*, SrbA is the SREBP homolog that controls sterol biosynthesis (Willger et al. 2008). SrbA influences cellular responses to azoles, as do genes implicated in SrbA regulation (Willger et al. 2008, 2012). The SREBP-like proteins of *C. neoformans* and *A. fumigatus* influence not only sterol biosynthesis but are also implicated in virulence in animal models.

Increased Drug Efflux

A pervasive mechanism of drug resistance is overexpression of drug efflux transporters leading to reduced intracellular drug concentration. In terms of antifungal drugs, increased efflux has the greatest impact on resistance to azoles (Cannon et al. 2009; Morschhauser 2010). In *C. albicans*, the ATP-dependent transporters Cdr1 and Cdr2 and the major facilitator Mdr1 are key for azole efflux. Transcriptional upregulation of *CDR1* and *CDR2* can be achieved by gain-of-function mutations in the transcription factor encoded by *TAC1*; such mutations are often homozygous in azole-resistant clinical isolates (Coste et al. 2006, 2004). Activation of *CDR1* transcription is also influenced by the transcription factor Ndt80 (Wang et al. 2006), while *MDR1* expression is controlled by the transcription factor Mrr1 (Dunkel et al. 2008b). Considerable advances have been made in understanding the

Fig. 2 (continued) resistance, while dimmed images are those mechanisms that have little impact on resistance to the relevant drug class (Reproduced by permission from Copyright © American Society for Microbiology [Microbiology and Molecular Biology Reviews, 75, 2011, 213–67 and ▸ 10.1128/MMBR.00045-10] (Shapiro et al. 2011)) circuitry through which transcriptional control of drug efflux transporters is achieved in *C. albicans* (Mogavero et al. 2011; Sasse et al. 2012a; Schubert et al. 2011; Dhamgaye et al. 2012; Shukla et al. 2011).

Increased efflux of antifungal drugs is also a prevalent resistance mechanism in other fungi. In *C. neoformans*, reduced azole susceptibility can be attributed to overexpression of the efflux transporters encoded by *AFR1* and *MDR1* (Heilmann et al. 2010). In *A. fumigatus* overexpression of *atrF*, which encodes an ABC transporter, is associated with azole resistance (Sionov et al. 2010). Reduced intracellular azole accumulation may also arise from reduced drug import, as azoles enter fungal cells by facilitated diffusion and some azole-resistant clinical isolates have reduced azole import relative to the majority of susceptible isolates (Mansfield et al. 2010).

Genomic Plasticity

The emergence of antifungal drug resistance is associated with multiple genomic alterations, likely due to the resulting increase in dosage of relevant resistance determinants. *C. albicans* azole-resistant clinical isolates have an elevated incidence of aneuploidies, the most common of which involves chromosome 5. Recombination events at a breakpoint in repetitive sequences flanking the centromere generate an isochromosome with two left arms of chromosome 5, i5L (Selmecki et al. 2006). Azole resistance due to i5L is attributable to duplication of *ERG11* and *TAC1*, which are located on the left arm of chromosome 5 (Selmecki et al. 2008). Azole resistance in *C. neoformans* can also arise by duplication of chromosome 1, where the drug target gene *ERG11* and drug transporter gene *AFR1* reside (Sionov et al. 2010).

Activation of Cellular Stress Responses

Cellular stress response pathways have a profound impact on the evolution of antifungal drug resistance. Diverse signaling pathways are crucial for sensing and responding to the stress exerted by antifungal drug exposure (Cowen and Steinbach 2008; Cannon et al. 2007). One of the key examples of a global regulator of cellular stress responses required for basal tolerance and resistance to antifungal drugs is the molecular chaperone Hsp90. Inhibition of Hsp90 abrogates resistance to azoles and echinocandins in diverse fungi and can block the evolution of drug resistance (Cowen et al. 2006, 2009; Cowen and Lindquist 2005; Singh et al. 2009; Singh-Babak et al. 2012). The molecular details have been studied most extensively in *C. albicans*, where Hsp90 regulates drug resistance by stabilizing signal transducers including the protein phosphatase calcineurin and the terminal mitogen-activated protein kinase in the Pkc1-mediated cell wall integrity pathway, Mkc1 (Fig. 3) (Singh et al. 2009; LaFayette et al. 2010). Inhibition of Hsp90, calcineurin, or Pkc1 reduces drug resistance of *C. albicans* that evolved resistance in a human host (Singh et al. 2009; LaFayette et al. 2010; Cruz et al. 2002). Hsp90 function is

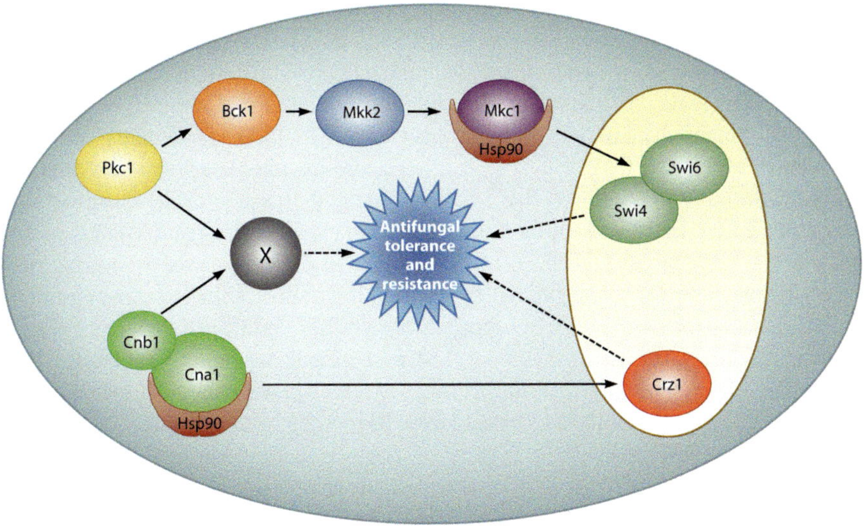

Fig. 3 Hsp90's role in *C. albicans* drug resistance. Schematic of the mechanisms by which Hsp90 regulates basal tolerance and resistance to antifungal drugs that target the cell membrane and the cell wall. Hsp90 physically interacts with and confers stability to the catalytic subunit of calcineurin (Cna1), thereby supporting stress responses mediated by calcineurin and its downstream effector protein Crz1 as well as through an additional target. Stress induced by antifungal drug exposure also activates signaling through the Pkc1 cell wall integrity pathway. Hsp90 stabilizes the terminal kinase Mkc1. Pkc1 also influences antifungal drug resistance and tolerance through a distinct pathway in common with calcineurin (Adapted by permission from Copyright © American Society for Microbiology [Microbiology and Molecular Biology Reviews, 75, 2011, 213–67 and ► 10.1128/MMBR.00045-10] (Shapiro et al. 2011))

itself regulated by acetylation such that hyperacetylation of Hsp90 compromises its function, thereby impairing the evolution of drug resistance and reversing resistance that had already evolved (Robbins et al. 2012). Targeting these cellular stress response pathways enhances antifungal efficacy in diverse models of infection including biofilm and systemic infections and attenuates virulence (Cowen et al. 2009; Singh et al. 2009; Singh-Babak et al. 2012; LaFayette et al. 2010; Robbins et al. 2011, 2012; Shapiro et al. 2009; Uppuluri et al. 2008; Sanglard et al. 2003; Steinbach et al. 2006, 2007a; Chen et al. 2011, 2012; Reedy et al. 2010). These signaling pathways are critical components of the cellular circuitry regulating the emergence and maintenance of drug resistance.

Evolution of Drug Resistance in the Human Host

The human host provides the most clinically relevant context to study microevolutionary processes by examining fungal specimens isolated from an infected individual over the course of treatment. Antifungal drug resistance can arise in a patient due to replacement of the susceptible strain with a resistant strain or species

(White et al. 1998). Resistance can also evolve as mutations accumulate in a susceptible population under drug selection, as is the focus of this section.

The evolution of drug resistance in the human host is most often accompanied by a stepwise increase in resistance due to the acquisition of multiple resistance mutations. A classic example is with a set of 17 *C. albicans* isolates collected from an HIV-infected patient over 2 years of azole treatment for recurrent oropharyngeal candidiasis (White 1997b). The progressive increase in drug resistance was accompanied by increased expression of the efflux transporter gene *MDR1*, mutations in the drug target gene *ERG11*, a mutation in *UPC2* causing transcriptional upregulation of *ERG11*, and ultimately a *TAC1* mutation leading to transcriptional upregulation of the drug efflux transporter genes *CDR1* and *CDR2* (White 1997a, b; Hoot et al. 2011; White et al. 1997). The first global analysis of mutations that accompany the evolution of antifungal drug resistance in a human host focused on a series of 7 *C. glabrata* isolates recovered over 10 months from a patient with Crohn's disease who received multiple rounds of echinocandin treatment for recurrent bloodstream candidemia (Singh-Babak et al. 2012). Whole genome sequencing revealed a mutation in the drug target gene *FKS2* that coincided with the largest increase in resistance, as well as 8 additional non-synonymous mutations (Fig. 4). A mutation in *CDC6*, whose product contributes to DNA replication initiation, was acquired at an earlier time point and was associated with a small increase in resistance (Singh-Babak et al. 2012). With advances in sequencing technologies, it is now feasible to sequence fungal genomes on a much larger scale to refine our appreciation of the dynamics of the evolution of antifungal drug resistance in the human host.

Experimental Evolution of Drug Resistance

A powerful complement to studying the evolution of drug resistance in the human host is the analysis of experimental populations that evolved under controlled laboratory conditions. This approach can overcome some of the limitations inherent to the analysis of clinical isolates, including the inability to control population parameters such as the genotype of the initial strain, the number of generations, the effective population size, and the strength of selection. Experimental evolution typically involves a population initiated from a single progenitor that is propagated for numerous generations, such that the evolution of new traits can be monitored and evolutionary intermediates can be archived (Elena and Lenski 2003). As a model for the evolution of drug resistance, this approach enables high levels of replication and fine-scale analysis of factors influencing the evolution of drug resistance. Despite the fact that experimental evolution does not capture complexities of evolution in the host where organisms face microenvironments, nutrient limitation, spatial structure, and competition with other pathogens, there is often a concordance of resistance mechanisms that evolve in the host and those that evolve in the test tube (Cowen et al. 2000; MacLean et al. 2010; Scully and Bidochka 2005).

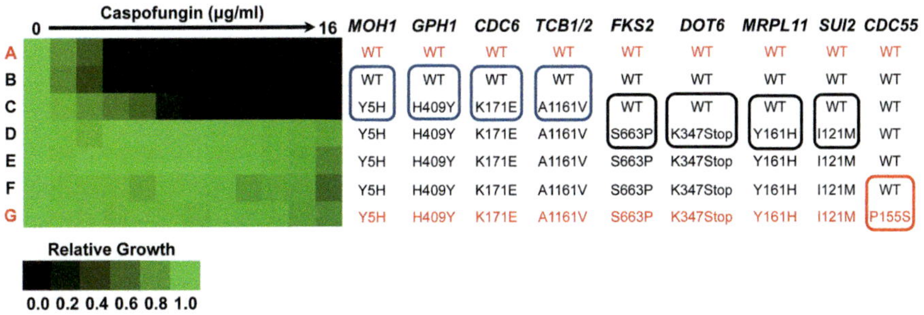

Fig. 4 The evolution of echinocandin resistance in *C. glabrata* clinical isolates is accompanied by multiple non-synonymous mutations. Isolates are arranged in the order they were recovered from the patient, with isolate A recovered prior to treatment and isolate G recovered after multiple rounds of treatment with the echinocandin caspofungin. Resistance increases in a stepwise manner. The nine non-synonymous mutations identified in isolate G compared to isolate A using whole genome sequencing were mapped in isolates B to F. Mutations in *MOH1*, *GPH1*, *CDC6*, and *TCB1/2* were identified between isolates B and C, accompanying a small increase in resistance (*blue outline*). Mutations in *DOT6*, *MRPL11*, *FKS2*, and *SUI2* were identified between isolates C and D, accompanying a sharp increase in echinocandin resistance (*black outline*). A mutation in *CDC55* was identified between isolates F and G (*red outline*) (Reproduced by permission from PLoS Pathogens, 8(5), 2012, e1002718. doi:10.1371/journal.ppat.1002718 (Singh-Babak et al. 2012))

The majority of experimental evolution studies of antifungal drug resistance have been performed with *C. albicans*. Evolutionary dynamics were monitored in replicate *C. albicans* populations propagated for 330 generations in the presence of fluconazole (Cowen et al. 2000). The populations evolved cross-resistance to multiple azoles following distinct trajectories with different expression levels of four resistance determinants: *ERG11*, *CDR1*, *CDR2*, and *MDR1*. Global analyses revealed three distinct gene expression profiles among the evolved lineages, profiles that were also observed among clinical isolates (Cowen et al. 2002). Aneuploidy was prevalent in the populations evolved with fluconazole, evidenced by the rapid emergence of i5L (Selmecki et al. 2006). Population dynamics can differ considerably in mouse models from test tubes, with increased genotypic and phenotypic variation in mouse-evolved strains (Forche et al. 2009), suggesting that infection models may provide an attractive system experimental evolution with more commonalities to the human host.

There have been a limited number of studies focused on experimental evolution of drug resistance in other human fungal pathogens. Replicate experimental populations of *A. fumigatus* evolved resistance to itraconazole by distinct mechanisms including overexpression of efflux pumps and mutations in the drug targets encoded by *cyp51A* and *cyp51B* (da Silva Ferreira et al. 2004). Multiple resistance mutations accumulated within populations, as is often the case with clinical isolates. Experimental evolution of *C. neoformans* in the presence of increasing concentrations of arsenite yielded highly resistant strains with amplification of a subtelomeric region that includes the arsenite efflux transporter encoded by *ARR3* to over 50 copies, accounting for up to ~1 % of the whole genome (Chow et al. 2012).

The model yeast *Saccharomyces cerevisiae* has provided a tractable system to study the mechanisms underpinning the evolution of antifungal drug resistance. In one study, the mode of selection was determined to have a profound impact on the mechanisms by which resistance emerges (Anderson et al. 2003). *S. cerevisiae* populations exposed to a single high dose of fluconazole evolved resistance by loss-of-function mutations in the ergosterol biosynthetic gene *ERG3*, while those propagated for 400 generations in the presence of increasing concentrations of azole acquired mutations in *PDR1* and *PDR3*, which encode transcription factors that control the expression of multidrug efflux transporters (Anderson et al. 2003). There is antagonism between the resistance mechanisms favored by the different selection regimes, as hybrids with both resistance determinants have impaired growth in the presence of fluconazole (Anderson et al. 2006). Experimental evolution studies with *S. cerevisiae* have also identified factors that enable the evolution of drug resistance and the impact of ploidy on adaptation. For example, deletion of *PDR16*, which is involved in lipid metabolism, caused extinction during selection with azoles (Anderson et al. 2009). Further, different ploidies were found to favor the emergence of distinct resistance mechanisms; recessive, loss-of-function mutations in *ERG3* were recovered in haploids, while mutations in *PDR1* and *PDR3* were favored in diploids as a result of the larger mutational target with twice the number of genes as haploids (Anderson et al. 2004).

Fitness Consequences of Drug Resistance

The ultimate fate of a drug-resistant pathogen is contingent on its fitness relative to its drug-sensitive counterparts. If resistance mutations are associated with a fitness cost that reduces growth and reproduction in the absence of drug, then discontinuing the use of the drug may allow susceptible isolates to outcompete those that are resistant. If there is no cost of resistance or if any cost is mitigated by the accumulation of compensatory mutations, then the resistant population will likely persist.

The fitness effects of resistance mutations in human fungal pathogens have been studied most extensively in *C. albicans*. Fitness of experimental populations that evolved azole resistance was measured by monitoring growth rates and by competing the evolved strains against their progenitor, in the presence and absence of azole. Some populations demonstrated no cost of resistance, while for others that had a fitness disadvantage in the absence of drug at earlier points, this cost was ameliorated with further evolution (Cowen et al. 2001). In some of these populations, the isochromosome i5L was associated with improved fitness both in the presence and absence of the drug (Selmecki et al. 2009). In contrast to populations that evolved azole resistance in response to drug selection, introduction of specific resistance mutations individually or in combination without the opportunity for compensatory evolution can be costly. This was investigated by introducing activating mutations in the *C. albicans* transcription factors genes *MRR1*, *TAC1*, and *UPC2* that control the expression of azole resistance determinants, individually and in combinations, and monitoring the impact on azole resistance and fitness (Sasse et al. 2012b). The multiple resistance mutations resulted in an incremental increase in azole resistance that was associated with reduced fitness in the absence of drug in vitro as well as in a mammalian host (Sasse et al. 2012b). Together, this suggests that compensatory mutations are key for reducing the cost of azole resistance that may be associated with resistance mechanisms such as constitutive changes in gene expression.

Recent work has identified the premier compensatory mutation that mitigates the cost of antifungal drug resistance. The most well-characterized echinocandin resistance mechanism is amino acid substitutions in the target (1,3)-β-D-glucan synthase that reduce the sensitivity of the enzyme to echinocandins (Garcia-Effron et al. 2009). These substitutions also reduce catalytic capacity of the enzyme even in the absence of echinocandin, imparting a cost of resistance (Ben-Ami and Kontoyiannis 2012). In a *C. glabrata* lineage that evolved echinocandin resistance in a human host, the acquisition of resistance by mutation of the drug target gene was associated with a fitness cost that was ameliorated with further evolution in the host (Singh-Babak et al. 2012). Whole genome sequencing identified a mutation in *CDC55*, which encodes the regulatory subunit of protein phosphatase 2A, that conferred a fitness increase evident in vitro and in the host (Singh-Babak et al. 2012). Cdc55 is involved in meiotic spindle assembly, mitotic exit, pseudohyphal growth, and chromosome disjunction, though the mechanism by which it mitigates the cost of echinocandin resistance remains unknown. Other studies with *C. glabrata* have established that drug resistance mechanisms may not always be costly. For example, gain-of-function mutations in *C. glabrata* Pdr1 cause azole resistance due to upregulation of multidrug transporters and are also associated with increased virulence (Ferrari et al. 2011). Given that a cost to antifungal drug resistance is not ubiquitous and that compensatory evolution can readily overcome any cost of resistance, it is likely that once resistance has evolved it will remain a persistent problem.

Drug Combinations to Thwart the Evolution of Drug Resistance

The evolution of drug resistance far outpaces the development of new antifungal drugs, demanding new strategies to block the evolution of drug resistance and render existing antifungal drugs more effective. Drug combinations have emerged as a powerful therapeutic strategy to extend the life of current antimicrobial agents (Torella et al. 2010). They can impair the emergence of drug resistance by more effectively eliminating pathogen populations and by necessitating multiple mutations to confer resistance to both drugs simultaneously (zur Wiesch et al. 2011). Drug combinations can also enhance the efficacy of either agent and can create cidal combinations with static agents. Combination therapy is fundamental for the treatment of HIV (Martin et al. 2003; Pfaller and Diekema 2007; Brown et al. 2012a), and it is the recommended therapeutic strategy for tuberculosis and malaria (Brown et al. 2012b; Ostrosky-Zeichner et al. 2010).

Combination therapies have been less well explored in the clinic for fungal pathogens. One clinically relevant example of combination therapy for fungal

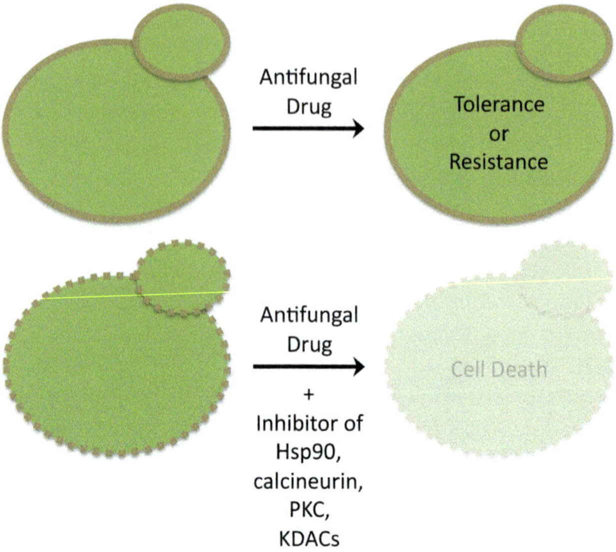

Fig. 5 Inhibition of cellular stress response regulators reduces basal tolerance and resistance to antifungal drugs such as azoles and echinocandins, transforms fungistatic agents to a fungicidal combination, and impairs the evolution of drug resistance. Examples of relevant inhibitors include those that target Hsp90, calcineurin, protein kinase C (PKC), and lysine deacetylases (KDACs)

infections is the treatment of patients with cryptococcal meningitis with the combination of 5-flucytosine and amphotericin B (Johnson and Perfect 2010). The rapid emergence of resistance to 5-flucytosine precludes its use as a single agent, though it has efficacy in combination with polyenes or azoles (White et al. 1998).

Targeting regulators of cellular stress responses has emerged as a promising strategy to enhance the efficacy of azoles and echinocandins and to minimize the emergence of resistance to these agents (Fig. 5). Multiple cellular signaling pathways are required for fungal pathogens to mount crucial responses to the cellular stress exerted by exposure to antifungal drugs. One of the most promising examples of a global regulator of cellular stress responses with broad antifungal potential is the molecular chaperone Hsp90. Hsp90 enables the evolution of drug resistance by stabilizing regulators of cellular stress responses and thereby allows for basal tolerance as well as the phenotypic effects of resistance mutations (Cowen 2008, 2009). In *S. cerevisiae* and *C. albicans*, compromise of Hsp90 function impairs the evolution of resistance to azoles and abrogates azole resistance that had already been acquired by diverse mutations (Cowen et al. 2006; Cowen and Lindquist 2005). Inhibiting *C. albicans* Hsp90 function also impairs biofilm growth, blocks biofilm dispersal, and abolishes biofilm azole resistance (Robbins et al. 2011). In *C. albicans*, *C. glabrata*, and *A. fumigatus*, Hsp90 inhibition also abrogates echinocandin resistance acquired by diverse mutations and renders echinocandins fungicidal against azole-resistant *A. fumigatus* strains (Cowen and Lindquist 2005; Cowen et al. 2009; Singh et al. 2009; Singh-Babak et al. 2012; Lamoth et al. 2012).

Hsp90 compromise also reduces echinocandin resistance of *A. fumigatus* biofilms (Robbins et al. 2011).

The therapeutic promise of targeting Hsp90 is corroborated by multiple infection models. Inhibiting Hsp90 with molecules that are well tolerated in humans and in clinical development for cancer transforms the therapeutic efficacy of azoles against *C. albicans*, rescuing infections that are otherwise lethal in the invertebrate *Galleria mellonella* (Cowen et al. 2009). Although these Hsp90 inhibitors are generally well tolerated in mice, their therapeutic utility is compromised by toxicity observed in the context of acute fungal infections (Cowen et al. 2009). Genetic reduction of *C. albicans* Hsp90 enhances the efficacy of azoles and echinocandins in a murine model of disseminated candidiasis, providing further proof-of-principle that Hsp90 is an attractive target for combination therapy (Cowen et al. 2009; Singh et al. 2009). Notably, Hsp90 inhibitors in clinical development transform azoles from largely ineffective to highly efficacious in a rat model of central venous catheter infection, where the infection and drug delivery remain more localized (Robbins et al. 2011). Current efforts focus on development of fungal-selective Hsp90 inhibitors for the treatment of systemic fungal infections.

Many of the other regulators of cellular stress responses that show promise for thwarting drug resistance are integral components of the Hsp90 chaperone network. The best example is the Hsp90 client protein calcineurin. Hsp90 physically interacts with and stabilizes the catalytic subunit of the protein phosphatase calcineurin; consequently, depletion of Hsp90 leads to depletion of calcineurin, thereby blocking calcineurin-mediated stress responses required for survival during the stress induced by antifungal drug exposure (Singh et al. 2009). Inhibition of calcineurin with agents used widely in the clinic as immunosuppressants, tacrolimus (FK506) or cyclosporin A, enhances the efficacy of azoles and echinocandins against diverse fungal pathogens and creates fungicidal combinations (Singh et al. 2009; Cruz et al. 2002; Sanglard et al. 2003; Lamoth et al. 2012; Onyewu et al. 2003; Steinbach et al. 2007b). Calcineurin inhibitors also act synergistically with azoles against fungal biofilms both in vitro and in vivo (Uppuluri et al. 2008). As with Hsp90 inhibitors, current efforts focus on identifying fungal-selective calcineurin inhibitors that lack the immunosuppressive effects on the host. PKC signaling intersects with calcineurin signaling and provides another downstream effector of Hsp90 with a key role in drug resistance (LaFayette et al. 2010). Upstream regulators of Hsp90 function also serve to modulate the evolution and maintenance of antifungal drug resistance with broad therapeutic potential, as is the case with lysine deacetylases (Robbins et al. 2012). Additional regulators that may be independent of the Hsp90 chaperone network have also emerged as promising targets to block drug resistance (Wurtele et al. 2010). Chemical and genomic screens promise to reveal many diverse molecules and genes that control antifungal drug resistance, offering possibility for therapeutic exploitation (LaFayette et al. 2010; Spitzer et al. 2011; Epp et al. 2010; Zhang et al. 2007).

While drug combinations should theoretically minimize the evolution of drug resistance, there has been a paucity of experimental studies that address this directly. The impact of drug combinations on the evolution of resistance has recently been explored with experimental populations of *S. cerevisiae* and *C. albicans* (Hill et al. 2013). Populations that were resistant to azoles due to loss of function of Erg3 were evolved with a combination of an azole and an inhibitor of Hsp90 or calcineurin, in order to recapitulate a clinical context where inhibitors of Hsp90 or calcineurin could be administered in combination with an azole to render azole-resistant pathogenes responsive to treatment. Of 290 lineages initiated, the majority went extinct, consistent with the inherent challenge of evolving resistance to drug combinations (Hill et al. 2013). Genome sequencing and genetic analyses revealed diverse resistance mutations including mutations in genes encoding: the target of the inhibitor of Hsp90 (Hsp90) or calcineurin (Fpr1, the immunophilin that binds to FK506 to form the protein-drug complex that inhibits calcineurin); a transcriptional activator of drug efflux pumps, Pdr1; a regulator of sphingolipid biosynthesis, Lcb1; the catalytic subunit of calcineurin; and a repressor of ergosterol biosynthesis genes, Mot3 (Hill et al. 2013). Numerous mutations conferred resistance to the inhibitor of Hsp90 or calcineurin, while others rendered azole resistance independent of calcineurin. Extensive aneuploidy was also identified in several of the *C. albicans* lineages (Hill et al. 2013). This approach integrating experimental evolution and genome-scale analyses provides a framework for predicting and preventing the evolution of antifungal drug resistance.

Conclusion

The evolution of drug resistance is inevitable, but there are effective strategies to delay this ubiquitous process. While resistance to drug combinations can evolve by multiple mechanisms, there is limited evidence in the clinic. For example, ~40 % of transplant recipients suffer from invasive fungal infections, including those that receive a calcineurin inhibitor as an immunosuppressant; however, resistance to calcineurin inhibitors has not been observed in fungal pathogens recovered from patients receiving this immunosuppressive therapy (Blankenship et al. 2005; Reedy et al. 2006). Consistent with this, target-based resistance to Hsp90 inhibitors has yet to emerge in Hsp90 inhibitor clinical trials. That resistance has not been observed in the clinic suggests that these mutations may be associated with a fitness cost in conditions relevant to the human host. Given that there may be ample possibility for compensatory evolution to ameliorate the fitness costs, there is strong impetus to invest in the discovery of a multitude of strategies to improve clinical outcome for patients with invasive fungal infections.

Approaching antifungal drug resistance as an evolutionary problem has great potential to improve our capacity to predict and prevent it (Antonovics et al. 2007). Many of the paradigms for the evolution of drug resistance in fungal pathogens of humans also pertain to the evolution of fungicide resistance in fungal pathogens of plants, which have a staggering impact on agriculture. In fact, the processes may be intimately related. Drug resistance can be selected for with the prophylactic administration of antifungal drugs for high-risk patients and with the agricultural deployment of fungicides, and there is potential for pathogens to be transmitted between these environments (Verweij et al. 2009; Mortensen et al. 2010). This is illustrated by the finding that environmental isolates of azole-resistant *A. fumigatus* show greater genetic similarity to azole-resistant clinical isolates than to those that are susceptible, suggesting that patients are being colonized with isolates that acquired azole resistance in the field (Snelders et al. 2009). In the broader context, it is clear that many parallels exist in the evolution of resistance to diverse agents by fungi, bacteria, protozoan parasites, insects, and even mammalian cancer cells. An interdisciplinary approach is poised to accelerate our understanding of the principles and mechanisms governing the evolution of drug resistance, which should ultimately manifest in novel and effective strategies to keep pace with the rapid evolution of resistance across the kingdoms.

References

Alastruey-Izquierdo A, Castelli MV, Cuesta I, Zaragoza O, Monzon A et al (2009) In vitro activity of antifungals against Zygomycetes. Clin Microbiol Infect 15(Suppl 5):71–76

Alcazar-Fuoli L, Mellado E, Cuenca-Estrella M, Sanglard D (2011) Probing the role of point mutations in the *cyp51A* gene from *Aspergillus fumigatus* in the model yeast *Saccharomyces cerevisiae*. Med Mycol 49:276–284

Allen HK, Donato J, Wang HH, Cloud-Hansen KA, Davies J et al (2010) Call of the wild: antibiotic resistance genes in natural environments. Nat Rev Microbiol 8:251–259

Anderson JB (2005) Evolution of antifungal-drug resistance: mechanisms and pathogen fitness. Nat Rev Microbiol 3:547–556

Anderson JB, Sirjusingh C, Parsons AB, Boone C, Wickens C et al (2003) Mode of selection and experimental evolution of antifungal drug resistance in *Saccharomyces cerevisiae*. Genetics 163:1287–1298

Anderson JB, Sirjusingh C, Ricker N (2004) Haploidy, diploidy and evolution of antifungal drug resistance in *Saccharomyces cerevisiae*. Genetics 168:1915–1923

Anderson JB, Ricker N, Sirjusingh C (2006) Antagonism between two mechanisms of antifungal drug resistance. Eukaryot Cell 5:1243–1251

Anderson JB, Sirjusingh C, Syed N, Lafayette S (2009) Gene expression and evolution of antifungal drug resistance. Antimicrob Agents Chemother 53:1931–1936

Antonovics J, Abbate JL, Baker CH, Daley D, Hood ME et al (2007) Evolution by any other name: antibiotic resistance and avoidance of the E-word. PLoS Biol 5:e30

Ben-Ami R, Kontoyiannis DP (2012) Resistance to echinocandins comes at a cost: the impact of *FKS1* hotspot mutations on *Candida albicans* fitness and virulence. Virulence 3:95–97

Bien CM, Espenshade PJ (2010) Sterol regulatory element binding proteins in fungi: hypoxic transcription factors linked to pathogenesis. Eukaryot Cell 9:352–359

Blankenship JR, Mitchell AP (2006) How to build a biofilm: a fungal perspective. Curr Opin Microbiol 9:588–594

Blankenship JR, Singh N, Alexander BD, Heitman J (2005) *Cryptococcus neoformans* isolates from transplant recipients are not selected for resistance to calcineurin inhibitors by current immunosuppressive regimens. J Clin Microbiol 43:464–467

Brown GD, Denning DW, Gow NA, Levitz SM, Netea MG et al (2012a) Hidden killers: human fungal infections. Sci Transl Med 4:165rv113

Brown GD, Denning DW, Levitz SM (2012b) Tackling human fungal infections. Science 336:647

Cannon RD, Lamping E, Holmes AR, Niimi K, Tanabe K et al (2007) *Candida albicans* drug resistance another way to cope with stress. Microbiology 153:3211–3217

Cannon RD, Lamping E, Holmes AR, Niimi K, Baret PV et al (2009) Efflux-mediated antifungal drug resistance. Clin Microbiol Rev 22:291–321

Chen YL, Brand A, Morrison EL, Silao FG, Bigol UG et al (2011) Calcineurin controls drug tolerance, hyphal growth, and virulence in *Candida dubliniensis*. Eukaryot Cell 10:803–819

Chen YL, Konieczka JH, Springer DJ, Bowen SE, Zhang J et al (2012) Convergent evolution of calcineurin pathway roles in thermotolerance and virulence in *Candida glabrata*. G3 (Bethesda) 2:675–691

Chow EW, Morrow CA, Djordjevic JT, Wood IA, Fraser JA (2012) Microevolution of *Cryptococcus neoformans* driven by massive tandem gene amplification. Mol Biol Evol 29:1987–2000

Cifani C, Costantino S, Massi M, Berrino L (2012) Commercially available lipid formulations of amphotericin B: are they bioequivalent and therapeutically equivalent? Acta Biomed 83:154–163

Coste AT, Karababa M, Ischer F, Bille J, Sanglard D (2004) *TAC1*, transcriptional activator of *CDR* genes, is a new transcription factor involved in the regulation of *Candida albicans* ABC transporters *CDR1* and *CDR2*. Eukaryot Cell 3:1639–1652

Coste A, Turner V, Ischer F, Morschhauser J, Forche A et al (2006) A mutation in Tac1p, a transcription factor regulating *CDR1* and *CDR2*, is coupled with loss of heterozygosity at chromosome 5 to mediate antifungal resistance in *Candida albicans*. Genetics 172:2139–2156

Cowen LE (2008) The evolution of fungal drug resistance: modulating the trajectory from genotype to phenotype. Nat Rev Microbiol 6:187–198

Cowen LE (2009) Hsp90 orchestrates stress response signaling governing fungal drug resistance. PLoS Pathog 5:e1000471

Cowen LE, Lindquist S (2005) Hsp90 potentiates the rapid evolution of new traits: drug resistance in diverse fungi. Science 309:2185–2189

Cowen LE, Steinbach WJ (2008) Stress, drugs, and evolution: the role of cellular signaling in fungal drug resistance. Eukaryot Cell 7:747–764

Cowen LE, Sanglard D, Calabrese D, Sirjusingh C, Anderson JB et al (2000) Evolution of drug resistance in experimental populations of *Candida albicans*. J Bacteriol 182:1515–1522

Cowen LE, Kohn LM, Anderson JB (2001) Divergence in fitness and evolution of drug resistance in experimental populations of *Candida albicans*. J Bacteriol 183:2971–2978

Cowen LE, Nantel A, Whiteway MS, Thomas DY, Tessier DC et al (2002) Population genomics of drug resistance in *Candida albicans*. Proc Natl Acad Sci U S A 99:9284–9289

Cowen LE, Carpenter AE, Matangkasombut O, Fink GR, Lindquist S (2006) Genetic architecture of Hsp90-dependent drug resistance. Eukaryot Cell 5:2184–2188

Cowen LE, Singh SD, Kohler JR, Collins C, Zaas AK et al (2009) Harnessing Hsp90 function as a powerful, broadly effective therapeutic strategy for fungal infectious disease. Proc Natl Acad Sci U S A 106:2818–2823

Cruz MC, Goldstein AL, Blankenship JR, Del Poeta M, Davis D et al (2002) Calcineurin is essential for survival during membrane stress in *Candida albicans*. EMBO J 21:546–559

da Silva Ferreira ME, Capellaro JL, dos Reis Marques E, Malavazi I, Perlin D et al (2004) In vitro evolution of itraconazole resistance in *Aspergillus fumigatus* involves multiple mechanisms of resistance. Antimicrob Agents Chemother 48:4405–4413

Davies J, Davies D (2010) Origins and evolution of antibiotic resistance. Microbiol Mol Biol Rev 74:417–433

d'Enfert C (2006) Biofilms and their role in the resistance of pathogenic *Candida* to antifungal agents. Curr Drug Targets 7:465–470

Denning DW (2003) Echinocandin antifungal drugs. Lancet 362:1142–1151

Dhamgaye S, Bernard M, Lelandais G, Sismeiro O, Lemoine S et al (2012) RNA sequencing revealed novel actors of the acquisition of drug resistance in *Candida albicans*. BMC Genomics 13:396

Dunkel N, Liu TT, Barker KS, Homayouni R, Morschhauser J et al (2008a) A gain-of-function mutation in the transcription factor Upc2p causes upregulation of ergosterol biosynthesis genes and increased fluconazole resistance in a clinical *Candida albicans* isolate. Eukaryot Cell 7:1180–1190

Dunkel N, Blass J, Rogers PD, Morschhauser J (2008b) Mutations in the multi-drug resistance regulator *MRR1*, followed by loss of heterozygosity, are the main cause of *MDR1* overexpression in fluconazole-resistant *Candida albicans* strains. Mol Microbiol 69:827–840

Elena SF, Lenski RE (2003) Evolution experiments with microorganisms: the dynamics and genetic bases of adaptation. Nat Rev Genet 4:457–469

Epp E, Vanier G, Harcus D, Lee AY, Jansen G et al (2010) Reverse genetics in *Candida albicans* predicts ARF cycling is essential for drug resistance and virulence. PLoS Pathog 6:e1000753

Fanos V, Cataldi L (2000) Amphotericin B-induced nephrotoxicity: a review. J Chemother 12:463–470

Ferrari S, Sanguinetti M, Torelli R, Posteraro B, Sanglard D (2011) Contribution of *CgPDR1*-regulated genes in enhanced virulence of azole-resistant *Candida glabrata*. PLoS One 6:e17589

Forche A, Magee PT, Selmecki A, Berman J, May G (2009) Evolution in *Candida albicans* populations during a single passage through a mouse host. Genetics 182:799–811

Garcia-Effron G, Lee S, Park S, Cleary JD, Perlin DS (2009) Effect of *Candida glabrata FKS1* and *FKS2* mutations on echinocandin sensitivity and kinetics of 1,3-beta-D-glucan synthase: implication for the existing susceptibility breakpoint. Antimicrob Agents Chemother 53:3690–3699

Gruszecki WI, Gagos M, Herec M, Kernen P (2003) Organization of antibiotic amphotericin B in model lipid membranes. A mini review. Cell Mol Biol Lett 8:161–170

Heilmann CJ, Schneider S, Barker KS, Rogers PD, Morschhauser J (2010) An A643T mutation in the transcription factor Upc2p causes constitutive *ERG11* upregulation and increased fluconazole resistance in *Candida albicans*. Antimicrob Agents Chemother 54:353–359

Hill JA, Hoot SJ, White TC, Cowen LE (2012) Evolution of drug resistance in fungi. In: Sibley LD, Howlett BJ, Heitman J (eds) Evolution of virulence in eukaryotic microbes. Wiley Blackwell, Somerset

Hill JA, Ammar R, Torti D, Nislow C, Cowen LE (2013) Genetic and genomic architecture of the evolution of resistance to antifungal drug combinations. PLoS Genet 9:e1003390

Hoot SJ, Smith AR, Brown RP, White TC (2011) An A643V amino acid substitution in Upc2p contributes to azole resistance in well-characterized clinical isolates of *Candida albicans*. Antimicrob Agents Chemother 55:940–942

Johnson MD, Perfect JR (2010) Use of antifungal combination therapy: agents, order, and timing. Curr Fungal Infect Rep 4:87–95

LaFayette SL, Collins C, Zaas AK, Schell WA, Betancourt-Quiroz M et al (2010) PKC signaling regulates drug resistance of the fungal pathogen *Candida albicans* via circuitry comprised of Mkc1, calcineurin, and Hsp90. PLoS Pathog 6:e1001069

LaFleur MD, Kumamoto CA, Lewis K (2006) *Candida albicans* biofilms produce antifungal-tolerant persister cells. Antimicrob Agents Chemother 50:3839–3846

Lamb DC, Kelly DE, Schunck WH, Shyadehi AZ, Akhtar M et al (1997) The mutation T315A in *Candida albicans* sterol 14alpha-demethylase causes reduced enzyme activity and fluconazole resistance through reduced affinity. J Biol Chem 272:5682–5688

Lamoth F, Juvvadi PR, Gehrke C, Steinbach WJ (2012) In vitro activity of calcineurin and heat-shock protein 90 (Hsp90) inhibitors against *Aspergillus fumigatus* azole- and echinocandin-resistant strains. Antimicrob Agents Chemother 51:2979–2981

MacCallum DM, Coste A, Ischer F, Jacobsen MD, Odds FC et al (2010) Genetic dissection of azole resistance mechanisms in *Candida albicans* and their validation in a mouse model of disseminated infection. Antimicrob Agents Chemother 54:1476–1483

MacLean RC, Hall AR, Perron GG, Buckling A (2010) The population genetics of antibiotic resistance: integrating molecular mechanisms and treatment contexts. Nat Rev Genet 11:405–414

Mansfield BE, Oltean HN, Oliver BG, Hoot SJ, Leyde SE et al (2010) Azole drugs are imported by facilitated diffusion in *Candida albicans* and other pathogenic fungi. PLoS Pathog 6:e1001126

Marr KA, Lyons CN, Ha K, Rustad TR, White TC (2001) Inducible azole resistance associated with a heterogeneous phenotype in *Candida albicans*. Antimicrob Agents Chemother 45:52–59

Martin GS, Mannino DM, Eaton S, Moss M (2003) The epidemiology of sepsis in the United States from 1979 through 2000. N Engl J Med 348:1546–1554
Mogavero S, Tavanti A, Senesi S, Rogers PD, Morschhauser J (2011) Differential requirement of the transcription factor Mcm1 for activation of the *Candida albicans* multidrug efflux pump *MDR1* by its regulators Mrr1 and Cap1. Antimicrob Agents Chemother 55:2061–2066
Morschhauser J (2010) Regulation of multidrug resistance in pathogenic fungi. Fungal Genet Biol 47:94–106
Mortensen KL, Mellado E, Lass-Florl C, Rodriguez-Tudela JL, Johansen HK et al (2010) Environmental study of azole-resistant *Aspergillus fumigatus* and other aspergilli in Austria, Denmark, and Spain. Antimicrob Agents Chemother 54:4545–4549
Nagi M, Nakayama H, Tanabe K, Bard M, Aoyama T et al (2011) Transcription factors *CgUPC2A* and *CgUPC2B* regulate ergosterol biosynthetic genes in *Candida glabrata*. Genes Cells 16:80–89
Netea MG, Brown GD, Kullberg BJ, Gow NA (2008) An integrated model of the recognition of *Candida albicans* by the innate immune system. Nat Rev Microbiol 6:67–78
Niimi K, Monk BC, Hirai A, Hatakenaka K, Umeyama T et al (2010) Clinically significant micafungin resistance in *Candida albicans* involves modification of a glucan synthase catalytic subunit *GSC1* (*FKS1*) allele followed by loss of heterozygosity. J Antimicrob Chemother 65:842–852
Odds FC, Brown AJ, Gow NA (2003) Antifungal agents: mechanisms of action. Trends Microbiol 11:272–279
Onyewu C, Blankenship JR, Del Poeta M, Heitman J (2003) Ergosterol biosynthesis inhibitors become fungicidal when combined with calcineurin inhibitors against *Candida albicans*, *Candida glabrata*, and *Candida krusei*. Antimicrob Agents Chemother 47:956–964
Ostrosky-Zeichner L, Casadevall A, Galgiani JN, Odds FC, Rex JH (2010) An insight into the antifungal pipeline: selected new molecules and beyond. Nat Rev Drug Discov 9:719–727
Palumbi SR (2001) Humans as the world's greatest evolutionary force. Science 293:1786–1790
Perlin DS (2007) Resistance to echinocandin-class antifungal drugs. Drug Resist Updat 10:121–130
Pfaller MA (2012) Antifungal drug resistance: mechanisms, epidemiology, and consequences for treatment. Am J Med 125:S3–S13
Pfaller MA, Diekema DJ (2004) Rare and emerging opportunistic fungal pathogens: concern for resistance beyond *Candida albicans* and *Aspergillus fumigatus*. J Clin Microbiol 42:4419–4431
Pfaller MA, Diekema DJ (2007) Epidemiology of invasive candidiasis: a persistent public health problem. Clin Microbiol Rev 20:133–163
Pfaller MA, Diekema DJ (2010) Epidemiology of invasive mycoses in North America. Crit Rev Microbiol 36:1–53
Pitman SK, Drew RH, Perfect JR (2011) Addressing current medical needs in invasive fungal infection prevention and treatment with new antifungal agents, strategies and formulations. Expert Opin Emerg Drugs. [Epub ahead of print]
Ramage G, Mowat E, Jones B, Williams C, Lopez-Ribot J (2009) Our current understanding of fungal biofilms. Crit Rev Microbiol 35:340–355
Reedy JL, Husain S, Ison M, Pruett TL, Singh N et al (2006) Immunotherapy with tacrolimus (FK506) does not select for resistance to calcineurin inhibitors in *Candida albicans* isolates from liver transplant patients. Antimicrob Agents Chemother 50:1573–1577
Reedy JL, Filler SG, Heitman J (2010) Elucidating the *Candida albicans* calcineurin signaling cascade controlling stress response and virulence. Fungal Genet Biol 47:107–116
Robbins N, Uppuluri P, Nett J, Rajendran R, Ramage G et al (2011) Hsp90 governs dispersion and drug resistance of fungal biofilms. PLoS Pathog 7:e1002257
Robbins N, Leach MD, Cowen LE (2012) Lysine deacetylases Hda1 and Rpd3 regulate Hsp90 function thereby governing fungal drug resistance. Cell Rep 2:878–888
Sanglard D, Ischer F, Marchetti O, Entenza J, Bille J (2003) Calcineurin A of *Candida albicans*: involvement in antifungal tolerance, cell morphogenesis and virulence. Mol Microbiol 48:959–976

Sasse C, Schillig R, Reimund A, Merk J, Morschhauser J (2012a) Inducible and constitutive activation of two polymorphic promoter alleles of the *Candida albicans* multidrug efflux pump *MDR1*. Antimicrob Agents Chemother 56:4490–4494

Sasse C, Dunkel N, Schafer T, Schneider S, Dierolf F et al (2012b) The stepwise acquisition of fluconazole resistance mutations causes a gradual loss of fitness in *Candida albicans*. Mol Microbiol 86:539–556

Schubert S, Barker KS, Znaidi S, Schneider S, Dierolf F et al (2011) Regulation of efflux pump expression and drug resistance by the transcription factors Mrr1, Upc2, and Cap1 in *Candida albicans*. Antimicrob Agents Chemother 55:2212–2223

Scully LR, Bidochka MJ (2005) Serial passage of the opportunistic pathogen *Aspergillus flavus* through an insect host yields decreased saprobic capacity. Can J Microbiol 51:185–189

Selmecki A, Forche A, Berman J (2006) Aneuploidy and isochromosome formation in drug-resistant *Candida albicans*. Science 313:367–370

Selmecki A, Gerami-Nejad M, Paulson C, Forche A, Berman J (2008) An isochromosome confers drug resistance in vivo by amplification of two genes, *ERG11* and *TAC1*. Mol Microbiol 68:624–641

Selmecki AM, Dulmage K, Cowen LE, Anderson JB, Berman J (2009) Acquisition of aneuploidy provides increased fitness during the evolution of antifungal drug resistance. PLoS Genet 5: e1000705

Shapiro RS, Uppuluri P, Zaas AK, Collins C, Senn H et al (2009) Hsp90 orchestrates temperature-dependent *Candida albicans* morphogenesis via Ras1-PKA signaling. Curr Biol 19:621–629

Shapiro RS, Robbins N, Cowen LE (2011) Regulatory circuitry governing fungal development, drug resistance, and disease. Microbiol Mol Biol Rev 75:213–267

Shukla S, Yadav V, Mukhopadhyay G, Prasad R (2011) Ncb2 is involved in activated transcription of *CDR1* in azole-resistant clinical isolates of *Candida albicans*. Eukaryot Cell 10:1357–1366

Singh SD, Robbins N, Zaas AK, Schell WA, Perfect JR et al (2009) Hsp90 governs echinocandin resistance in the pathogenic yeast *Candida albicans* via calcineurin. PLoS Pathog 5:e1000532

Singh-Babak SD, Babak T, Diezmann S, Hill JA, Xie JL et al (2012) Global analysis of the evolution and mechanism of echinocandin resistance in *Candida glabrata*. PLoS Pathog 8: e1002718

Sionov E, Chang YC, Garraffo HM, Kwon-Chung KJ (2009) Heteroresistance to fluconazole in *Cryptococcus neoformans* is intrinsic and associated with virulence. Antimicrob Agents Chemother 53:2804–2815

Sionov E, Lee H, Chang YC, Kwon-Chung KJ (2010) *Cryptococcus neoformans* overcomes stress of azole drugs by formation of disomy in specific multiple chromosomes. PLoS Pathog 6: e1000848

Sionov E, Chang YC, Garraffo HM, Dolan MA, Ghannoum MA et al (2012) Identification of a *Cryptococcus neoformans* cytochrome P450 lanosterol 14alpha-demethylase (Erg11) residue critical for differential susceptibility between fluconazole/voriconazole and itraconazole/ posaconazole. Antimicrob Agents Chemother 56:1162–1169

Snelders E, Huis In 't Veld RA, Rijs AJ, Kema GH, Melchers WJ et al (2009) Possible environmental origin of resistance of *Aspergillus fumigatus* to medical triazoles. Appl Environ Microbiol 75:4053–4057

Spitzer M, Griffiths E, Blakely KM, Wildenhain J, Ejim L et al (2011) Cross-species discovery of syncretic drug combinations that potentiate the antifungal fluconazole. Mol Syst Biol 7:499

Steinbach WJ, Cramer RA Jr, Perfect BZ, Asfaw YG, Sauer TC et al (2006) Calcineurin controls growth, morphology, and pathogenicity in *Aspergillus fumigatus*. Eukaryot Cell 5:1091–1103

Steinbach WJ, Reedy JL, Cramer RA Jr, Perfect JR, Heitman J (2007a) Harnessing calcineurin as a novel anti-infective agent against invasive fungal infections. Nat Rev Microbiol 5:418–430

Steinbach WJ, Cramer RA Jr, Perfect BZ, Henn C, Nielsen K et al (2007b) Calcineurin inhibition or mutation enhances cell wall inhibitors against *Aspergillus fumigatus*. Antimicrob Agents Chemother 51:2979–2981

Tada R, Latge JP, Aimanianda V (2013) Undressing the fungal cell wall/cell membrane - the antifungal drug targets. Curr Pharm Des 19:3738–3747

Torella JP, Chait R, Kishony R (2010) Optimal drug synergy in antimicrobial treatments. PLoS Comput Biol 6:e1000796

Turner MS, Drew RH, Perfect JR (2006) Emerging echinocandins for treatment of invasive fungal infections. Expert Opin Emerg Drugs 11:231–250

Uppuluri P, Nett J, Heitman J, Andes D (2008) Synergistic effect of calcineurin inhibitors and fluconazole against *Candida albicans* biofilms. Antimicrob Agents Chemother 52:1127–1132

Verweij PE, Snelders E, Kema GH, Mellado E, Melchers WJ (2009) Azole resistance in *Aspergillus fumigatus*: a side-effect of environmental fungicide use? Lancet Infect Dis 9:789–795

Vincent BM, Lancaster AK, Scherz-Shouval R, Whitesell L, Lindquist S (2013) Fitness trade-offs restrict the evolution of resistance to amphotericin B. PLoS Biol 11:e1001692

Wang JS, Yang YL, Wu CJ, Ouyang KJ, Tseng KY et al (2006) The DNA-binding domain of CaNdt80p is required to activate *CDR1* involved in drug resistance in *Candida albicans*. J Med Microbiol 55:1403–1411

White TC (1997a) The presence of an R467K amino acid substitution and loss of allelic variation correlate with an azole-resistant lanosterol 14alpha demethylase in *Candida albicans*. Antimicrob Agents Chemother 41:1488–1494

White TC (1997b) Increased mRNA levels of *ERG16*, *CDR*, and *MDR1* correlate with increases in azole resistance in *Candida albicans* isolates from a patient infected with human immunodeficiency virus. Antimicrob Agents Chemother 41:1482–1487

White TC, Oliver BG (2004) Antifungal drug resistance: pumps and permutations. In: Domer JE, Kobyashi GS (eds) Human fungal pathogens. Springer, Heidelberg

White TC, Pfaller MA, Rinaldi MG, Smith J, Redding SW (1997) Stable azole drug resistance associated with a substrain of *Candida albicans* from an HIV-infected patient. Oral Dis 3(Suppl 1):S102–S109

White TC, Marr KA, Bowden RA (1998) Clinical, cellular, and molecular factors that contribute to antifungal drug resistance. Clin Microbiol Rev 11:382–402

Willger SD, Puttikamonkul S, Kim KH, Burritt JB, Grahl N et al (2008) A sterol-regulatory element binding protein is required for cell polarity, hypoxia adaptation, azole drug resistance, and virulence in *Aspergillus fumigatus*. PLoS Pathog 4:e1000200

Willger SD, Cornish EJ, Chung D, Fleming BA, Lehmann MM et al (2012) Dsc orthologs are required for hypoxia adaptation, triazole drug responses, and fungal virulence in *Aspergillus fumigatus*. Eukaryot Cell 11:1557–1567

Wright GD (2007) The antibiotic resistome: the nexus of chemical and genetic diversity. Nat Rev Microbiol 5:175–186

Wright GD (2012) The origins of antibiotic resistance. Handb Exp Pharmacol 211:13–30

Wurtele H, Tsao S, Lepine G, Mullick A, Tremblay J et al (2010) Modulation of histone H3 lysine 56 acetylation as an antifungal therapeutic strategy. Nat Med 16:774–780

Zhang L, Yan K, Zhang Y, Huang R, Bian J et al (2007) High-throughput synergy screening identifies microbial metabolites as combination agents for the treatment of fungal infections. Proc Natl Acad Sci U S A 104:4606–4611

zur Wiesch PA, Kouyos R, Engelstadter J, Regoes RR, Bonhoeffer S (2011) Population biological principles of drug-resistance evolution in infectious diseases. Lancet Infect Dis 11:236–247

The Role of Biofilm Matrix in Mediating Antifungal Resistance

Jeniel E. Nett and David Andes

Contents

Abstract

Fungal pathogens can adhere to medical devices and other surfaces, forming resilient biofilms. One of the hallmark features of biofilm formation is the production of a polymeric extracellular matrix which encases the cells within the biofilm. This protective covering has been linked to a mulit-drug resistant phenotype for a variety of fungi, including *Candida* spp. and *Aspergillus* spp.

J.E. Nett
Department of Medicine, Department of Medical Microbiology and Immunology, University of Wisconsin, School of Medicine and Public Health, Madison, WI, USA
e-mail: jenett@medicine.wisc.edu

D. Andes (✉)
Department of Medicine, Department of Medical Microbiology and Immunology, University of Wisconsin, School of Medicine and Public Health, Madison, WI, USA

UW Medical Foundation Centennial Building, Madison, WI, USA
e-mail: dra@medicine.wisc.edu

M. Gotte et al. (eds.), *Handbook of Antimicrobial Resistance*,
DOI 10.1007/978-1-4939-0694-9_20

Here we describe environmental and genetic factors governing manufacture of the fungal biofilm matrix. We also highlight key matrix components, including β-1,3 glucan and extracellular DNA, which have been specifically shown to be instrumental for production the biofilm drug-resistant phenotype.

Keywords
Candida • Aspergillus • Biofilm • Matrix • Glucan • DNA • Antifungal • Drug resistance

Introduction

Candida albicans, the most common hospital-acquired fungal pathogen, frequently grows as a community of adherent cells encased in an extracellular matrix (Donlan 2001a). The majority of *Candida* infections are now thought to involve growth in this biofilm lifestyle, including virtually all infections associated with medical devices, such as vascular and urinary catheters (Douglas 2002; Kojic and Darouiche 2004). The susceptibility of medical devices to infection has been increasingly appreciated. There are estimated to be more than 45 million medical devices implanted in patients in the USA per year, and at least 50 % of all nosocomial infections are associated with these devices (Raad et al. 1992; Groeger et al. 1993; Kralovicova et al. 1997; Richards et al. 1999; Schmitt et al. 1990). The consequences of device infections can be disastrous, including life-threatening infection and device malfunction necessitating device removal (Donlan 2001b). Successful treatment of foreign-body infections requires device removal in most instances (Anaissie et al. 1998; Lecciones et al. 1992; Rex et al. 1995; Andes et al. 2012). These infections are extremely difficult to cure without removal of the medical device, in part due to the drug resistance associated with biofilm growth.

The ability to live as a fungal biofilm was first described for *Candida*, and the most common pathogenic species, including *C. albicans*, C. *dubliniensis*, *C. glabrata*, *C. krusei*, *C. tropicalis*, and *C. parapsilosis*, have now been shown to cause biofilm infections (Shin et al. 2002). As *C. albicans* is the most frequently encountered fungal biofilm infection, this species has been used as a model pathogen for many investigations regarding biofilm pathogenesis and drug resistance. However, more recent findings suggest that numerous medically important fungi may also adopt a biofilm lifestyle, including filamentous fungi (*Aspergillus*, *Zygomycetes*), *Pneumocystis*, and other yeasts (*Blastoschizomyces*, *Saccharomyces*, *Malassezia*, *Trichosporon*, and *Cryptococcus*) (Ramage et al. 2012; Loussert et al. 2010; Seidler et al. 2008; Davis et al. 2002; Singh et al. 2011; D'Antonio et al. 2004; Reynolds and Fink 2001; Cannizzo et al. 2007; Di Bonaventura et al. 2006; Walsh et al. 1986). These fungi have been shown to exhibit properties similar to those described for *Candida* biofilms, including the ability to adhere to medical devices and an increased tolerance of antifungal therapy (Ramage et al. 2009). As much of our knowledge of fungal biofilms and drug resistance was learned from investigations of *Candida*, it will be the focus of this chapter.

Candida biofilms have characteristic architecture and phenotypic traits distinct from free-floating or planktonic cells (Chandra et al. 2001; Costerton et al. 1999; O'Toole 2003; Ramage et al. 2001). Perhaps the most clinically relevant biofilm-specific property is the development of profound drug resistance, allowing biofilm cells to withstand antifungal concentrations up to 1,000-fold higher than those required to inhibit planktonic cells (Chandra et al. 2001; O'Toole 2003; Hawser and Douglas 1994; Mah et al. 2003). This characteristic of biofilms makes them extremely difficult, if not impossible to control in the medical setting. *Candida* biofilms have been shown to be resistant to various antifungals, including amphotericin B, triazoles, echinocandins, and flucytosine, the most commonly used drugs for treatment of *Candida* infections (Chandra et al. 2001; Hawser and Douglas 1994; Baillie and Douglas 1998; Lewis et al. 2002; Mukherjee et al. 2003; Ramage et al. 2002a). Similarly, both *Aspergillus* and *Cryptococcus* biofilms have shown to be less susceptible to multiple drug classes (Seidler et al. 2008; Martinez and Casadevall 2006; Mowat et al. 2008; Beauvais et al. 2007).

Key investigations have explored the mechanisms underlying biofilm-associated drug resistance (Mukherjee et al. 2003; Ramage et al. 2002b; Kumamoto 2005; Khot et al. 2006; LaFleur et al. 2006; Al-Fattani and Douglas 2006; Mitchell et al. 2013). These studies suggest that multiple factors contribute to development of this resilient phenotype. Furthermore, the influence of the individual mechanisms varies throughout the phases of biofilm development and is specific to the antifungal drug class. Factors contributing to *Candida* biofilm resistance include an increase in efflux pump activity, alterations in cell membrane ergosterol content, development of resistant "persister cells," activation of stress responses, an increase in cell density, and the presence of the extracellular matrix (Mukherjee et al. 2003; Ramage et al. 2002b; Kumamoto 2005; Khot et al. 2006; LaFleur et al. 2006; Perumal et al. 2007; Uppuluri et al. 2008; Robbins et al. 2011). Likewise, the *Aspergillus* biofilm phenotype has been linked to increased efflux pump activity and production of an extracellular matrix (Mowat et al. 2008; Rajendran et al. 2013; Bugli et al. 2013). Manufacture of biofilm matrix, a defining biofilm property, is one of the most influential resistance mechanisms, promoting resistance to multiple drug classes for *Candida* biofilms formed by a variety of species (Al-Fattani and Douglas 2006; Mitchell et al. 2013; Hawser et al. 1998; Nett et al. 2007, 2010a; Taff et al. 2012; Martins et al. 2012). The focus of this chapter is the role of extracellular matrix in resistance to antifungals during biofilm growth. The following sections describe pioneering investigations that examined the content of biofilm matrix and established its role in drug resistance. More recent studies have discovered key matrix components, identified a mechanism of resistance, and characterized several factors governing this process.

Extracellular Matrix of Fungal Biofilms

Production of an extracellular matrix is one of the distinguishing characteristics of both eukaryotic and prokaryotic biofilms (O'Toole 2003; Hawser et al. 1998; Donlan and Costerton 2002). This material is critical for biofilm formation, providing the scaffold for surface adhesion and cellular aggregation to maintain the biofilm architecture (Flemming and Wingender 2010). Extracellular matrix has also been shown to assist with retention of water and sorption of nutrients. In addition, the material may be degraded during nutrient-limiting conditions by microbial produced enzymes, providing a carbon or nitrogen source (Flemming and Wingender 2010). One of the most medically important attributes of the matrix is the ability to provide protection from environmental insults, including host defenses and antimicrobial therapies (Donlan 2001b; Costerton et al. 1999).

Candida Biofilm Matrix

Candida frequently causes disease by forming biofilm on the surface of medical devices and has become the most commonly used model for study of fungal biofilms. Hawser et al. initially described the presence of matrix material for *C. albicans* biofilms (Hawser et al. 1998). The extent and character of matrix production was found to vary with environmental conditions. Compared to statically grown biofilms, those formed under rotary shaking conditions produced a denser, canopy-like, extracellular material when imaged by scanning electron microscopy. Also, *C. albicans* biofilms appear to produce less matrix under hypoxic conditions (Stichternoth and Ernst 2009). The clinical relevance of this material is evident by its presence on the catheters of patients with *Candida* biofilm (Paulitsch et al. 2009). Animal models of device-associated infections also reveal abundant biofilm matrix material and provide a means to study the function of this material in vivo (Fig. 1) (Andes et al. 2004; Nett et al. 2010b; Johnson et al. 2012). In vivo, the matrix is postulated to contain both the microbial-derived components identified in vitro and host proteins, such as plasma and salivary proteins that adsorb to the surface of medical devices (Nett and Andes 2006).

The Douglas group has performed several key investigations to examine the content of *Candida* biofilm matrix, including the description of a technique to extract and isolate the matrix of in vitro biofilms (Baillie and Douglas 2000). Quantitative analysis of the *C. albicans* matrix material removed by sonication showed a composition of carbohydrate (41 %, including 15.9 % glucose), protein (5.2 %), and hexosamine (3.4 %). As a complementary method to explore the matrix content, the Douglas group also exposed biofilms to various enzymatic treatments and measured cellular detachment (Al-Fattani and Douglas 2006). This study suggested that protein, chitin, DNA, and β-1,3 glucan are present in the extracellular matrix and contribute to surface adhesion or cellular cohesion (Table 1). Further studies have corroborated these findings and have linked two of these components, β-1,3 glucan and DNA, to the biofilm-specific drug-resistant phenotype, as described in the following section "*Candida* Biofilm Matrix and Drug Resistance" (Table 2) (Nett et al. 2007; Martins et al. 2010, 2012).

To examine the protein content of *C. albicans* biofilm matrix, the Lopez-Ribot group employed 2-D PAGE followed by mass spectrometry (Thomas et al. 2006).

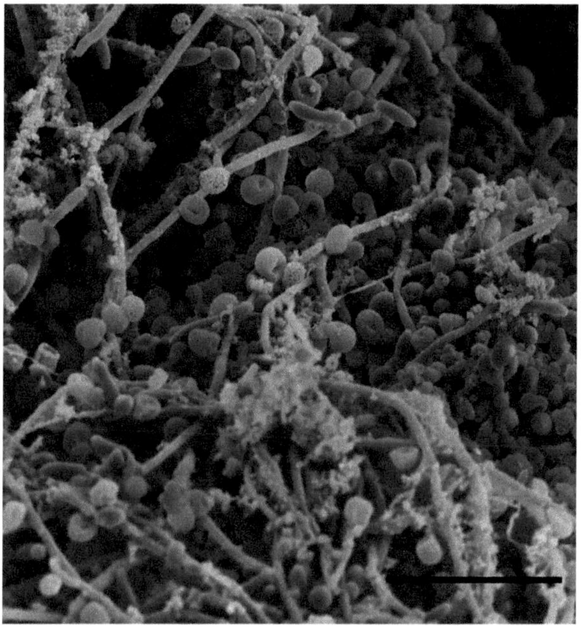

Fig. 1 Extracellular matrix of an in vivo *Candida* biofilm SEM and model

Table 1 Components of fungal biofilm matrix

C. albicans	*A. fumigatus*
Glucose	Galactomannan
Protein	Galactosaminogalactan
Hexosamine	α-1,3 glucan
DNA	Monosaccharides
β-1,3 glucan	Polyols
	Melanin
	Protein

Table 2 *C. albicans* and *A. fumigatus* matrix components influencing antifungal drug resistance

C. albicans	*A. fumigatus*	
β-1,3 glucan		
Fluconazole		
Amphotericin B		
Flucytosine		
DNA	DNA	
Amphotericin B	Amphotericin	
	C. albicans	*A. fumigatus*
β-1,3 glucan	Fluconazole	
	Amphotericin B	
	Flucytosine	
DNA	Amphotericin B	Amphotericin B

Surprisingly, the proteins found in the biofilm matrix were very similar to those identified in the supernatants of non-biofilm cultures. This suggests that in vitro, the proteins that are normally secreted during non-biofilm growth become incorporated into the extracellular matrix during biofilm growth. Several of the identified proteins had previously been shown to be part of the *C. albicans* secretome, including Cht3p, Mp65p, and Mp58p. However, others were not predicted secretory proteins. The role of the individual matrix proteins in biofilm function is not well understood.

Interestingly, the matrix content appears to vary significantly among *Candida* species (Al-Fattani and Douglas 2006; Silva et al. 2009). For example, compared to *C. albicans*, *C. tropicalis* biofilms were found to have a higher hexosamine content (27 %) and were not disrupted by DNase treatment (Al-Fattani and Douglas 2006). Also, the matrix composition is dependent on environmental and media conditions. The matrix of *C. albicans* biofilms formed in RPMI has a nearly a 1,000×-fold higher concentration of DNA when compared to YNB conditions (Martins et al. 2010). Although the concentration of individual matrix components varies among these conditions, *Candida* biofilms uniformly remain resistant to antifungals when adopting a biofilm lifestyle.

Aspergillus Biofilm Matrix

Although *Candida* has been the most commonly studied fungal biofilm pathogen, the role of *Aspergillus* biofilms in clinical disease has become increasingly recognized (Loussert et al. 2010; Ramage et al. 2009). Like *Candida*, *Aspergillus* biofilms have been linked to infection of medical devices (Ramage et al. 2011). However, biofilm growth has also been associated with the most common *Aspergillus* infections, including invasive pulmonary aspergillosis and aspergilloma (Loussert et al. 2010). As a clinical niche, the lung varies greatly from the environments for most *Candida* biofilm infections. Here, fungal biofilms proliferate under static, aerial conditions. The ability of the most common *Aspergillus* sp., *A. fumigatus*, to form a multicellular community with a surrounding extracellular matrix material has been demonstrated both in vitro and in vivo (Loussert et al. 2010; Beauvais et al. 2007). For this organism, biofilm formation and matrix production are greatest under static, aerial conditions. Ultrastructure analysis shows that these biofilms are composed of hyphae coalescing into a three-dimensional structure covered in dense extracellular material with embedded air channels (Beauvais et al. 2007).

Beauvais et al. analyzed the extracellular matrix of in vitro *A. fumigatus* biofilms and found this material to be composed of galactomannan, α-1,3 glucan, monosaccharides, polyols, melanin, and protein (Table 1) (Beauvais et al. 2007). Using immunolabeling, they were able to show galactomannan throughout the cell wall and matrix. In contrast, the labeling of α-1,3 glucan was the highest in the amorphous extracellular matrix material near the hyphal surface. Only a small portion of the matrix contained protein (2 %). Identified proteins included several major secreted antigens, as well as a group of hydrophobins. These hydrophobic surface active proteins, commonly associated with aerial growth, are presumed to play a role in cell-cell adhesion required for mycelial colony formation during biofilm growth. Recent analysis has also shown that DNA accumulates in the matrix of *A. fumigatus* biofilms in vitro (Rajendran et al. 2013; Shopova et al. 2013). This extracellular DNA is identical to genomic DNA and is proposed to be released to the matrix following autolysis (Rajendran et al. 2013). The role of matrix DNA in *Aspergillus* biofilm resistance will be discussed in the following section "*Aspergillus* Biofilm Matrix and Drug Resistance."

By studying the resected aspergillomas of several patients, Loussert et al. shed light on the in vivo composition of *A. fumigatus* biofilms (Loussert et al. 2010). Similar to in vitro biofilms, galactomannan was identified throughout the fungal cell wall and extracellular matrix of in vivo biofilms upon immunolabeling. Also, α-1,3 glucan was found in the matrix material located closest to the cell wall surface. Compared to in vitro biofilms, in vivo biofilms appeared to have a higher concentration of the recently identified cell wall polysaccharide galactosaminogalactan. The presence of melanin in the biofilm matrix was confirmed in vivo, while antigenic proteins were not as apparent in vivo. When comparing the aspergillomas of patients with a murine model of invasive pulmonary aspergillosis, many similarities were noted, including the presence of both matrix galactomannan and galactosaminogalactan (Loussert et al. 2010). However, unlike in vitro biofilms and the aspergilloma biofilm, the extracellular matrix of the pulmonary aspergillosis biofilms did not appear to have a high concentration of α-1,3 glucan.

Candida Biofilm Matrix and Drug Resistance

Linking Matrix to Biofilm Drug Resistance

Several investigations have examined the contribution of the biofilm extracellular matrix to the drug-resistant phenotype associated with the *Candida* biofilm lifestyle (Al-Fattani and Douglas 2004, 2006; Baillie and Douglas 2000; Samaranayake et al. 2005). These studies have used various experimental designs to test the hypothesis that matrix may prevent access of antifungals to the cells embedded in the biofilm, postulating that the material may either slow the rate of drug transport or specifically bind antifungals extracellularly. Together, these investigations show that an intact matrix is one of most influential factors promoting the drug resistance of biofilms formed by various *Candida* species.

The Douglas group performed several of the initial studies exploring *Candida* biofilm matrix and drug resistance (Al-Fattani and Douglas 2004, 2006; Baillie and Douglas 2000). They took advantage of the variable matrix observed under flow and static conditions to determine its impact on drug resistance. *C. albicans* biofilms formed under laminar flow produced an extensive extracellular matrix as observed by scanning electron microscopy (Al-Fattani and Douglas 2006). Compared to biofilms with minimal matrix following growth in static conditions, the dense matrix biofilms were significantly more resistant to amphotericin B. This suggests that the character of the matrix may influence its ability to impede antifungals. However, the

Douglas group also examined the drug susceptibility of biofilms produced under shaking conditions. Although these biofilms produced more matrix than those grown under static conditions, a difference in drug susceptibility was not detected (Baillie and Douglas 2000).

To correlate matrix production with biofilm drug resistance, Samaranayake et al. utilized an antifungal diffusion apparatus (Samaranayake et al. 2005). Biofilms were grown on filter disks, and the penetration of antifungal through the biofilm to a fresh filter was measured by a zone-of-inhibition assay. *C. albicans* biofilms inhibited the penetration of all antifungals tested, including fluconazole, amphotericin B, and flucytosine. *C. parapsilosis* and *C. krusei* biofilms were also found to impede amphotericin B, but flucytosine and fluconazole penetration was higher than for *C. albicans* biofilms. Findings from this investigation support a role for matrix in biofilm antifungal resistance. However, the finding that antifungal concentrations exceeding the amount needed to kill planktonic cells traversed the biofilm questions the importance of the results. One study limitation was the use of a filter substrate which is anticipated to have properties distinct from common device substrates, such as vascular catheters or dentures. Unlike the filter, these confluent surfaces support an adjacent basal layer of cells deep within the biofilm. It is quite possible that antifungal penetration to these cells would be even less than that measured for the filter biofilms in the study.

Matrix Glucan and Drug Sequestration

Several key observations led to the discovery of a drug sequestration activity for the *Candida* biofilm matrix. The Andes group added isolated *Candida* biofilm matrix to planktonic MIC assays and found that this material was able to provide a degree of antifungal resistance to the non-biofilm cells (Nett et al. 2007). To test the hypothesis that matrix was interacting with an antifungal, preventing drug penetration into the cells, radiolabeled fluconazole was tracked through biofilm. The vast majority of the drug was found in association with matrix, suggesting drug sequestration. To explore the contribution of individual matrix components, the biofilm matrix was exposed to enzymes targeting the constituents. Degradation of matrix β-1,3 glucan impaired the biofilm-associated resistance mechanism, indicating a role for this matrix component in protecting biofilms from antifungal drugs. The role for matrix β-1,3 glucan in biofilm drug resistance during clinical infection was supported by the synergistic action of glucanase and fluconazole on rat venous catheters infected with *C. albicans* (Nett et al. 2007).

While investigating the impact of drug treatment on *Candida* biofilm transcription, Vediyappan et al. noted a very interesting finding (Vediyappan et al. 2010). Upon exposure to amphotericin B, biofilms rapidly converted to the yellow color of the drug. After DMSO extraction of biofilms, active amphotericin B was recovered. A similar drug binding pattern was observed for several preparations of β-1,3 glucan, suggesting that this component of the matrix may be binding amphotericin B as well, trapping the antifungal and preventing its activity on cells within the biofilm.

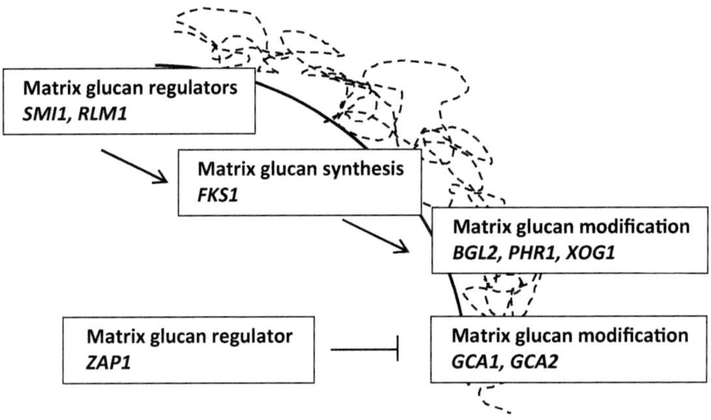

Fig. 2 Genetic regulation of *C. albicans* biofilm matrix productions

Linking matrix β-1,3 glucan to resistance with a second antifungal in a distinct drug class points to a multidrug mechanism specific to the biofilm lifestyle. A similar resistance mechanism has also been shown for flucytosine (Nett et al. 2010a). Furthermore, this mechanism does not appear to be unique to *C. albicans*. Biofilms formed by other common *Candida* species, including *C. glabrata*, *C. parapsilosis*, and *C. tropicalis*, also have been shown to produce matrix β-1,3 glucan that sequesters antifungal and enhances drug resistance (Mitchell et al. 2013).

Matrix Glucan Production and Modification

Uncovering the genetic basis underlying matrix antifungal sequestration has been of great interest. As β-1,3 glucan was found to be the matrix component most closely linked to biofilm drug resistance, gene products capable of synthesizing and modifying this polysaccharide were ideal suspects (Fig. 2). In *C. albicans*, *FKS1* encodes a glucan synthase responsible for manufacture of cell wall β-1,3 glucan during planktonic growth. By employing a set of genetic mutants, Nett et al. linked this gene to the production of matrix β-1,3 glucan, matrix sequestration of antifungal, and multidrug resistance (Nett et al. 2010a, c). The finding was described both in vitro and in a rat venous catheter model of biofilm infection. The enhanced drug resistance related to *FKS1* appears to be specific to the biofilm lifestyle. During biofilm growth, *C. albicans* mutants with *FKS1* disruption were significantly more susceptible to fluconazole while this mutation did not impact planktonic susceptibility.

To delineate the process by which glucan is modified and delivered to the extracellular biofilm matrix, Taff et al. employed a candidate gene approach, examining a set of mutants based on transcriptional profiling of *C. albicans* in a rat venous catheter biofilm (Taff et al. 2012). They identified a role for two predicted glucan transferases (Bgl2p and Phr1p) and an exo-glucanase (Xog1p) in both delivery of biofilm matrix and the development of the resistance to antifungals during biofilm growth. Mutants with disruption of one of these genes produced significantly less matrix β-1,3 glucan, ultimately resulting in disruption of matrix function. During biofilm growth, the mutants were approximately 50–70 % more susceptible to azole drugs compared to the parent strain both in vitro and in a rat venous catheter biofilm model. The isolated matrix of the mutant strains exhibited decreased capacity for antifungal sequestration. The gene products appear to have partially redundant functions as the phenotype was augmented in strains with two of the three genes deleted. Furthermore, studies support a role for Bgl2p, Phr1p, and Xog1p downstream of Fks1p, the primary glucan synthase for biofilm matrix β-1,3 glucan. These gene products are proposed to cooperate in modification of matrix glucan for development of functional matrix capable of sequestering antifungal drugs and promoting biofilm antifungal drug resistance.

Regulation of Matrix Glucan

Several pathways have now been shown to be involved in regulating production of *Candida* biofilm matrix and drug resistance. Nobile et al. discovered a critical negative regulator of *C. albicans* biofilm matrix glucan production both in vitro and in vivo (Nobile et al. 2009). In a screen of transcription factor mutants, the *zap1−/−* mutant was noted to have a glistening appearance that correlated with abundant matrix glucan. Through transcription profiling and chromatin immunoprecipitation, several groups of target genes were identified. First, Zap1p was found to repress transcription of two glucoamylases (*GCA1* and *GCA2*). These enzymes are postulated to have a positive role in matrix production, likely by hydrolyzing insoluble carbohydrates for release into the matrix. However, their specific role has not been further identified. A second group of Zap1p targets includes three alcohol dehydrogenases (*ADH5*, *CSH1*, and *LFD6*). These gene products are proposed to participate in production of alcohols, influencing biofilm formation and matrix glucan production through quorum signal pathways. However, further investigation is needed to establish this link. Interestingly, the enzymes required for matrix glucan modification do not appear to be under Zap1p control (Taff et al. 2012). Transcription of *XOG1*, *PHR1*, and *BGL2* was not altered in the *zap1−/−* mutant, suggesting that Zap1 governs matrix production through an independent pathway.

The Cowen group discovered heat shock protein, Hsp90p, as novel regulator *of C. albicans* biofilm matrix production and drug resistance (Robbins et al. 2011). Disruption of this pathway increased the effectiveness of triazole drugs both in vitro and in a rat venous catheter model. Unlike planktonic conditions, this pathway was not modulated via calcineurin or Mkc1 pathways. The finding that inhibition of Hsp90p activity led to decreased β-1,3 glucan in the matrix of *C. albicans* biofilms suggests that Hsp90p is a key player in the production of drug-sequestering matrix. How Hsp90p specifically modulates this activity is unknown, but it is hypothesized to stabilize one or more of the proteins involved in production and regulation of matrix production, such as Fks1p or Zap1p.

A search for additional regulators of biofilm matrix-associated drug resistance identified downstream components of the yeast PKC pathway (Nett et al. 2011). *C. albicans* mutants with disruption of either *SMI1* or *RLM1* were deficient in both matrix glucan production and susceptibility to azole drugs. These factors are thought to govern matrix-associated drug resistance through *FKS1*, as overexpression of this glucan synthase gene restored the biofilm-associated drug-resistant phenotype. Surprisingly, upstream PKC pathway components do not appear to be involved in regulation of biofilm matrix production and drug resistance. This suggests that matrix-associated drug resistance and cell wall integrity are networked, but that the biofilm drug resistance is triggered through a pathway distinct from the PKC pathway.

Matrix Extracellular DNA and Drug Resistance

Extracellular DNA is one of the *Candida* biofilm matrix components critical for biofilm integrity and maintenance (Martins et al. 2010). Degradation of matrix DNA not only destroys the biofilm architecture, but the addition of exogenous DNA promotes biofilm growth (Martins et al. 2010). To determine the contribution of matrix DNA to biofilm drug resistance, Martins et al. treated *C. albicans* biofilms with DNase and measured the impact on drug susceptibility (Martins et al. 2012). Degradation of extracellular DNA significantly improved the activity of amphotericin B against *Candida* biofilms. However, biofilms treated with DNase remained resistant to both fluconazole and caspofungin. This suggests that the mechanism involves a specific DNA-amphotericin B interaction. An alternative possibility is that the matrix DNA may interact with a variety of antifungals, but other resistance processes in play maintain biofilm resistance upon DNA degradation. The mechanism underlying how matrix DNA contributes to *Candida* biofilm resistance remains unknown. It is also a mystery if the biofilm resistance phenotypes linked to matrix glucan and matrix DNA are intertwined.

Aspergillus Biofilm Matrix and Drug Resistance

Considerably less is known about the process of *Aspergillus* biofilm matrix production and how it impacts drug susceptibility during biofilm growth. Based upon findings from bacterial and *Candida* biofilm investigations, the matrix of *Aspergillus* biofilms is similarly thought to contribute to antimicrobial resistance, perhaps through impairing drug diffusion to the fungal cells, either by slow transit or by binding the drugs (Beauvais et al. 2007; Rajendran et al. 2013; Bugli et al. 2013). As the extracellular matrix content increases as *A. fumigatus* biofilms mature, this material is thought to play a role in drug resistance during the later phases of biofilm growth (Beauvais et al. 2007).

One recently recognized matrix component shown to impact drug resistance is extracellular DNA. Rajendran et al. showed that the content of DNA in the matrix increased as in vitro *A. fumigatus* biofilms matured from 8 to 48 h (Rajendran et al. 2013). Using RAPD, they were able to confirm that this extracellular DNA was identical to genomic DNA. The finding that this DNA release was linked to chitinase activity suggests autolysis as the underlying process. The matrix DNA of *A. fumigatus* biofilms appears to be important for both biofilm structural integrity and resistance to antifungals. Degradation of this material by DNase decreases the biomass of the biofilm and renders biofilms more susceptible to both amphotericin B and the echinocandin, caspofungin. Interestingly, exogenous DNA also promotes structural integrity and increases biofilm matrix carbohydrate production, suggesting a potential role for host DNA during in vivo *Aspergillus* biofilm formation (Rajendran et al. 2013; Shopova et al. 2013).

Much remains unknown about *Aspergillus* biofilm drug resistance and how the various components of the biofilm matrix influence this phenotype. An intriguing study by Bugli et al. found that administration of alginate lyase increased in vitro *A. fumigatus* biofilm susceptibility to amphotericin B (Bugli et al. 2013). This enzyme degrades uronic acid-containing carbohydrates and is anticipated to be acting on the extracellular matrix carbohydrates of *Aspergillus* biofilms. This study suggests that a previously unidentified matrix carbohydrate is contributing to antifungal drug resistance during biofilm growth. Further investigation is of interest to characterize this material and its specific role in resistance to antifungal therapy.

Conclusions

The most common nosocomial fungal pathogens produce disease by growing as drug-resistant, multicellular, biofilm communities. Production of an extracellular matrix, one of the distinguishing biofilm traits, is not only critical for adhesion and structural support but confers resistance to antimicrobials (Fig. 3). In *Candida*, the presence of β-1,3 glucan has been linked to the ability of the matrix material to sequester antifungals and prevent them from reaching their cellular targets. For both *Candida* and *Aspergillus*, extracellular DNA in the biofilm matrix has been shown to be instrumental in maintaining the biofilm drug resistance. Whether the matrix carbohydrates and DNA cooperate for this process remains unknown. Several key regulators of *C. albicans* biofilm matrix and drug resistance have been identified, while regulation of this pathway in *Aspergillus* has been relatively unexplored.

With the increasing prevalence of immunosuppressed patients with invasive fungal infections, further understanding of this drug resistance mechanism is a logical step to identification of novel drug targets and therapeutic strategies. However, delivery of novel compounds targeting biofilms cells may prove a challenge, as the matrix often impedes or sequesters drugs extracellularly. Potential strategies to overcome this phenomenon include identification of matrix-degrading compounds, development of matrix-permeable compounds, and combination therapy targeting both the matrix and biofilm cells.

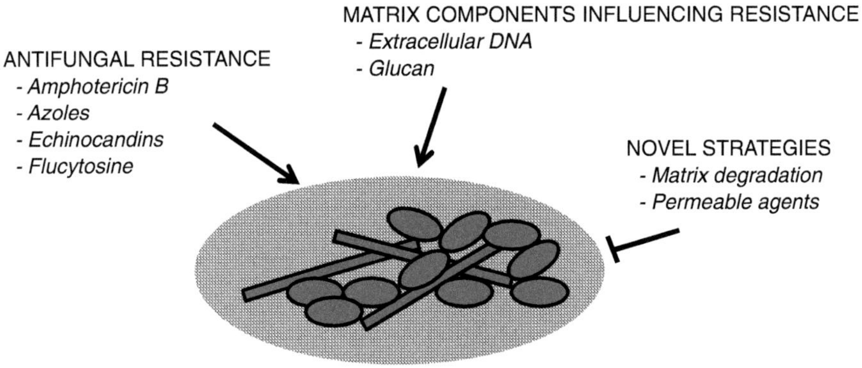

Fig. 3 Overview of fungal biofilm matrix and drug resistance

References

Al-Fattani MA, Douglas LJ (2004) Penetration of *Candida* biofilms by antifungal agents. Antimicrob Agents Chemother 48:3291–3297

Al-Fattani MA, Douglas LJ (2006) Biofilm matrix of *Candida albicans* and *Candida tropicalis*: chemical composition and role in drug resistance. J Med Microbiol 55:999–1008

Anaissie EJ, Rex JH, Uzun O, Vartivarian S (1998) Predictors of adverse outcome in cancer patients with candidemia. Am J Med 104:238–245

Andes D, Nett J, Oschel P, Albrecht R, Marchillo K, Pitula A (2004) Development and characterization of an in vivo central venous catheter *Candida albicans* biofilm model. Infect Immun 72:6023–6031

Andes DR, Safdar N, Baddley JW et al (2012) Impact of treatment strategy on outcomes in patients with candidemia and other forms of invasive candidiasis: a patient-level quantitative review of randomized trials. Clin Infect Dis 54:1110–1122

Baillie GS, Douglas LJ (1998) Effect of growth rate on resistance of *Candida albicans* biofilms to antifungal agents. Antimicrob Agents Chemother 42:1900–1905

Baillie GS, Douglas LJ (2000) Matrix polymers of *Candida biofilms* and their possible role in biofilm resistance to antifungal agents. J Antimicrob Chemother 46:397–403

Beauvais A, Schmidt C, Guadagnini S et al (2007) An extracellular matrix glues together the aerial-grown hyphae of *Aspergillus fumigatus*. Cell Microbiol 9:1588–1600

Bugli F, Posteraro B, Papi M et al (2013) In vitro interaction between alginate lyase and amphotericin B against *Aspergillus fumigatus* biofilm determined by different methods. Antimicrob Agents Chemother 57:1275–1282

Cannizzo FT, Eraso E, Ezkurra PA et al (2007) Biofilm development by clinical isolates of *Malassezia pachydermatis*. Med Mycol 45:357–361

Chandra J, Kuhn DM, Mukherjee PK, Hoyer LL, McCormick T, Ghannoum MA (2001) Biofilm formation by the fungal pathogen *Candida albicans*: development, architecture, and drug resistance. J Bacteriol 183:5385–5394

Costerton JW, Stewart PS, Greenberg EP (1999) Bacterial biofilms: a common cause of persistent infections. Science 284:1318–1322

D'Antonio D, Parruti G, Pontieri E et al (2004) Slime production by clinical isolates of *Blastoschizomyces capitatus* from patients with hematological malignancies and catheter-related fungemia. Eur J Clin Microbiol Infect Dis 23:787–789

Davis LE, Cook G, Costerton JW (2002) Biofilm on ventriculo-peritoneal shunt tubing as a cause of treatment failure in coccidioidal meningitis. Emerg Infect Dis 8:376–379

Di Bonaventura G, Pompilio A, Picciani C, Iezzi M, D'Antonio D, Piccolomini R (2006) Biofilm formation by the emerging fungal pathogen *Trichosporon asahii*: development, architecture, and antifungal resistance. Antimicrob Agents Chemother 50:3269–3276

Donlan RM (2001a) Biofilm formation: a clinically relevant microbiological process. Clin Infect Dis 33:1387–1392

Donlan RM (2001b) Biofilms and device-associated infections. Emerg Infect Dis 7:277–281

Donlan RM, Costerton JW (2002) Biofilms: survival mechanisms of clinically relevant microorganisms. Clin Microbiol Rev 15:167–193

Douglas LJ (2002) Medical importance of biofilms in *Candida* infections. Rev Iberoam Micol 19:139–143

Flemming HC, Wingender J (2010) The biofilm matrix. Nat Rev 8:623–633

Groeger JS, Lucas AB, Thaler HT et al (1993) Infectious morbidity associated with long-term use of venous access devices in patients with cancer. Ann Intern Med 119:1168–1174

Hawser SP, Douglas LJ (1994) Biofilm formation by *Candida* species on the surface of catheter materials in vitro. Infect Immun 62:915–921

Hawser SP, Baillie GS, Douglas LJ (1998) Production of extracellular matrix by *Candida albicans* biofilms. J Med Microbiol 47:253–256

Johnson CC, Yu A, Lee H, Fidel PL Jr, Noverr MC (2012) Development of a contemporary animal model of *Candida albicans*-associated denture stomatitis using a novel intraoral denture system. Infect Immun 80:1736–1743

Khot PD, Suci PA, Miller RL, Nelson RD, Tyler BJ (2006) A small subpopulation of blastospores in *Candida albicans* biofilms exhibit resistance to amphotericin B associated with differential regulation of ergosterol and beta-1,6-glucan pathway genes. Antimicrob Agents Chemother 50:3708–3716

Kojic EM, Darouiche RO (2004) *Candida* infections of medical devices. Clin Microbiol Rev 17:255–267

Kralovicova K, Spanik S, Oravcova E et al (1997) Fungemia in cancer patients undergoing chemotherapy versus surgery: risk factors, etiology and outcome. Scand J Infect Dis 29:301–304

Kumamoto CA (2005) A contact-activated kinase signals *Candida albicans* invasive growth and biofilm development. Proc Natl Acad Sci U S A 102:5576–5581

LaFleur MD, Kumamoto CA, Lewis K (2006) *Candida albicans* biofilms produce antifungal-tolerant persister cells. Antimicrob Agents Chemother 50:3839–3846

Lecciones JA, Lee JW, Navarro EE et al (1992) Vascular catheter-associated fungemia in patients with cancer: analysis of 155 episodes. Clin Infect Dis 14:875–883

Lewis RE, Kontoyiannis DP, Darouiche RO, Raad II, Prince RA (2002) Antifungal activity of amphotericin B, fluconazole, and voriconazole in an in vitro model of *Candida* catheter-related bloodstream infection. Antimicrob Agents Chemother 46:3499–3505

Loussert C, Schmitt C, Prevost MC et al (2010) In vivo biofilm composition of *Aspergillus fumigatus*. Cell Microbiol 12:405–410

Mah TF, Pitts B, Pellock B, Walker GC, Stewart PS, O'Toole GA (2003) A genetic basis for *Pseudomonas aeruginosa* biofilm antibiotic resistance. Nature 426:306–310

Martinez LR, Casadevall A (2006) Susceptibility of *Cryptococcus neoformans* biofilms to antifungal agents in vitro. Antimicrob Agents Chemother 50:1021–1033

Martins M, Uppuluri P, Thomas DP et al (2010) Presence of extracellular DNA in the *Candida albicans* biofilm matrix and its contribution to biofilms. Mycopathologia 169:323–331

Martins M, Henriques M, Lopez-Ribot JL, Oliveira R (2012) Addition of DNase improves the in vitro activity of antifungal drugs against *Candida albicans* biofilms. Mycoses 55:80–85

Mitchell KF, Taff HT, Cuevas MA, Reinicke EL, Sanchez H, Andes DR (2013) Role of matrix beta-1,3 glucan in antifungal resistance of non-albicans *Candida* biofilms. Antimicrob Agents Chemother 57:1918–1920

Mowat E, Lang S, Williams C, McCulloch E, Jones B, Ramage G (2008) Phase-dependent antifungal activity against *Aspergillus fumigatus* developing multicellular filamentous biofilms. J Antimicrob Chemother 62:1281–1284

Mukherjee PK, Chandra J, Kuhn DM, Ghannoum MA (2003) Mechanism of fluconazole resistance in *Candida albicans* biofilms: phase-specific role of efflux pumps and membrane sterols. Infect Immun 71:4333–4340

Nett J, Andes D (2006) *Candida albicans* biofilm development, modeling a host-pathogen interaction. Curr Opin Microbiol 9:340–345

Nett J, Lincoln L, Marchillo K et al (2007) Putative role of beta-1,3 glucans in *Candida albicans* biofilm resistance. Antimicrob Agents Chemother 51:510–520

Nett JE, Crawford K, Marchillo K, Andes DR (2010a) Role of Fks1p and matrix glucan in *Candida albicans* biofilm resistance to an echinocandin, pyrimidine, and polyene. Antimicrob Agents Chemother 54:3505–3508

Nett JE, Marchillo K, Spiegel CA, Andes DR (2010b) Development and validation of an in vivo *Candida albicans* biofilm denture model. Infect Immun 78:3650–3659

Nett JE, Sanchez H, Cain MT, Andes DR (2010c) Genetic basis of *Candida* biofilm resistance due to drug-sequestering matrix glucan. J Infect Dis 202:171–175

Nett JE, Sanchez H, Cain MT, Ross KM, Andes DR (2011) Interface of *Candida albicans* biofilm matrix-associated drug resistance and cell wall integrity regulation. Eukaryot Cell 10:1660–1669

Nobile CJ, Nett JE, Hernday AD et al (2009) Biofilm matrix regulation by *Candida albicans* Zap1. PLoS Biol 7:e1000133

O'Toole GA (2003) To build a biofilm. J Bacteriol 185:2687–2689

Paulitsch AH, Willinger B, Zsalatz B, Stabentheiner E, Marth E, Buzina W (2009) In-vivo *Candida* biofilms in scanning electron microscopy. Med Mycol 47:690–696

Perumal P, Mekala S, Chaffin WL (2007) Role for cell density in antifungal drug resistance in *Candida albicans* biofilms. Antimicrob Agents Chemother 51:2454–2463

Raad II, Sabbagh MF, Rand KH, Sherertz RJ (1992) Quantitative tip culture methods and the diagnosis of central venous catheter-related infections. Diagn Microbiol Infect Dis 15:13–20

Rajendran R, Williams C, Lappin DF, Millington O, Martins M, Ramage G (2013) Extracellular DNA release acts as an antifungal resistance mechanism in mature *Aspergillus fumigatus* biofilms. Eukaryot Cell 12:420–429

Ramage G, Vandewalle K, Wickes BL, Lopez-Ribot JL (2001) Characteristics of biofilm formation by *Candida albicans*. Rev Iberoam Micol 18:163–170

Ramage G, VandeWalle K, Bachmann SP, Wickes BL, Lopez-Ribot JL (2002a) In vitro pharmacodynamic properties of three antifungal agents against preformed *Candida albicans* biofilms determined by time-kill studies. Antimicrob Agents Chemother 46:3634–3636

Ramage G, Bachmann S, Patterson TF, Wickes BL, Lopez-Ribot JL (2002b) Investigation of multidrug efflux pumps in relation to fluconazole resistance in *Candida albicans* biofilms. J Antimicrob Chemother 49:973–980

Ramage G, Mowat E, Jones B, Williams C, Lopez-Ribot J (2009) Our current understanding of fungal biofilms. Crit Rev Microbiol 35:340–355

Ramage G, Rajendran R, Gutierrez-Correa M, Jones B, Williams C (2011) *Aspergillus* biofilms: clinical and industrial significance. FEMS Microbiol Lett 324:89–97

Ramage G, Rajendran R, Sherry L, Williams C (2012) Fungal biofilm resistance. Int J Microbiol 2012:528521

Rex JH, Bennett JE, Sugar AM et al (1995) Intravascular catheter exchange and duration of candidemia. NIAID Mycoses Study Group and the Candidemia Study Group. Clin Infect Dis 21:994–996

Reynolds TB, Fink GR (2001) Bakers' yeast, a model for fungal biofilm formation. Science 291:878–881

Richards MJ, Edwards JR, Culver DH, Gaynes RP (1999) Nosocomial infections in medical intensive care units in the United States. National Nosocomial Infections Surveillance System. Crit Care Med 27:887–892

Robbins N, Uppuluri P, Nett J et al (2011) Hsp90 governs dispersion and drug resistance of fungal biofilms. PLoS Pathog 7:e1002257

Samaranayake YH, Ye J, Yau JY, Cheung BP, Samaranayake LP (2005) In vitro method to study antifungal perfusion in *Candida* biofilms. J Clin Microbiol 43:818–825

Schmitt ME, Brown TA, Trumpower BL (1990) A rapid and simple method for preparation of RNA from *Saccharomyces cerevisiae*. Nucleic Acids Res 18:3091–3092

Seidler MJ, Salvenmoser S, Muller FM (2008) *Aspergillus fumigatus* forms biofilms with reduced antifungal drug susceptibility on bronchial epithelial cells. Antimicrob Agents Chemother 52:4130–4136

Shin JH, Kee SJ, Shin MG et al (2002) Biofilm production by isolates of *Candida* species recovered from nonneutropenic patients: comparison of bloodstream isolates with isolates from other sources. J Clin Microbiol 40:1244–1248

Shopova I, Bruns S, Thywissen A, Kniemeyer O, Brakhage AA, Hillmann F (2013) Extrinsic extracellular DNA leads to biofilm formation and colocalizes with matrix polysaccharides in the human pathogenic fungus *Aspergillus fumigatus*. Front Microbiol 4:141

Silva S, Henriques M, Martins A, Oliveira R, Williams D, Azeredo J (2009) Biofilms of non-*Candida albicans Candida* species: quantification, structure and matrix composition. Med Mycol 47:681–689

Singh R, Shivaprakash MR, Chakrabarti A (2011) Biofilm formation by zygomycetes: quantification, structure and matrix composition. Microbiology 157:2611–2618

Stichternoth C, Ernst JF (2009) Hypoxic adaptation by Efg1 regulates biofilm formation by *Candida albicans*. Appl Environ Microbiol 75:3663–3672

Taff HT, Nett JE, Zarnowski R et al (2012) A *Candida* biofilm-induced pathway for matrix glucan delivery: implications for drug resistance. PLoS Pathog 8:e1002848

Thomas DP, Bachmann SP, Lopez-Ribot JL (2006) Proteomics for the analysis of the *Candida albicans* biofilm lifestyle. Proteomics 6:5795–5804

Uppuluri P, Nett J, Heitman J, Andes D (2008) Synergistic effect of calcineurin inhibitors and fluconazole against *Candida albicans* biofilms. Antimicrob Agents Chemother 52:1127–1132

Vediyappan G, Rossignol T, d'Enfert C (2010) Interaction of *Candida albicans* biofilms with antifungals: transcriptional response and binding of antifungals to beta-glucans. Antimicrob Agents Chemother 54:2096–2111

Walsh TJ, Schlegel R, Moody MM, Costerton JW, Salcman M (1986) Ventriculoatrial shunt infection due to *Cryptococcus neoformans*: an ultrastructural and quantitative microbiological study. Neurosurgery 18:373–375

Use of Novel Tools to Probe Drug Resistance in Fungi

Yanan Zhao and David S. Perlin

Contents

Abstract

Antifungal drug resistance threatens therapeutic effectiveness and needs to be diagnosed in a timely manner. Currently, recognition of antifungal resistance still relies on culture-based susceptibility testing. Yet, antifungal susceptibility testing is not routinely performed and often comes too late to influence a timely decision on patient management. With the quantum leap of molecular technology and accrued insights on basic fungal cell biology and antifungal drug resistance mechanisms, some novel molecular techniques are now available to provide a faster and more accurate assessment of both primary and secondary resistance than classical methodologies. Validated targets for echinocandin resistance in *Candida* spp. and triazole resistance in *Aspergillus fumigatus* and *Candida* spp. are particularly well suited for molecular detection. Yet, implementation of a

Y. Zhao • D.S. Perlin (✉)
Department of Microbiology and Molecular Genetics, Public Health Research Institute, New Jersey Medical School, Rutgers, The State University of New Jersey, Newark, NJ, USA
e-mail: zhaoy1@njms.rutgers.edu; perlinds@njms.rutgers.edu

M. Gotte et al. (eds.), *Handbook of Antimicrobial Resistance*,
DOI 10.1007/978-1-4939-0694-9_21

molecular diagnosis for drug resistance into the clinical settings requires validation in well-designed clinical trials, as well as improved methods for highly efficient primary sample preparation.

Keywords
Invasive fungal infections • Molecular diagnosis • Species identification • Susceptibility • Triazole • Echinocandin • Antifungal drug resistance • Primary resistance • Secondary resistance • *Candida* spp. • *Aspergillus* spp. • Efflux pumps • *CYP51A* • 1,3-β-D-glucan synthase • *FKS*

Introduction

Opportunistic fungal infections are widespread in immunosuppressed individuals and are a growing concern for the management of such patients. In the past two decades, the frequency of invasive fungal infections (IFIs) has risen (Pfaller and Diekema 2010) and the high mortality rate poses challenges for clinicians. The treatment options for IFIs are limited since there are relatively few chemical classes and targets represented by existing antifungal drugs. Triazole and/or echinocandin antifungal drugs are widely used as first-line antifungal therapy, depending on the pathogen, disease, and host status. Antifungal agents are often prescribed for prophylaxis and empiric or preemptive therapy for patients at risk of developing IFIs. Both facts have raised concern about the emergence of antifungal drug resistance. Antifungal resistance is generally classified as either primary (present before exposure to antifungals) or secondary (develops after exposure to antifungals). Primary resistance is observed as a shift toward colonization with inherently less susceptible organisms, while secondary resistance involves the emergence of cell-specific resistance mechanisms in normally susceptible strains. In both cases, antifungal-resistant strains threaten therapeutic effectiveness and need to be diagnosed in a timely manner. Delays in the administration of appropriate therapy beyond 12 h can increase the apparent mortality for *Candida* bloodstream infections by threefold (Morrell et al. 2005).

Currently, recognition of antifungal resistance still relies on culture-based susceptibility testing. Antifungal susceptibility is normally measured by broth microdilution using the minimum inhibitory concentration (MIC) or disk diffusion assays in accordance with guidelines of the Clinical Laboratory Standards Institute (CLSI) standard and European Committee on Antimicrobial Susceptibility Testing (EUCAST) Definitive Document (2008a, b; CLSI 2008a, b). Yet, antifungal susceptibility testing is not routinely performed and requires 48–72 h following identification, which often comes too late to influence a timely decision on patient management. In the meantime, with the quantum leap of molecular technology and accrued insights on basic fungal cell biology and antifungal drug mechanisms, some novel and robust molecular techniques are now available to provide a faster and more accurate assessment of both primary and secondary resistance than classical methodologies.

Primary Resistance Assessment by Molecular Methods

As primary resistance occurs due to inherently less susceptible fungal species, a rapid and accurate identification of fungal pathogen to the species level provides a workable inference of drug susceptibility that guides treatment choices. For example, serious infection due to *C. krusei* would not be expected to be treated effectively with triazoles like fluconazole or itraconazole because of the well-known intrinsic resistance. Using culture-based identification, the gold standard of IFI diagnosis, such information is available in 48 ~ 72 h after blood draw. However, in the case of *Candida* infections, the mortality rate increases steeply from 11.1 % if antifungal treatment is initiated within 12 h following the first culture-positive blood draw to 33.1 % at 48 h (Morrell et al. 2005). Whereas it seems formidable to fit culture-based identification into this narrow time window, molecular methods offer a promising alternative to facilitate rapid and accurate diagnosis. In principle, a primary sample like blood or tissue specimen can be analyzed in a matter of hours to generate species-specific information, which predominantly involves amplification-detection platforms, including polymerase chain reaction (PCR) (DNA amplification) and nucleic acid sequence-based amplification (RNA amplification)-based assays. Various molecular tools, in particular, post-amplification reporting methods like allele-specific molecular beacon (MB) technology, DNA sequencing, and melt curve analysis have been incorporated with these amplification techniques for species identification (Al-Wathiqi et al. 2013; Loeffler et al. 2000a; Park et al. 2000). Of note, some new high-throughput technologies seem more attractive, such as Luminex xMAP technology, which utilizes microbeads and specific capture probe hybridization to identify up to 100 different target sequences in a single reaction vessel (Loeffler et al. 2000b). The assay permits rapid identification of a broad spectrum of fungal pathogens, including 10 fungal genera and 29 fungal species, covering both commonly occurring and emerging fungi (Landlinger et al. 2009). PCR/electrospray ionization mass spectrometry (PCR/ESI-MS) is another robust tool, which is capable of identifying nearly all known human pathogens, including previously unknown or unculturable organisms directly from primary clinical samples such as blood or respiratory specimen (Ecker et al. 2010; Wolk et al. 2012). By identifying minute quantities and mixtures of nucleic acids without the need for a detection probe, PCR/ESI-MS offers a critical advantage of discovering unusual or unculturable pathogens and mixed infections. This was evidenced by a recent study finding *Aspergillus terreus* in culture-negative bronchoalveolar lavage (BAL) fluid from a myelogenous leukemia patient who was on empiric amphotericin B therapy (Modi et al. 2012).

Molecular Diagnosis of Acquired Triazole Resistance

Triazole antifungal drugs (fluconazole, voriconazole, itraconazole, and posaconazole) have been in clinical use since early 1980s. Acquired azole resistance was rare during the first decade of clinical use, but it became a significant problem in the 1990s when more and more azole-resistant *Candida* spp. isolates were reported in patients with compromised immune systems (Heald et al. 1996; Rautemaa et al. 2007; Rex et al. 1995). Later, a global antifungal surveillance study involving more than 140,000 *Candida* spp. isolates collected over the period of 1997–2005 showed that the overall resistance to fluconazole and voriconazole was 6.2 % and 3.1 %, respectively (Pfaller et al. 2007). Similarly, it is increasingly recognized that *Aspergillus fumigatus* has been rapidly acquiring resistance to triazole agents (Verweij et al. 2007), the first-line therapy for all forms of aspergillosis and the only orally active group of antifungal drugs within the limited therapeutic options (Walsh et al. 2008). The frequency of azole resistance in clinical *A. fumigatus* isolates by patient was 0 % in 2002 and 2003, significantly increased to 17 % in 2007, 14 % in 2008, and 20 % in 2009 at a referral center for chronic aspergillosis in Manchester, United Kingdom (Bueid et al. 2010; Howard et al. 2009). Given the fact that *Candida* spp. are the most common overall invasive fungal infection, and *Aspergillus* infections are the most predominant invasive mold infection, and collectively they account for 90 % of all nosocomial fungal infections (Fridkin and Jarvis 1996), triazole resistance is a serious issue. Going forward, effective management of invasive fungal infections requires rapid diagnosis of both the infecting organism and associated drug resistance, as well as discovery of new drugs with novel mechanisms of action.

The target of triazole drugs is lanosterol 14α-demethylase, a key enzyme in ergosterol biosynthesis. The action of triazole agents on this target enzyme results in depletion of ergosterol, which disrupts the structure and alters the functional properties of the fungal plasma membrane leading to inhibition of fungal growth. Triazole resistance is well characterized and several principal mechanisms have been described in *Candida* species (MacCallum et al. 2010; Perlin 2009; Verweij et al. 2009a) (Table 1). One prominent mechanism is the acquisition of point mutations in the gene encoding for the target enzyme (*ERG11*), resulting in an altered drug-binding domain with reduced affinity for or incapacity to bind azoles. Another mechanism related is the overexpression or upregulation of the target enzyme. The third prominent mechanism involves upregulation of a variety of multidrug efflux pumps including the ATP-binding cassette (ABC) transporters encoded by *CDR* genes (*CDR1* and *CDR2*) and major facilitator superfamily (MFS) encoded by *MDR* genes (*MDR1*). Upregulation of the *CDR* gene-encoded efflux pumps appears to confer resistance to multiple triazole drugs, while induction of that encoded by *MDR* genes are more closely associated with fluconazole resistance (Pfaller 2012). The increased mRNA level of these genes are further observed to be associated with alterations on global transcriptional regulators such as *TAC1*, *PDR1*, and *UPC2* (Coste et al. 2006; Flowers et al. 2012; Nagi et al. 2011; Oliver et al. 2007; Sanglard and Odds 2002; Vermitsky and Edlind 2004). Another mechanism of azole resistance in *Candida* species is revealed by the observation that growth inhibition of *Candida* cells can be circumvented by the accumulation of 14α-methylfecosterol if cells are deficient in sterol $\Delta^{5,6}$-desaturase, encoded by *ERG3* (Kelly et al. 1997; Martel et al. 2010). Last, chromosomal aneuploidy

Table 1 Summary of potential targets for acquired triazole and echinocandin resistance

	Molecular mechanism	Organism	Genetic target	References	Suitable detection methods
Triazoles	1. Target site mutations	*C. albicans*	*ERG11*	MacCallum et al. 2010; Morio et al. 2010; White et al. 2002	DNA sequencing; real-time PCR with allele-specific molecular beacon probe or melting curve analysis
		C. glabrata	*ERG11*	Hull et al. 2012; Sanguinetti et al. 2005	
		A. fumigatus	*CYP51A*	Bueid et al. 2010; Howard et al. 2009; Verweij et al. 2009a	
	2. Overexpression of target site	*C. albicans*	*ERG11*	Pancholi et al. 2004; Perea et al. 2001	Quantitative RT-PCR; microarray
		C. glabrata	*ERG11*	Henry et al. 2000	
		A. fumigatus	*CYP51A*	Arendrup et al. 2010	
	3. Drug efflux pumps				
	ABC	*C. albicans*	*CDR1, CDR2*	Chau et al. 2004; Holmes et al. 2008; Karababa et al. 2004	Quantitative RT-PCR; microarray
		C. glabrata	*CDR1, CDR2, SNQ2*	Sanguinetti et al. 2005	
		A. fumigatus	*MDR1, MDR4, CDR1B*	Ferreira et al. 2005; Fraczek et al. 2013; Nascimento et al. 2003; Slaven et al. 2002	
	MFS	*C. albicans*	*MDR1*	Chau et al. 2004; Karababa et al. 2004	
		A. fumigatus	*MDR3*	Ferreira et al. 2005; Nascimento et al. 2003	
	4. Transcription factors				
	ABC	*C. albicans*	*TAC1, CZF1*	Coste et al. 2006; Dhamgaye et al. 2012	Microarray; DNA sequencing; real-time PCR; RNA sequencing

(*continued*)

Table 1 (continued)

	Molecular mechanism	Organism	Genetic target	References	Suitable detection methods
		C. glabrata	*PDR1*	Ferrari et al. 2011	
	MFS	*C. albicans*	*MRR1, CAP1*	Mogavero et al. 2011	
	ERG	*C. albicans*	*UPC2*	Flowers et al. 2012; Oliver et al. 2007; Schubert et al. 2011	
	5. Accumulation of alternative sterols	*C. albicans*	*ERG*	Kelly et al. 1997; Morio et al. 2012	DNA sequencing
		C. glabrata	*ERG3*	Geber et al. 1995	
	6. Chromosomal aneuploidy	*C. albicans*	Chromosome 5	Selmecki et al. 2006	Comparative genome hybridization
		C. glabrata	Chromosome D, E, F, M	Polakova et al. 2009	
Echinocandins	Target site mutations	*C. albicans*	*FKS1*	Park et al. 2005	DNA sequencing; real-time PCR
		C. glabrata	*FKS1, FKS2*	Garcia-Effron et al. 2010; Katiyar et al. 2006	
		A. fumigatus	*FKS1*	Gardiner et al. 2005; Lewis et al. 2011; Rocha et al. 2007	

which presents as chromosome missegregation has been linked to azole resistance in *C. albicans* by comparative genome hybridization analysis (Selmecki et al. 2006).

With increased insights into these resistance mechanisms, molecular detection of azole resistance in *Candida* species seems feasible under certain circumstances. In particular, resistance due to drug target gene mutations can be easily detected by DNA sequencing (Sanguinetti et al. 2005), allele-specific real-time molecular probes (Park and Perlin 2005), LightCycler melt curve analysis (Loeffler et al. 2000a), or DNA microarray technology (Yan et al. 2008). However, these target gene mutations do not seem to be the dominant mechanism of azole resistance in *Candida* in the clinic. Instead, prominent resistance arises from overexpression of the sterol pathway genes and upregulation of efflux pumps (Perea et al. 2001; White et al. 2002). Quantitative reverse transcription PCR (RT-PCR) has been the mainstream of expression profiling in assessing such overexpression and upregulation associated with secondary triazole resistance (Gygax et al. 2008; Kofla and Ruhnke 2007; Park and Perlin 2005). However, measurement of gene expression levels requires cell cultures grown in the presence/absence of drug, and primary specimens are not suitable for such assessment. A quantitative correlation must be made that links an overall level of expression with a resistance phenotype to establish a threshold level of overexpression (Park and Perlin 2005). Such measurements can be complicated when resistance is a product of multiple mechanisms operating in tandem. This problem can be effectively overcome by evaluating gain-of-function mutations in transcription factors like *CgPDR1*, *TAC1*, *MRR1*, *UPC2*, and *CAP1*, as predictive markers for upregulation of efflux pumps. These mutations can be directly targeted without cell culture by real-time PCR, high-throughput sequencing, or microarray analysis for rapid identification (Perlin 2009). Nevertheless, the variety of resistance mechanisms prominent in *Candida* spp. can make direct molecular detection of triazole resistance difficult to interpret. Clinical studies are needed to relate such markers to existing gold-standard culture-based technology to assess their relative importance for therapeutic response. It remains to be seen whether profiling a single target mechanism among a multitude of potentially operative mechanisms in a single organism is sufficient to assess the azole resistance phenotype.

In contrast, triazole resistance in *A. fumigatus* appears more limited and predominantly involves mutations in the gene (*CYP51A*) encoding the protein sterol 14-α-demethylase. Mutational hot spots confirmed to cause resistance have been characterized at Gly54, Met220, Leu98, Gly138, and Gly448; and other mutations in *CYP51A* have been reported (Bueid et al. 2010; Howard et al. 2009; Verweij et al. 2009a). In the Netherlands, most resistance is due to tandem mutations in Leu98 and the promoter region of *CYP51A*, which arise as a consequence of azole use in agriculture (Snelders et al. 2009; Verweij et al. 2009b). This specific resistance mechanism has been detected in many countries in Europe and Asia (Arikan-Akdagli 2012; Chowdhary et al. 2012), although it has not been observed in patients that acquired resistance during therapy. Overexpression of ABC and MFS drug transporters has been described more recently in 15–20 % of isolates, as they confer resistance to itraconazole, voriconazole, and posaconazole (Bowyer et al. 2012; Fraczek et al. 2013). Most recently, high-level expression of the alternative gene

CYP51B was observed in two clinical azole-resistant strains which did not carry mutations in *CYP51A* (Buied et al. 2013). Finally, in a small percentage of isolates, the mechanism of triazole resistance is unclear and may be novel.

Modification of *CYP51A* remains the most dominant mechanism, and a limited number of mutations have been proven to confer resistance, which makes it ideal as a detection target for the development of real-time PCR assays to assess triazole resistance in *A. fumigatus* (Balashov et al. 2005; Garcia-Effron et al. 2008; Klaassen et al. 2010). An early comprehensive molecular diagnostic assay combined allele-specific molecular beacon technology and associations between specific *CYP51A* mutations and different triazole drug resistance to distinguish azole-resistant *A. fumigatus* from susceptible strains. Furthermore, it provided possible therapeutic options depending on the mutation detected, as some mutations confer limited resistance to the triazole class of drugs (Garcia-Effron et al. 2008). In this assay, strains that harbor mutations associated with azole resistance in the first tier of screening enter the next tier which was composed of multiple MB probes to pinpoint specific mutations as well as to reveal the relationship with different triazole antifungal drugs. In another study, a novel mixed-format real-time PCR assay was used to detect the most frequent mutations occurred at codons G54, L98, G138, and M220 and the existence of tandem repeat (TR) in the *CYP51A* promoter region (Klaassen et al. 2010). This assay mixed fluorescence resonance energy transfer (FRET) probes, melting curve analysis, and asymmetric PCR together and successfully identified four triazole-resistant strains from a random collection of 209 clinical isolates of *A. fumigatus*. Success of these molecular detections has shed light on faster diagnosis of azole resistance in *Aspergillus* and holds the promise of resolving infections with cryptic azole-resistant *Aspergillus* where culture isolation is not feasible or available.

Molecular Diagnosis of Resistance in Unculturable Cryptic Infections

Aspergilli are frequently not cultured from primary samples obtained from chronic pulmonary aspergillosis (CPA) patients, and molecular methods hold promise for the rapid detection of triazole resistance. Yet fungal burdens are usually very low and sample preparation is often inefficient. This makes it difficult to directly detect azole resistance in single-copy genes like *CYP51A* from the primary samples using standard real-time PCR assays. To enhance sensitivity, nested PCR with subsequent sequencing of the entire *CYP51A* gene was adopted by Denning et al. to investigate the triazole resistance in bronchoalveolar lavage (BAL) and sputum samples from patients with chronic fungal diseases (Denning et al. 2011). The high-frequency triazole resistance found in unculturable *A. fumigatus* in this study indicated that nested PCR/sequencing approach is a useful tool for rapid detection of triazole-resistant *Aspergillus* from the primary clinical samples. This method was also successfully applied on BAL fluids collected from patients with aspergillosis (Zhao et al. 2013). The study showed 4.3 % azole resistance rate in cultured *Aspergillus* isolates, but 14.8 % *CYP51A* PCR-positive samples were found to have mutations resulting in amino acid substitutions, including two confirmed azole resistance-associated mutations M220V and P216L. Both cases highlight the potential of detecting cryptic resistant *A. fumigatus* with the aid of molecular diagnostic tools.

Molecular Detection of Acquired Echinocandin Resistance

Echinocandin-class antifungals target the fungal cell wall by inhibiting the synthesis of β-1,3-D-glucan, a critical cell wall component of most pathogenic fungi. It has been over a decade since caspofungin was approved for clinical use as the first echinocandin, followed by micafungin and anidulafungin. Echinocandins are highly effective against a wide range of *Candida* spp., including azole-resistant strains and biofilms (Bowman et al. 2002; Denning 2003; Ferreira et al. 2009; Morrison 2006; Wiederhold and Lewis 2003), and are increasingly being used as first-line therapy in many hospitals to treat mucosal and invasive forms of candidiasis (Kartsonis et al. 2002; Pappas et al. 2007). On a limited basis, echinocandins are also used to treat invasive aspergillosis, as they are fungicidal against actively growing hyphal tips but less effective against nongrowing subapical cells (Bowman et al. 2002). In general, resistance to echinocandin drugs remains low, but reports of clinical failure due to echinocandin-resistant *Candida* spp. are rising with the expanding drug use (Arendrup et al. 2009; Castanheira et al. 2010; Pfaller et al. 2011, 2012; Zimbeck et al. 2010), and it was reported to be >13 % isolates at one high-risk center (Alexander et al. 2013).

Just like other antifungals, detection of echinocandin resistance still largely relies on in vitro antifungal susceptibility testing. The CLSI has defined laboratory standards to determine MICs for wild-type (WT) susceptible strains and clinical breakpoints (CBP) for echinocandin drugs (Pfaller et al. 2011). It is now well recognized that amino acid substitutions in the catalytic subunits (Fks1p and/or Fks2p) of the 1,3-β-D-glucan synthase confer reduced echinocandin susceptibility and are associated with clinical failure (Perlin 2007) (Table 1). However, the degree of MIC elevation and reduced sensitivity of glucan synthase (the kinetic parameters 50 % inhibitory concentration IC_{50}/K_i) to various echinocandins can vary by 50 to several 1,000-fold relative to those for the WT, depending on the specific amino acid substitution (Garcia-Effron et al. 2009a, b). With numerous studies on clinical isolates with echinocandin resistance, the dominant point mutations have been localized in two highly conserved "hot spot" regions of *FKS1* of all *Candida* spp. (Park et al. 2005) or both *FKS1* and *FKS2* of *C. glabrata* (Garcia-Effron et al. 2010; Katiyar et al. 2006). The limited spectrum of mutations conferring resistance is ideal for detection by molecular diagnostic tools. One of a few pioneer studies assessed caspofungin resistance in *C. albicans* by developing a multiplex real-time PCR assay with molecular beacons targeting a range of prominent *FKS1* mutations (Balashov et al. 2006). It must be pointed out that the three amino acid alterations occurred at codon Ser645 (S645P, S645Y, S645F) targeted by this multiplex assay along with alterations at codon Phe641 (F641S and F641L) are indeed the most prominent amino acid changes in *C. albicans*, which can lead to 2–3 logs shifts in the enzyme sensitivity to drug (Garcia-Effron et al. 2009b; Park et al. 2005). These mutations not only account for nearly 80 % of the *FKS1*-mediated resistance in our database ($n >$ 180) but also have stronger phenotypes associated with resistance and much higher IC_{50}/Ki values than mutations occurred at other positions within hot spots (Perlin 2011).

Now that kinetic inhibition studies of glucan synthase have revealed a strong correlation between specific *FKS* mutations, elevated MICs, and pharmacodynamic behavior in animal models (Arendrup et al. 2012; Garcia-Effron et al. 2009a, b; Howard et al. 2011; Slater et al. 2011; Wiederhold et al. 2011), ranking *FKS* mutations based on enzyme sensitivity to drug seems to be a reasonable way to predict resistant phenotypes and, more importantly, to help guide appropriate antifungal treatment. In general, the greater the ability of an *FKS* mutation to confer reduced drug sensitivity on glucan synthase, the more pronounced the resistance observed. In *C. albicans*, the rank order of relative resistance conferred from Fks1p amino acid substitutions has been suggested as: S645, F641 >> L642, T643, L644, R647, D648 > P649 (Perlin 2011). This is consistent with what was observed by pharmacodynamic (PD) study and drug dose escalation experiment on animal models, where conventional dosing of echinocandins cannot elicit an antifungal response in animals infected with S645 and F641 *C. albicans* mutants (Slater et al. 2011; Wiederhold et al. 2011). Similarly, in *C. glabrata*, amino acid substitutions at S663 in Fks2p, which is equivalent to S645 in Fks1p in *C. albicans*, cause the most prominent resistance observed in clinical isolates resulting in high MICs and remarkably reduced glucan synthase sensitivity to all three echinocandin drugs (Garcia-Effron et al. 2009a). Other mutations occurred at F659 in Fks1p and S629, F625, and D632 in Fks2p in *C. glabrata* also had similar rank order of resistance comparable to that in *C. albicans* (Perlin 2011). The key aspect of such ranking is to reflect the pattern of antifungal response in resistance caused by different *FKS* mutations and to further assist finding the most effective therapeutic options. In fact, a recent study demonstrated the superiority of detection of *FKS* mutations to MICs in predicting echinocandin therapeutic responses among patients with invasive candidiasis (Shields et al. 2012). In the meantime, another study, from pharmacodynamic perspective, revealed a dose–response relationship between *FKS* mutations and echinocandin drug exposure (Lepak et al. 2012).

Although the limited spectrum and genetic clustering of *FKS* mutations conferring echinocandin resistance for the major *Candida* species seems amenable to real-time PCR techniques, there are only limited published studies that applied these techniques to characterization of clinical echinocandin-resistant isolates (Balashov et al. 2006; Ben-Ami et al. 2011). Until now, no study has reported direct detection of echinocandin resistance using molecular methods from primary clinical samples such as tissue specimen or blood.

As aforementioned, echinocandin drugs have a largely fungistatic effect against filamentous fungi such as *Aspergillus* spp. The deficiency of having complete growth inhibition has resulted in an alternative susceptibility endpoint testing method known as the minimum effective concentration (MEC) to determine the activity of echinocandins against filamentous fungi. The MEC is defined as the lowest drug concentration at which short, stubby, highly branched hyphae are observed (Arikan et al. 2001; Espinel-Ingroff 2003; Imhof et al. 2003). MEC testing demonstrated that echinocandin susceptibility profiles are varying in different *Aspergillus* species (Antachopoulos et al. 2008; Imhof et al. 2003). Overall, *A. fumigatus*, *A. flavus*, and *A. terreus* have comparable susceptibilities to all three echinocandins, but *A. niger* seems more susceptible to caspofungin than *A. fumigatus*. Much less is known about echinocandin resistance in *Aspergillus*, although the upregulated expression level of *FKS1* gene was observed in *A. fumigatus* clinical isolate with the reduced susceptibility to caspofungin (Arendrup et al. 2008) and in vitro studies with manipulated laboratory strains indicate that modification of Fks1p confers high-level resistance (Gardiner et al. 2005; Rocha et al. 2007). To date, only a few clinical isolates associated with echinocandin treatment failures have been investigated so far. Limited experience along with insufficient insight of molecular mechanism has made molecular detection of echinocandin resistance in *Aspergillus* spp. a challenging task.

Challenges and Future Perspectives

At the present time, culture-based methods still dominate diagnosis of fungal infections and related antifungal resistance. Yet, molecular diagnostics have the potential to transform the modern clinical microbiology laboratory by providing rapid identification of infecting organisms while profiling the presence of inherently resistant species or acquired genetic mechanisms that alter susceptibility to antifungal drugs. However, molecular diagnosis of antifungal drug resistance must overcome a few hurdles to open up the door for routine clinical use. A key to the successful application of molecular technology for antifungal resistance is a strong association between genetic mechanisms, in vitro reduced susceptibility, and clinical outcome. Fully elucidating genetic mechanisms of various antifungal drugs in different fungal species is a prerequisite to utilize novel molecular tools to probe drug resistance. In addition, a systematic evaluation relationship between specific molecular mechanisms of resistance and clinical outcome in well-designed clinical trials is critical to establish the value of molecular diagnosis in the clinical settings. Another challenge is the inefficient sample preparation, which must be improved and automated. The difficulties of efficient extraction from the primary samples exist in two aspects: first, the low circulating levels of pathogens or naked DNA for most IFIs, especially invasive aspergillosis, and, second, the relatively large amount of human DNA compared to target fungal DNA present in the extracts that may either inhibit downstream detection or cross-react with fungal primers/probes to cause false-positive results. Considerations to address the unfavorable pathogen-human DNA ratio have involved novel technologies for pathogen DNA enrichment. One uses selective lysis of blood cells to reduce the human DNA background in an extracted blood sample (Molzym). The manual version of this sample preparation is known as MolYsis, and the automated platform is named as SelectNA™.

The MolYsis method showed good performance with whole blood from patients with candidemia (Wellinghausen et al. 2009), but there was no head-to-head study to measure the exact benefit in terms of extraction efficiency of fungal DNA from using this particular method. Another technology called LOOXSTER® (SIRS-Lab) utilizes the methylation differences between bacterial/fungal DNA to enrich pathogen DNA in the clinical sample by affinity chromatography, but the performance on antifungal resistance has not been evaluated. Clearly, novel and practical approaches and massive evaluation in clinical settings of these methods are urgently needed for sample preparation. The full potential of molecular diagnosis of both primary and secondary antifungal resistance will not be fully reached until a phenomenal advance in specimen preparation is achieved.

Conclusion

In summary, molecular diagnostic platforms are ideal for rapid detection of drug resistance in fungal pathogens. However, more comprehensive and deeper insights into genetic mechanisms of antifungal resistance, extensive validation in well-designed clinical trials, as well as innovative methods for highly efficient and selective fungal nucleic acid extraction from primary samples are needed for the implementation of molecular diagnosis of drug resistance into the clinical settings serving as the guidance of antifungal therapy.

References

Alexander BD et al (2013) Increasing echinocandin resistance in candida glabrata: clinical failure correlates with presence of FKS mutations and elevated minimum inhibitory concentrations. Clin Infect Dis 56:1724

Al-Wathiqi F, Ahmad S, Khan Z (2013) Molecular identification and antifungal susceptibility profile of Aspergillus flavus isolates recovered from clinical specimens in Kuwait. BMC Infect Dis 13:126

Antachopoulos C, Meletiadis J, Sein T, Roilides E, Walsh TJ (2008) Comparative in vitro pharmacodynamics of caspofungin, micafungin, and anidulafungin against germinated and nongerminated Aspergillus conidia. Antimicrob Agents Chemother 52:321

Arendrup MC, Perkhofer S, Howard SJ, Garcia-Effron G, Vishukumar A, Perlin D, Lass-Florl C (2008) Establishing in vitro-in vivo correlations for Aspergillus fumigatus: the challenge of azoles versus echinocandins. Antimicrob Agents Chemother 52:3504

Arendrup MC et al (2009) Breakthrough Aspergillus fumigatus and Candida albicans double infection during caspofungin treatment: laboratory characteristics and implication for susceptibility testing. Antimicrob Agents Chemother 53:1185

Arendrup MC et al (2010) Development of azole resistance in Aspergillus fumigatus during azole therapy associated with change in virulence. PLoS One 5:e10080

Arendrup MC, Perlin DS, Jensen RH, Howard SJ, Goodwin J, Hope W (2012) Differential in vivo activities of anidulafungin, caspofungin, and micafungin against Candida glabrata isolates with and without FKS resistance mutations. Antimicrob Agents Chemother 56:2435

Arikan S, Lozano-Chiu M, Paetznick V, Rex JH (2001) In vitro susceptibility testing methods for caspofungin against Aspergillus and Fusarium isolates. Antimicrob Agents Chemother 45:327

Arikan-Akdagli S (2012) Azole resistance in Aspergillus: global status in Europe and Asia. Ann N Y Acad Sci 1272:9

Balashov SV, Gardiner R, Park S, Perlin DS (2005) Rapid, high-throughput, multiplex, real-time PCR for identification of mutations in the cyp51A gene of Aspergillus fumigatus that confer resistance to itraconazole. J Clin Microbiol 43:214

Balashov SV, Park S, Perlin DS (2006) Assessing resistance to the echinocandin antifungal drug caspofungin in Candida albicans by profiling mutations in FKS1. Antimicrob Agents Chemother 50:2058

Ben-Ami R, Garcia-Effron G, Lewis RE, Gamarra S, Leventakos K, Perlin DS, Kontoyiannis DP (2011) Fitness and virulence costs of Candida albicans FKS1 hot spot mutations associated with echinocandin resistance. J Infect Dis 204:626

Bowman JC, Hicks PS, Kurtz MB, Rosen H, Schmatz DM, Liberator PA, Douglas CM (2002) The antifungal echinocandin caspofungin acetate kills growing cells of Aspergillus fumigatus in vitro. Antimicrob Agents Chemother 46:3001

Bowyer P, Mosquera J, Anderson M, Birch M, Bromley M, Denning DW (2012) Identification of novel genes conferring altered azole susceptibility in Aspergillus fumigatus. FEMS Microbiol Lett 332:10

Bueid A, Howard SJ, Moore CB, Richardson MD, Harrison E, Bowyer P, Denning DW (2010) Azole antifungal resistance in Aspergillus fumigatus: 2008 and 2009. J Antimicrob Chemother 65:2116

Buied A, Moore CB, Denning DW, Bowyer P (2013) High-level expression of cyp51B in azole-resistant clinical Aspergillus fumigatus isolates. J Antimicrob Chemother 68:512

Castanheira M, Woosley LN, Diekema DJ, Messer SA, Jones RN, Pfaller MA (2010) Low prevalence of fks1 hot spot 1 mutations in a worldwide collection of Candida strains. Antimicrob Agents Chemother 54:2655

Chau AS, Mendrick CA, Sabatelli FJ, Loebenberg D, McNicholas PM (2004) Application of real-time quantitative PCR to molecular analysis of Candida albicans strains exhibiting reduced susceptibility to azoles. Antimicrob Agents Chemother 48:2124

Chowdhary A et al (2012) Clonal expansion and emergence of environmental multiple-triazole-resistant Aspergillus fumigatus strains carrying the TR(3)(4)/L98H mutations in the cyp51A gene in India. PLoS One 7:e52871

CLSI (2008a) CLSI document M28-A2. Clinical and Laboratory Standards Institute, Wayne

CLSI (2008b) CLSI document M27-A3. Clinical and Laboratory Standards Institute, Wayne

Coste A et al (2006) A mutation in Tac1p, a transcription factor regulating CDR1 and CDR2, is coupled with loss of heterozygosity at chromosome 5 to mediate antifungal resistance in Candida albicans. Genetics 172:2139

Denning DW (2003) Echinocandin antifungal drugs. Lancet 362:1142

Denning DW et al (2011) High-frequency triazole resistance found In nonculturable Aspergillus fumigatus from lungs of patients with chronic fungal disease. Clin Infect Dis 52:1123

Dhamgaye S et al (2012) RNA sequencing revealed novel actors of the acquisition of drug resistance in Candida albicans. BMC Genomics 13:396

Ecker DJ et al (2010) New technology for rapid molecular diagnosis of bloodstream infections. Expert Rev Mol Diagn 10:399

Espinel-Ingroff A (2003) Utility of mould susceptibility testing. Curr Opin Infect Dis 16:527

Ferrari S, Sanguinetti M, Torelli R, Posteraro B, Sanglard D (2011) Contribution of CgPDR1-Regulated Genes in Enhanced Virulence of Azole-Resistant Candida glabrata. PLoS One 6: e17589

Ferreira ME et al (2005) The ergosterol biosynthesis pathway, transporter genes, and azole resistance in Aspergillus fumigatus. Med Mycol 43(Suppl 1):S313

Ferreira JA, Carr JH, Starling CE, de Resende MA, Donlan RM (2009) Biofilm formation and effect of caspofungin on biofilm structure of Candida species bloodstream isolates. Antimicrob Agents Chemother 53:4377

Flowers SA et al (2012) Gain-of-function mutations in UPC2 are a frequent cause of ERG11 upregulation in azole-resistant clinical isolates of Candida albicans. Eukaryot Cell 11:1289

Fraczek MG et al (2013) The cdr1B efflux transporter is associated with non-cyp51a-mediated itraconazole resistance in Aspergillus fumigatus. J Antimicrob Chemother 68:1486
Fridkin SK, Jarvis WR (1996) Epidemiology of nosocomial fungal infections. Clin Microbiol Rev 9:499
Garcia-Effron G, Dilger A, Alcazar-Fuoli L, Park S, Mellado E, Perlin DS (2008) Rapid detection of triazole antifungal resistance in Aspergillus fumigatus. J Clin Microbiol 46:1200
Garcia-Effron G, Lee S, Park S, Cleary JD, Perlin DS (2009a) Effect of Candida glabrata FKS1 and FKS2 mutations on echinocandin sensitivity and kinetics of 1,3-beta-D-glucan synthase: implication for the existing susceptibility breakpoint. Antimicrob Agents Chemother 53:3690
Garcia-Effron G, Park S, Perlin DS (2009b) Correlating echinocandin MIC and kinetic inhibition of fks1 mutant glucan synthases for Candida albicans: implications for interpretive breakpoints. Antimicrob Agents Chemother 53:112
Garcia-Effron G, Chua DJ, Tomada JR, DiPersio J, Perlin DS, Ghannoum M, Bonilla H (2010) Novel FKS mutations associated with echinocandin resistance in Candida species. Antimicrob Agents Chemother 54:2225
Gardiner RE, Souteropoulos P, Park S, Perlin DS (2005) Characterization of Aspergillus fumigatus mutants with reduced susceptibility to caspofungin. Med Mycol 43(Suppl 1):S299
Geber A, Hitchcock CA, Swartz JE, Pullen FS, Marsden KE, Kwon-Chung KJ, Bennett JE (1995) Deletion of the Candida glabrata ERG3 and ERG11 genes: effect on cell viability, cell growth, sterol composition, and antifungal susceptibility. Antimicrob Agents Chemother 39:2708
Gygax SE et al (2008) Antifungal resistance of Candida glabrata vaginal isolates and development of a quantitative reverse transcription-PCR-based azole susceptibility assay. Antimicrob Agents Chemother 52:3424
Heald AE, Cox GM, Schell WA, Bartlett JA, Perfect JR (1996) Oropharyngeal yeast flora and fluconazole resistance in HIV-infected patients receiving long-term continuous versus intermittent fluconazole therapy. AIDS 10:263
Henry KW, Nickels JT, Edlind TD (2000) Upregulation of ERG genes in Candida species by azoles and other sterol biosynthesis inhibitors. Antimicrob Agents Chemother 44:2693
Holmes AR et al (2008) ABC transporter Cdr1p contributes more than Cdr2p does to fluconazole efflux in fluconazole-resistant Candida albicans clinical isolates. Antimicrob Agents Chemother 52:3851
Howard SJ et al (2009) Frequency and evolution of Azole resistance in Aspergillus fumigatus associated with treatment failure. Emerg Infect Dis 15:1068
Howard SJ et al (2011) Pharmacodynamics of echinocandins against Candida glabrata: requirement for dosage escalation to achieve maximal antifungal activity in neutropenic hosts. Antimicrob Agents Chemother 55:4880
Hull CM et al (2012) Facultative sterol uptake in an ergosterol-deficient clinical isolate of Candida glabrata harboring a missense mutation in ERG11 and exhibiting cross-resistance to azoles and amphotericin B. Antimicrob Agents Chemother 56:4223
Imhof A, Balajee SA, Marr KA (2003) New methods to assess susceptibilities of Aspergillus isolates to caspofungin. J Clin Microbiol 41:5683
Karababa M, Coste AT, Rognon B, Bille J, Sanglard D (2004) Comparison of gene expression profiles of Candida albicans azole-resistant clinical isolates and laboratory strains exposed to drugs inducing multidrug transporters. Antimicrob Agents Chemother 48:3064
Kartsonis N, DiNubile MJ, Bartizal K, Hicks PS, Ryan D, Sable CA (2002) Efficacy of caspofungin in the treatment of esophageal candidiasis resistant to fluconazole. J Acquir Immune Defic Syndr 31:183
Katiyar S, Pfaller M, Edlind T (2006) Candida albicans and Candida glabrata clinical isolates exhibiting reduced echinocandin susceptibility. Antimicrob Agents Chemother 50:2892
Kelly SL et al (1997) Resistance to fluconazole and cross-resistance to amphotericin B in Candida albicans from AIDS patients caused by defective sterol delta5,6- desaturation. FEBS Lett 400:80
Klaassen CH, de Valk HA, Curfs-Breuker IM, Meis JF (2010) Novel mixed-format real-time PCR assay to detect mutations conferring resistance to triazoles in Aspergillus fumigatus and

prevalence of multi-triazole resistance among clinical isolates in the Netherlands. J Antimicrob Chemother 65:901
Kofla G, Ruhnke M (2007) Development of a new real-time TaqMan PCR assay for quantitative analyses of Candida albicans resistance genes expression. J Microbiol Methods 68:178
Landlinger C, Preuner S, Willinger B, Haberpursch B, Racil Z, Mayer J, Lion T (2009) Species-specific identification of a wide range of clinically relevant fungal pathogens by use of Luminex xMAP technology. J Clin Microbiol 47:1063
Lepak A, Castanheira M, Diekema D, Pfaller M, Andes D (2012) Optimizing Echinocandin dosing and susceptibility breakpoint determination via in vivo pharmacodynamic evaluation against Candida glabrata with and without fks mutations. Antimicrob Agents Chemother 56:5875
Lewis RE, Liao G, Hou J, Prince RA, Kontoyiannis DP (2011) Comparative in vivo dose-dependent activity of caspofungin and anidulafungin against echinocandin-susceptible and -resistant Aspergillus fumigatus. J Antimicrob Chemother 66:1324
Loeffler J, Hagmeyer L, Hebart H, Henke N, Schumacher U, Einsele H (2000a) Rapid detection of point mutations by fluorescence resonance energy transfer and probe melting curves in Candida species. Clin Chem 46:631
Loeffler J, Henke N, Hebart H, Schmidt D, Hagmeyer L, Schumacher U, Einsele H (2000b) Quantification of fungal DNA by using fluorescence resonance energy transfer and the light cycler system. J Clin Microbiol 38:586
MacCallum DM, Coste A, Ischer F, Jacobsen MD, Odds FC, Sanglard D (2010) Genetic dissection of azole resistance mechanisms in Candida albicans and their validation in a mouse model of disseminated infection. Antimicrob Agents Chemother 54:1476
Martel CM et al (2010) Identification and characterization of four azole-resistant erg3 mutants of Candida albicans. Antimicrob Agents Chemother 54:4527
Modi DA, Farrell JJ, Sampath R, Bhatia NS, Massire C, Ranken R, Bonomo RA (2012) Rapid identification of Aspergillus terreus from Bronchoalverolar lavage fluid by PCR and Electrospray-Ionization with Mass Spectrometry (PCR/ESI-MS). J Clin Microbiol 50:2529
Mogavero S, Tavanti A, Senesi S, Rogers PD, Morschhauser J (2011) Differential Requirement of the Transcription Factor Mcm1 for Activation of the Candida albicans Multidrug Efflux Pump MDR1 by Its Regulators Mrr1 and Cap1. Antimicrob Agents Chemother 55:2061
Morio F, Loge C, Besse B, Hennequin C, Le Pape P (2010) Screening for amino acid substitutions in the Candida albicans Erg11 protein of azole-susceptible and azole-resistant clinical isolates: new substitutions and a review of the literature. Diagn Microbiol Infect Dis 66:373
Morio F, Pagniez F, Lacroix C, Miegeville M, Le Pape P (2012) Amino acid substitutions in the Candida albicans sterol Delta5,6-desaturase (Erg3p) confer azole resistance: characterization of two novel mutants with impaired virulence. J Antimicrob Chemother 67:2131
Morrell M, Fraser VJ, Kollef MH (2005) Delaying the empiric treatment of candida bloodstream infection until positive blood culture results are obtained: a potential risk factor for hospital mortality. Antimicrob Agents Chemother 49:3640
Morrison VA (2006) Echinocandin antifungals: review and update. Expert Rev Anti Infect Ther 4:325
Nagi M et al (2011) Transcription factors CgUPC2A and CgUPC2B regulate ergosterol biosynthetic genes in Candida glabrata. Genes Cells 16:80
Nascimento AM et al (2003) Multiple Resistance Mechanisms among Aspergillus fumigatus Mutants with High-Level Resistance to Itraconazole. Antimicrob Agents Chemother 47:1719
Oliver BG, Song JL, Choiniere JH, White TC (2007) cis-Acting elements within the Candida albicans ERG11 promoter mediate the azole response through transcription factor Upc2p. Eukaryot Cell 6:2231
Pancholi P, Park S, Perlin D, Kubin C, Della-Latta P (2004) Molecular characterization of fluconazole resistance in a case of Candida albicans ocular infection. J Clin Microbiol 42:5938
Pappas PG et al (2007) Micafungin versus caspofungin for treatment of candidemia and other forms of invasive candidiasis. Clin Infect Dis 45:883

Park S, Perlin DS (2005) Establishing surrogate markers for fluconazole resistance in Candida albicans. Microb Drug Resist 11:232
Park S et al (2000) Rapid identification of Candida dubliniensis using a species-specific molecular beacon. J Clin Microbiol 38:2829
Park S et al (2005) Specific substitutions in the echinocandin target Fks1p account for reduced susceptibility of rare laboratory and clinical Candida sp. isolates. Antimicrob Agents Chemother 49:3264
Perea S et al (2001) Prevalence of molecular mechanisms of resistance to azole antifungal agents in Candida albicans strains displaying high-level fluconazole resistance isolated from human immunodeficiency virus-infected patients. Antimicrob Agents Chemother 45:2676
Perlin DS (2007) Resistance to echinocandin-class antifungal drugs. Drug Resist Updat 10:121
Perlin DS (2009) Antifungal drug resistance: do molecular methods provide a way forward? Curr Opin Infect Dis 22:568
Perlin DS (2011) Current perspectives on echinocandin class drugs. Future Microbiol 6:441
Pfaller MA (2012) Antifungal drug resistance: mechanisms, epidemiology, and consequences for treatment. Am J Med 125:S3
Pfaller MA, Diekema DJ (2010) Epidemiology of invasive mycoses in North America. Crit Rev Microbiol 36:1
Pfaller MA et al (2007) Results from the ARTEMIS DISK Global Antifungal Surveillance study, 1997 to 2005: an 8.5-year analysis of susceptibilities of Candida species and other yeast species to fluconazole and voriconazole determined by CLSI standardized disk diffusion testing. J Clin Microbiol 45:1735
Pfaller MA et al (2011) Clinical breakpoints for the echinocandins and Candida revisited: integration of molecular, clinical, and microbiological data to arrive at species-specific interpretive criteria. Drug Resist Updat 14:164
Pfaller MA, Castanheira M, Lockhart SR, Ahlquist AM, Messer SA, Jones RN (2012) Frequency of decreased susceptibility and resistance to echinocandins among fluconazole-resistant bloodstream isolates of Candida glabrata. J Clin Microbiol 50:1199
Polakova S, Blume C, Zarate JA, Mentel M, Jorck-Ramberg D, Stenderup J, Piskur J (2009) Formation of new chromosomes as a virulence mechanism in yeast Candida glabrata. Proc Natl Acad Sci U S A 106:2688
Rautemaa R, Richardson M, Pfaller M, Koukila-Kahkola P, Perheentupa J, Saxen H (2007) Decreased susceptibility of Candida albicans to azole antifungals: a complication of long-term treatment in autoimmune polyendocrinopathy-candidiasis-ectodermal dystrophy (APECED) patients. J Antimicrob Chemother 60:889
Rex JH, Rinaldi MG, Pfaller MA (1995) Resistance of Candida species to fluconazole. Antimicrob Agents Chemother 39:1
Rocha EM, Garcia-Effron G, Park S, Perlin DS (2007) A Ser678Pro substitution in Fks1p confers resistance to echinocandin drugs in Aspergillus fumigatus. Antimicrob Agents Chemother 51:4174
Sanglard D, Odds FC (2002) Resistance of Candida species to antifungal agents: molecular mechanisms and clinical consequences. Lancet Infect Dis 2:73
Sanguinetti M, Posteraro B, Fiori B, Ranno S, Torelli R, Fadda G (2005) Mechanisms of azole resistance in clinical isolates of Candida glabrata collected during a hospital survey of antifungal resistance. Antimicrob Agents Chemother 49:668
Schubert S et al (2011) Regulation of Efflux Pump Expression and Drug Resistance by the Transcription Factors Mrr1, Upc2, and Cap1 in Candida albicans. Antimicrob Agents Chemother 55:2212
Selmecki A, Forche A, Berman J (2006) Aneuploidy and isochromosome formation in drug-resistant Candida albicans. Science 313:367
Shields RK, Nguyen MH, Press EG, Kwa AL, Cheng S, Du C, Clancy CJ (2012) The presence of an FKS mutation rather than MIC is an independent risk factor for failure of echinocandin therapy

among patients with invasive candidiasis due to Candida glabrata. Antimicrob Agents Chemother 56:4862

Slater JL et al (2011) Disseminated Candidiasis caused by Candida albicans with amino acid substitutions in Fks1 at position Ser645 cannot be successfully treated with micafungin. Antimicrob Agents Chemother 55:3075

Slaven JW, Anderson MJ, Sanglard D, Dixon GK, Bille J, Roberts IS, Denning DW (2002) Increased expression of a novel Aspergillus fumigatus ABC transporter gene, atrF, in the presence of itraconazole in an itraconazole resistant clinical isolate. Fungal Genet Biol 36:199

Snelders E, Huis In't Veld RA, Rijs AJ, Kema GH, Melchers WJ, Verweij PE (2009) Possible environmental origin of resistance of Aspergillus fumigatus to medical triazoles. Appl Environ Microbiol 75:4053

Subcommittee on Antifungal Susceptibility Testing (AFST) of the ESCMID European Committee for Antimicrobial Susceptibility Testing (EUCAST) (2008a) EUCAST definitive document EDef 7.1: method for the determination of broth dilution MICs of antifungal agents for fermentative yeasts. Clin Microbiol Infect 14:398

Subcommittee on Antifungal Susceptibility Testing of the ESCMID European Committee for Antimicrobial Susceptibility Testing (2008b) EUCAST Technical Note on the method for the determination of broth dilution minimum inhibitory concentrations of antifungal agents for conidia-forming moulds. Clin Microbiol Infect 14:982

Vermitsky JP, Edlind TD (2004) Azole resistance in Candida glabrata: coordinate upregulation of multidrug transporters and evidence for a Pdr1-like transcription factor. Antimicrob Agents Chemother 48:3773

Verweij PE, Mellado E, Melchers WJ (2007) Multiple-triazole-resistant aspergillosis. N Engl J Med 356:1481

Verweij PE, Howard SJ, Melchers WJ, Denning DW (2009a) Azole-resistance in Aspergillus: proposed nomenclature and breakpoints. Drug Resist Updat 12:141

Verweij PE, Snelders E, Kema GH, Mellado E, Melchers WJ (2009b) Azole resistance in Aspergillus fumigatus: a side-effect of environmental fungicide use? Lancet Infect Dis 9:789

Walsh TJ et al (2008) Treatment of aspergillosis: clinical practice guidelines of the Infectious Diseases Society of America. Clin Infect Dis 46:327

Wellinghausen N, Siegel D, Winter J, Gebert S (2009) Rapid diagnosis of candidaemia by real-time PCR detection of Candida DNA in blood samples. J Med Microbiol 58:1106

White TC, Holleman S, Dy F, Mirels LF, Stevens DA (2002) Resistance mechanisms in clinical isolates of Candida albicans. Antimicrob Agents Chemother 46:1704

Wiederhold NP, Lewis RE (2003) The echinocandin antifungals: an overview of the pharmacology, spectrum and clinical efficacy. Expert Opin Investig Drugs 12:1313

Wiederhold NP, Najvar LK, Bocanegra RA, Kirkpatrick WR, Patterson TF (2011) Caspofungin dose escalation for invasive candidiasis due to resistant Candida albicans. Antimicrob Agents Chemother 55:3254

Wolk DM, Kaleta EJ, Wysocki VH (2012) PCR-Electrospray Ionization Mass Spectrometry: The Potential to Change Infectious Disease Diagnostics in Clinical and Public Health Laboratories. J Mol Diagn 14:295

Yan L et al (2008) DNA microarray analysis of fluconazole resistance in a laboratory Candida albicans strain. Acta Biochim Biophys Sin (Shanghai) 40:1048

Zhao Y, Stensvold CR, Perlin DS, Arendrup MC (2013) Azole resistance in Aspergillus fumigatus from bronchoalveolar lavage fluid samples of patients with chronic diseases. J Antimicrob Chemother 68:1497

Zimbeck AJ, Iqbal N, Ahlquist AM, Farley MM, Harrison LH, Chiller T, Lockhart SR (2010) FKS mutations and elevated echinocandin MIC values among Candida glabrata isolates from U.S. population-based surveillance. Antimicrob Agents Chemother 54:5042

Azole Resistance in *Aspergillus fumigatus*: Mechanisms, Route of Resistance Selection, and Clinical Implications

Seyedmojtaba Seyedmousavi and Paul E. Verweij

Contents

Abstract

The medical triazoles, itraconazole, voriconazole, and posaconazole, are the most widely used drugs for the management of infections caused by the saprophytic mold *Aspergillus fumigatus*. However, acquired azole resistance in *A. fumigatus* is an emerging problem that compromises the clinical efficacy of azole antifungals. Several mutations in the cyp51A gene of *A. fumigatus* affect the activity of

S. Seyedmousavi (✉)
Department of Medical Microbiology, Radboud University Medical Center, Nijmegen, The Netherlands

Department of Medical Microbiology and Infectious Diseases, Erasmus MC, Rotterdam, The Netherlands
e-mail: S.Seyedmousavi@gmail.com

P.E. Verweij (✉)
Department of Medical Microbiology, Radboud University Medical Center, Nijmegen, The Netherlands
e-mail: Paul.Verweij@radboudumc.nl

M. Gotte et al. (eds.), *Handbook of Antimicrobial Resistance*,
DOI 10.1007/978-1-4939-0694-9_22

all mold-active antifungal azoles. These mutations result in the complete loss of activity of a specific azole and are commonly associated with cross-resistance to other azoles. While azole resistance may emerge during antifungal therapy of individual azole-treated patients, selection of resistance can also occur in the environment. The selection for azole resistance within the environment poses an emerging global threat as mutations associated with environmental resistance have now been detected with increasing frequency in multiple European countries, Asia, the Middle East, and Africa.

Keywords
Aspergillus fumigatus • Azole- resistance • Epidemiology • Clinical implications

Introduction

Aspergillus spp. are cosmopolitan filamentous fungi often found in soil, where they thrive as saprophytes, but occasionally they infect living hosts including plants, insects, and mammals (Pitt 1994; Heitman 2011). Aspergillosis is an umbrella term coined by Hinson, Moon, and Plummer in 1952, encompassing a range of conditions from localized to fatal disseminated infections caused by fungi belonging to the genus *Aspergillus*.

In humans, *Aspergillus fumigatus* is the most common and life-threatening airborne fungal pathogen, especially among immunocompromised hosts (Kwon-Chung and Sugui 2013). *A. fumigatus* was first described as a pathogen by Fresenius in 1863 when it was isolated from the bronchi and alveoli of a great bustard (*Otis tarda*) (Fresenius 1863). It has been recognized for most of this century as a pathogen, capable of invading the human lungs, brain, paranasal sinuses, eyes, pharynx, skin, and open wounds, but most commonly this has been observed in immunocompromised individuals (Latge 1999; Meersseman et al. 2004; Denning 1998; Segal and Romani 2009; Patterson and Strek 2010; DeLone et al. 1999; Gefter 1992; Germaud and Tuchais 1995; Galimberti et al. 1998; Garrett et al. 1999). The potential of *Aspergillus* spp. to cause severe disease in humans was recognized by Young and colleagues in 1966 when a series of 98 patients was described with invasive aspergillosis (Young et al. 1970).

Depending on the immunological status of the host, inhalation of *A. fumigatus* spores (conidia) into the lungs can cause multiple diseases (Latge 1999; Greub and Bille 1998; Henriet et al. 2013; Gallin and Zarember 2007). Healthy hosts are able to ward off infections, so that severe illness usually results only from massive or long-term exposure (Pitt 1994; Arne et al. 2011). It can cause acute and subacute invasive disease in immunocompromised patients and chronic pulmonary aspergillosis (CPA) and aspergilloma in immunocompetent patients with underlying lung disease (Smith and Denning 2011). In CPA, *Aspergillus* gradually destroys lung tissue, resulting in the formation and expansion of cavities as well as the formation of fungal balls (aspergilloma) within these cavities (Smith and Denning 2011; Saraceno et al. 1997; Soubani and Chandrasekar 2002).

Notably, the population at risk for invasive aspergillosis (IA) is expanding due to recent advances in human medicine including patients on steroids and chemotherapy treatment resulting in severe neutropenia, stem cell and solid organ transplantation, and advances in the development of immunosuppressive and myeloablative therapies for autoimmune and neoplastic disease, later stages of AIDS, and hereditary immunodeficiencies such as chronic granulomatous disease (Brown et al. 2012; Patterson 2005). Approximately 300,000 people are estimated to develop IA annually, 1.5–10 % of the millions of highly immunocompromised patients at risk worldwide (Brown et al. 2012). The global burden of CPA has recently been estimated at three million patients (Brown et al. 2012; Denning et al. 2011).

Phylogeny and Subgeneric Taxonomy of *Aspergillus* spp.

Polyphasic taxonomy has had a major impact on species concepts in the genus *Aspergillus* (Peterson et al. 2008; Peterson 2008), as shown in Fig. 1. The genus has been subdivided into 22 distinct sections, of which *Fumigati, Circumdati, Terrei, Nidulantes, Ornati, Warcupi, Candidi, Restricti, Usti, Flavipedes*, and *Versicolores* contain clinically relevant species (Peterson et al. 2008). Although there are more than 200 known species in the genus, only a small number is associated with infection. Among them, *A. fumigatus* (subgenus *Fumigati*, section *Fumigati*), *A. flavus* (subgenus *Circumdati*, section *Flavi*), and *A. niger* (subgenus *Circumdati*, section *Nigri*) are the most frequently encountered species (Greub and Bille 1998; Peterson et al. 2008; de Hoog et al. 2009). Others, such as *A. terreus* (subgenus *Terrei*, section *Terrei*), *A. versicolor* (subgenus *Nidulantes*, section *Versicolores*), and *A. nidulans* (subgenus *Nidulantes*, section *Nidulantes*), are occasionally isolated from clinical specimens (Balajee 2009). The impact of new taxonomy of *Aspergillus* spp. on antifungal susceptibility profiles will be discussed below.

Treatment of *A. fumigatus* Diseases in Humans

Triazole antifungals play an important role in the management of *Aspergillus* diseases (Herbrecht et al. 2002; Walsh et al. 2008). These agents exert their antifungal activity by blocking the demethylation of lanosterol, thereby inhibiting the synthesis of ergosterol, a key lipid in the cell membrane of fungi. They have an expanded spectrum with fungicidal activity against a wide spectrum of molds as well as enhanced activity against *Candida* spp. and other yeasts (Denning 1998). Three triazole compounds (itraconazole, voriconazole, and posaconazole) have been clinically licensed for and are currently in use for the prevention and treatment of invasive aspergillosis (EMA 2012a, b). A fourth triazole, isavuconazole, is currently in phase III clinical development for treatment of aspergillosis and expected to be licensed in the near future (Seyedmousavi et al. 2015). Itraconazole, voriconazole, posaconazole, and isavuconazole have been shown to be fungicidal against *Aspergillus* spp. (Mohr et al. 2008; Guinea et al. 2008; Pfaller et al. 2002). Itraconazole is

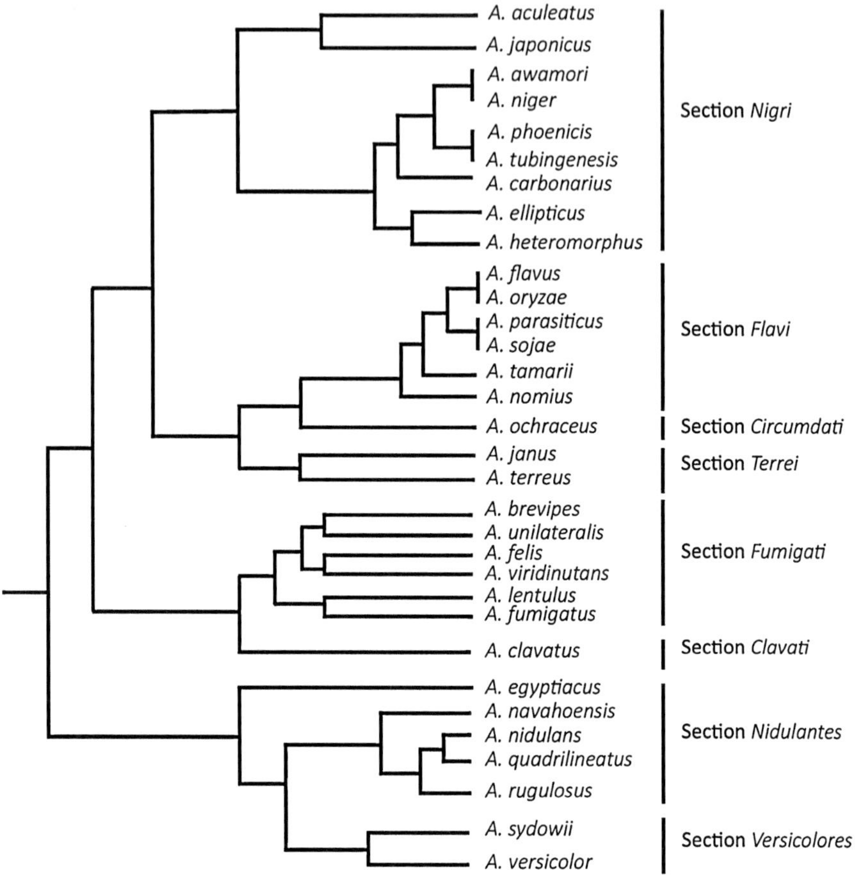

Fig. 1 The phylogenetic relationships of ten gene regions of *Aspergillus* species

commonly used for the treatment of chronic pulmonary disease (EMA 2012a, b), while voriconazole is the treatment of choice for IA (EMA 2012b). Posaconazole is licensed for prophylaxis in patients receiving remission induction chemotherapy for acute myelogenous leukemia (AML) or myelodysplastic syndromes (MDS) and in hematopoietic stem cell transplant (HSCT) recipients who are undergoing high-dose immunosuppressive therapy for graft-versus-host disease. It is also licensed in some countries for salvage therapy of IA in patients with disease that is refractory to amphotericin B or itraconazole or in patients who are intolerant of these agents (Herbrecht et al. 2002; Walsh et al. 2008; Cornely et al. 2007; Ullmann et al. 2007).

Besides azoles, only amphotericin B and the echinocandins (caspofungin, micafungin, and anidulafungin) have demonstrated clinical activity against *Aspergillus* diseases. None of these agents however have been directly compared with azoles in randomized controlled clinical trials, and they are therefore considered as alternative agents for the therapy of IA (Walsh et al. 2008).

Table 1 Examples of intrinsic resistance against antifungals in *fumigatus* and non-*fumigatus Aspergillus* species

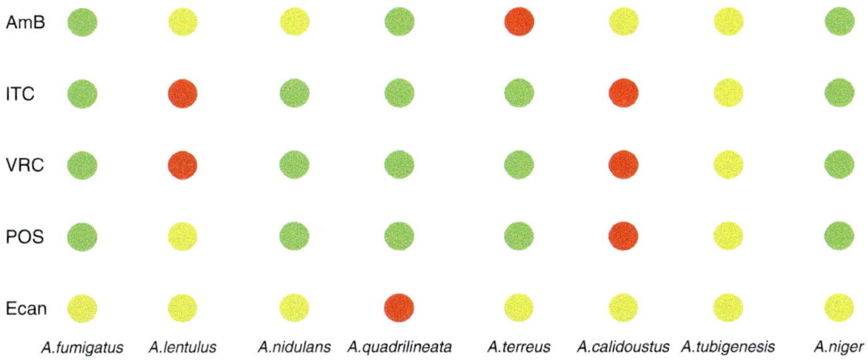

AmB amphotericin B, *ITC* itraconazole, *VRC* voriconazole, *POS* posaconazole, *Ecan* echinocandins. *Green*, sensitive; *yellow*, intermediate susceptibility; *red*, no sensitivity

Intrinsic Versus Acquired Azole Resistance in *A. fumigatus*

Although *Aspergillus* spp. are generally susceptible to the medical triazoles, intrinsic and acquired resistance has been documented. In general there are two types of resistance: microbiological versus clinical. Microbiological resistance relates to an in vitro susceptibility test, which indicates that the activity of a certain drug against the pathogen is low or absent and corresponds with a high probability of treatment failure. In vitro resistance can be primary (intrinsic) or secondary (acquired). Primary resistance occurs naturally, without prior exposure to the drug. Secondary resistance is generated following exposure to an antifungal and may be associated with altered gene expression or with the acquisition of mutations (Diekema et al. 2009; Verweij et al. 2009a). Clinical resistance, however, occurs when a patient fails to respond to antimicrobial therapy despite the administration of an antifungal. Clinical resistance may indicate microbiological resistance of the pathogen but can also be a consequence of other factors such as drug pharmacokinetics or the immune status of the host (Diekema et al. 2009).

Recent changes in the taxonomy of *Aspergillus* spp. have had major implications on our understanding of intrinsic drug susceptibility profiles (Van Der Linden et al. 2011a). New sibling species of *A. fumigatus* exhibit in vitro susceptibility profiles that differ significantly from that of *A. fumigatus*. While acquired azole resistance is an emerging problem in *A. fumigatus* (Verweij et al. 2007, 2009b), some other *Aspergillus* spp. are intrinsically more resistant to specific classes of antifungal agents (Table 1). Minimum inhibitory concentrations (MICs) of amphotericin B and azoles for some of the non-*fumigatus Aspergillus* spp. are elevated compared to *A. fumigatus* (Van Der Linden et al. 2011a). The MICs of *A. flavus* clinical isolates to amphotericin B are consistently twofold dilution steps higher than those of *A. fumigatus* (Gomez-Lopez et al. 2003). Using Clinical Laboratory Standards Institute (CLSI) methodology (CLSI 2008), *A. nidulans* was shown to have MIC values of 1–2 mg/L of amphotericin B, which is higher than commonly observed with *A. fumigatus* (van der Linden et al. 2013). In the section *Usti*, the azoles are not active against *A.calidoustus* with MICs of ≥8 mg/L, and the other classes of antifungal drugs also appear less active as compared with their activity against *A. fumigatus*. For example, the MICs of amphotericin B were found to range from 1 to 2 mg/L, which is relatively high (Varga et al. 2008). Resistance of *A. terreus* to amphotericin B is well recognized (Lass-Florl et al. 2009). The black aspergilli, *Aspergillus* section *Nigri*, exhibit three different azole susceptibility patterns: low azole MICs, high MICs, and a less common paradoxical effect. However, the classification of these fungi by azole MICs does not match with their species classification making it difficult to determine if these alterations in drug susceptibility represent intrinsic or acquired properties of these molds (Alcazar-Fuoli et al. 2009).

Azole Resistance Phenotypes in *A. fumigatus*

Antifungal drug resistance is normally quantified by MIC determination. Both the CLSI and European Committee on Antimicrobial Susceptibility Testing-Subcommittee on Antifungal Susceptibility Testing (EUCAST-AFST) have developed and standardized phenotypic methods that enable the reliable and reproducible determination of the MIC for conidia-forming molds such as *Aspergillus* spp. (CLSI 2008; Subcommittee on Antifungal Susceptibility Testing of the EECfAST 2008). The MIC represents the lowest drug concentration resulting either a significant reduction or complete lack of fungal growth (European Committee on Antimicrobial Susceptibility Testing-Subcommittee on Antifungal Susceptibility T 2008). Interpretation of resistance from the results of MIC testing requires the application of breakpoints. There are currently three sets of breakpoints and epidemiological cutoff values available. The first was published in 2009 by Verweij et al. based on clinical experience and the available knowledge at that time (Verweij et al. 2009b). More recently, the CLSI (Espinel-Ingroff et al. 2010) and the EUCAST-AFST (Arendrup et al. 2012a; Hope et al. 2013) have published guidelines in which strains with MICs <2 mg/L are considered susceptible for itraconazole and voriconazole, while those >2 mg/L are considered resistant; while for posaconazole strains with an MIC ≤0.25 are considered susceptible, those with an MIC >0.5 mg/L are considered resistant.

Azole-Resistant Genotypes in *A. fumigatus*

Several mechanisms of acquired resistance have been described in *Aspergillus* spp. Azole resistance has most commonly been associated with alterations in cyp51A, which represents the target enzyme of the azoles (Verweij et al. 2007). The corresponding phenotype depends on the particular mutation and may affect the activity of multiple triazoles. The most frequently characterized polymorphisms associated with resistance are found at codons 54, 98, 138, 220, and 448, although other single nucleotide polymorphisms (SNPs) have been reported (Verweij et al. 2007; Snelders et al. 2008; Mellado et al. 2004, 2007; Chen et al. 2005;

Howard et al. 2006). In addition to coding SNPs, other mutations have been described in azole-resistant *A. fumigatus* isolates which increase cyp51A expression (Verweij et al. 2007; Snelders et al. 2008; Mellado et al. 2004, 2007). At the present time, three common genetic variants associated with resistance to azoles have been described: a 34 base pair tandem repeat combined with a L98H substitution in the Cyp51A gene (TR_{34}/L98H) (Mellado et al. 2007), a 53 bp tandem repeat without substitutions in the Cyp51A gene (TR_{53}) (Camps et al. 2012a), and recently a 46 bp tandem repeat with two substitutions in the cyp51A gene (TR_{46}/Y121F/T289A)(van der Linden et al. 2013).

Notably, there are several studies indicating that mutations unrelated to Cyp51A might be associated with azole resistance in *Aspergillus* spp. Buied et al. reported that Cyp51B overexpression was associated with azole resistance mechanism in *A. fumigatus* (Buied et al. 2013). Other researchers demonstrated that the changes in a drug efflux pump of *Aspergillus* spp. can also contribute to the emergence of microbiological resistance. Overexpression of the *cdr1B* efflux transporter genes (Fraczek et al. 2013), modifications in AfuMDR1 and AfuMDR2 genes (da Silva Ferreira et al. 2004), and changes in expression of AfuMDR3 and AfuMDR4 (da Silva Ferreira et al. 2004; Nascimento et al. 2003) were all linked to high-level azole resistance in *A. fumigatus*. Similarly, Krishan-Natesan et al. showed that overexpression of ATP-binding cassette transporters and changes in major facilitator superfamily class efflux pumps contribute to voriconazole resistance in *A. flavus* (Natesan et al. 2013). Camps et al. reported a novel resistance mechanism, consisting of a mutation in the CCAAT-binding transcription factor complex subunit HapE (Camps et al. 2012b). A substitution was found in P88L within the exonic region of HapE gene resulting in an azole-resistant phenotype. Unlike cyp51A-mediated resistance mechanisms, HapE was associated with a fitness cost (Arendrup et al. 2010). Finally, as is the case for *A. fumigatus*, azole resistance in other species of *Aspergillus*, such as *A. flavus* (Liu et al. 2012) and *A. terreus* (Arendrup et al. 2012b), may be also caused by alterations and overexpression of the azole target 14α-demethylase (Buied et al. 2013). Collectively these observations indicate that acquired azole resistance is a clinical challenge that is not restricted to *A. fumigatus*, and multiple mechanisms may contribute to this resistance.

Routes of Azole Resistance Development: Clinical Versus Environmental

In *A. fumigatus* two routes of resistance selection have been reported. First, resistance may develop in patients treated with azole antifungal agents. Azole resistance has been reported in patients with chronic cavitating *Aspergillus* diseases, such as aspergilloma, that received long-term azole therapy (Howard et al. 2009). In these patients the initial infection was caused by an azole-susceptible isolate, but through therapy azole-resistant isolates were cultured. Azole resistance in isolates from these patients has been associated with point mutations only. Until recently, this mode of resistance development was believed to account for the majority of cases of acquired resistance.

A second route of selection for acquired resistance has recently been suggested. The exposure of *A. fumigatus* to azole 14α-demethylase inhibitors (DMIs) in the environment (Verweij et al. 2009a; Snelders et al. 2008, 2009, 2012), although still controversial, has been linked to the emergence of azole resistance (Enserink 2009). Azole fungicides inhibit fungal Cyp51A activity and are used abundantly for crop protection and material preservation. *A. fumigatus*, which is a saprophytic fungus, is thus hypothesized to develop azole resistance in response to environmental exposure to azole fungicides (Verweij et al. 2009a). In support of this hypothesis, five DMI fungicides were identified with in vitro activity against *A. fumigatus* and with molecule structures that are highly similar to that of the medical triazoles (Verweij et al. 2009a; Snelders et al. 2012).

Molecular Basis of Environmental Resistance

The first strains that were reported to be associated with environmental acquisition of resistance were found to contain TR_{34}/L98H in the Cyp51A gene (Snelders et al. 2008). Duplication of the 34 bp sequence in the promoter region was found to significantly increase the expression of Cyp51A gene; however it was not sufficient for the full azole-resistant phenotype. Similarly isolates harboring the L89H mutation only were not fully azole resistant. Introduction of both mutations into the same strain was required to reproduce the multi-azole-resistant phenotype (Mellado et al. 2007).

More recently a second set of mutations associated with presumed environmental acquisition of resistance was described (TR_{46}/Y121F/T289A) (van der Linden et al. 2013; Chowdhary et al. 2014; Vermeulen et al. 2012). TR_{46}/Y121F/T289A conferred high resistance to voriconazole and was associated with treatment failure in patients with IA. Interestingly, both sets of mutations consist of a combination of genomic changes that include a tandem repeat in the promotor region of CYP51a in addition to point mutations within the gene itself. The TR_{46}/Y121F/T289A resistance mechanism included three genomic changes, and it appears unlikely that these would have evolved independently during azole therapy in all the reported cases (van der Linden et al. 2013).

Epidemiology of Azole Resistance in *A. fumigatus*

Acquired triazole resistance among *Aspergillus* spp. is an emerging phenomenon (Pfaller et al. 2008, 2011; Verweij et al. 2002) that has now been reported across multiple continents (Snelders et al. 2008; Howard et al. 2009; Mellado et al. 2013; Lockhart et al. 2011; Rath et al. 2012; Seyedmousavi et al. 2013a; van der Linden et al. 2011b; Chowdhary et al. 2012a; Tashiro et al. 2012). A number of studies report that azole resistance in *A. fumigatus* has increased in recent years, with both intrinsic and acquired resistances having been documented in different regions and patient groups. Therefore, knowledge of the local epidemiology of azole-resistant *Aspergillus* diseases is important with respect to the development of management strategies.

The overall incidence of azole resistance has been increasing. Reports from the Netherlands and Manchester, United Kingdom, display an alarming increase of azole resistance in *A. fumigatus* since 1998 (Fig. 2; Verweij et al. 2009b). The widespread increase of azole resistance in Manchester is primarily related to long-term azole treatment in patients (Howard et al. 2009). In Manchester, the first published case of itraconazole resistance in *A. fumigatus* appeared in 1997 (the isolate originated from the late 1980s) (Denning et al. 1997), then in 2000 epidemiological surveys showed a 2 % prevalence of itraconazole resistance (Moore et al. 2000), and in 2007 the percentage of patients with an azole-resistant *A. fumigatus* increased up to 15 % (Verweij et al. 2007; Pfaller et al. 2008).

In the Netherlands azole resistance increased dramatically from 2.5 % in 2000, to 4.9 % in 2002, to 6.6 % in 2004, to 10 % in 2009 (van der Linden et al. 2011b). TR_{34}/L98H first emerged in clinical *A. fumigatus* isolates from the Netherlands in 1998 and is now endemic in Dutch hospitals (van der Linden et al. 2015). This change in epidemiology is of major importance as >90 % of Dutch clinical azole-resistant isolates are believed to share this molecular mechanism of resistance (Verweij et al. 2009a; Snelders et al. 2008). Both invasive and noninvasive aspergillosis

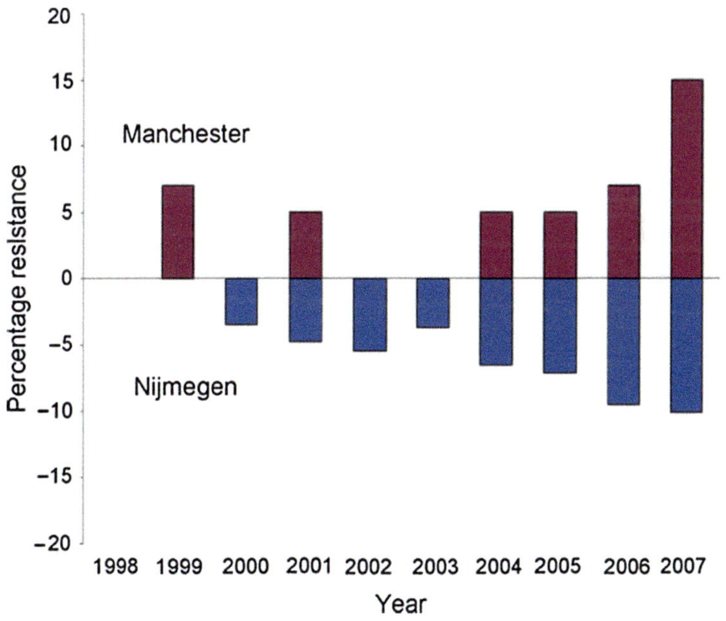

Fig. 2 The percentage of patients with azole-resistant *A. fumigatus* strains in Manchester (United Kingdom) and Nijmegen (the Netherlands) between 1998 and 2007 (Adapted from Verweij et al. (2009b))

infections due to TR_{34}/L98H have been reported in azole-treated as well as in azole-naive patients (Snelders et al. 2008; van der Linden et al. 2011b). Importantly, the geographic area where TR_{34}/L98H strains have been reported coincides with the region with the most intensive use of fungicides, suggesting that an environmental source is very likely (Snelders et al. 2008, 2009). Azole resistance, due to the TR_{34}/L98H resistance mechanism, has also been reported in clinical *A. fumigatus* isolates from other European countries and more recently from China and India (Snelders et al. 2008; Howard et al. 2009; Mellado et al. 2013; Lockhart et al. 2011; Rath et al. 2012; Seyedmousavi et al. 2013a; Chowdhary et al. 2012a, b; Burgel et al. 2012; Morio et al. 2012; Mortensen et al. 2010; Lagrou et al. 2008). Genotyping studies indicate that in Europe, TR_{34}/L98H isolates represent offspring of a common ancestor (Camps et al. 2012c) and could have developed locally, possibly in the Netherlands, and then subsequently spread across countries through wind-dispersed conidia or ascospores.

Similar findings have been observed with the newly emerging TR_{46}/Y121F/T289A mutation which is spreading rapidly in Dutch hospitals (van der Linden et al. 2013; Chowdhary et al. 2014). Strains bearing this TR_{46}/Y121F/T289A mutation have been recovered from epidemiologically unrelated patients, most of whom were azole naive, as well as from the environment. Furthermore, genetic typing of isolates bearing these mutations showed clustering of these strains in separate clades from wild-type (azole-susceptible) isolates.

As with strains bearing the TR_{34}/L98H mutation, the rapid geographical migration of TR_{46}/Y121F/T289A strains in Dutch hospitals indicates that this resistance mechanism will likely spread more widely. Indeed, a lethal case of azole-resistant invasive aspergillosis due to TR_{46}/Y121F/T289A was recently reported in a patient from Belgium, suggesting that this strain has already spread beyond the borders of the Netherlands (Vermeulen et al. 2012). The presence of TR_{46}/Y121F/T289A mutation has also been reported in environmental *A. fumigatus* strains in India, which were also cross-resistant to commonly used azole fungicides (Chowdhary et al. 2013, 2014). From a global perspective, fungicide use is second highest in the Asia-Pacific regions (24 %), preceded only by Western Europe (37 %) (Christen Rune Stensvold et al. 2012).

Clinical Implications of Azole Resistance and Impact of Underlying Diseases

The clinical implications of azole resistance depend on the route of resistance selection (Table 2). The patient profiles are very different with patients with chronic lung diseases, cavitary pulmonary lesions, and chronic azole therapy at risk for resistance selection through patient therapy. However, azole-resistant aspergillosis can occur in *any* patient if infected through the environmental route, causing any kind of *Aspergillus* disease, including ABPA and IA. For the environmental route, there are no clear clinical risk factors other than living in an area where environmental azole resistance is found. Both environmental sampling of soil or ambient air

Table 2 Implications for the patient and environmental routes of azole resistance selection in *A. fumigatus*

Patient route	Environmental route
Chronic *Aspergillus* diseases (usually with chronic lung disease)	All *Aspergillus* diseases including IA
Cavitary lesion	No specific lesion
(Previous) azole therapy in all patients	(Previous) azole therapy in one third of patients
High diversity of mutations; both Cyp51A mediated and others	Low diversity of azole resistance mutations associated with the Cyp51A gene
Cyp51A point mutations	Tandem repeat
Both azole-susceptible and azole-resistant phenotypes simultaneously present	Both azole-susceptible and azole-resistant phenotypes simultaneously present
High genetic diversity between azole-resistant isolates from unrelated patients	Low genetic diversity between azole-resistant isolates from unrelated patients
A. fumigatus colonies may show an abnormal phenotype, sporulation, and growth rate	No apparent fitness cost

for the presence of azole-resistant *A. fumigatus* and testing collection of clinical isolates will help to determine if azole resistance is an issue in the patient population. Previous studies indicate that at least 70 isolates need to be tested in order to detect azole-resistant isolates (van der Linden et al. 2011b).

There are currently no controlled trials that have evaluated the effect of azole resistance on the probability of treatment success. However, case series of patients with azole-resistant chronic *Aspergillus* diseases and azole-resistant IA have found that the recovery of an azole-resistant isolate is associated with a higher probability of azole treatment failure (Snelders et al. 2008; Howard et al. 2009; Mellado et al. 2013; Rath et al. 2012; Hodiamont et al. 2009; van der Linden et al. 2009; van Leer-Buter et al. 2007; Warris et al. 2002; Hamprecht et al. 2012).

In patients receiving chronic azole therapy, a wide range of mutations was found in azole-resistant *Aspergillus* spp. isolates (Howard et al. 2009). Consistent with these findings, cross-resistance among the azoles varied between isolates. Of 34 itraconazole-resistant isolates studied, 65 % (Soubani and Chandrasekar 2002) were cross-resistant to voriconazole and 74 % (Denning et al. 2011) were cross-resistant to posaconazole, likely reflecting the similarity in structure between itraconazole and posaconazole. Thirteen of 14 evaluable patients had prior azole exposure; eight infections failed therapy, and five failed to improve (Howard et al. 2009).

Two case series of patients with environmentally acquired azole-resistant IA were reported from the Netherlands (van der Linden et al. 2011b, 2013). In the first study, seven of eight (88 %) patients with proven or probable, culture-positive IA due to *A. fumigatus* harboring the TR_{34}/L98H resistance mechanism died at 12 weeks. Voriconazole was the initial treatment choice in most patients. In a second study the emergence of a voriconazole resistance associated with the TR_{46}/Y121F/T289A mutation was reported (van der Linden et al. 2013). At 12 weeks after recovery of the TR_{46}/Y121F/T289A isolate, four of eight patients with IA had died and two patients had persisting infection. In addition, a number of single cases have been described harboring TR_{34}/L98H (Snelders et al. 2008; Howard et al. 2009; Mellado et al. 2013; Rath et al. 2012; Hodiamont et al. 2009; van der Linden et al. 2009; van Leer-Buter et al. 2007; Warris et al. 2002; Hamprecht et al. 2012) or TR_{46}/Y121F/T289A mutations (Vermeulen et al. 2012). In all cases, patients with infection due to an azole-resistant isolate failed to respond to azole therapy. Primary invasive infections due to resistant *A. fumigatus* isolates have been reported involving the lung (Verweij et al. 2007; Howard et al. 2009), bone (Hodiamont et al. 2009), and brain (Howard et al. 2009; van der Linden et al. 2009) as well as from respiratory isolates in allergic bronchopulmonary aspergillosis (Howard et al. 2006). Importantly, there is no apparent risk of spread of azole-resistant isolates to other patients, consistent with the observation that *A. fumigatus* does not sporulate in the human host during invasive infection.

These data notwithstanding, it must be recognized that there are numerous other factors that can impact treatment success in *Aspergillus* infection. Patients with refractory underlying malignancy are prone to failure of therapy, even if the infection is caused by an azole-susceptible isolate. Azole exposure might have been insufficient in patients failing therapy, and as most patients were culture positive, treatment might have been initiated relatively late in the course of the infection. Furthermore, azole-resistant infection might occur predominantly in patients in poor clinical condition, compared to wild-type isolates.

In the absence of robust clinical evidence, experimental models of *Aspergillus* infection may help us to understand the implications of azole resistance on treatment efficacy. In animal models of IA, the MIC has been found to be a powerful predictor of the efficacy of voriconazole and posaconazole (Mavridou et al. 2010a; Howard et al. 2011; Seyedmousavi et al. 2014). There was a clear association between the MIC and efficacy in the animal model, with increasing MIC corresponding with decreasing efficacy (Mavridou et al. 2010a, b; Seyedmousavi et al. 2014). The results of combination therapy also suggested that a combination of voriconazole or posaconazole with an echinocandin may be effective (Seyedmousavi et al. 2013b, c; Lepak et al. 2013). However, the synergistic interaction may be lost when an azole-resistant isolate (voriconazole MIC, 4 mg/L) is the infectious agent.

These results highlight a significant clinical problem. With the increased use of non-culture diagnostics and imaging studies for the early detection of IA, the isolation of *A. fumigatus* by culture is relatively uncommon. As voriconazole resistance rates increase (van der Linden et al. 2013; Snelders et al. 2008), the choice of empiric therapy in culture-negative patients is difficult. While preclinical studies suggest that the efficacy of liposomal amphotericin B (L-AmB) is preserved in azole-resistant infections (Seyedmousavi et al. 2013d), some post-marketing studies suggest that L-AmB may be less active than voriconazole against *Aspergillus* (Nivoix et al. 2008; Baddley et al. 2010; Denning and Bowyer 2013). Balancing the benefits of voriconazole therapy against the chance of a resistant isolate requires up-to-date knowledge of local resistance rates, which is often not available to clinicians.

Concluding Remarks

Azole-resistant *Aspergillus* infection is commonly associated with treatment failure. Although azole resistance may emerge during antifungal therapy of individual azole-treated patients, selection of resistance may also occur in the environment. The evolving epidemiology of strains bearing TR_{34}/L98H and TR_{46}/Y121F/T289A mutations indicates that these resistance mechanisms will be increasingly observed in European Union member states and outside Europe. Given the prominent role of azoles in the management of *Aspergillus* diseases, successful management of azole-resistant *Aspergillus* diseases in patients with infection caused by *A. fumigatus* is a challenge and suggests a need to critically examine our use of azole-type antifungals in agriculture.

References

Alcazar-Fuoli L, Mellado E, Alastruey-Izquierdo A, Cuenca-Estrella M, Rodriguez-Tudela JL (2009) Species identification and antifungal susceptibility patterns of species belonging to *Aspergillus* section Nigri. Antimicrob Agents Chemother 53:4514–4517

Arendrup MC, Mavridou E, Mortensen KL, Snelders E, Frimodt-Moller N, Khan H, Melchers WJ, Verweij PE (2010) Development of azole resistance in *Aspergillus fumigatus* during azole therapy associated with change in virulence. PLoS One 5, e10080

Arendrup MC, Cuenca-Estrella M, Lass-Florl C, Hope WW, European Committee on Antimicrobial Susceptibility Testing Subcommittee on Antifungal Susceptibility T (2012a) EUCAST technical note on *Aspergillus* and amphotericin B, itraconazole, and posaconazole. Clin Microbiol Infect 18:E248–E250

Arendrup MC, Jensen RH, Grif K, Skov M, Pressler T, Johansen HK, Lass-Florl C (2012b) In vivo emergence of *Aspergillus terreus* with reduced azole susceptibility and a Cyp51a M217I alteration. J Infect Dis 206:981–985

Arne P, Thierry S, Wang D, Deville M, Le Loc'h G, Desoutter A, Femenia F, Nieguitsila A, Huang W, Chermette R, Guillot J (2011) Aspergillus fumigatus in Poultry. Int J Microbiol 2011:746356

Baddley JW, Andes DR, Marr KA, Kontoyiannis DP, Alexander BD, Kauffman CA, Oster RA, Anaissie EJ, Walsh TJ, Schuster MG, Wingard JR, Patterson TF, Ito JI, Williams OD, Chiller T, Pappas PG (2010) Factors associated with mortality in transplant patients with invasive aspergillosis. Clin Infect Dis 50:1559–1567

Balajee SA (2009) Aspergillus terreus complex. Med Mycol 47(Suppl 1):S42–S46

Brown GD, Denning DW, Gow NA, Levitz SM, Netea MG, White TC (2012) Hidden killers: human fungal infections. Sci Transl Med 4:165rv113

Buied A, Moore CB, Denning DW, Bowyer P (2013) High-level expression of cyp51B in azole-resistant clinical *Aspergillus fumigatus* isolates. J Antimicrob Chemother 68:512–514

Burgel PR, Baixench MT, Amsellem M, Audureau E, Chapron J, Kanaan R, Honore I, Dupouy-Camet J, Dusser D, Klaassen CH, Meis JF, Hubert D, Paugam A (2012) High prevalence of azole-resistant *Aspergillus fumigatus* in adults with cystic fibrosis exposed to itraconazole. Antimicrob Agents Chemother 56:869–874

Camps SM, van der Linden JW, Li Y, Kuijper EJ, van Dissel JT, Verweij PE, Melchers WJ (2012a) Rapid induction of multiple resistance mechanisms in *Aspergillus fumigatus* during azole therapy: a case study and review of the literature. Antimicrob Agents Chemother 56:10–16

Camps SM, Dutilh BE, Arendrup MC, Rijs AJ, Snelders E, Huynen MA, Verweij PE, Melchers WJ (2012b) Discovery of a HapE mutation that causes azole resistance in *Aspergillus fumigatus* through whole genome sequencing and sexual crossing. PLoS One 7, e50034

Camps SM, Rijs AJ, Klaassen CH, Meis JF, O'Gorman CM, Dyer PS, Melchers WJ, Verweij PE (2012c) Molecular epidemiology of *Aspergillus fumigatus* isolates harboring the TR34/L98H azole resistance mechanism. J Clin Microbiol 50:2674–2680

Chen J, Li H, Li R, Bu D, Wan Z (2005) Mutations in the cyp51A gene and susceptibility to itraconazole in *Aspergillus fumigatus* serially isolated from a patient with lung Aspergilloma. J Antimicrob Chemother 55:31–37

Chowdhary A, Kathuria S, Randhawa HS, Gaur SN, Klaassen CH, Meis JF (2012a) Isolation of multiple-triazole-resistant *Aspergillus fumigatus* strains carrying the TR/L98H mutations in the cyp51A gene in India. J Antimicrob Chemother 67:362–366

Chowdhary A, Kathuria S, Xu J, Sharma C, Sundar G, Singh PK, Gaur SN, Hagen F, Klaassen CH, Meis JF (2012b) Clonal expansion and emergence of environmental multiple-triazole-resistant *Aspergillus fumigatus* strains carrying the TR(3)(4)/L98H mutations in the cyp51A gene in India. PLoS One 7, e52871

Chowdhary A, Kathuria S, Xu J, Meis JF (2013) Emergence of azole-resistant *Aspergillus fumigatus* strains due to agricultural azole use creates an increasing threat to human health. PLoS Pathog 9, e1003633

Chowdhary A, Sharma C, Kathuria S, Hagen F, Meis JF (2014) Azole-resistant *Aspergillus fumigatus* with the environmental TR46/Y121F/T289A mutation in India. J Antimicrob Chemother 69:555–557

Christen Rune Stensvold CR, Jørgensen LN, Arendrup MC (2012) Azole-resistant invasive Aspergillosis: relationship to agriculture. Curr Fungal Infect Rep 6:178–191

CLSI (2008) Reference method for broth dilution antifungal susceptibility testing of filamentous fungi; Approved standard-Second Edition. CLSI Document. M38-A2., vol 28 no 16. Clinical and laboratory Standards Institute, Wane

Cornely OA, Maertens J, Winston DJ, Perfect J, Ullmann AJ, Walsh TJ, Helfgott D, Holowiecki J, Stockelberg D, Goh YT, Petrini M, Hardalo C, Suresh R, Angulo-Gonzalez D (2007) Posaconazole vs. fluconazole or itraconazole prophylaxis in patients with neutropenia. N Engl J Med 356:348–359

da Silva Ferreira ME, Capellaro JL, dos Reis ME, Malavazi I, Perlin D, Park S, Anderson JB, Colombo AL, Arthington-Skaggs BA, Goldman MH, Goldman GH (2004) In vitro evolution of itraconazole resistance in *Aspergillus fumigatus* involves multiple mechanisms of resistance. Antimicrob Agents Chemother 48:4405–4413

de Hoog GS, Guarro J, Gene J, Figueras MJ (2009) Atlas of clinical fungi: the ultimate benchtool for diagnostics, A pilot version of the 3rd edition ed, vol. CD-ROM. Centraalbureau voor Schimmelcultures, KNAW Fungal Biodiversity Centre / Universitat Rovira i Virgili Utrecht/Reus

DeLone DR, Goldstein RA, Petermann G, Salamat MS, Miles JM, Knechtle SJ, Brown WD (1999) Disseminated Aspergillosis involving the brain: distribution and imaging characteristics. AJNR Am J Neuroradiol 20:1597–1604

Denning DW (1998) Invasive Aspergillosis. Clin Infect Dis 26:781–803; quiz 804–785

Denning DW, Bowyer P (2013) Voriconazole resistance in *Aspergillus fumigatus*: should we be concerned? Clin Infect Dis 57:521–523

Denning DW, Radford SA, Oakley KL, Hall L, Johnson EM, Warnock DW (1997) Correlation between in-vitro susceptibility testing to itraconazole and in-vivo outcome of *Aspergillus fumigatus* infection. J Antimicrob Chemother 40:401–414

Denning DW, Pleuvry A, Cole DC (2011) Global burden of chronic pulmonary Aspergillosis as a sequel to pulmonary tuberculosis. Bull World Health Organ 89:864–872

Diekema DJ, Messer SA, Hollis RJ, Boyken L, Tendolkar S, Kroeger J, Jones RN, Pfaller MA (2009) A global evaluation of voriconazole activity tested against recent clinical isolates of *Candida* spp. Diagn Microbiol Infect Dis 63:233–236

EMA (2012a) European public assessment report (EPAR) for Noxafil, 06/09/2012 ed. European Medicines Agency

EMA (2012b) European public assessment report (EPAR) for Vfend, 04/12/2012 ed. European Medicines Agency

Enserink M (2009) Infectious diseases. Farm fungicides linked to resistance in a human pathogen. Science 326:1173

Espinel-Ingroff A, Diekema DJ, Fothergill A, Johnson E, Pelaez T, Pfaller MA, Rinaldi MG, Canton E, Turnidge J (2010) Wild-type MIC distributions and epidemiological cutoff values for the triazoles and six *Aspergillus* spp. for the CLSI broth microdilution method (M38-A2 document). J Clin Microbiol 48:3251–3257

European Committee on Antimicrobial Susceptibility Testing-Subcommittee on Antifungal Susceptibility T (2008) EUCAST technical note on fluconazole. Clin Microbiol Infect 14:193–195

Fraczek MG, Bromley M, Buied A, Moore CB, Rajendran R, Rautemaa R, Ramage G, Denning DW, Bowyer P (2013) The cdr1B efflux transporter is associated with non-cyp51a-mediated itraconazole resistance in *Aspergillus fumigatus*. J Antimicrob Chemother 68:1486–1496

Fresenius GW (1863) Beiträge zur Mykologie. Brönner Frankfurt, Frankfurt a. M, pp 81–82

Galimberti R, Kowalczuk A, Hidalgo Parra I, Gonzalez Ramos M, Flores V (1998) Cutaneous Aspergillosis: a report of six cases. Br J Dermatol 139:522–526

Gallin JI, Zarember K (2007) Lessons about the pathogenesis and management of Aspergillosis from studies in chronic granulomatous disease. Trans Am Clin Climatol Assoc 118:175–185

Garrett DO, Jochimsen E, Jarvis W (1999) Invasive *Aspergillus* spp infections in rheumatology patients. J Rheumatol 26:146–149

Gefter WB (1992) The spectrum of pulmonary Aspergillosis. J Thorac Imaging 7:56–74

Germaud P, Tuchais E (1995) Allergic bronchopulmonary Aspergillosis treated with itraconazole. Chest 107:883

Gomez-Lopez A, Garcia-Effron G, Mellado E, Monzon A, Rodriguez-Tudela JL, Cuenca-Estrella M (2003) In vitro activities of three licensed antifungal agents against Spanish clinical isolates of *Aspergillus* spp. Antimicrob Agents Chemother 47:3085–3088

Greub G, Bille J (1998) *Aspergillus* species isolated from clinical specimens: suggested clinical and microbiological criteria to determine significance. Clin Microbiol Infect 4:710–716

Guinea J, Pelaez T, Recio S, Torres-Narbona M, Bouza E (2008) In vitro antifungal activities of isavuconazole (BAL4815), voriconazole, and fluconazole against 1,007 isolates of *zygomycete*, *Candida*, *Aspergillus*, *Fusarium*, and *Scedosporium* species. Antimicrob Agents Chemother 52:1396–1400

Hamprecht A, Buchheidt D, Vehreschild JJ, Cornely OA, Spiess B, Plum G, Halbsguth TV, Kutsch N, Stippel D, Kahl P, Persigehl T, Steinbach A, Bos B, Hallek M, Vehreschild MJ (2012) Azole-resistant invasive aspergillosis in a patient with acute myeloid leukaemia in Germany. Euro Surveill 17:20262

Heitman J (2011) Microbial pathogens in the fungal kingdom. Fungal Biol Rev 25:48–60

Henriet S, Verweij PE, Holland SM, Warris A (2013) Invasive fungal infections in patients with chronic granulomatous disease. Adv Exp Med Biol 764:27–55

Herbrecht R, Denning DW, Patterson TF, Bennett JE, Greene RE, Oestmann JW, Kern WV, Marr KA, Ribaud P, Lortholary O, Sylvester R, Rubin RH, Wingard JR, Stark P, Durand C, Caillot D, Thiel E, Chandrasekar PH, Hodges MR, Schlamm HT, Troke PF, de Pauw B, Invasive Fungal Infections Group of the European Organisation for R, Treatment of C, the Global Aspergillus Study G (2002) Voriconazole versus amphotericin B for primary therapy of invasive Aspergillosis. N Engl J Med 347:408–415

Hodiamont CJ, Dolman KM, Ten Berge IJ, Melchers WJ, Verweij PE, Pajkrt D (2009) Multiple-azole-resistant *Aspergillus fumigatus* osteomyelitis in a patient with chronic granulomatous disease successfully treated with long-term oral posaconazole and surgery. Med Mycol 47:217–220

Hope WW, Cuenca-Estrella M, Lass-Florl C, Arendrup MC, European Committee on Antimicrobial Susceptibility Testing-Subcommittee on Antifungal Susceptibility T (2013) EUCAST technical note on voriconazole and *Aspergillus* spp. Clin Microbiol Infect 19:E278–E280

Howard SJ, Webster I, Moore CB, Gardiner RE, Park S, Perlin DS, Denning DW (2006) Multi-azole resistance in *Aspergillus fumigatus*. Int J Antimicrob Agents 28:450–453

Howard SJ, Cerar D, Anderson MJ, Albarrag A, Fisher MC, Pasqualotto AC, Laverdiere M, Arendrup MC, Perlin DS, Denning DW (2009) Frequency and evolution of Azole resistance in *Aspergillus fumigatus* associated with treatment failure. Emerg Infect Dis 15:1068–1076

Howard SJ, Lestner JM, Sharp A, Gregson L, Goodwin J, Slater J, Majithiya JB, Warn PA, Hope WW (2011) Pharmacokinetics and pharmacodynamics of posaconazole for invasive pulmonary aspergillosis: clinical implications for antifungal therapy. J Infect Dis 203:1324–1332

Kwon-Chung KJ, Sugui JA (2013) Aspergillus fumigatus–what makes the species a ubiquitous human fungal pathogen? PLoS Pathog 9, e1003743

Lagrou K, Vleeschouwer J, Meersseman W, Dupont L, Verleden GM, Melchers WJG, Verweij PE, Martens J (2008) 3rd Adv. Against Aspergillosis. Miami, p 33

Lass-Florl C, Alastruey-Izquierdo A, Cuenca-Estrella M, Perkhofer S, Rodriguez-Tudela JL (2009) In vitro activities of various antifungal drugs against *Aspergillus terreus*: global assessment using the methodology of the European committee on antimicrobial susceptibility testing. Antimicrob Agents Chemother 53:794–795

Latge JP (1999) Aspergillus fumigatus and Aspergillosis. Clin Microbiol Rev 12:310–350

Lepak AJ, Marchillo K, VanHecker J, Andes DR (2013) Impact of in vivo triazole and echinocandin combination therapy for invasive pulmonary aspergillosis: enhanced efficacy against Cyp51 mutant isolates. Antimicrob Agents Chemother 57:5438–5447

Liu W, Sun Y, Chen W, Liu W, Wan Z, Bu D, Li R (2012) The T788G mutation in the cyp51C gene confers voriconazole resistance in *Aspergillus flavus* causing Aspergillosis. Antimicrob Agents Chemother 56:2598–2603

Lockhart SR, Frade JP, Etienne KA, Pfaller MA, Diekema DJ, Balajee SA (2011) Azole resistance in *Aspergillus fumigatus* isolates from the ARTEMIS global surveillance study is primarily due to the TR/L98H mutation in the cyp51A gene. Antimicrob Agents Chemother 55:4465–4468

Mavridou E, Bruggemann RJ, Melchers WJ, Mouton JW, Verweij PE (2010a) Efficacy of posaconazole against three clinical *Aspergillus fumigatus* isolates with mutations in the cyp51A gene. Antimicrob Agents Chemother 54:860–865

Mavridou E, Bruggemann RJ, Melchers WJ, Verweij PE, Mouton JW (2010b) Impact of cyp51A mutations on the pharmacokinetic and pharmacodynamic properties of voriconazole in a murine model of disseminated aspergillosis. Antimicrob Agents Chemother 54:4758–4764

Meersseman W, Vandecasteele SJ, Wilmer A, Verbeken E, Peetermans WE, Van Wijngaerden E (2004) Invasive Aspergillosis in critically ill patients without malignancy. Am J Respir Crit Care Med 170:621–625

Mellado E, Garcia-Effron G, Alcazar-Fuoli L, Cuenca-Estrella M, Rodriguez-Tudela JL (2004) Substitutions at methionine 220 in the 14alpha-sterol demethylase (Cyp51A) of *Aspergillus fumigatus* are responsible for resistance in vitro to azole antifungal drugs. Antimicrob Agents Chemother 48:2747–2750

Mellado E, Garcia-Effron G, Alcazar-Fuoli L, Melchers WJ, Verweij PE, Cuenca-Estrella M, Rodriguez-Tudela JL (2007) A new *Aspergillus fumigatus* resistance mechanism conferring in vitro cross-resistance to azole antifungals involves a combination of cyp51A alterations. Antimicrob Agents Chemother 51:1897–1904

Mellado E, De La Camara R, Buendia B, Rodriguez-Tudela JL, Cuenca-Estrella M (2013) Breakthrough pulmonary *Aspergillus fumigatus* infection with multiple triazole resistance in a Spanish patient with chronic myeloid leukemia. Rev Iberoam Micol 30:64–68

Mohr J, Johnson M, Cooper T, Lewis JS, Ostrosky-Zeichner L (2008) Current options in antifungal pharmacotherapy. Pharmacotherapy 28:614–645

Moore CB, Walls CM, Denning DW (2000) In vitro activity of the new triazole BMS-207147 against *Aspergillus* species in comparison with itraconazole and amphotericin B. Antimicrob Agents Chemother 44:441–443

Morio F, Aubin GG, Danner-Boucher I, Haloun A, Sacchetto E, Garcia-Hermoso D, Bretagne S, Miegeville M, Le Pape P (2012) High prevalence of triazole resistance in *Aspergillus fumigatus*, especially mediated by TR/L98H, in a French cohort of patients with cystic fibrosis. J Antimicrob Chemother 67:1870–1873

Mortensen KL, Mellado E, Lass-Florl C, Rodriguez-Tudela JL, Johansen HK, Arendrup MC (2010) Environmental study of azole-resistant *Aspergillus fumigatus* and other Aspergilli in Austria, Denmark, and Spain. Antimicrob Agents Chemother 54:4545–4549

Nascimento AM, Goldman GH, Park S, Marras SA, Delmas G, Oza U, Lolans K, Dudley MN, Mann PA, Perlin DS (2003) Multiple resistance mechanisms among *Aspergillus fumigatus* mutants with high-level resistance to itraconazole. Antimicrob Agents Chemother 47:1719–1726

Natesan SK, Lamichchane AK, Swaminathan S, Wu W (2013) Differential expression of ATP-binding cassette and/or major facilitator superfamily class efflux pumps contributes to voriconazole resistance in *Aspergillus flavus*. Diagn Microbiol Infect Dis 76:458–463

Nivoix Y, Velten M, Letscher-Bru V, Moghaddam A, Natarajan-Ame S, Fohrer C, Lioure B, Bilger K, Lutun P, Marcellin L, Launoy A, Freys G, Bergerat JP, Herbrecht R (2008) Factors associated with overall and attributable mortality in invasive aspergillosis. Clin Infect Dis 47:1176–1184

Patterson TF (2005) Advances and challenges in management of invasive mycoses. Lancet 366:1013–1025

Patterson K, Strek ME (2010) Allergic bronchopulmonary Aspergillosis. Proc Am Thorac Soc 7:237–244

Peterson SW (2008) Phylogenetic analysis of *Aspergillus* species using DNA sequences from four loci. Mycologia 100:205–226

Peterson SW, Varga J, Frisvad JC, Samson RA (2008) Phylogeny and subgeneric taxonomy of *Aspergillus*. Wageningen Academic Publishers, Wageningen

Pfaller MA, Messer SA, Hollis RJ, Jones RN, Group SP (2002) Antifungal activities of posaconazole, ravuconazole, and voriconazole compared to those of itraconazole and amphotericin B against 239 clinical isolates of *Aspergillus* spp. and other filamentous fungi: report from SENTRY Antimicrobial Surveillance Program, 2000. Antimicrob Agents Chemother 46:1032–1037

Pfaller MA, Messer SA, Boyken L, Rice C, Tendolkar S, Hollis RJ, Diekema DJ (2008) In vitro survey of triazole cross-resistance among more than 700 clinical isolates of *Aspergillus* species. J Clin Microbiol 46:2568–2572

Pfaller M, Boyken L, Hollis R, Kroeger J, Messer S, Tendolkar S, Diekema D (2011) Use of epidemiological cutoff values to examine 9-year trends in susceptibility of *Aspergillus* species to the triazoles. J Clin Microbiol 49:586–590

Pitt JI (1994) The current role of *Aspergillus* and *Penicillium* in human and animal health. J Med Vet Mycol 32(Suppl 1):17–32

Rath PM, Buchheidt D, Spiess B, Arfanis E, Buer J, Steinmann J (2012) First reported case of azole-resistant aspergillus fumigatus due to the TR/L98H mutation in Germany. Antimicrob Agents Chemother 56:6060–6061

Saraceno JL, Phelps DT, Ferro TJ, Futerfas R, Schwartz DB (1997) Chronic necrotizing pulmonary Aspergillosis: approach to management. Chest 112:541–548

Segal BH, Romani LR (2009) Invasive Aspergillosis in chronic granulomatous disease. Med Mycol 47(Suppl 1):S282–S290

Seyedmousavi S, Hashemi SJ, Zibafar E, Zoll J, Hedayati MT, Mouton JW, Melchers WJ, Verweij PE (2013a) Azole-resistant *Aspergillus fumigatus*, Iran. Emerg Infect Dis 19:832–834

Seyedmousavi S, Meletiadis J, Melchers WJ, Rijs AJ, Mouton JW, Verweij PE (2013b) In vitro interaction of voriconazole and anidulafungin against triazole-resistant *Aspergillus fumigatus*. Antimicrob Agents Chemother 57:796–803

Seyedmousavi S, Bruggemann RJ, Melchers WJ, Rijs AJ, Verweij PE, Mouton JW (2013c) Efficacy and pharmacodynamics of voriconazole combined with anidulafungin in azole-resistant invasive aspergillosis. J Antimicrob Chemother 68:385–393

Seyedmousavi S, Melchers WJ, Mouton JW, Verweij PE (2013d) Pharmacodynamics and dose–response relationships of liposomal amphotericin B against different azole-resistant *Aspergillus fumigatus* isolates in a murine model of disseminated aspergillosis. Antimicrob Agents Chemother 57:1866–1871

Seyedmousavi S, Mouton JW, Melchers WJ, Bruggemann RJ, Verweij PE (2014) The role of azoles in the management of azole-resistant aspergillosis: from the bench to the bedside. Drug Resist Updat 17:37–50

Seyedmousavi S, Verweij PE, Mouton JW (2015) Isavuconazole, a broad-spectrum triazole for the treatment of systemic fungal diseases. Expert Rev Anti Infect Ther 13:9–27

Smith NL, Denning DW (2011) Underlying conditions in chronic pulmonary Aspergillosis including simple Aspergilloma. Eur Respir J 37:865–872

Snelders E, van der Lee HA, Kuijpers J, Rijs AJ, Varga J, Samson RA, Mellado E, Donders AR, Melchers WJ, Verweij PE (2008) Emergence of azole resistance in *Aspergillus fumigatus* and spread of a single resistance mechanism. PLoS Med 5, e219

Snelders E, Huis In 't Veld RA, Rijs AJ, Kema GH, Melchers WJ, Verweij PE (2009) Possible environmental origin of resistance of *Aspergillus fumigatus* to medical triazoles. Appl Environ Microbiol 75:4053–4057

Snelders E, Camps SM, Karawajczyk A, Schaftenaar G, Kema GH, van der Lee HA, Klaassen CH, Melchers WJ, Verweij PE (2012) Triazole fungicides can induce cross-resistance to medical triazoles in *Aspergillus fumigatus*. PLoS One 7, e31801

Soubani AO, Chandrasekar PH (2002) The clinical spectrum of pulmonary Aspergillosis. Chest 121:1988–1999

Subcommittee on Antifungal Susceptibility Testing of the EECfAST (2008) EUCAST Technical Note on the method for the determination of broth dilution minimum inhibitory concentrations of antifungal agents for conidia-forming moulds. Clin Microbiol Infect 14:982–984

Tashiro M, Izumikawa K, Minematsu A, Hirano K, Iwanaga N, Ide S, Mihara T, Hosogaya N, Takazono T, Morinaga Y, Nakamura S, Kurihara S, Imamura Y, Miyazaki T, Nishino T, Tsukamoto M, Kakeya H, Yamamoto Y, Yanagihara K, Yasuoka A, Tashiro T, Kohno S (2012) Antifungal susceptibilities of *Aspergillus fumigatus* clinical isolates obtained in Nagasaki, Japan. Antimicrob Agents Chemother 56:584–587

Ullmann AJ, Lipton JH, Vesole DH, Chandrasekar P, Langston A, Tarantolo SR, Greinix H, Morais de Azevedo W, Reddy V, Boparai N, Pedicone L, Patino H, Durrant S (2007) Posaconazole or fluconazole for prophylaxis in severe graft-versus-host disease. N Engl J Med 356:335–347

van der Linden JW, Jansen RR, Bresters D, Visser CE, Geerlings SE, Kuijper EJ, Melchers WJ, Verweij PE (2009) Azole-resistant central nervous system aspergillosis. Clin Infect Dis 48:1111–1113

Van Der Linden JW, Warris A, Verweij PE (2011a) *Aspergillus* species intrinsically resistant to antifungal agents. Med Mycol 49(Suppl 1):S82–S89

van der Linden JW, Snelders E, Kampinga GA, Rijnders BJ, Mattsson E, Debets-Ossenkopp YJ, Kuijper EJ, Van Tiel FH, Melchers WJ, Verweij PE (2011b) Clinical implications of azole resistance in *Aspergillus fumigatus*, The Netherlands, 2007–2009. Emerg Infect Dis 17:1846–1854

van der Linden JW, Arendrup MC, Warris A, Lagrou K, Pelloux H, Hauser PM, Chryssanthou E, Mellado E, Kidd SE, Tortorano AM, Dannaoui E, Gaustad P, Baddley JW, Uekötter A, Lass-Flörl C, Klimko N, Moore CB, Denning DW, Pasqualotto AC, Kibbler C, Arikan-Akdagli S, Andes D, Meletiadis J, Naumiuk L, Nucci M, Melchers WJ, Verweij PE (2015) Prospective multicenter international surveillance of azole resistance in Aspergillus fumigatus. Emerg Infect

Dis; 21(6):1041-4. doi: 10.3201/eid2106.140717. http://www.ncbi.nlm.nih.gov/pubmed/25988348

van der Linden JW, Camps SM, Kampinga GA, Arends JP, Debets-Ossenkopp YJ, Haas PJ, Rijnders BJ, Kuijper EJ, van Tiel FH, Varga J, Karawajczyk A, Zoll J, Melchers WJ, Verweij PE (2013) Aspergillosis due to voriconazole highly resistant *Aspergillus fumigatus* and recovery of genetically related resistant isolates from domiciles. Clin Infect Dis 57:513–520

van Leer-Buter C, Takes RP, Hebeda KM, Melchers WJ, Verweij PE (2007) Aspergillosis–and a misleading sensitivity result. Lancet 370:102

Varga J, Houbraken J, Van Der Lee HA, Verweij PE, Samson RA (2008) *Aspergillus calidoustus* sp. nov., causative agent of human infections previously assigned to *Aspergillus ustus*. Eukaryot Cell 7:630–638

Vermeulen E, Maertens J, Schoemans H, Lagrou K (2012) Azole-resistant *Aspergillus fumigatus* due to TR46/Y121F/T289A mutation emerging in Belgium, July 2012. Euro Surveill 17

Verweij PE, Te Dorsthorst DT, Rijs AJ, De Vries-Hospers HG, Meis JF (2002) Nationwide survey of in vitro activities of itraconazole and voriconazole against clinical *Aspergillus fumigatus* isolates cultured between 1945 and 1998. J Clin Microbiol 40:2648–2650

Verweij PE, Mellado E, Melchers WJ (2007) Multiple-triazole-resistant Aspergillosis. N Engl J Med 356:1481–1483

Verweij PE, Snelders E, Kema GH, Mellado E, Melchers WJ (2009a) Azole resistance in *Aspergillus fumigatus*: a side-effect of environmental fungicide use? Lancet Infect Dis 9:789–795

Verweij PE, Howard SJ, Melchers WJ, Denning DW (2009b) Azole-resistance in *Aspergillus*: proposed nomenclature and breakpoints. Drug Resist Updat 12(6):141–147

Walsh TJ, Anaissie EJ, Denning DW, Herbrecht R, Kontoyiannis DP, Marr KA, Morrison VA, Segal BH, Steinbach WJ, Stevens DA, van Burik JA, Wingard JR, Patterson TF, Infectious Diseases Society of A (2008) Treatment of Aspergillosis: clinical practice guidelines of the Infectious Diseases Society of America. Clin Infect Dis 46:327–360

Warris A, Weemaes CM, Verweij PE (2002) Multidrug resistance in *Aspergillus fumigatus*. N Engl J Med 347:2173–2174

Young RC, Bennett JE, Vogel CL, Carbone PP, DeVita VT (1970) Aspergillosis. The spectrum of the disease in 98 patients. Medicine 49:147–173

The Ins and Outs of Azole Antifungal Drug Resistance: Molecular Mechanisms of Transport

Martin Zavrel, Brooke D. Esquivel, and Theodore C. White

Contents

Abstract

Azoles are a major class of antifungal drugs commonly used to treat pathogenic fungi. Azole antifungals are relatively inexpensive, share similar chemical structures, and are effective against most fungal species. Azoles target a crucial enzyme in the ergosterol biosynthesis pathway whose inhibition leads to reduced

M. Zavrel
Institute of Organic Chemistry and Biochemistry, Prague 6, Czech Republic
e-mail: zavrel@uochb.cas.cz

B.D. Esquivel • T.C. White (✉)
Division of Cell Biology and Biophysics, School of Biological Sciences, University of Missouri-Kansas City, Kansas City, MO, USA
e-mail: bdp3k9@mail.umkc.edu; whitetc@umkc.edu

M. Gotte et al. (eds.), *Handbook of Antimicrobial Resistance*,
DOI 10.1007/978-1-4939-0694-9_29

fungal growth. Azole treatment, combined with the host's immune system, results in the elimination of the fungus from the host. Since azoles are fungistatic instead of fungicidal, their prolonged use and abuse often results in the development of resistance, which is a serious clinical problem in antifungal therapy. The main mechanisms by which fungi become resistant to azoles are increased efflux of the drug from the fungal cell, and modifications in the sterol biosynthesis pathway, especially in the azole target enzyme. In general, all known fungal pathogens share these two basic types of resistance mechanisms, although the specific efflux pumps or mutations in the sterol pathway may be unique for each fungus. This chapter summarizes the development of azole resistance in the major human fungal pathogen, *Candida albicans*, and compares these mechanisms to those in other fungal pathogens. Resistance to other non-azole antifungal drugs is also discussed.

Keywords
Azoles • Antifungal drug resistance • Drug efflux • Membrane transporters • Pathogenic fungi

Introduction

The frequency of patients with immune deficiency has grown dramatically in the last three decades due to the AIDS epidemic, increased organ and bone marrow transplants, as well as aggressive cancer chemotherapy. All of these conditions compromise the immune system of the host and have led to an increased emergence of opportunistic fungal pathogen infections as a result of these natural or artificially induced immune deficiencies. Not surprisingly, there has also been a dramatic increase in the use of antifungals to treat these infections. As a result of this increased antifungal use, strains resistant to each of the classes of antifungals are emerging. In medicine, the most widely used antifungals are polyenes, azoles, allylamines, echinocandins, and 5-flucytosine. The most common antifungals and their targets are summarized in Fig. 1.

Antifungal drug resistance is difficult to define. Its threshold is set up individually for each drug, organism, and site of infection, respectively. Antifungal drug resistance can be categorized as intrinsic or acquired. Intrinsic resistance is an inherited characteristic of a species or strain that causes antifungal drug therapy to fail. The fungal species and strain will clearly determine which drugs are effective. The main human fungal pathogens and the effectiveness of antifungals to each are presented in Table 1. Acquired resistance, on the other hand, occurs when a previously susceptible isolate develops a resistant phenotype, usually as a result of prolonged treatment with antifungals.

While resistance is a clinical problem, the "90–60" rule states that susceptible isolates respond to appropriate therapy approximately 90 % of the time, while resistant isolates respond to therapy about 60 % of the time, despite their drug resistance (Rex and Pfaller 2002). The 90–60 rule applies to most microbes, including fungal and bacterial pathogens.

There are several factors that affect treatment outcome of a fungal infection, including a variety of characteristics associated with the host, the drug, and the

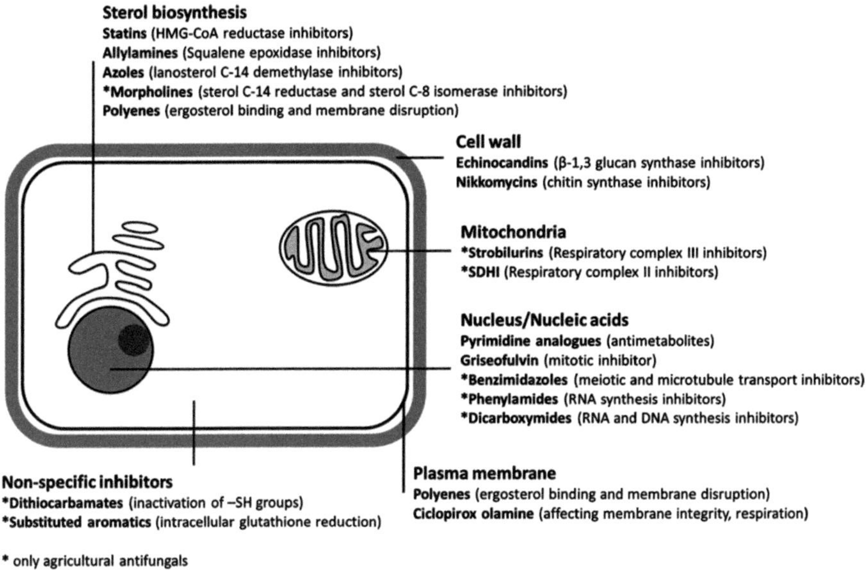

Fig. 1 Antifungal drugs and their site of action

fungus. Generally, antifungal drugs work alongside the host immune system to control the infection. Infections in immunocompromised patients are generally more recalcitrant to treatment because of the lost additive effect from the host immune system. The infection location (systemic, skin, oral mucosa, vaginal mucosa, eye, brain, etc.) is also an important factor in drug resistance, as some infection sites may be less accessible to drug therapy.

Finally, the cell type or morphological stage of the fungi can alter drug efficacy. Most antifungals are effective only against actively growing fungi, while dormant stages with minimal metabolic activity are usually not responsive to drug. Most fungi exist as various cell types or morphologies, including yeast stages (blastospores), pseudohyphae, hyphae, chlamydospores, and conidiospores, each of which can have a specific susceptibility to antifungal drugs. In some *Candida albicans* strains, yeast forms can further switch between additional phenotypes, including white and opaque. Besides phenotypic switching, some fungi also exist in different serotypes. These phenotypic switches or different serotypes are usually distinguished by different cell surface markers and display alterations in their transcriptional profiles, often effecting genes involved in antifungal resistance.

In general, the organism's susceptibility to an antifungal is expressed as a minimal inhibitory concentration (MIC). The MIC can be presented as MIC_{50} or MIC_{80}, which is drug concentration leading to 50 % or 80 % reduction in fungal growth, respectively. Protocols for drug susceptibility testing in different organisms have been standardized by the Clinical and Laboratory Standards Institute (CLSI) and by the European Committee on Antimicrobial Susceptibility Testing (EUCAST). Both organizations define the specific growth media and conditions for testing of each organism.

Table 1 Antifungal spectrum of activity against common fungi

Organism	Antifungal agent								
	AmB[a,b]	Flu[c]	Itr[c]	Vor[c]	Pos[c]	Anid[d]	Casp[d]	Mica[d]	5-FC
***Aspergillus* species**	+	–	+	+	+	+	+	+	–
A. flavus	±	–	+	+	+	+	+	+	–
A. fumigatus	+	–	+	+	+	+	+	+	–
A. niger	+	–	±	+	+	+	+	+	–
A. terreus	–	–	+	+	+	+	+	+	–
***Candida* species**	+	+	+	+	+	+	+	+	+
C. albicans	+	+	+	+	+	+	+	+	+
C. glabrata	+	±	±	+	+	+	+	+	+
C. krusei	+	–	±	+	+	+	+	+	±
C. lusitaniae	–	+	+	+	+	+	+	+	+
C. parapsilosis	+	+	+	+	+	±	±	±	+
C. tropicalis	+	+	+	+	+	+	+	+	+
Cryptococcus neoformans	+	+	+	+	+	–	–	–	+
***Coccidioides* species**	+	+	+	+	+	±[e]	±[e]	±[e]	–
Blastomyces	+	+	+	+	+	±[e]	±[e]	±[e]	–
***Histoplasma* species**	+	+	+	+	+	±[e]	±[e]	±[e]	–
***Fusarium* species**	±	–	–	+	+	–	–	–	–
Scedosporium apiospermum	±	–	±	+	+	–	–	–	–
Scedosporium prolificans	–	–	–	±	±	–	–	–	–
Zygomycetes	±	–	–	–	+	–	–	–	–

AmB amphotericin B, Flu fluconazole, Itr itraconazole, Vor voriconazole, Pos posaconazole, Anid anidulafungin, Casp caspofungin, Mica micafungin, 5-FC 5-fluorocytosine
[a]Polyenes
[b]Includes lipid formulations
[c]Azoles
[d]Echinocandins
[e]*In vitro* data show that the echinocandins (specifically micafungin) may have variable activity against the dimorphic fungi, depending on whether they are in the mycelial or yeastlike form. Reproduced from "Dodds Ashley et al., Pharmacology of systemic antifungal agents, 2006, Clin. Infect. Dis. 43, pp. S28–S39" with permission from Oxford University Press (Dodds Ashley et al. 2006)

Azole Antifungal Drugs

Ergosterol is a fungal-specific sterol that is homologous to cholesterol and similar sterols found in the membranes of other eukaryotic cells. Ergosterol is an essential component of fungal plasma membranes and its metabolism is tightly regulated by fungal cells. Alterations in ergosterol levels significantly affect the susceptibility of fungal cells to a variety of environmental stresses. Although similar to plant and animal sterol biosynthesis pathways, ergosterol biosynthesis is unique to fungi, and so its metabolism is a prime target of antifungal therapy with minimal negative effects on the animal or plant host. Currently, there are four classes of drugs that target enzymes in the sterol biosynthesis pathway (Fig. 1), including statins (HMG-CoA reductase inhibitors; used in mammalian cells), allylamines (squalene epoxidase inhibitors), azoles (lanosterol 14α-demethylase inhibitors), and morpholines (sterol C-14 reductase and sterol C-8 isomerase inhibitors; only used agriculturally). One additional class of drugs, polyenes, directly targets ergosterol in fungal membranes and negatively affects the native membrane structure.

Azole antifungals, such as fluconazole, are one of the most commonly used drugs to treat fungal infections. Azoles are fungistatic drugs, which do not kill the cells, and are thus more likely to allow cells to develop resistance. Azole antifungals are a class of organic compounds consisting of a five-membered nitrogen-containing heterocyclic ring (imidazole or triazole), and a halogenated benzene ring. These two prerequisites are crucial for their antifungal activity, as well as their successful import into the fungal cells (Mansfield et al. 2010; Esquivel et al. 2015). Apart from having a nitrogen-containing ring and a halogenated benzene ring, each azole antifungal has a distinctive chemical structure that dictates its pharmacological properties.

Once in the fungal cell, azoles target and inhibit the endoplasmic reticulum (ER)-located cytochrome P450-dependent enzyme, lanosterol 14α-demethylase (*ERG11* in *C. albicans*; see Table 2). At the moment there are numerous azoles on the market, both for medical and agricultural use. The medical azoles are highly specific to the fungal enzyme and generally not effective at inhibiting the human homolog. This is important because these drugs are capable of entering both the host mammalian cells as well as the fungal pathogen cells (Campoli et al. 2013). In contrast, agricultural azoles have less selectivity for the fungal lanosterol 14α-demethylase over its human homolog, which has led to concerns over agricultural azole side effects on humans and animals (Verweij et al. 2009; Warrilow et al. 2013).

Azole Resistance

Many fungal species display intrinsic resistance to azoles, making azole treatment ineffective against such fungi. Their mechanisms of resistance are probably the same as those acquired in other fungal species (see below), but in this case they are naturally occurring. These fungi include *Candida krusei*, most strains of *Candida glabrata*, *Fusarium* species, and the Zygomycetes. Both *C. krusei* and *C. glabrata* are increasing in frequency in oral and systemic candidiasis in patient populations that use azole drugs for treatment or prophylaxis. There are also clear differences in azole susceptibility among strains within one species, due to randomly occurring genetic differences.

Table 2 Genes encoding proteins involved in azole resistance

Organism	*Ca*	*Cg*	*Sc*	*Af*	*Cn*
Lanosterol 14α-demethylase	*ERG11*	*ERG11*	*ERG11*	*cyp51A*	*ERG11*
				cyp51B	
Sterol metabolism regulators	*UPC2*	*UPC2A*	*UPC2*	*srbA*	*SRE1*
		UPC2B	*ECM22*		
MFS transporters	*MDR1*	*FLR1*	*QDR2*	*mdr3* (?)	
	FLU1	*QDR2*	*FLR1* (?)		
Regulators of MFS transporters	*MRR1*	*YAP1*	*GCN4*		
		PDR1	*YAP1* (?)		
ABC transporters	*CDR1*	*CDR1*	*PDR5*	*abcC*	*AFR1*
	CDR2	*PDH1*		*mdr1*	
		SNQ2		*atrF* (?)	
				mdr4 (?)	
Regulators of ABC transporters	*TAC1*	*PDR1*	*PDR1*		
			PDR3		

Ca Candida albicans, Cg Candida glabrata, Sc Saccharomyces cerevisiae, Af Aspergillus fumigatus, Cn Cryptococcus neoformans

Acquired azole resistance was rare in the 1980s, when azoles were primarily used to treat patients with chronic mucocutaneous candidiasis. However, with AIDS epidemic in the 1990s, azole resistance in *C. albicans* became a significant problem as oral candidiasis occurred in over 90 % of all HIV-positive individuals. In recent years, highly active antiretroviral therapy, which restores the patient's immune response, is reducing the frequency of most opportunistic fungal infections and also the need for azole prophylaxis. In addition to *Candida* species, acquired azole resistance has been detected in isolates of *Cryptococcus neoformans* from AIDS patients on prophylactic azole therapy to prevent the recurrence of cryptococcal meningitis and in isolates of *Aspergillus fumigatus* from patients who have received regular treatment with itraconazole or voriconazole. Azoles are also used in surgical wards to prevent systemic candidiasis and as nonprescription drugs to treat fungal skin infections, including athlete's foot. The use of azoles in the environment to treat and prevent fungal pathogens of plant crops is a concern. It has been correlated with an increasing number of agricultural azole-resistant *A. fumigatus* isolates occurring in azole-naïve human patients, and unfortunately these isolates are also resistant to medical azoles such as itraconazole, posaconazole, and voriconazole.

In fungal pathogens naturally susceptible to azoles, there are several mechanisms of azole resistance that can develop as a result of azole treatment (Fig. 2). These mechanisms include (1) reduced azole import; (2) increased azole efflux; (3) import of sterols from host, replacing endogenous ergosterol biosynthesis; (4) increased expression of lanosterol 14α-demethylase, the azole target enzyme; (5) mutation of lanosterol 14α-demethylase, altering its azole affinity; (6) alteration of the ergosterol biosynthetic pathway; and (7) additional nonspecific metabolic adjustments. There are additional possible drug resistance mechanisms that have not yet been observed,

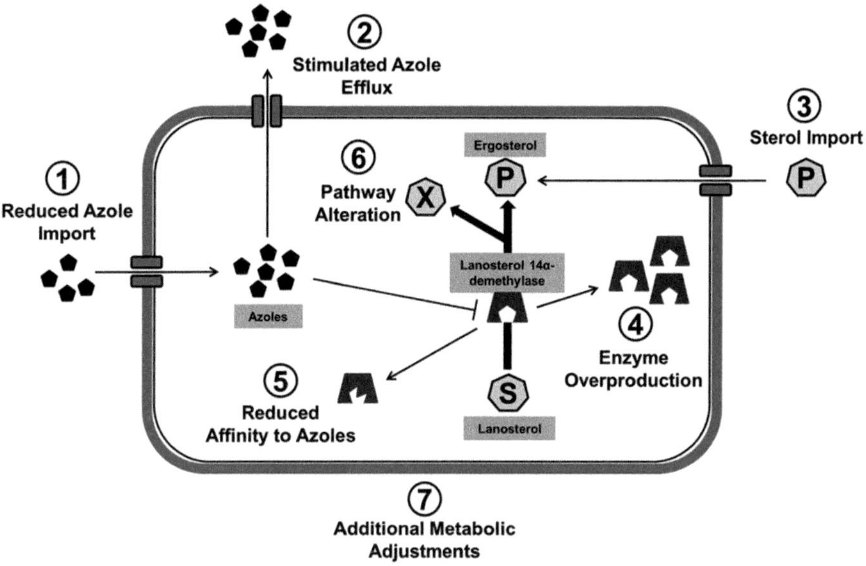

Fig. 2 Potential and actual azole resistance mechanisms in fungi. Actual mechanisms include *2*, *3*, *4*, *5*, *6*, and *7*. A potential mechanism is represented by 1

including intracellular drug sequestration into vesicles/vacuole or azole degradation. Table 2 lists the gene homologs involved in these mechanisms of azole resistance in the most prevalent fungal pathogens and in the model organism *Saccharomyces cerevisiae*.

Resistance in *C. albicans* clinical isolates is not usually the result of a single alteration. The resistance is gradually developed through a series of independent steps. Each acquired mutation decreases azole susceptibility and increases the fitness of the cell under the drug-selective pressure. As a result, this newly acquired allele allows the corresponding clone to outgrow the rest of the population, becoming the new major strain. A series of such steps result in the development of a highly azole-resistant phenotype, where each alteration only partially contributes to the resulting phenotype. This has been well documented in a series of sequential isolates from a single patient during azole treatment (White et al. 1998). All the acquired resistance mechanisms are described in detail in the latter parts of this chapter, but they include mutation and overexpression of the azole target enzyme and efflux of the drug from the fungal cells with two types of efflux pumps. The timing and the order in which each of these changes occurred are unlikely to be critical to the development of resistance, but the sum of each of these alterations results in the resistant phenotype.

Molecular analyses of antifungal drug resistance have focused mainly on *C. albicans*, which is at the moment the best understood, but have included studies in *C. glabrata*, *C. neoformans*, and *A. fumigatus*. This chapter will concentrate mainly on the mechanisms identified in *C. albicans*, with the discussion of mechanisms identified in other fungi when applicable.

Azole Import

Azole accumulation within a fungal cell is the result of a balance among drug import, retention, and efflux. Azole drug accumulation has been studied primarily in *C. albicans* but has also been described for *S. cerevisiae*, *C. glabrata*, *C. krusei*, *C. neoformans*, and *A. fumigatus* ((Mansfield et al. 2010; Denning et al. 1997; Manavathu et al. 1999; Tsai et al. 2004) and our unpublished results Esquivel et al. 2015). In general, all fungal species susceptible to azoles are expected to import these drugs.

Based on the information obtained from studies on *C. albicans*, azole import into fungi is independent of ATP or pH. It follows a concentration gradient, is saturable, and proceeds via facilitated diffusion through a yet unknown transporter. All analyzed azoles seem to utilize the same import mechanism. The drug import depends strictly on the chemical structure of azoles, requiring both a halogenated benzene ring and an imidazole or triazole ring in one molecule. Omitting either one results in the failure of the molecule to be imported ((Mansfield et al. 2010) and our unpublished results). Additional structures, as well as molecule size, seem rather insignificant. In *C. albicans*, conditions that favor the maximum rate of import include an optimal temperature of 30 °C, cells harvested from exponential phase of growth, and cells grown anaerobically. Hyphae also display a higher import rate than yeast cells.

So far, no natural environmental compounds have been identified that utilize the same import mechanism and thus compete with azoles for import. Thus, the origin and evolutional importance of the import mechanism are unclear. Due to the failure of genetic screens to identify the transporter, it is likely to be either essential for cell viability or part of a multimember family of transporters with overlapping function. Import is specific for fungi, since bacteria (*Escherichia coli*) are incapable of fluconazole import (Mansfield et al. 2010). Import into mammalian cells has been reported as well, with azoles accumulating in their cellular membranes (Campoli et al. 2013).

Drug import into the fungal cell by facilitated diffusion is a mechanism that might be manipulated by the fungal cell to confer drug resistance and may play a role in azole-resistant isolates. However, direct evidence for this is lacking. Clinical isolates of *C. albicans* and other species show high variability in the rate of azole import, as well as different end points for saturation with azoles. Although reduced azole import can be involved in azole resistance, the reduced import levels cannot always be correlated with the individual strain's azole susceptibilities ((Mansfield et al. 2010) and our unpublished results).

Experiments in *A. fumigatus* using itraconazole also showed that drug import is saturable and time and concentration dependent (Manavathu et al. 1999). The correlation between increased itraconazole resistance and its decreased intracellular accumulation has been reported (Denning et al. 1997; Manavathu et al. 1999); however, this was most likely due to increased azole efflux, since the cells were not depleted of an energy source.

Finally, in *C. glabrata*, reduced activity of squalene epoxidase (Erg1; another enzyme in the ergosterol biosynthesis pathway) results in the disruption of ergosterol biosynthesis and stimulates azole import. Even import of exogenous ergosterol in this strain does not revert the phenotype (Tsai et al. 2004). Thus, this phenomenon cannot be attributed to lower ergosterol content in membranes. Upc2 is the transcription factor that regulates sterol metabolism in yeasts, and the *UPC2* null mutants in *C. albicans*, *C. glabrata*, and *S. cerevisiae* all have decreased ergosterol content, but do not display significant changes in azole import from their respective parents (our unpublished work).

As mentioned, the concentration of azoles within the cells is saturable. This saturation level can be partially correlated with the level of the azole binding target, Erg11 (our unpublished work). Also, the levels of *A. fumigatus* lanosterol 14-α-demethylase (*cyp51A and cyp51B*, two homologs of *C. albicans ERG11* (Mellado et al. 2001)) and resulting ergosterol levels both seem to partially correlate with intracellular itraconazole concentration (Denning et al. 1997). Since mutations in *cyp51A* seem to be the major resistance mechanism in *A. fumigatus* (discussed later), the reduced affinity of this enzyme to azoles may partially result in the observed lower azole levels in the azole-resistant cells (Denning et al. 1997; Manavathu et al. 1999). Also in the case of *C. glabrata*, the reduced Erg1 activity might result in the upregulation of ergosterol biosynthesis pathway, including *ERG11*, thus resulting in higher azole retention (Tsai et al. 2004).

ERG11 Mutation

In *C. albicans*, once the azoles have been imported, they target the ER-located enzyme Erg11, which is an essential enzyme for ergosterol biosynthesis. Erg11 is a P450-dependent enzyme containing a heme moiety in its active site. The azoles bind to the heme iron through an unhindered nitrogen, thus inhibiting the Erg11-catalyzed enzymatic reaction. The second nitrogen of the azoles interacts directly with the apoprotein. The position of the second nitrogen is thought to modulate the affinity of different azoles (Hitchcock 1991). The inhibited Erg11 fails to remove methyl groups at the 14α-carbon of ergosterol precursors, resulting in an accumulation of 14α-methyl sterols, which are further processed into toxic intermediates by sterol C5-desaturase (Erg3) (Odds et al. 2003). These intermediates affect the fluidity and function of the fungal plasma membrane, resulting in higher susceptibility to environmental stress, including host immune system defense mechanisms.

One way of developing azole resistance is mutation of *ERG11* that decreases its affinity for azoles. Depending on the location of the mutation and the amino acid change, the reduced susceptibility can be specific for all azoles or only a subset of them. Gene conversion/mitotic recombination in diploid *C. albicans* can also occur, increasing the azole resistance even further (see below). Permanent *ERG11* upregulation is the second way of gaining azole resistance through *ERG11*. This could be mediated through mutations in transcription factors such as *UPC2*, through mutations in *ERG11* promoter, or through *ERG11* gene amplification.

The Erg11 amino acid structure is crucial for azole susceptibility or resistance in different fungal species. *ERG11* in intrinsically azole-resistant fungi have lower affinity to azoles, as shown, for example, in *C. krusei* (Venkateswarlu et al. 1997). In azole-susceptible fungi, mutation of *ERG11* can result in a high level of resistance. A list of different Erg11 amino acid exchanges in *C. albicans* has been provided by numerous studies; some of them have summarized these changes (Morschhauser 2002; Marichal et al. 1999). Unique amino acid substitutions in *ERG11* resulting in an azole-resistant phenotype have been reported from all over the world. In general, the amino acid (AA) substitutions can be found all over the enzyme, but they are enriched in three regions, called hotspots. These regions include AA 105–165, which is exposed to the substrate access channel, AA 266–287, which forms the substrate entry site, and AA 405–488, which forms the active site and docks the cytochrome (Marichal et al. 1999).

In *A. fumigatus*, mutations have rarely been detected in *cyp51B* and have rarely been shown to be related to azole resistance (Snelders et al. 2011). On the other hand, mutations identified in *cyp51A* correspond with azole resistance (Diaz-Guerra et al. 2003; Howard et al. 2006; Mellado et al. 2004). The most common mutations are reported in AA positions G54, L98, and M220 (Howard and Arendrup 2011). *cyp51A* resistance mutations also include tandem repeats in the promoter, increasing *cyp51* expression. This is often combined with mutations in the *cyp51A* coding region itself (most common is a mutation termed "TR/L98H" with 36-base tandem repeat in the promoter and an L98H substitution in Cyp51A) (Verweij et al. 2009; Warrilow et al. 2013; Camps et al. 2012a; Snelders et al. 2008, 2012; Mellado et al. 2007). Mutations in *cyp51A* are often correlated with the use of agricultural azoles. Tebuconazole, a common agricultural azole, has been shown to induce a tandem repeat mutation in the *cyp51A* promoter (Snelders et al. 2012).

ERG11 mutation has also been shown to cause azole resistance in *C. neoformans* (Rodero et al. 2003), although further analyses are warranted.

ERG11 Overexpression

Another way of gaining resistance through *ERG11* is by its overexpression, which results in an increased production of the encoded enzyme. Increased amounts of enzyme require increased amounts of drug for the same level of inhibition. Normally, as a response to azole treatment (or other ergosterol biosynthesis inhibitors), *ERG11* expression is increased above normal in many *Candida* species (Henry et al. 2000). This upregulation often includes other *ERG* genes in the pathway. In certain cases, the upregulation of the *ERG11* or the whole pathway can be permanent, leading to the resistant phenotype. The permanent upregulation in *C. albicans* can happen basically by two mechanisms: (1) duplication of chromosome 5, increasing the copy number of the *ERG11* gene located on it (see below), and (2) a gain-of-function (GOF) mutation in Upc2 (Table 2).

GOF mutations in Upc2 lead to the overexpression of many ergosterol biosynthesis genes, including the already mentioned *ERG11* (MacPherson et al. 2005; Silver et al. 2004). Upc2 is a Zn_2–Cys_6 transcriptional factor and central regulator of the ergosterol biosynthesis pathway in *C. albicans*. In the model organism, *S. cerevisiae*, constitutively active mutants of the two paralogs Upc2 (G888D) and Ecm22 (G790D) only induce sterol uptake under aerobic conditions (Crowley et al. 1998; Davies et al. 2005; Lewis et al. 1988; Shianna et al. 2001). However, in *C. albicans*, Upc2 constitutively active mutants in the C-terminus (Y642F, A643V/T, A646W, and G648D/S) or additional areas (G304R and W478C) increase resistance to the azoles by direct *ERG11* upregulation (Dunkel et al. 2008a; Flowers et al. 2012; Heilmann et al. 2010; Hoot et al. 2011). Upc2 forms dimers (our unpublished data) and these GOF mutations can express their full potential in diploid *C. albicans* only when found in the homozygous state (Heilmann et al. 2010; Coste et al. 2004, 2007; Dunkel et al. 2008b; Schubert et al. 2011). Homozygous GOF Upc2 (G648D) stimulates *ERG11* promoter expression approximately fourfold resulting in a fourfold increase in MIC (Schubert et al. 2011; Sasse et al. 2011).

Distantly related fungi (e.g., *Aspergillus* and *Cryptococcus*) are missing Upc2 homologs but have genes that regulate ergosterol biosynthesis that are functional homologs of the *s*terol *r*egulatory *e*lement-*b*inding *p*rotein (SREBP) of higher eukaryotes. The genes are *srbA* in *Aspergillus* and *SRE1* in *Cryptococcus*. These proteins belong to helix-loop-helix transcriptional factors, are structurally unrelated to Upc2, and also have a different mechanism of activation. No GOF mutations have been identified in these proteins to date. However, the *A. fumigatus srbA* deletion results in azole hypersusceptibility similar to *upc2* mutants in *Candida* (Willger et al. 2008). Recently, increased expression of *Aspergillus cyp51A* has been linked to a P88L mutation in the unrelated transcription factor HapE (Camps et al. 2012b), which may interact with SrbA. Finally, *ERG11* overexpression has been shown to affect azole susceptibility in *C. glabrata* (Marichal et al. 1997) and *C. neoformans* (Lamb et al. 1995), but the mechanisms for this overexpression have not yet been identified.

Alterations in Ergosterol Biosynthesis

Besides Erg11, alterations in other enzymes involved in ergosterol biosynthesis can affect azole susceptibility. One of these is the inactivation of the enzyme sterol C5-desaturase, encoded by *ERG3*, which introduces a double bond in sterol substrate molecules between carbons C5 and C6. Normally, after Erg11 inhibition, Erg3 converts nontoxic 14α-methylated sterol intermediates (mostly 14-α-methylfecosterol) into the toxic 14α-methylergosta-8,24(28)-dien-3β,6α-diol. Thus, *ERG3* inactivation in *C. albicans* undergoing azole treatment allows the cells to bypass the synthesis of toxic sterols and leads to azole resistance (Watson et al. 1989; Kelly et al. 1995, 1997). However, this type of resistance is rather uncommon in clinical isolates, probably due to the fact that the inactive *ERG3* allele has to be homozygous to manifest the reduced azole susceptibility (Miyazaki et al. 2006) and the inactive *ERG3* alleles in *C. albicans* lead to the loss of filamentation and attenuated virulence (Chau et al. 2005). Interestingly, azole treatment is still effective against *ERG3* mutants in vivo (Miyazaki et al. 2006). Surprisingly, the *ERG3* mutation does not result in azole resistance in *C. glabrata* (Geber et al. 1995), although in its closely related *S. cerevisiae* it does (Watson et al. 1989). Studies in *A. fumigatus* (deletion of *erg3A* and *erg3B*) also demonstrated that neither of the two genes is implicated in azole resistance (Alcazar-Fuoli et al. 2006).

In *S. cerevisiae*, the loss of function of *ERG6* (sterol C24-methyltransferase) or *ERG28* (a scaffold protein mediating the interaction between Erg26, Erg27, and possibly Erg6) has been shown to decrease azole susceptibility (Anderson et al. 2003). However, the *ERG6* mutation has no such effect in either *C. albicans* (Jensen-Pergakes et al. 1998) or *C. glabrata* (Vandeputte et al. 2008). The *ERG28* deletion in these species has not been reported to date.

As illustrated above, the *ERG* gene deletion phenotypes work very differently in different fungal species. This suggests high plasticity of the ergosterol biosynthesis pathway and its regulation among different fungi. Thus, it is highly probable that mutations in other ergosterol biosynthesis enzymes will be isolated from azole-resistant fungal pathogens in the future.

Azole Efflux

In *C. albicans*, there are several transporters involved in azole efflux – the major ones are Cdr1, Cdr2, and Mdr1 and minor ones are Pdr16 and Flu1. The upregulation of *CDR1* and *CDR2* (*Candida* *d*rug *r*esistance) is the most frequent azole resistance mechanism in *C. albicans* (Perea et al. 2001). Pdr16 (*p*leiotropic *d*rug *r*esistance), which is induced together with Cdr1 and Cdr2, is also involved in azole resistance, although indirectly – it acts as phosphatidylinositol transfer protein (Saidane et al. 2006). While Pdr16, Cdr1, and Cdr2 belong to the class of ABC (ATP-binding cassette) transporters using ATP for transport, Mdr1 (*m*ulti*d*rug *r*esistance) and Flu1 (*flu*conazole resistance) are representatives of the major facilitator superfamily (MFS), which use a membrane proton (H^+) gradient for drug/H^+ antiport. Interestingly, *C. albicans* Mdr1 is specific only for fluconazole and not for other azoles (Sanglard et al. 1995). Although Flu1 has been shown to be involved in fluconazole resistance (Calabrese et al. 2000), it is not considered a major azole transporter. And although there are other ABC and MSF transporters in *C. albicans* genome, none of them have been shown to date to participate in azole resistance.

All the above mentioned transporters are naturally expressed in response to toxic substances in the environment and are associated with efflux of small hydrophobic or lipophilic molecules. In general, the efflux pump genes *CDR1*, *CDR2*, *PDR16*, *MDR1*, and *FLU1* are not induced in response to azole drugs, but they do respond to steroids, fluphenazine, benomyl, and stress inducers including oxidizing agents.

Mrr1 and Tac1 are two transcriptional activators in *C. albicans* whose GOF mutations affect azole resistance through the upregulation of the abovementioned efflux pumps. Mrr1 and Tac1 both belong to Zn_2–Cys_6 type of zinc cluster transcription factors, similar to Upc2. In clinically resistant *C. albicans* isolates, the mutations in Mrr1 and Tac1 are often combined with each other and with the already mentioned GOF Upc2 version. The azole resistance in these strains is significantly higher than it is in strains containing a single GOF mutation in one of these three transcriptional factors (Sasse et al. 2012). Additional transcription factors that are known to regulate the expression of *CDR1* and *CDR2* include Ndt80, Fcr1, and Fcr3, but to date, none of these has been shown to be able to induce azole resistance *in vivo*. The *C. albicans MDR1* gene is also transcriptionally regulated by the transcription factors Cap1 and Mcm1, but these factors have not been linked to azole resistance in clinical isolates either. Only Cap1 has been shown to be able to increase azole resistance *in vitro*, when its cysteine-rich C-terminus is truncated (Alarco and Raymond 1999).

GOF mutations (P683S, P683H) in Mrr1 promote the overexpression of *MDR1* (Dunkel et al. 2008b; Morschhauser et al. 2007; Schubert et al. 2008). Similar mutations were also identified in the *C. dubliniensis* Mrr1 homolog, proving that GOF mutations affect the activity of Mrr1 similarly in both closely related species (Schubert et al. 2008). Upc2 (mentioned above) is also capable of binding to the *MDR1* promoter and stimulating its expression, although the effect of GOF Upc2 is minimal, with roughly twofold *MDR1* induction (Schubert et al. 2011). GOF Upc2 might be further involved in increased azole efflux by inducing a not yet characterized efflux pump *CDR11* (Flowers et al. 2012).

Tac1 is perhaps the most important transcription factor involved in azole resistance of clinical isolates. It is the transcriptional activator of *CDR1*, *CDR2*, and *PDR16*, which binds to the *d*rug *r*esponse *e*lement (DRE) sequence in the promoters of these genes (Coste et al. 2004; de Micheli et al. 2002). Interestingly, the *TAC1* gene is located on the left arm of chromosome 5, 15 kb from mating-type locus (MTL) in the area where *ERG11* is also located. Constitutively active alleles of *TAC1* contain GOF mutations resulting in amino acid substitutions T225A, V736A, N972D, N977D, G980E, and G980W or deletions ΔM677 and Δ962-969. T225A appears to be located in the transcriptional inhibitory domain and the other mutations in the transcriptional activation domain. Each mutation causes increased expression of many responsive genes including the already mentioned *CDR1*, *CDR2*, and *PDR16* (Coste et al. 2006, 2007, 2009; Znaidi et al. 2007). As in the case of *MDR1*, Upc2 also seems to slightly induce *CDR1* expression (Znaidi et al. 2008). In addition to transcriptional regulation, recent studies have demonstrated increased mRNA stability and increased transcriptional initiation for the *CDR1* gene in resistant isolates, possibly the result of altered sequences in the 3′ untranslated region of the mRNA (Manoharlal et al. 2008).

The ABC transporters Cdr1 and Cdr2, whose expression is controlled by Tac1, are more efficient fluconazole efflux pumps than the major facilitator Mdr1 (Lamping et al. 2007). However, strains with the hyperactive Mrr1 are slightly more resistant to fluconazole than strains with the hyperactive Tac1, pointing out the significant contribution of additional Mrr1 target genes to fluconazole resistance (Schubert et al. 2011; Sasse et al. 2012). The combination of both transcription factors has only a minor additive effect (Sasse et al. 2012). Like GOF Upc2, both GOF Mrr1 and GOF Tac1 increase their effect with homozygosity, selecting for the loss of heterozygosity under azole-selective pressure (Dunkel et al. 2008b; Sasse et al. 2011; Morschhauser et al. 2007). In the presence of homozygous GOF Mrr1 (P683S), the *MDR1* promoter displays approximately 50-fold induction. Homozygous GOF Tac1 (G980E) stimulates the *CDR1* promoter approximately 8-fold and *CDR2* promoter 10-fold. The increase in MICs for homozygous GOF alleles is 8-fold for *TAC1* and 16-fold for *MRR1* (Schubert et al. 2011; Sasse et al. 2011).

Although intrinsically highly azole resistant, an increase in azole resistance in *C. glabrata*, based on the ABC drug efflux pumps Cdr1, Pdh1, and Snq2, has been described (Torelli et al. 2008; Tsai et al. 2006; Sanglard et al. 2001). Members of the MFS transporter family Flr1 (Chen et al. 2007) and Qdr2 (Costa et al. 2013) are also involved in azole efflux in *C. glabrata*. GOF mutations in the transcription factor Pdr1 induce the overexpression of the ABC efflux pumps Cdr1, Snq2, and Pdh1 (Torelli et al. 2008; Tsai et al. 2006; Ferrari et al. 2009) and may also overexpress the MFS transporter Qdr2, since the *QDR2* gene has been shown to be induced through Pdr1 in the presence of azoles (Costa et al. 2013). GOF mutations in the transcription factor Pdr1 in *C. glabrata* are another proof of induced azole export through mutation of an efflux pump transcription factor. Interestingly, also mitochondrial loss in *C. glabrata* is connected to increased azole resistance through the upregulation of *CDR1*, *PDH1*, and possibly other genes (Sanglard et al. 2001). The loss of mitochondria has been reported even in clinical isolates (Bouchara et al. 2000), despite their reduced virulence (Brun et al. 2005). An effect of mitochondrial loss on increased azole resistance has not been reported for any other organism yet.

Compared to the other studied species, the fungal pathogen *A. fumigatus* contains unusually high number of genes encoding ABC (close to 50) and MFS (close to 300) transporters, which are mostly uncharacterized to date (Nierman et al. 2005). Although several ABC and MFS transporters have been proposed to be involved in azole resistance (Slaven et al. 2002), only *abcC*/*cdr1B* and *mdr1* have been shown to play a direct role in azole efflux (Fraczek et al. 2013). In contrast to *C. albicans*, and similar to *C. glabrata*, some ABC and MFS transporters are induced in the presence of azoles (Fraczek et al. 2013; da Silva Ferreira et al. 2006). Many transporters are also induced in biofilms (Rajendran et al. 2011), possibly playing similar role in azole resistance similar to azole transporters in *C. albicans* (see below).

Although less studied, *C. neoformans* also connects azole efflux to the acquired azole resistance (Joseph-Horne et al. 1995). To date, only the ABC transporter Afr1 has been shown to be capable of fluconazole efflux (Posteraro et al. 2003), although mutants in this transporter regulation have never been reported in clinical isolates. However, *AFR1* duplication, caused by chromosome 1 disomy, leads to an increase in azole resistance (Sionov et al. 2010).

Finally, in the intrinsically highly azole-resistant *C. krusei*, azole export can also be involved in increased resistance. This organism contains the main azole transporter Abc1 that is induced in the presence of azoles (Lamping et al. 2009).

Sterol Import

Sterol import is a potential azole resistance mechanism described relatively recently. To date, this phenomenon is related only to two fungal species – the model organism *S. cerevisiae* (Andreasen and Stier 1953) and the closely related pathogen *C. glabrata* (Zavrel et al. 2013; Bard et al. 2005; Nakayama et al. 2007; Nagi et al. 2013). Although *C. albicans* is also capable of sterol import, the rate is insufficient to replace the endogenous ergosterol biosynthesis (Zavrel et al. 2013). *S. cerevisiae* and *C. glabrata* are the only two described species able to import extracellular sterols in quantities sufficient to replace endogenous ergosterol biosynthesis in the presence of azoles. The difference from other fungi is the presence of *AUS1/PDR11* ABC type of sterol importers (Nakayama et al. 2007; Wilcox et al. 2002), which have not been identified in any other fungal species. In *S. cerevisiae*, sterols are imported exclusively anaerobically (Andreasen and Stier 1953) or in strains that mimic anaerobic conditions because of heme biosynthesis defects (*HEM1* mutations) or containing GOF Upc2/Ecm22 allele (Crowley et al. 1998; Lewis et al. 1985). Like *S. cerevisiae*, *C. glabrata* also imports sterols anaerobically and in mutants with defective *HEM1* (Bard et al. 2005). Additionally, sterol import is observed in mutants in early steps of ergosterol biosynthesis (*ERG1*, squalene epoxidase, or *ERG7*, lanosterol synthase) (Bard et al. 2005). *C. glabrata* also imports small amounts of sterols aerobically, and this can be greatly stimulated in the presence of blood serum together with a block in ergosterol biosynthesis caused by azoles (Zavrel et al. 2013; Nagi et al. 2013). Thus, an azole-induced block in ergosterol biosynthesis can be compensated *in vivo* by sterol import from its host. Similarly, a defect in the ergosterol biosynthesis pathway can also trigger sterol import in host.

Finally, sterol import has also been reported for *A. fumigatus* (Xiong et al. 2005). The presence of cholesterol or blood serum in the growth medium, and the subsequent cholesterol uptake, reduces the susceptibility to itraconazole and voriconazole. However, compared to *C. glabrata*, the rescue is only partial, suggesting that the rate of sterol import is insufficient for complete replacement of endogenous ergosterol biosynthesis. The sterol transporter in *A. fumigatus* has not been identified yet, but there is no direct homolog of the *AUS1/PDR11* type of sterol transporter in its genome.

Gene Conversions and Aneuploidy

The azole resistance mechanisms described above can be facilitated by chromosomal recombination and/or duplication of resistant alleles, which can involve either whole chromosome or segmental aneuploidy. Because *C. albicans* is diploid, the GOF alleles of transcription factors *TAC1*, *MRR1*, and *UPC2*, as well as an azole-resistant allele of *ERG11*, can be present either in a heterozygous or homozygous state. All of the mentioned transcription factors are likely to form dimers, a common characteristic of zinc cluster proteins. The loss of heterozygosity (LOH), through allele gene conversion, resulting in the presence of GOF transcription factor alleles or mutated

ERG11 alleles in two identical copies, contributes to azole resistance (Heilmann et al. 2010; Coste et al. 2004, 2006, 2007; Dunkel et al. 2008b; Schubert et al. 2011; Selmecki et al. 2006).

Azole resistance can be increased also through isochromosome 5 L [i(5 L)] formation. This results in an artificial chromosome containing two left arms of chromosome 5, where both *TAC1* and *ERG11* genes are located (Coste et al. 2007). Such aneuploidy is not well tolerated; it is unstable; and it can be easily lost in the absence of drugs, resulting in partial loss of the drug resistance. The mechanism by which these isochromosomes are created is not known in detail, but it has been suggested that they are created by recombination at an inverted repeat in the centrosome region of the chromosome (Coste et al. 2007; Selmecki et al. 2006). There is indirect evidence that chromosome 5 duplication and subsequent loss may occur relatively often during stepwise acquisition of azole resistance. Besides *ERG11* and *TAC1*, the MTL mating locus is also localized at chromosome 5. Compared to azole-susceptible strains, there is an increase in MTL locus homozygosity among azole-resistant isolates (Rustad et al. 2002). This might be indicative of frequent duplication of "azole-resistant" chromosome 5, leading to trisomy, and subsequent loss of the "susceptible" third chromosome, reverting the chromosome 5 back to disomy.

An additional possibility for decreased azole susceptibility is in vivo in-host mating of two strains with opposite mating types, both carrying different alleles contributing to decreased azole susceptibility. As described about a decade ago, *C. albicans* is able to mate; however, instead of sporulation, the tetraploid cells revert back to diploids by continuous chromosome loss (Bennett and Johnson 2003). This is more theoretical option for gaining azole resistance and it has not yet been reported.

Chromosome duplication has also been reported in *C. glabrata*, increasing the copy number of efflux pump encoding genes (Polakova et al. 2009). A fluconazole-resistant clinical isolate was found to contain an additional minichromosome, consisting of a duplicated portion of chromosome F, where ABC transporter gene, *CDR2*, is located. This minichromosome was also stable in the presence of fluconazole but again was frequently lost in drug-free medium. *ERG11* gene amplification through chromosome duplication has also been identified in this organism, although this isolate demonstrated other resistance mechanisms (Marichal et al. 1997). Again, the duplicated chromosome was unstable and was lost in the absence of azoles.

In *C. neoformans*, chromosome duplication is a very common azole resistance mechanism, known as heteroresistance. It is caused by disomy of chromosome 1, sometimes in combination with other chromosomes (Sionov et al. 2010). Chromosome 1 contains both known genes involved in resistance, *ERG11* and *AFR1*. This phenomenon is strain dependent and the aneuploidy is induced in the presence of fluconazole and does not seem to be spontaneous due to its unusually high frequency. However, the chromosome 1 disomy has a growth disadvantage and is reduced in virulence in animal models. Again, without fluconazole-selective pressure, the additional chromosomes are lost like in other organisms.

Biofilms

Another mechanism of resistance is the formation of a biofilm, the predominant mode of growth of many microorganisms in nature. The presence of foreign objects, including catheters, dentures, and artificial heart valves, can contribute to a recalcitrant infection, as the fungus can attach to and invade these objects, creating a source of constant inoculation and protection from drug therapy.

Candida infections primarily begin with adherence and colonization on a biotic or an artificial host surface. This process leads to the formation of biofilms – surface-attached communities encased in a matrix of secreted polymeric substances. The matrix encased cells forming the biofilm display unique characteristics over their planktonic or free-floating counterparts. In many *Candida* species, drug resistance is a common characteristic of biofilms (Lewis et al. 2002). In general, these biofilms require 5–8 times higher drug concentrations for a similar reduction in metabolic activity compared to their planktonic cells, and their MICs can differ up to four orders of magnitude (Hawser and Douglas 1995). Mechanisms that explain this higher antifungal resistance include the presence of extracellular matrix, a robust architecture with reduced drug diffusion, decreased cellular metabolic activity, the existence of "persistent cells," altered gene expression including the overexpression of efflux pumps and stress genes, and finally higher anti-oxidative capacities (Lopez-Ribot 2005; Nobile and Mitchell 2006; Ramage et al. 2002). Efflux pump activity plays a contributory role in biofilm azole resistance but is not the principal mechanism. *C. albicans* biofilms formed by *MDR* and *CDR* deletions still display the resistant phenotype despite high susceptibility of planktonic cells to fluconazole (Ramage et al. 2002). Recent evidence suggests that the extracellular matrix material in the biofilm, partially formed by glucans, can act as a chelator for antifungal drugs, so that the cell is not exposed to high drug concentrations (Nett et al. 2007). The glucan is produced by β-1,3-glucan synthase, Fks1, and its reduced activity results in increased biofilm azole susceptibility (Nett et al. 2010).

A. fumigatus and *C. glabrata* also form biofilms. *A. fumigatus* seems to exploit the same resistance mechanisms as *C. albicans*, including the overexpression of numerous transporters (Rajendran et al. 2011). However, compared to *C. albicans* and *A. fumigatus* biofilms, formed mostly by hyphae, *C. glabrata* biofilms are exclusively composed of yeast cells. These *C. glabrata* biofilms are also highly antifungal resistant compared to the planktonic cells, and this may be partially caused by an induced stress response (Seneviratne et al. 2009).

Heat Shock Proteins

Cellular stress conditions, including drug treatment, high temperatures, starvation, mutations, and oxidative stress, can negatively affect intracellular homeostasis and cause protein unfolding and aggregation leading to cell death. *H*eat *s*hock *p*roteins (HSPs) are dramatically upregulated during times of stress to act in part as chaperones to regulate the folding, transport, and degradation of many important proteins

(Cowen and Lindquist 2005; Lamoth et al. 2013; Mayer et al. 2013). *C. albicans* contains multiple HSPs including Hsp104, Hsp90, Hsp78, Hsp70, and Hsp60, which all function in the heat shock response either with unique functions or in response to specific stressors (Mayer et al. 2013). Hsp90 is the major HSP in *C. albicans* and in other fungi that is involved in drug resistance and virulence among its other functions (Cowen and Lindquist 2005; Mayer et al. 2013).

The main role of Hsp90 in drug resistance is to buffer the negative effects induced by drug treatment including the buildup of toxic protein aggregates. Its role is to unfold, refold, or stabilize proteins damaged in response to the stresses. Hsp90 activation following azole treatment allows cells to adapt to the resulting stress, including altered sterol biosynthesis and membrane composition.

Hsp90 is also critical for adaptation to newly acquired resistance mechanisms. In conditions of high cellular stress when the amount of damaged proteins outnumber the available Hsp90s, the *absence* of Hsp90 regulation can also benefit the cell by allowing protein mutations to go unchecked, such as those mutations that alter sterol biosynthesis and membrane composition. The exposure of a variety of new mutations offers the stressed cell a new repertoire of selectable variants for overcoming the stress agent and developing resistance.

Hsp90 is crucial for toleration of *ERG3* mutations as an azole-resistant mechanism (Cowen and Lindquist 2005). In cells, Hsp90 functions in drug resistance through the calcineurin pathway, which is known to be implicated in virulence of several pathogenic fungi and also enables fungal cells to tolerate ergosterol biosynthesis inhibitors (Cowen and Lindquist 2005). Exposure of cells to stress leads to elevated cytosolic Ca^{2+} concentrations and activation of calcineurin, a protein phosphatase whose primary function in yeast is to dephosphorylate and activate the transcription factor Crz1p. Calcineurin itself is an Hsp90 substrate and Hsp90 stabilizes its catalytic domain. Screens in *C. albicans* have also identified another gene involved in calcineurin signaling, *CKA2*, encoding casein kinase II (Bruno and Mitchell 2005). Recently, a new link between calcineurin signaling and iron homeostasis has been reported (Hameed et al. 2011). Iron deprivation results in reduced expression of the catalytic subunit of calcineurin, *CMP1*, plus several of the *ERG* genes, disrupting ergosterol biosynthesis.

cAMP signaling also plays a role in azole susceptibility. Deletion of enzymes involved in cAMP synthesis results in increased susceptibility to azoles and other sterol biosynthesis inhibitors (Jain et al. 2003). Cyclic AMP-dependent protein kinase A (PKA) in *S. cerevisiae* phosphorylates and negatively regulates Crz1 activity by inhibiting its nuclear import (Kafadar and Cyert 2004). Otherwise, PKA regulates the general stress response in yeast and coordinates this response with nutrient availability. In contrast, calcineurin regulates the cellular response to a restricted set of environmental insults.

Not surprisingly, Hsp90 inactivation leads to increased susceptibility to environmental stress including exposure to azoles. In general, a compromised Hsp90 or calcineurin transforms the fungistatic effect of many antifungals to fungicidal. Thus, HSP response in the evolution of fungal drug resistance has broad therapeutic implications and so has become a promising drug target (see below).

Resistance to Other Drugs

The mechanisms of resistance to the other three clinically used classes of drugs (echinocandins, polyenes, and 5-fluorocytosine) are limited. *C. albicans* strains can develop resistance to echinocandins (caspofungin, micafungin, and anidulafungin) due to mutations in the target enzyme β-1,3-glucan synthase (Gcsl/Fks1). This enzyme produces β-1,3-glucan and is essential for cell wall synthesis and fungal viability (Perlin 2007). There are two other Gscl homologs in *C. albicans*, Gsl1 and Gs12/Fks2, however they cannot completely compensate for Gscl loss of function. Mutations in the plasma membrane (PM)-localized Gsc1 enzyme usually occur in two hotspots (AA regions 641–649 and 1345–1365) and reduce the enzyme's affinity for the echinocandins. The drugs bind to Gsc1/Fks1 from the extracellular side of the PM and reduce its enzymatic activity. The same mechanism of resistance is employed in *C. glabrata* (Garcia-Effron et al. 2009) and *A. fumigatus* (Arendrup et al. 2009). However, in *A. fumigatus*, resistance due to the *FKS1* overexpression has also been reported (Arendrup et al. 2008). *C. albicans* cells respond to echinocandin treatment with an increase in chitin levels, and strains with higher chitin content in the cell wall (including those naturally occurring) are less echinocandin susceptible (Plaine et al. 2008; Lee et al. 2012). In some *C. albicans* isolates, the "paradoxical effect" is observed, where cell growth is stimulated at concentrations of echinocandin significantly above the MIC (Stevens et al. 2004). This is most likely due to the induction of cell wall stress response, resulting in increased chitin levels (Stevens et al. 2006).

Resistance to polyenes, like amphotericin B or nystatin, is usually associated with lowered levels of ergosterol in the plasma membrane (Dick et al. 1980). Polyenes bind to the ergosterol in fungal membranes resulting in pores that affect the membrane integrity and lead to the loss of the membrane potential. The molecular mechanisms of resistance to polyenes are poorly understood; however, resistance is associated with alterations in *ERG* genes (Sanglard et al. 2003) as well as an increase in resistance to oxidative stress (Sokol-Anderson et al. 1986).

The last medically important drug, 5-fluorocytosine (flucytosine; 5-FC), is metabolized via the pyrimidine salvage pathway, where it acts as a substrate with the subsequent production of toxic nucleotides and disruption of DNA and protein synthesis. After being actively transported into the cell by the permease Fcy2, 5-FC is converted to 5-fluoro-uridylate (5-FU) with the help of the enzymes cytosine deaminase (Fca1) and uracil phosphoribosyltransferase (Fur1). 5-FU is then processed and incorporated into RNA. 5-FU by-products also inhibit the enzyme thymidylate synthase (Cdc21) and thus DNA synthesis by decreasing the available nucleotide pool. 5-FC resistance mechanisms include mutation of enzymes, Fur1 (R101C) and Fca1 (G28D) (Hope et al. 2004). Both mutant alleles must be in homozygous state. These mutations most likely lead to reduced activity or even complete inactivation of the enzymes, since both genes are nonessential. In *Candida lusitaniae*, deletion of the cytosine permease Fcy2, as well as deletions of Fur1 and Fca1, leads to increased 5-FC resistance (Chapeland-Leclerc et al. 2005). However, the effect of the inactivation of *C. albicans* Fcy2 permease has not been reported to date.

Drug Combinations and Perspectives

In recent years, multiple drugs have been reported to have a synergistic effect with azoles, which provides new hope for combined therapy that will be less likely to result in rapid drug resistance development. One treatment combination would be to use antifungal drugs from different drug classes/families. For example, the composition and genetic regulation of *Candida* biofilm matrix are a promising target for the development of treatment of medical device-associated infections. The synergistic effect of azoles and echinocandins would be expected to negatively affect biofilms that were previously unresponsive to a single-drug treatment alone (Nett et al. 2010).

Calcineurin and Hsp90 inhibitors are another group of drugs displaying a synergistic effect with azoles and other antifungals. Since the cell wall integrity is connected to calcineurin signaling, there is a synergistic effect of echinocandins with HSP90/calcineurin inhibitors creating a fungicidal combination (Singh et al. 2009). There are several drugs with an inhibitory effect on calcineurin signaling. First, tacrolimus (FK506) forms a complex with peptidyl-prolyl cis-trans isomerase, Fpr1, a binding partner of calcineurin (Kissinger et al. 1995). Another drug, cyclosporine A, binds to another calcineurin partner – the peptidyl-prolyl cis-trans isomerase Cpr1 (Etzkorn et al. 1994). There are also two direct Hsp90 inhibitors, geldanamycin and radicicol, both docking into Hsp90's nucleotide-binding pocket (Schulte et al. 1998; Stebbins et al. 1997). Although these drugs exhibit their own direct antifungal activity (Lamoth et al. 2013), they also significantly increase in vitro susceptibility of *Candida* and *Aspergillus* species to azoles and other antifungals (Lamoth et al. 2013; Cruz et al. 2002; Onyewu et al. 2003). These drug combinations induce a better response in drug-resistant pathogens, turning fungistatic drugs to fungicidal and delaying or disrupting the acquisition of new resistance mechanisms. Their potential is also in the sensitization of biofilms to other antifungals (Shinde et al. 2012). Moreover, tacrolimus has been shown to work directly as a *C. albicans CDR1* inhibitor (Schuetzer-Muehlbauer et al. 2003).

Depletion of iron, an important part of heme present in Erg11 and Erg25 enzymes, also has a negative effect on calcineurin signaling, as mentioned above. Recently, doxycycline and to a lesser extent tetracycline have been shown to act synergistically with azoles in *C. albicans* in vitro through iron chelation (Fiori and Van Dijck 2012). The involvement of calcineurin signaling is likely, since the cyclins shift the azole effect from fungistatic to fungicidal and since the combination of azoles and doxycycline does not allow cells to develop resistance to this combination. Another proof of synergism between azole and iron chelation is lactoferrin, a transferrin present in milk and in body secretory fluids and part of innate immunity (Kobayashi et al. 2011).

Another group of drugs that might be considered for combined therapy are efflux pump inhibitors. Several have been identified to date. Two inhibitors, clorgyline (monoamine oxidase A inhibitor) and ebselen (antioxidant under investigation for several medical uses), were described to inhibit several efflux pumps including the *C. albicans* pumps Cdr1 and Cdr2, the *C. glabrata* pump Cdr1, and the *C. krusei* pump Abc1 (Holmes et al. 2012). Clorgyline is also active against and shows better potency with the *C. albicans* pump Mdr1. It displays synergistic effect with azoles against azole-resistant strains of both *C. albicans* and *C. glabrata* in vitro. On the other hand, ebselen is known to have antifungal activity by inhibition of Pma1, the main plasma membrane H^+-ATPase (Billack et al. 2009). Other potent ABC pump inhibitors are the milbemycins (antiparasitic agents of macrolide type) (Lamping et al. 2007), unnarmicins (bacterial cyclic peptides) (Tanabe et al. 2007), tetrandrine (anti-inflammatory calcium channel blocker) (Zhang et al. 2009), enniatins (cyclic depsipeptides) (Hiraga et al. 2005), and ofloxacin and grepafloxacin (both synthetic fluoroquinolone antibiotics) (Sasaki et al. 2000). Ibuprofen also displays synergistic effect with azoles against azole-resistant strains of *C. albicans* (Ricardo et al. 2009). Although ibuprofen's mechanism of action has not been proven directly, it is suspected to be another ABC pump inhibitor. Another drug showing synergy with the azoles is amiodarone (an antiarrhythmic drug) (Guo et al. 2008). Although its mode of action is unknown, it is suggested to either affect cellular Ca^{2+} membrane transport, consistent with its antiarrhythmic use, or to inhibit ABC transporters. Lastly, several analogs of cerulenin (an inhibitor of fungal sterol synthesis and fatty acid synthesis) have been described to block the *C. albicans* Mdr1 major facilitator (Diwischek et al. 2009).

Several of the above drugs are already marketed for medical use. Therefore, clinical trials are needed to show efficacy, but not to ascertain their safety in humans. Synergy *in vivo* is not guaranteed due to the limits in physiological concentrations and possible alterations in metabolism. Several of the efflux pump inhibitors are used in traditional medicine and clearly warrant clinical trials for safety and efficacy. It is clear that as we learn about mechanisms of resistance in the fungi, we are also identifying strategies to interfere with these mechanisms.

Conclusion

Prolonged exposure of human fungal pathogens to azoles and other classes of antifungals often results in the development of resistance to these drugs. Every organism contains numerous pathways that can contribute to drug resistance. Azole resistance is best understood in the human fungal pathogen *C. albicans*, where the upregulation of the three major transporters responsible for azole efflux, Cdr1, Cd2, and Mdr1, is the most common resistance mechanism. This is usually accomplished by the acquisition of a GOF mutation in transcription factors Mrr1 and Tac1 that regulate these pumps, resulting in pump overexpression. A second major mechanism of resistance involves alterations in the ergosterol biosynthesis pathway. This includes the overexpression of *ERG11*, altering the affinity of Erg11 for azoles or inactivating the *ERG3* gene, which is responsible for synthesis of toxic intermediates after azole inhibition of Erg11. Further increases in resistance can be accomplished by copying the resistant allele into the susceptible allele in a diploid fungus, either by gene conversion or gene duplication.. All the above-described mechanisms can be combined, resulting in strains completely nonresponsive to therapeutic doses of azoles. Other fungi share identical mechanisms of azole resistance, although *C. glabrata* and *A. fumigatus* appear to be capable of exogenous sterol import, which can eliminate the importance of endogenous ergosterol biosynthesis. This fact might lead to an alteration of the conditions for antifungal susceptibility testing in the future.

New antifungal treatments in the near future may require the combination of existing antifungal drugs with the development of new compounds. Numerous drugs approved for other clinical uses display antifungal activity, often acting as efflux inhibitors. Combined therapy with two drugs, attacking two different targets in the cell, has a lower probability of developing resistance to both drugs than the probability of developing resistance to a single drug. One major target of this strategy is the HSP90/calcineurin pathway. The inactivation of this pathway results in the inability of fungal cells to deal with some of the newly acquired mutations involved in azole resistance. Specificity of these drugs for fungal cell targets is important because the current HSP90/calcineurin-targeting drugs can act as immunosuppressants in humans. Therefore, their use in a human host and subsequent immune suppression often results in the acquisition of a fungal infection.

To prevent the development of antifungal drug resistance in the future, it is crucial to identify new fungal drug targets and to create drugs that are fungicidal. One of these new targets might be cell wall assembly and cell wall remodeling enzymes. These drugs work on the exterior of the cell, thus omitting the need for the drug to be imported into the fungal cells. This is similar to the bacterial transpeptidases for β-lactam antibiotics that also work outside of the cell. The future of antifungal drug development lies in using the information we currently have to develop therapies that inhibit or kill the fungal cells while minimizing the possibility of drug resistance.

References

Alarco AM, Raymond M (1999) The bZip transcription factor Cap1p is involved in multidrug resistance and oxidative stress response in *Candida albicans*. J Bacteriol 181:700–708

Alcazar-Fuoli L, Mellado E, Garcia-Effron G, Buitrago MJ, Lopez JF, Grimalt JO, Cuenca-Estrella JM, Rodriguez-Tudela JL (2006) *Aspergillus fumigatus* C-5 sterol desaturases Erg3A and Erg3B: role in sterol biosynthesis and antifungal drug susceptibility. Antimicrob Agents Chemother 50:453–460

Anderson JB, Sirjusingh C, Parsons AB, Boone C, Wickens C, Cowen LE, Kohn LM (2003) Mode of selection and experimental evolution of antifungal drug resistance in *Saccharomyces cerevisiae*. Genetics 163:1287–1298

Andreasen AA, Stier TJ (1953) Anaerobic nutrition of *Saccharomyces cerevisiae*. I Ergosterol requirement for growth in a defined medium. J Cell Physiol 41:23–36

Arendrup MC, Perkhofer S, Howard SJ, Garcia-Effron G, Vishukumar A, Perlin D, Lass-Florl C (2008) Establishing in vitro-in vivo correlations for *Aspergillus fumigatus*: the challenge of azoles versus echinocandins. Antimicrob Agents Chemother 52:3504–3511

Arendrup MC, Garcia-Effron G, Buzina W, Mortensen KL, Reiter N, Lundin C, Jensen HE, Lass-Florl C, Perlin DS, Bruun B (2009) Breakthrough *Aspergillus fumigatus* and *Candida albicans* double infection during caspofungin treatment: laboratory characteristics and implication for susceptibility testing. Antimicrob Agents Chemother 53:1185–1193

Bard M, Sturm AM, Pierson CA, Brown S, Rogers KM, Nabinger S, Eckstein J, Barbuch R, Lees ND, Howell SA, Hazen KC (2005) Sterol uptake in *Candida glabrata*: rescue of sterol auxotrophic strains. Diagn Microbiol Infect Dis 52:285–293

Bennett RJ, Johnson AD (2003) Completion of a parasexual cycle in *Candida albicans* by induced chromosome loss in tetraploid strains. Embo J 22:2505–2515

Billack B, Santoro M, Lau-Cam C (2009) Growth inhibitory action of ebselen on fluconazole-resistant *Candida albicans*: role of the plasma membrane H^{+} – ATPase. Microb Drug Resist 15:77–83

Bouchara JP, Zouhair R, Le Boudouil S, Renier G, Filmon R, Chabasse D, Hallet JN, Defontaine A (2000) In-vivo selection of an azole-resistant petite mutant of *Candida glabrata*. J Med Microbiol 49:977–984

Brun S, Dalle F, Saulnier P, Renier G, Bonnin A, Chabasse D, Bouchara JP (2005) Biological consequences of petite mutations in *Candida glabrata*. J Antimicrob Chemother 56:307–314

Bruno VM, Mitchell AP (2005) Regulation of azole drug susceptibility by *Candida albicans* protein kinase CK2. Mol Microbiol 56:559–573

Calabrese D, Bille J, Sanglard D (2000) A novel multidrug efflux transporter gene of the major facilitator superfamily from *Candida albicans* (*FLU1*) conferring resistance to fluconazole. Microbiology 146(Pt 11):2743–2754

Campoli P, Perlin DS, Kristof AS, White TC, Filler SG, Sheppard DC (2013) Pharmacokinetics of posaconazole within epithelial cells and fungi: insights into potential mechanisms of action during treatment and prophylaxis. J Infect Dis 208:1717–1728

Camps SM, Rijs AJ, Klaassen CH, Meis JF, O'Gorman CM, Dyer PS, Melchers WJ, Verweij PE (2012a) Molecular epidemiology of *Aspergillus fumigatus* isolates harboring the TR34/L98H azole resistance mechanism. J Clin Microbiol 50:2674–2680

Camps SM, Dutilh BE, Arendrup MC, Rijs AJ, Snelders E, Huynen MA, Verweij PE, Melchers WJ (2012b) Discovery of a HapE mutation that causes azole resistance in *Aspergillus fumigatus* through whole genome sequencing and sexual crossing. PLoS One 7:e50034

Chapeland-Leclerc F, Bouchoux J, Goumar A, Chastin C, Villard J, Noel T (2005) Inactivation of the *FCY2* gene encoding purine-cytosine permease promotes cross-resistance to flucytosine and fluconazole in *Candida lusitaniae*. Antimicrob Agents Chemother 49:3101–3108

Chau AS, Gurnani M, Hawkinson R, Laverdiere M, Cacciapuoti A, McNicholas PM (2005) Inactivation of sterol Delta5,6-desaturase attenuates virulence in *Candida albicans*. Antimicrob Agents Chemother 49:3646–3651

Chen KH, Miyazaki T, Tsai HF, Bennett JE (2007) The bZip transcription factor Cgap1p is involved in multidrug resistance and required for activation of multidrug transporter gene *CgFLR1* in *Candida glabrata*. Gene 386:63–72

Costa C, Pires C, Cabrito TR, Renaudin A, Ohno M, Chibana H, Sa-Correia I, Teixeira MC (2013) *Candida glabrata* drug:H^{+} antiporter CgQdr2 confers imidazole drug resistance, being activated by transcription factor CgPdr1. Antimicrob Agents Chemother 57:3159–3167

Coste AT, Karababa M, Ischer F, Bille J, Sanglard D (2004) *TAC1*, transcriptional activator of *CDR* genes, is a new transcription factor involved in the regulation of *Candida albicans* ABC transporters *CDR1* and *CDR2*. Eukaryot Cell 3:1639–1652

Coste A, Turner V, Ischer F, Morschhauser J, Forche A, Selmecki A, Berman J, Bille J, Sanglard D (2006) A mutation in Tac1p, a transcription factor regulating *CDR1* and *CDR2*, is coupled with loss of heterozygosity at chromosome 5 to mediate antifungal resistance in *Candida albicans*. Genetics 172:2139–2156

Coste A, Selmecki A, Forche A, Diogo D, Bougnoux ME, D'Enfert C, Berman J, Sanglard D (2007) Genotypic evolution of azole resistance mechanisms in sequential *Candida albicans* isolates. Eukaryot Cell 6:1889–1904

Coste AT, Crittin J, Bauser C, Rohde B, Sanglard D (2009) Functional analysis of cis- and trans-acting elements of the *Candida albicans CDR2* promoter with a novel promoter reporter system. Eukaryot Cell 8:1250–1267

Cowen LE, Lindquist S (2005) Hsp90 potentiates the rapid evolution of new traits: drug resistance in diverse fungi. Science 309:2185–2189

Crowley JH, Leak FW Jr, Shianna KV, Tove S, Parks LW (1998) A mutation in a purported regulatory gene affects control of sterol uptake in *Saccharomyces cerevisiae*. J Bacteriol 180:4177–4183

Cruz MC, Goldstein AL, Blankenship JR, Del Poeta M, Davis D, Cardenas ME, Perfect JR, McCusker JH, Heitman J (2002) Calcineurin is essential for survival during membrane stress in *Candida albicans*. Embo J 21:546–559

da Silva Ferreira ME, Malavazi I, Savoldi M, Brakhage AA, Goldman MH, Kim HS, Nierman WC, Goldman GH (2006) Transcriptome analysis of *Aspergillus fumigatus* exposed to voriconazole. Curr Genet 50:32–44

Davies BS, Wang HS, Rine J (2005) Dual activators of the sterol biosynthetic pathway of *Saccharomyces cerevisiae*: similar activation/regulatory domains but different response mechanisms. Mol Cell Biol 25:7375–7385

de Micheli M, Bille J, Schueller C, Sanglard D (2002) A common drug-responsive element mediates the upregulation of the *Candida albicans* ABC transporters *CDR1* and *CDR2*, two genes involved in antifungal drug resistance. Mol Microbiol 43:1197–1214

Denning DW, Venkateswarlu K, Oakley KL, Anderson MJ, Manning NJ, Stevens DA, Warnock DW, Kelly SL (1997) Itraconazole resistance in *Aspergillus fumigatus*. Antimicrob Agents Chemother 41:1364–1368

Diaz-Guerra TM, Mellado E, Cuenca-Estrella M, Rodriguez-Tudela JL (2003) A point mutation in the 14alpha-sterol demethylase gene *cyp51A* contributes to itraconazole resistance in *Aspergillus fumigatus*. Antimicrob Agents Chemother 47:1120–1124

Dick JD, Merz WG, Saral R (1980) Incidence of polyene-resistant yeasts recovered from clinical specimens. Antimicrob Agents Chemother 18:158–163

Diwischek F, Morschhauser J, Holzgrabe U (2009) Cerulenin analogues as inhibitors of efflux pumps in drug-resistant *Candida albicans*. Arch Pharm (Weinheim) 342:150–164

Dodds Ashley ES, Lewis R, Lewis JS, Martin C, Andes D (2006) Pharmacology of systemic antifungal agents. Clin Infect Dis 43:S28–S39

Dunkel N, Liu TT, Barker KS, Homayouni R, Morschhauser J, Rogers PD (2008a) A gain-of-function mutation in the transcription factor Upc2p causes upregulation of ergosterol biosynthesis genes and increased fluconazole resistance in a clinical *Candida albicans* isolate. Eukaryot Cell 7:1180–1190

Dunkel N, Blass J, Rogers PD, Morschhauser J (2008b) Mutations in the multi-drug resistance regulator *MRR1*, followed by loss of heterozygosity, are the main cause of *MDR1* overexpression in fluconazole-resistant *Candida albicans* strains. Mol Microbiol 69:827–840

Esquivel BE, Smith AR, Zavrel M, White TC (2015) Azole drug import into the pathogenic fungus *Aspergillus fumigatus*. Antimicrob Agents and Chemother. 59-3390-3398

Etzkorn FA, Chang ZY, Stolz LA, Walsh CT (1994) Cyclophilin residues that affect noncompetitive inhibition of the protein serine phosphatase activity of calcineurin by the cyclophilin.cyclosporin A complex. Biochemistry 33:2380–2388

Ferrari S, Ischer F, Calabrese D, Posteraro B, Sanguinetti M, Fadda G, Rohde B, Bauser C, Bader O, Sanglard D (2009) Gain of function mutations in *CgPDR1* of *Candida glabrata* not only mediate antifungal resistance but also enhance virulence. PLoS Pathog 5:e1000268

Fiori A, Van Dijck P (2012) Potent synergistic effect of doxycycline with fluconazole against *Candida albicans* is mediated by interference with iron homeostasis. Antimicrob Agents Chemother 56:3785–3796

Flowers SA, Barker KS, Berkow EL, Toner G, Chadwick SG, Gygax SE, Morschhauser J, Rogers PD (2012) Gain-of-function mutations in *UPC2* are a frequent cause of *ERG11* upregulation in azole-resistant clinical isolates of *Candida albicans*. Eukaryot Cell 11:1289–1299

Fraczek MG, Bromley M, Buied A, Moore CB, Rajendran R, Rautemaa R, Ramage G, Denning DW, Bowyer P (2013) The *cdr1B* efflux transporter is associated with non-cyp51a-mediated itraconazole resistance in *Aspergillus fumigatus*. J Antimicrob Chemother 68:1486–1496

Garcia-Effron G, Lee S, Park S, Cleary JD, Perlin DS (2009) Effect of *Candida glabrata FKS1* and *FKS2* mutations on echinocandin sensitivity and kinetics of 1,3-beta-D-glucan synthase: implication for the existing susceptibility breakpoint. Antimicrob Agents Chemother 53:3690–3699

Geber A, Hitchcock CA, Swartz JE, Pullen FS, Marsden KE, Kwon-Chung KJ, Bennett JE (1995) Deletion of the *Candida glabrata ERG3* and *ERG11* genes: effect on cell viability, cell growth, sterol composition, and antifungal susceptibility. Antimicrob Agents Chemother 39:2708–2717

Guo Q, Sun S, Yu J, Li Y, Cao L (2008) Synergistic activity of azoles with amiodarone against clinically resistant *Candida albicans* tested by chequerboard and time-kill methods. J Med Microbiol 57:457–462

Hameed S, Dhamgaye S, Singh A, Goswami SK, Prasad R (2011) Calcineurin signaling and membrane lipid homeostasis regulates iron mediated multidrug resistance mechanisms in *Candida albicans*. PLoS One 6:e18684

Hawser SP, Douglas LJ (1995) Resistance of *Candida albicans* biofilms to antifungal agents in vitro. Antimicrob Agents Chemother 39:2128–2131

Heilmann CJ, Schneider S, Barker KS, Rogers PD, Morschhauser J (2010) An A643T mutation in the transcription factor Upc2p causes constitutive *ERG11* upregulation and increased fluconazole resistance in *Candida albicans*. Antimicrob Agents Chemother 54:353–359

Henry KW, Nickels JT, Edlind TD (2000) Upregulation of *ERG* genes in *Candida* species by azoles and other sterol biosynthesis inhibitors. Antimicrob Agents Chemother 44:2693–2700

Hiraga K, Yamamoto S, Fukuda H, Hamanaka N, Oda K (2005) Enniatin has a new function as an inhibitor of Pdr5p, one of the ABC transporters in *Saccharomyces cerevisiae*. Biochem Biophys Res Commun 328:1119–1125

Hitchcock CA (1991) Cytochrome P-450-dependent 14 alpha-sterol demethylase of *Candida albicans* and its interaction with azole antifungals. Biochem Soc Trans 19:782–787

Holmes AR, Keniya MV, Ivnitski-Steele I, Monk BC, Lamping E, Sklar LA, Cannon RD (2012) The monoamine oxidase A inhibitor clorgyline is a broad-spectrum inhibitor of fungal ABC and MFS transporter efflux pump activities which reverses the azole resistance of *Candida albicans* and *Candida glabrata* clinical isolates. Antimicrob Agents Chemother 56:1508–1515

Hoot SJ, Smith AR, Brown RP, White TC (2011) An A643V amino acid substitution in Upc2p contributes to azole resistance in well-characterized clinical isolates of *Candida albicans*. Antimicrob Agents Chemother 55:940–942

Hope WW, Tabernero L, Denning DW, Anderson MJ (2004) Molecular mechanisms of primary resistance to flucytosine in *Candida albicans*. Antimicrob Agents Chemother 48:4377–4386

Howard SJ, Arendrup MC (2011) Acquired antifungal drug resistance in *Aspergillus fumigatus*: epidemiology and detection. Med Mycol 49(Suppl 1):S90–S95

Howard SJ, Webster I, Moore CB, Gardiner RE, Park S, Perlin DS, Denning DW (2006) Multi-azole resistance in *Aspergillus fumigatus*. Int J Antimicrob Agents 28:450–453

Jain P, Akula I, Edlind T (2003) Cyclic AMP signaling pathway modulates susceptibility of *Candida* species and *Saccharomyces cerevisiae* to antifungal azoles and other sterol biosynthesis inhibitors. Antimicrob Agents Chemother 47:3195–3201

Jensen-Pergakes KL, Kennedy MA, Lees ND, Barbuch R, Koegel C, Bard M (1998) Sequencing, disruption, and characterization of the *Candida albicans* sterol methyltransferase (*ERG6*) gene: drug susceptibility studies in *erg6* mutants. Antimicrob Agents Chemother 42:1160–1167

Joseph-Horne T, Hollomon D, Loeffler RS, Kelly SL (1995) Cross-resistance to polyene and azole drugs in *Cryptococcus neoformans*. Antimicrob Agents Chemother 39:1526–1529

Kafadar KA, Cyert MS (2004) Integration of stress responses: modulation of calcineurin signaling in *Saccharomyces cerevisiae* by protein kinase A. Eukaryot Cell 3:1147–1153

Kelly SL, Lamb DC, Corran AJ, Baldwin BC, Kelly DE (1995) Mode of action and resistance to azole antifungals associated with the formation of 14 alpha-methylergosta-8,24(28)-dien-3 beta,6 alpha-diol. Biochem Biophys Res Commun 207:910–915

Kelly SL, Lamb DC, Kelly DE, Manning NJ, Loeffler J, Hebart H, Schumacher U, Einsele H (1997) Resistance to fluconazole and cross-resistance to amphotericin B in *Candida albicans* from AIDS patients caused by defective sterol delta5,6-desaturation. FEBS Lett 400:80–82

Kissinger CR, Parge HE, Knighton DR, Lewis CT, Pelletier LA, Tempczyk A, Kalish VJ, Tucker KD, Showalter RE, Moomaw EW et al (1995) Crystal structures of human calcineurin and the human FKBP12-FK506-calcineurin complex. Nature 378:641–644

Kobayashi T, Kakeya H, Miyazaki T, Izumikawa K, Yanagihara K, Ohno H, Yamamoto Y, Tashiro T, Kohno S (2011) Synergistic antifungal effect of lactoferrin with azole antifungals against *Candida albicans* and a proposal for a new treatment method for invasive candidiasis. Jpn J Infect Dis 64:292–296

Lamb DC, Corran A, Baldwin BC, Kwon-Chung J, Kelly SL (1995) Resistant P45051A1 activity in azole antifungal tolerant *Cryptococcus neoformans* from AIDS patients. FEBS Lett 368:326–330

Lamoth F, Juvvadi PR, Gehrke C, Steinbach WJ (2013) In vitro activity of calcineurin and heat shock protein 90 Inhibitors against *Aspergillus fumigatus* azole- and echinocandin-resistant strains. Antimicrob Agents Chemother 57:1035–1039

Lamping E, Monk BC, Niimi K, Holmes AR, Tsao S, Tanabe K, Niimi M, Uehara Y, Cannon RD (2007) Characterization of three classes of membrane proteins involved in fungal azole resistance by functional hyperexpression in *Saccharomyces cerevisiae*. Eukaryot Cell 6:1150–1165

Lamping E, Ranchod A, Nakamura K, Tyndall JD, Niimi K, Holmes AR, Niimi M, Cannon RD (2009) Abc1p is a multidrug efflux transporter that tips the balance in favor of innate azole resistance in *Candida krusei*. Antimicrob Agents Chemother 53:354–369

Lee KK, Maccallum DM, Jacobsen MD, Walker LA, Odds FC, Gow NA, Munro CA (2012) Elevated cell wall chitin in *Candida albicans* confers echinocandin resistance in vivo. Antimicrob Agents Chemother 56:208–217

Lewis TA, Taylor FR, Parks LW (1985) Involvement of heme biosynthesis in control of sterol uptake by *Saccharomyces cerevisiae*. J Bacteriol 163:199–207

Lewis TL, Keesler GA, Fenner GP, Parks LW (1988) Pleiotropic mutations in *Saccharomyces cerevisiae* affecting sterol uptake and metabolism. Yeast 4:93–106

Lewis RE, Kontoyiannis DP, Darouiche RO, Raad II, Prince RA (2002) Antifungal activity of amphotericin B, fluconazole, and voriconazole in an in vitro model of *Candida* catheter-related bloodstream infection. Antimicrob Agents Chemother 46:3499–3505

Lopez-Ribot JL (2005) *Candida albicans* biofilms: more than filamentation. Curr Biol 15: R453–R455

MacPherson S, Akache B, Weber S, De Deken X, Raymond M, Turcotte B (2005) *Candida albicans* zinc cluster protein Upc2p confers resistance to antifungal drugs and is an activator of ergosterol biosynthetic genes. Antimicrob Agents Chemother 49:1745–1752

Manavathu EK, Vazquez JA, Chandrasekar PH (1999) Reduced susceptibility in laboratory-selected mutants of *Aspergillus fumigatus* to itraconazole due to decreased intracellular accumulation of the antifungal agent. Int J Antimicrob Agents 12:213–219

Manoharlal R, Gaur NA, Panwar SL, Morschhauser J, Prasad R (2008) Transcriptional activation and increased mRNA stability contribute to overexpression of *CDR1* in azole-resistant *Candida albicans*. Antimicrob Agents Chemother 52:1481–1492

Mansfield BE, Oltean HN, Oliver BG, Hoot SJ, Leyde SE, Hedstrom L, White TC (2010) Azole drugs are imported by facilitated diffusion in *Candida albicans* and other pathogenic fungi. PLoS Pathog 6:e1001126

Marichal P, Vanden Bossche H, Odds FC, Nobels G, Warnock DW, Timmerman V, Van Broeckhoven C, Fay S, Mose-Larsen P (1997) Molecular biological characterization of an azole-resistant *Candida glabrata* isolate. Antimicrob Agents Chemother 41:2229–2237

Marichal P, Koymans L, Willemsens S, Bellens D, Verhasselt P, Luyten W, Borgers M, Ramaekers FC, Odds FC, Bossche HV (1999) Contribution of mutations in the cytochrome P450 14alpha-demethylase (Erg11p, Cyp51p) to azole resistance in *Candida albicans*. Microbiology 145 (Pt 10):2701–2713

Mayer FL, Wilson D, Hube B (2013) *Candida albicans* pathogenicity mechanisms. Virulence 4:119–128

Mellado E, Diaz-Guerra TM, Cuenca-Estrella M, Rodriguez-Tudela JL (2001) Identification of two different 14-alpha sterol demethylase-related genes (*cyp51A* and *cyp51B*) in *Aspergillus fumigatus* and other *Aspergillus* species. J Clin Microbiol 39:2431–2438

Mellado E, Garcia-Effron G, Alcazar-Fuoli L, Cuenca-Estrella M, Rodriguez-Tudela JL (2004) Substitutions at methionine 220 in the 14alpha-sterol demethylase (Cyp51A) of *Aspergillus fumigatus* are responsible for resistance in vitro to azole antifungal drugs. Antimicrob Agents Chemother 48:2747–2750

Mellado E, Garcia-Effron G, Alcazar-Fuoli L, Melchers WJ, Verweij PE, Cuenca-Estrella M, Rodriguez-Tudela JL (2007) A new *Aspergillus fumigatus* resistance mechanism conferring in vitro cross-resistance to azole antifungals involves a combination of *cyp51A* alterations. Antimicrob Agents Chemother 51:1897–1904

Miyazaki T, Miyazaki Y, Izumikawa K, Kakeya H, Miyakoshi S, Bennett JE, Kohno S (2006) Fluconazole treatment is effective against a *Candida albicans erg3/erg3* mutant in vivo despite in vitro resistance. Antimicrob Agents Chemother 50:580–586

Morschhauser J (2002) The genetic basis of fluconazole resistance development in *Candida albicans*. Biochim Biophys Acta 1587:240–248

Morschhauser J, Barker KS, Liu TT, Bla BWJ, Homayouni R, Rogers PD (2007) The transcription factor Mrr1p controls expression of the *MDR1* efflux pump and mediates multidrug resistance in *Candida albicans*. PLoS Pathog 3:e164

Nagi M, Tanabe K, Ueno K, Nakayama H, Aoyama T, Chibana H, Yamagoe S, Umeyama T, Oura T, Ohno H, Kajiwara S, Miyazaki Y (2013) The *Candida glabrata* sterol scavenging mechanism, mediated by the ATP-binding cassette transporter Aus1p, is regulated by iron limitation. Mol Microbiol 88:371–381

Nakayama H, Tanabe K, Bard M, Hodgson W, Wu S, Takemori D, Aoyama T, Kumaraswami NS, Metzler L, Takano Y, Chibana H, Niimi M (2007) The *Candida glabrata* putative sterol transporter gene *CgAUS1* protects cells against azoles in the presence of serum. J Antimicrob Chemother 60:1264–1272

Nett J, Lincoln L, Marchillo K, Massey R, Holoyda K, Hoff B, VanHandel M, Andes D (2007) Putative role of beta-1,3 glucans in *Candida albicans* biofilm resistance. Antimicrob Agents Chemother 51:510–520

Nett JE, Sanchez H, Cain MT, Andes DR (2010) Genetic basis of *Candida* biofilm resistance due to drug-sequestering matrix glucan. J Infect Dis 202:171–175

Nierman WC, Pain A, Anderson MJ, Wortman JR, Kim HS, Arroyo J, Berriman M, Abe K, Archer DB, Bermejo C, Bennett J, Bowyer P, Chen D, Collins M, Coulsen R, Davies R, Dyer PS, Farman M, Fedorova N, Feldblyum TV, Fischer R, Fosker N, Fraser A, Garcia JL, Garcia MJ, Goble A, Goldman GH, Gomi K, Griffith-Jones S, Gwilliam R, Haas B, Haas H, Harris D, Horiuchi H, Huang J, Humphray S, Jimenez J, Keller N, Khouri H, Kitamoto K, Kobayashi T, Konzack S, Kulkarni R, Kumagai T, Lafon A, Latge JP, Li W, Lord A, Lu C, Majoros WH, May GS, Miller BL, Mohamoud Y, Molina M, Monod M, Mouyna I, Mulligan S, Murphy L, O'Neil S, Paulsen I, Penalva MA, Pertea M, Price C, Pritchard BL, Quail MA, Rabbinowitsch E, Rawlins N, Rajandream MA, Reichard U, Renauld H, Robson GD, Rodriguez de Cordoba S, Rodriguez-Pena JM, Ronning CM, Rutter S, Salzberg SL, Sanchez M, Sanchez-Ferrero JC, Saunders D, Seeger K, Squares R, Squares S, Takeuchi M, Tekaia F, Turner G, Vazquez de Aldana CR, Weidman J, White O, Woodward J, Yu JH, Fraser C, Galagan JE, Asai K, Machida M, Hall N, Barrell B, Denning DW (2005) Genomic sequence of the pathogenic and allergenic filamentous fungus *Aspergillus fumigatus*. Nature 438:1151–1156

Nobile CJ, Mitchell AP (2006) Genetics and genomics of *Candida albicans* biofilm formation. Cell Microbiol 8:1382–1391

Odds FC, Brown AJ, Gow NA (2003) Antifungal agents: mechanisms of action. Trends Microbiol 11:272–279

Onyewu C, Blankenship JR, Del Poeta M, Heitman J (2003) Ergosterol biosynthesis inhibitors become fungicidal when combined with calcineurin inhibitors against *Candida albicans*, *Candida glabrata*, and *Candida krusei*. Antimicrob Agents Chemother 47:956–964

Perea S, Lopez-Ribot JL, Kirkpatrick WR, McAtee RK, Santillan RA, Martinez M, Calabrese D, Sanglard D, Patterson TF (2001) Prevalence of molecular mechanisms of resistance to azole antifungal agents in *Candida albicans* strains displaying high-level fluconazole resistance isolated from human immunodeficiency virus-infected patients. Antimicrob Agents Chemother 45:2676–2684

Perlin DS (2007) Resistance to echinocandin-class antifungal drugs. Drug Resist Updat 10:121–130

Plaine A, Walker L, Da Costa G, Mora-Montes HM, McKinnon A, Gow NA, Gaillardin C, Munro CA, Richard ML (2008) Functional analysis of *Candida albicans* GPI-anchored proteins: roles in cell wall integrity and caspofungin sensitivity. Fungal Genet Biol FG & B 45:1404–1414

Polakova S, Blume C, Zarate JA, Mentel M, Jorck-Ramberg D, Stenderup J, Piskur J (2009) Formation of new chromosomes as a virulence mechanism in yeast *Candida glabrata*. Proc Natl Acad Sci U S A 106:2688–2693

Posteraro B, Sanguinetti M, Sanglard D, La Sorda M, Boccia S, Romano L, Morace G, Fadda G (2003) Identification and characterization of a *Cryptococcus neoformans* ATP binding cassette (ABC) transporter-encoding gene, *CnAFR1*, involved in the resistance to fluconazole. Mol Microbiol 47:357–371

Rajendran R, Mowat E, McCulloch E, Lappin DF, Jones B, Lang S, Majithiya JB, Warn P, Williams C, Ramage G (2011) Azole resistance of *Aspergillus fumigatus* biofilms is partly associated with efflux pump activity. Antimicrob Agents Chemother 55:2092–2097

Ramage G, Bachmann S, Patterson TF, Wickes BL, Lopez-Ribot JL (2002) Investigation of multidrug efflux pumps in relation to fluconazole resistance in *Candida albicans* biofilms. J Antimicrob Chemother 49:973–980

Rex JH, Pfaller MA (2002) Has antifungal susceptibility testing come of age? Clin Infect Dis 35:982–989

Ricardo E, Costa-de-Oliveira S, Dias AS, Guerra J, Rodrigues AG, Pina-Vaz C (2009) Ibuprofen reverts antifungal resistance on *Candida albicans* showing overexpression of *CDR* genes. FEMS Yeast Res 9:618–625

Rodero L, Mellado E, Rodriguez AC, Salve A, Guelfand L, Cahn P, Cuenca-Estrella M, Davel G, Rodriguez-Tudela JL (2003) G484S amino acid substitution in lanosterol 14-alpha demethylase (*ERG11*) is related to fluconazole resistance in a recurrent *Cryptococcus neoformans* clinical isolate. Antimicrob Agents Chemother 47:3653–3656

Rustad TR, Stevens DA, Pfaller MA, White TC (2002) Homozygosity at the *Candida albicans* MTL locus associated with azole resistance. Microbiology 148:1061–1072

Saidane S, Weber S, De Deken X, St-Germain G, Raymond M (2006) PDR16-mediated azole resistance in *Candida albicans*. Mol Microbiol 60:1546–1562

Sanglard D, Kuchler K, Ischer F, Pagani JL, Monod M, Bille J (1995) Mechanisms of resistance to azole antifungal agents in *Candida albicans* isolates from AIDS patients involve specific multidrug transporters. Antimicrob Agents Chemother 39:2378–2386

Sanglard D, Ischer F, Bille J (2001) Role of ATP-binding-cassette transporter genes in high-frequency acquisition of resistance to azole antifungals in *Candida glabrata*. Antimicrob Agents Chemother 45:1174–1183

Sanglard D, Ischer F, Parkinson T, Falconer D, Bille J (2003) *Candida albicans* mutations in the ergosterol biosynthetic pathway and resistance to several antifungal agents. Antimicrob Agents Chemother 47:2404–2412

Sasaki E, Maesaki S, Miyazaki Y, Yanagihara K, Tomono K, Tashiro T, Kohno S (2000) Synergistic effect of ofloxacin and fluconazole against azole-resistant *Candida albicans*. J Infect Chemother 6:151–154

Sasse C, Schillig R, Dierolf F, Weyler M, Schneider S, Mogavero S, Rogers PD, Morschhauser J (2011) The transcription factor Ndt80 does not contribute to Mrr1-, Tac1-, and Upc2-mediated fluconazole resistance in *Candida albicans*. PLoS One 6:e25623

Sasse C, Dunkel N, Schafer T, Schneider S, Dierolf F, Ohlsen K, Morschhauser J (2012) The stepwise acquisition of fluconazole resistance mutations causes a gradual loss of fitness in *Candida albicans*. Mol Microbiol 86:539–556

Schubert S, Rogers PD, Morschhauser J (2008) Gain-of-function mutations in the transcription factor *MRR1* are responsible for overexpression of the *MDR1* efflux pump in fluconazole-resistant *Candida dubliniensis* strains. Antimicrob Agents Chemother 52:4274–4280

Schubert S, Barker KS, Znaidi S, Schneider S, Dierolf F, Dunkel N, Aid M, Boucher G, Rogers PD, Raymond M, Morschhauser J (2011) Regulation of efflux pump expression and drug resistance by the transcription factors Mrr1, Upc2, and Cap1 in *Candida albicans*. Antimicrob Agents Chemother 55:2212–2223

Schuetzer-Muehlbauer M, Willinger B, Egner R, Ecker G, Kuchler K (2003) Reversal of antifungal resistance mediated by ABC efflux pumps from *Candida albicans* functionally expressed in yeast. Int J Antimicrob Agents 22:291–300

Schulte TW, Akinaga S, Soga S, Sullivan W, Stensgard B, Toft D, Neckers LM (1998) Antibiotic radicicol binds to the N-terminal domain of Hsp90 and shares important biologic activities with geldanamycin. Cell Stress Chaperones 3:100–108

Selmecki A, Forche A, Berman J (2006) Aneuploidy and isochromosome formation in drug-resistant *Candida albicans*. Science 313:367–370

Seneviratne CJ, Wang Y, Jin L, Abiko Y, Samaranayake LP (2009) Proteomics of drug resistance in *Candida glabrata* biofilms. Proteomics 10:1444–1454

Shianna KV, Dotson WD, Tove S, Parks LW (2001) Identification of a *UPC2* homolog in *Saccharomyces cerevisiae* and its involvement in aerobic sterol uptake. J Bacteriol 183:830–834

Shinde RB, Chauhan NM, Raut JS, Karuppayil SM (2012) Sensitization of *Candida albicans* biofilms to various antifungal drugs by cyclosporine A. Ann Clin Microbiol Antimicrob 11:27

Silver PM, Oliver BG, White TC (2004) Role of *Candida albicans* transcription factor Upc2p in drug resistance and sterol metabolism. Eukaryot Cell 3:1391–1397

Singh SD, Robbins N, Zaas AK, Schell WA, Perfect JR, Cowen LE (2009) Hsp90 governs echinocandin resistance in the pathogenic yeast *Candida albicans* via calcineurin. PLoS Pathog 5:e1000532

Sionov E, Lee H, Chang YC, Kwon-Chung KJ (2010) *Cryptococcus neoformans* overcomes stress of azole drugs by formation of disomy in specific multiple chromosomes. PLoS Pathog 6: e1000848

Slaven JW, Anderson MJ, Sanglard D, Dixon GK, Bille J, Roberts IS, Denning DW (2002) Increased expression of a novel *Aspergillus fumigatus* ABC transporter gene, *atrF*, in the presence of itraconazole in an itraconazole resistant clinical isolate. Fungal Genet Biol 36:199–206

Snelders E, van der Lee HA, Kuijpers J, Rijs AJ, Varga J, Samson RA, Mellado E, Donders AR, Melchers WJ, Verweij PE (2008) Emergence of azole resistance in *Aspergillus fumigatus* and spread of a single resistance mechanism. PLoS Med 5:e219

Snelders E, Melchers WJ, Verweij PE (2011) Azole resistance in *Aspergillus fumigatus*: a new challenge in the management of invasive aspergillosis? Future Microbiol 6:335–347

Snelders E, Camps SM, Karawajczyk A, Schaftenaar G, Kema GH, van der Lee HA, Klaassen CH, Melchers WJ, Verweij PE (2012) Triazole fungicides can induce cross-resistance to medical triazoles in *Aspergillus fumigatus*. PLoS One 7:e31801

Sokol-Anderson ML, Brajtburg J, Medoff G (1986) Amphotericin B-induced oxidative damage and killing of *Candida albicans*. J Infect Dis 154:76–83

Stebbins CE, Russo AA, Schneider C, Rosen N, Hartl FU, Pavletich NP (1997) Crystal structure of an Hsp90-geldanamycin complex: targeting of a protein chaperone by an antitumor agent. Cell 89:239–250

Stevens DA, Espiritu M, Parmar R (2004) Paradoxical effect of caspofungin: reduced activity against *Candida albicans* at high drug concentrations. Antimicrob Agents Chemother 48:3407–3411

Stevens DA, Ichinomiya M, Koshi Y, Horiuchi H (2006) Escape of *Candida* from caspofungin inhibition at concentrations above the MIC (paradoxical effect) accomplished by increased cell wall chitin; evidence for beta-1,6-glucan synthesis inhibition by caspofungin. Antimicrob Agents Chemother 50:3160–3161

Tanabe K, Lamping E, Adachi K, Takano Y, Kawabata K, Shizuri Y, Niimi M, Uehara Y (2007) Inhibition of fungal ABC transporters by unnarmicin A and unnarmicin C, novel cyclic peptides from marine bacterium. Biochem Biophys Res Commun 364:990–995

Torelli R, Posteraro B, Ferrari S, La Sorda M, Fadda G, Sanglard D, Sanguinetti M (2008) The ATP-binding cassette transporter-encoding gene *CgSNQ2* is contributing to the *CgPDR1*-dependent azole resistance of *Candida glabrata*. Mol Microbiol 68:186–201

Tsai HF, Bard M, Izumikawa K, Krol AA, Sturm AM, Culbertson NT, Pierson CA, Bennett JE (2004) *Candida glabrata erg1* mutant with increased sensitivity to azoles and to low oxygen tension. Antimicrob Agents Chemother 48:2483–2489

Tsai HF, Krol AA, Sarti KE, Bennett JE (2006) *Candida glabrata PDR1*, a transcriptional regulator of a pleiotropic drug resistance network, mediates azole resistance in clinical isolates and petite mutants. Antimicrob Agents Chemother 50:1384–1392

Vandeputte P, Tronchin G, Larcher G, Ernoult E, Berges T, Chabasse D, Bouchara JP (2008) A nonsense mutation in the *ERG6* gene leads to reduced susceptibility to polyenes in a clinical isolate of *Candida glabrata*. Antimicrob Agents Chemother 52:3701–3709

Venkateswarlu K, Denning DW, Kelly SL (1997) Inhibition and interaction of cytochrome P450 of *Candida krusei* with azole antifungal drugs. J Med Vet Mycol 35:19–25

Verweij PE, Snelders E, Kema GH, Mellado E, Melchers WJ (2009) Azole resistance in *Aspergillus fumigatus*: a side-effect of environmental fungicide use? Lancet Infect Dis 9:789–795

Warrilow AG, Parker JE, Kelly DE, Kelly SL (2013) Azole affinity of sterol 14alpha-demethylase (*CYP51*) enzymes from *Candida albicans* and *Homo sapiens*. Antimicrob Agents Chemother 57:1352–1360

Watson PF, Rose ME, Ellis SW, England H, Kelly SL (1989) Defective sterol C5-6 desaturation and azole resistance: a new hypothesis for the mode of action of azole antifungals. Biochem Biophys Res Commun 164:1170–1175

White TC, Marr KA, Bowden RA (1998) Clinical, cellular, and molecular factors that contribute to antifungal drug resistance. Clin Microbiol Rev 11:382–402

Wilcox LJ, Balderes DA, Wharton B, Tinkelenberg AH, Rao G, Sturley SL (2002) Transcriptional profiling identifies two members of the ATP-binding cassette transporter superfamily required for sterol uptake in yeast. J Biol Chem 277:32466–32472

Willger SD, Puttikamonkul S, Kim KH, Burritt JB, Grahl N, Metzler LJ, Barbuch R, Bard M, Lawrence CB, Cramer RA Jr (2008) A sterol-regulatory element binding protein is required for cell polarity, hypoxia adaptation, azole drug resistance, and virulence in *Aspergillus fumigatus*. PLoS Pathog 4:e1000200

Xiong Q, Hassan SA, Wilson WK, Han XY, May GS, Tarrand JJ, Matsuda SP (2005) Cholesterol import by *Aspergillus fumigatus* and its influence on antifungal potency of sterol biosynthesis inhibitors. Antimicrob Agents Chemother 49:518–524

Zavrel M, Hoot SJ, White TC (2013) Comparison of sterol import under aerobic and anaerobic conditions in three fungal species, *Candida albicans*, *Candida glabrata*, and *Saccharomyces cerevisiae*. Eukaryot Cell 12:725–738

Zhang H, Gao A, Li F, Zhang G, Ho HI, Liao W (2009) Mechanism of action of tetrandrine, a natural inhibitor of *Candida albicans* drug efflux pumps. Yakugaku Zasshi 129:623–630

Znaidi S, De Deken X, Weber S, Rigby T, Nantel A, Raymond M (2007) The zinc cluster transcription factor Tac1p regulates *PDR16* expression in *Candida albicans*. Mol Microbiol 66:440–452

Znaidi S, Weber S, Al-Abdin OZ, Bomme P, Saidane S, Drouin S, Lemieux S, De Deken X, Robert F, Raymond M (2008) Genomewide location analysis of *Candida albicans* Upc2p, a regulator of sterol metabolism and azole drug resistance. Eukaryot Cell 7:836–847

Part V

HIV

Transmission of HIV-1 Drug Resistance

Laura Marije Hofstra, Jean-Claude Schmit, and Annemarie M. J. Wensing

Contents

L.M. Hofstra
Department of Infection and Immunity, Luxembourg Institute of Health, Luxembourg, Luxembourg

Department of Medical Microbiology, University Medical Center Utrecht, Utrecht, The Netherlands
e-mail: laura-marije.hofstra@lih.lu; L.M.Hofstra-2@umcutrecht.nl

J.-C. Schmit
Department of Infection and Immunity, Luxembourg Institute of Health, Luxembourg, Luxembourg
e-mail: jc.schmit@lih.lu

A.M.J. Wensing (✉)
Department of Medical Microbiology, University Medical Center Utrecht, Utrecht, The Netherlands
e-mail: a.m.j.wensing@umcutrecht.nl

M. Gotte et al. (eds.), *Handbook of Antimicrobial Resistance*,
DOI 10.1007/978-1-4939-0694-9_23

Abstract
Infection with an HIV strain harboring drug resistance-related mutations is referred to as transmitted drug resistance (TDR) or primary resistance. As transmitted drug resistance increases the risk of virological failure, current guidelines recommend to perform drug resistance testing at baseline in all newly diagnosed individuals to guide the choice of antiretroviral therapy.

The prevalence of TDR varies among regions, risk groups, and drug classes due to different exposure to antiretroviral therapy (ART), risk behavior, and access to therapy. Of concern in developed countries is the rising prevalence of mutations associated with NNRTI resistance, a drug class frequently used in first-line therapy which has a low genetic barrier for development of resistance. In resource-limited settings (RLS), rollout of ART with limited virological monitoring frequently results in the risk of prolonged virological failure with selection and accumulation of drug resistance mutations and subsequent transmission of drug resistance. Most surveys in RLS showed still low to moderate prevalence of TDR, but greater coverage of ART is associated with a higher prevalence of TDR. Also in RLS the rise in prevalence of TDR is mostly driven by NNRTI resistance, which is of particular concern as this drug class constitutes the foundation of current first-line ART regimens and prophylaxis for prevention of mother-to-child transmission.

Introduction

In the 1980s, soon after the introduction of the first antiretroviral drug zidovudine, the emergence of viral variants harboring mutations associated with decreased susceptibility to zidovudine was reported. In 1996, the development of viral load assays provided a tool for clinicians to monitor the efficacy of antiretroviral therapy (ART), and it became clear that the presence of drug resistance mutations was associated with therapy failure (Katzenstein and Holodniy 1995; Lorenzi et al. 1999).

The first case of transmission of drug resistance was described by Erice et al. (1993). A young homosexual man presented with a primary HIV-1 infection. Genotypic analysis of the virus before the start of zidovudine therapy showed the presence of a mutation at position 215 in reverse transcriptase, which is associated with decreased susceptibility to zidovudine. Phenotypic analysis confirmed the decreased susceptibility of the virus. The authors suggested that he acquired a zidovudine-resistant virus from a sexual partner who was receiving zidovudine and they already inferred that the possibility of horizontal transmission of resistance may have a great impact on the clinical approach to newly infected persons (Erice et al. 1993). More case reports followed that showed transmission of resistance via various routes such as injection drug use and vertical transmission (de Ronde et al. 1996) and transmission of resistance to other drugs than zidovudine, including multidrug resistance (Hecht et al. 1998).

Since these first case reports, many have studied the transmission of HIV drug resistance. In this chapter, we will discuss the current knowledge on the different aspects of transmitted drug resistance, including evolution, prevalence, and clinical significance.

Development of Drug Resistance and Viral Dynamics

HIV is an RNA virus, a retrovirus, characterized by the presence of a viral enzyme called reverse transcriptase. By reverse transcription of the viral RNA, this enzyme will form a DNA double helix, which subsequently is transversed to the cell nucleus and integrated into the host cell's genome by another viral enzyme: integrase. Transcription of proviral DNA results in the formation of new viral RNA and viral proteins that together will form a new viral particle. After budding and release of the viral particle, precursor polyproteins are cleaved by the viral enzyme protease, which results in the maturation of the particle to fully infectious virus. HIV replicates billions of times per day, but reverse transcriptase is lacking proofreading activity, thus introducing errors in each replication cycle (Perelson et al. 1996). As a result of these random mutations, a large number of slightly genetically distinct viral variants are circulating within a particular host, named quasispecies (Eigen 1993). However, mutations may affect the replicative capacity and thereby the fitness of the virus. In the absence of antiretroviral drugs, wild-type virus is considered the most fit variant and dominates the quasispecies.

Antiretroviral drugs that are currently available interfere with the different viral enzymes: reverse transcriptase (nucleoside reverse transcriptase inhibitors (NRTIs) and non-nucleoside reverse transcriptase inhibitors (NNRTIs)), protease (protease inhibitors (PIs)), and integrase (integrase inhibitors (INIs)). Entry inhibitors interfere at the level of binding and fusion of the viral membrane with the host cell membrane. It is important that ART sufficiently suppresses replication of the virus, because continued viral replication in the presence of antiretroviral drugs will often lead to the selection of viral variants with resistance mutations. In the presence of antiretroviral drugs, these resistance mutations provide a replication advantage, which will result in fixation of this mutation in the population. The drug-resistant variant will become the dominant variant in the quasispecies, since replication of wild-type virus is suppressed by the antiretroviral drugs. When ART is interrupted, the resistant variants suddenly no longer have a replication advantage but instead have an impaired fitness compared to wild-type virus. Over time, wild-type virus that is archived as proviral DNA in infected cells will emerge again and become the dominant variant (Fig. 1).

Resistance mutations appear in the quasispecies by random error. These mutations can become fixed and dominate the quasispecies in case of suboptimal treatment or incomplete adherence to therapy. This is called acquired or secondary resistance. Certain resistance mutations will only become fixed in the viral population in the presence of selective drug pressure, but other resistance mutations can be present as natural polymorphism and occur commonly in the absence of selective

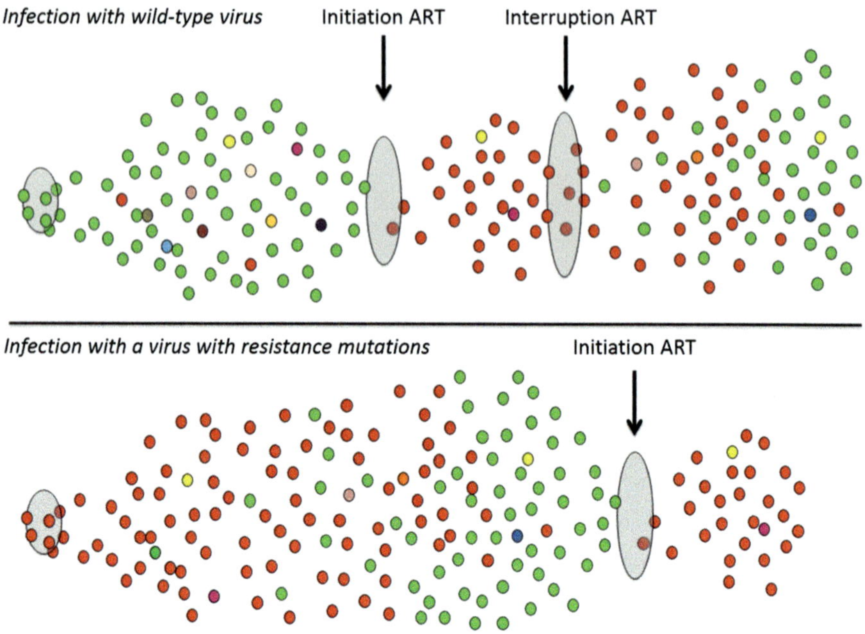

Fig. 1 Viral dynamics in acquired drug resistance (*top*) or transmitted drug resistance (*bottom*). *ART* antiretroviral therapy; *green variants* represent wild-type virus, *other colored variants* represent virus with mutations of which *red* variants represent virus with mutations that cause resistance to ART. Acquired drug resistance: after infection with wild-type virus, various variants with mutations emerge (quasispecies), but wild-type virus is the dominant variant. When ART is initiated but replication is not sufficiently suppressed, selection of variants with resistance mutations may occur, causing failure of therapy. When ART is interrupted, wild-type virus that is archived in proviral DNA will emerge and become the dominant variant again. Transmitted drug resistance: after infection with a virus with resistance mutations, reversion to wild type may occur over time. When ART is initiated, the initially transmitted variant with resistance mutations that is archived in proviral DNA may emerge and become the dominant variant, causing therapy failure

drug pressure. These resistance-associated natural polymorphisms only have a minor effect on susceptibility or only display an effect in a particular background. Resistance mutations can also be present in the dominant variant because the patient was initially infected with a drug-resistant strain, which is called primary resistance or transmitted drug resistance.

Evolution of Transmitted Drug Resistance

As described previously, in patients with acquired drug-resistant virus that emerged during therapy, a rapid reappearance of archived drug-susceptible virus has been observed at the time of treatment interruption as wild-type virus has a higher fitness than the resistant variants in absence of drug pressure. In contrast, in patients infected with a virus with resistance mutations, wild-type virus is usually not

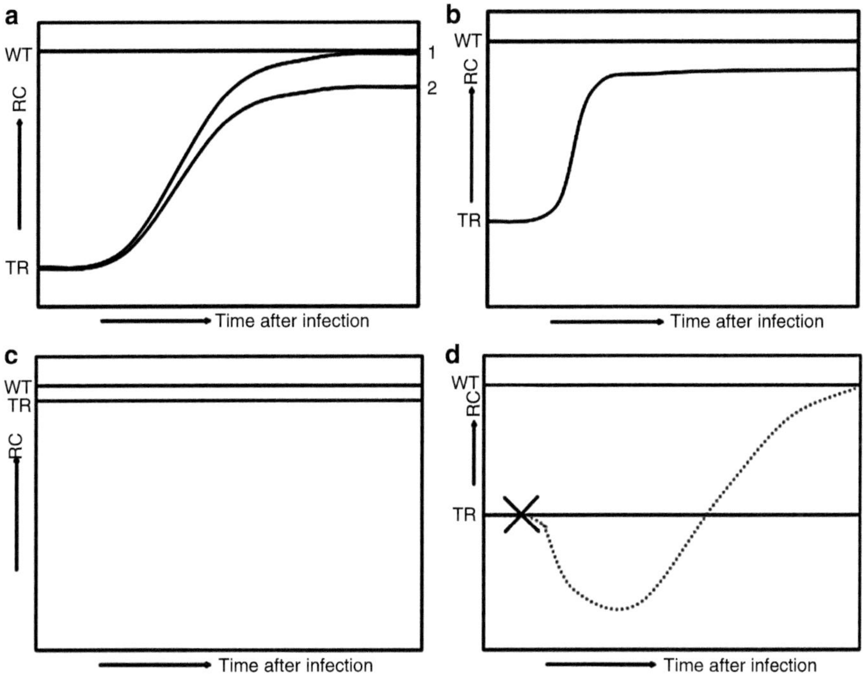

Fig. 2 Evolution of transmitted drug resistance. (**a**) Evolution to wild type. After transmission, the RC (y-axis) of the transmitted drug-resistant variant (*TR*) is lower than that of wild type (*WT*). Due to complete (1) or incomplete (2) reversion of the drug resistance mutation, the RC is restored or improved. (**b**) Selection of atypical mutations. After transmission of a drug-resistant HIV variant, atypical amino acids that are neither wild type nor intermediated may be selected, leading to improved RC. (**c**) Persistence because of a minimal reduction in RC. If the RC of the resistant variant (almost) equals the RC of wild type, persistence may occur for a considerable time. (**d**) Reversion is blocked by compensatory fixation. Due to compensatory mutations, multiple mutations are required for full reversion. The first mutation would decrease the RC, so reversion is blocked (Adapted from Pingen et al. JAC (2011))

co-transmitted and therefore not archived in latently infected cells. In the absence of drug pressure in the new host, transmitted viruses with resistance mutations may either (partly) revert to wild type, evolve to other variants, or persist in the viral population, depending on their relative fitness in the new environment. A recent review distinguished the particular pathways of evolution (Pingen et al. 2011) (Fig. 2).

Major drug resistance mutations may lower the replicative capacity of HIV. In the absence of drug pressure in a newly infected host, a virus with resistance mutations can revert rapidly to wild type if this has a substantial fitness benefit. A well-known example is the NRTI resistance mutation M184V/I, which has a significant negative effect on the replicative capacity. In a cohort of patients with acute HIV infection, the longitudinal follow-up of baseline mutations showed a markedly faster replacement of M184V/I than NNRTI mutations which only have a minor effect on replicative capacity (Jain et al. 2011). Since reversion from M184V/I to wild-type virus requires only one nucleotide change, a virus containing only M184V/I can rapidly revert to wild type with improved fitness.

Some resistance mutations require more than one mutation to revert to wild type, such as mutation T215Y/F in RT. Partial reversion to wild type results in intermediates (T215S/N/I). These intermediate variants have a replicative capacity similar to wild type and therefore tend to persist in the viral population. At position 215 in RT, also evolution toward atypical variants is often observed (T215C/D/L/V/G). A novel amino acid may be selected that is neither the wild-type amino acid nor an intermediate toward wild type. Due to the improved fitness compared to the originally transmitted variant, these atypical variants may persist for a long time. Both intermediate and atypical variants are called 215 revertants. Follow-up of ART-naïve patients showed that 215 revertants, in contrast to resistance mutation 215Y/F, were highly stable and are therefore often detected in treatment-naïve patients (Castro et al. 2013).

For some resistance mutations, it is known that they have a limited effect on the replicative capacity. There is no or only limited replicative advantage for wild-type virus; thus, the mutations may persist for years. Examples are NNRTI-resistance mutations, particularly K103N, and NRTI-resistance mutations L210W and K219R/G/Q/E (Little et al. 2008; Collins et al. 2004).

Persistence can also occur if reversion to wild type is not possible due to compensatory fixation by secondary mutations. This particular mechanism is seen if a primary resistance pattern is accompanied by one or more secondary (compensatory) mutations. These additional mutations have little or no contribution to the level of resistance, but (partly) compensate for the reduction in replicative capacity (Huigen et al. 2006). This process occurs in the drug-exposed host during therapy before the virus is transmitted, but has also been shown in vitro after transmission in absence of drug pressure. The pathway of reversion to wild type after the selection of compensatory mutations in the new host will include an initial decrease in fitness and therefore this pathway is blocked. As a result, viruses with drug resistance mutations may persist after transmission despite a lower replicative capacity than wild type.

First Insights in Prevalence of Transmitted Drug Resistance

After the first case reports of transmitted drug resistance, further analyses were performed to gain insight in the magnitude of this issue. The first studies on the prevalence of transmitted drug resistance were retrospectively performed in small cohorts of patients with primary HIV infection. During this time, patients were treated with mono- or dual therapy with thymidine analogues, which is now known to not sufficiently suppress the replication of HIV. A disturbing observation was the increasing prevalence of the resistance mutation at codon 215 in RT over time, from 1.4 % in 1988–1991 to 10.4 % in 1993–1994 (Mayers et al. 1995).

The increasing prevalence of transmitted resistance raised serious clinical and public health concerns and demonstrated the need to conduct epidemiologic surveys to monitor transmitted resistance. In the years when HAART (highly active antiretroviral therapy, a combination therapy with at least three drugs to sufficiently suppress HIV replication) became the standard of care, a study in a cohort of newly infected individuals, mostly homosexual men, from American urban areas showed a prevalence of 16.3 % (13/80), with multidrug resistance in three individuals (Boden et al. 1999). A Swiss study reported a prevalence of transmitted resistance of 11 % (9/82). The majority was infected with a virus harboring mutations associated with resistance to zidovudine. They observed an unexpected low prevalence of transmission of the M184V mutation, which causes high-level resistance to lamivudine and is frequently detected in patients failing on therapy that includes this compound (Yerly et al. 1999). The authors suggested that this supports the lower fitness of HIV-1 variants harboring the M184V mutation that had been shown in vitro (Schuurman et al. 1995). In 2002, two studies that only included patients with primary HIV infection showed that transmitted drug resistance was also increasing among recently infected patients (Little et al. 2002; Grant et al. 2002). One of the studies that was done in 10 American cities showed detection of genotypic resistance increasing to 22.7 % (Little et al. 2002). Both studies also reported a longer time to virological suppression after start of therapy in patients with transmitted drug resistance. This resulted in the first suggestions that clinicians could no longer rely on empirical treatment guidelines and that resistance testing should have a role in guiding antiretroviral therapy.

Guidelines on Drug Resistance

Due to the presumed lower replicative capacity of certain resistant viral variants, it was initially uncertain for how long the transmitted resistance mutations could be detected in the absence of drug pressure in the newly infected host. Therefore, guidelines first recommended drug resistance testing for subjects who are recently infected (Hirsch et al. 2003; Vandamme et al. 2004). A landmark study among more than 2000 individuals from 19 European countries showed that 10.4 % of patients who had never been exposed to ART carried HIV with ≥1 drug resistance mutation (Wensing et al. 2005a). A significant difference in prevalence was observed between recently infected patients (13.5 %) and patients infected for more than 1 year (8.7 %). This could either be due to a lower exposure to drug-resistant virus in the past or it is caused by reversion to wild-type viruses over time. Nevertheless, it was shown that drug resistance mutations could still be detected among a considerable percentage of chronically infected patients. As more evidence became available that variants with resistance mutations can persist, guidelines were updated and genotype testing was recommended for all newly diagnosed HIV patients at the moment of diagnosis (Hirsch et al. 2008). The routine use of baseline genotyping also allows large-scale surveillance of transmitted drug resistance.

In 1997, the International AIDS Society-USA assembled an independent panel of experts to review the data on antiretroviral drug resistance. They provided a first list summarizing common mutations selected by PIs, NRTIs, and NNRTIs

(Hirsch et al. 1998), which has been frequently updated since then with the latest published update in 2014 (Wensing et al. 2014). Periodically updates are also available online (www.iasusa.org). The current list includes 22 NRTI-resistance mutations, 34 NNRTI-resistance mutations, 75 PI-resistance mutations, 10 enfuvirtide resistance mutations, and 12 INI resistance mutations. The overview is designed to help clinicians identifying key mutations associated with viral resistance to antiretroviral drugs and to guide clinical decisions regarding antiretroviral therapy.

As previously explained, polymorphisms can occur in the absence of selective drug pressure. However for some polymorphisms it is known that they contribute to resistance to antiretroviral drugs. Since the IAS-USA list is used for clinical purposes, these particular polymorphisms are included in this list. But these polymorphic mutations should not be taken into account when one wants to monitor transmission of resistance, because presence of these polymorphisms before start of therapy is not an indication of drug pressure in a (previous) host. Including resistance-related polymorphisms in surveillance monitoring could lead to falsely elevated estimates of transmitted resistance (Wensing and Boucher 2003).

Many countries have implemented surveillance programs to monitor transmission of drug resistance. Study groups used different criteria to define transmitted drug resistance, resulting in widely varying estimates. In 2007, the WHO developed a consensus list of surveillance drug resistance mutations (SDRMs) (Bennett et al. 2009). A standard list of mutations would also allow comparison of prevalence of transmitted drug resistance from different times and regions. Four criteria were used to identify surveillance drug resistance mutations: (1) SDRMs should be recognized as causing or contributing to drug resistance, (2) mutations should be non-polymorphic and should not occur at highly polymorphic positions, (3) the mutation list had to be applicable to the eight most common HIV-1 subtypes, and (4) the list should be parsimonious, excluding mutations resulting exceedingly rarely from drug pressure. It is not a simple task to provide a list of mutations that are specific for transmitted drug resistance, since certain mutations associated with resistance in subtype B occur as polymorphisms in other subtypes. The list is subject of ongoing discussion and was last updated in 2009. It differs from the IAS-USA list in terms of number, position, and mutations and currently includes 93 mutations: 34 NRTI-resistance mutations at 15 RT positions, 19 NNRTI-resistance mutations at 10 RT positions, and 40 PI-resistance mutations at 18 protease positions (Fig. 3) (Bennett et al. 2009).

Current Trends

The prevalence of transmission of drug resistance varies among regions, risk groups, and drug classes, due to different exposure to ART, the use of diverse definitions of drug resistance mutations, varying sampling times after infection, and different risk behavior and access to therapy among risk groups.

NRTI		NNRTI		PI	
M41	L	L100	I	L23	I
K65	R	K101	E, P	L24	I
D67	N, G, E	K103	N, S	D30	N
T69	D, Ins	V106	M, A	V32	I
K70	R, E	V179	F	M46	I, L
L74	V, I	Y181	C, I, V	I47	V, A
V75	M, T, A, S	Y188	L, H, C	G48	V, M
F77	L	G190	A, S, E	I50	V, L
Y115	F	P225	H	F53	L, Y
F116	Y	M230	L	I54	V, L, M, A, T, S
Q151	M			G73	S, T, C, A
M184	V, I			L76	V
L210	W			V82	A, T, F, S, C, M, L
T215	Y, F, I, S, C, D, V, E			N83	D
K219	Q, E, N, R			I84	V, A, C
				I85	V
				N88	D, S
				L90	M

Fig. 3 Surveillance drug resistance mutations (SDRM) list of the WHO (Adapted from Bennett et al., PLoS One (2009))

Western Countries

In Europe, the overall prevalence of transmission of drug resistance seems to be stabilizing just below 10 % (Vercauteren et al. 2009; Hofstra et al. 2013a). A European surveillance cohort that includes newly diagnosed patients from 26 countries reported an overall prevalence of TDR of 9.2 % in 2008–2010. Mutations associated with resistance to NRTIs were observed most frequently (5.1 %), followed by resistance to NNRTIs (3.7 %). Regarding the different drug classes, no significant trends over time were observed (Hofstra et al. 2013a).

In the USA and Canada, an increasing prevalence of transmitted NNRTI resistance is observed. In a cohort of recently infected MSM in New York, enrolled from 1995 to 2010, the overall prevalence of resistance was 14.3 %. Over time NRTI resistance declined, but the prevalence of the NNRTI mutation K103N increased from 1.9 % to 8.0 % in 2010 (Castor et al. 2012). A cohort in San Francisco that included patients with acute HIV infection, mostly MSM, showed a rise in TDR from 2003 to 2007 to levels up to 24 %. Although this upward trend did not continue in 2008–2009, TDR remained substantial at 15 % (Jain et al. 2010). Convenience sampling of more than 18,000 newly diagnosed individuals of all risk groups in 2007–2010 from 10 surveillance areas in the USA showed an overall prevalence of 16.2 % transmitted drug resistance. The majority of transmitted drug resistance was due to mutations conferring drug resistance to a single drug class. Over time, NNRTI resistance significantly increased from 7.1 % in 2007 to 8.6 % in 2010, with K103N as the most frequent detected mutation (Kim et al. 2013). In a multi-site cohort of treatment-naïve individuals from Canada studied from 2002 to 2009, the overall prevalence was 13.6 %. An increase over time was observed which was driven by an increase in NRTI- and NNRTI-resistance mutations (Burchell et al. 2012).

This is likely due to the increased use of NNRTIs in first-line regimens. NNRTIs have a good efficacy and come with a low pill burden, but they have a low genetic barrier to resistance. A single amino acid change is sufficient to cause high-level resistance to most commonly used NNRTIs. These mutations (e.g., K103N) can be easily selected in patients failing on NNRTI-based regimens and can persist after transmission to a new host due to their limited effect on replicative capacity of the virus.

Transmission of PI resistance remains low in Europe (2.3 % in 2008–2010) (Hofstra et al. 2013a). In the different cohorts in the USA and Canada, prevalence of PI resistance varied between 2.7 % and 4.5 %. This is probably due to the preference of NNRTIs over PIs in first-line regimens. Furthermore, current PIs which are boosted with ritonavir have a high genetic barrier to resistance, rarely resulting in selection of PI-related resistance in protease in treated individuals.

In general, higher prevalence of transmitted drug resistance was reported in subtype B virus than in non-B viruses (Wensing et al. 2005a; Frentz et al. 2011). The question is whether this difference in prevalence can be attributed to the lack of exposure to drugs in countries with a high prevalence of non-B HIV or whether this is a result of specific viral characteristics. Furthermore, MSM infected with subtype B virus were more likely to be infected with drug-resistant HIV than other patients (Vercauteren et al. 2009). Risk behavior may play a role, although MSM may also be more exposed to antiretroviral drugs compared to patients from other risk groups.

Resource-Limited Setting

Sub-Saharan Africa has the largest number of people living with HIV/AIDS, an estimated 22.9 million people in 2010. This number is still increasing due to expanded access to antiretroviral therapy and care, currently reaching nearly 50 % of those in immediate need of therapy (World Health Organization et al. 2011). At the end of 2011, more than eight million people were receiving antiretroviral therapy in low- and middle-income countries, a dramatic 26-fold increase from December 2003 (World Health Organization 2012).

A consequence of ART scale-up is the possibility of treatment failure with the selection of drug-resistant HIV-1 variants (acquired drug resistance) and subsequent spread (transmitted drug resistance). In Europe and North America, the initial treatment with non-potent mono- and dual therapies resulted in high levels of acquired resistance and subsequent high levels of transmitted resistance. Due to increased potency of ART, virological monitoring, and baseline resistance testing to guide first-line therapy, the level of acquired resistance decreased and transmitted resistance stabilized. However, in resource-limited settings, both history and conditions of HIV treatment have been very different, making it difficult to predict trends for transmitted drug resistance in the developing world.

Antiretroviral drugs were initially introduced into African countries through preventing mother-to-child transmission (PMTCT) programs. Zidovudine was the first drug used in 1994, followed by nevirapine, lamivudine, efavirenz, tenofovir, and lopinavir. Single-dose usage of nevirapine resulted in a high prevalence of acquired nevirapine resistance in both mothers and infants. The public health approach of the WHO for the recent scale-up of ART is based on simplified treatment protocols, including standard first-line NNRTI-based regimens and second-line boosted PI-based regimens. A recognized limitation of NNRTI-based regimens is their relatively lower genetic barrier to resistance when compared to boosted PI regimens (World Health Organization 2012). Suboptimal regimens, such as the peripartum use of single-dose nevirapine in PMTCT, drug interactions (e.g., concomitant use of tuberculostatic therapy), inappropriate prescribing practices, and poor adherence can further increase the risk of acquiring drug resistance. Programmatic factors such as limited human resources, inadequate infrastructure, and weak supply management systems can negatively influence treatment adherence and retention in care and can result in drug stockouts (Hamers et al. 2013). A WHO survey showed that in 2004–2009, a large proportion of ART programs in 2107 clinics in more than 50 countries did not perform optimally regarding patient adherence, retention in care, and drug supply continuity, raising concern on potential increasing drug resistance (World Health Organization 2012). Abrupt interruption of combination therapy is of particular concern for selection of NNRTI resistance, since the longer plasma half-life of efavirenz results in functional efavirenz monotherapy with a low genetic barrier for resistance.

Plasma viral load testing is not generally available to monitor the efficacy of therapy and detect therapy failure. Instead, monitoring is often based on clinical staging and CD4 cell counts. However, it has been shown that virological failure precedes the WHO-defined immunological and clinical failure, often with detection of NNRTI resistance. Rapid accumulation of drug resistance (mostly NRTI resistance) occurred when ART was continued despite virological failure, resulting in the loss of treatment options (Barth et al. 2012). A randomized controlled trial at seven primary health clinics in rural Kenya showed that 6 monthly viral load testing of patients taking ART reduced the risk of virological failure at 18 months of follow-up with 46 % (Sawe et al. 2013). New guidelines of the WHO advise viral load testing at 6 months after initiating therapy and every 12 months thereafter (World Health Organization 2013).

Baseline resistance testing is not readily available and is mainly performed within studies and WHO surveys to monitor transmitted drug resistance. The WHO survey method is intended to classify transmitted resistance as low (<5 %), moderate (5–15 %), or high (>15 %) and is not meant as representative surveillance for the entire country.

In 2004–2010, 72 WHO surveys have been conducted in 26 countries, of which 52 (72.2 %) had a low prevalence classification to all drug classes (World Health Organization 2012). Twenty surveys showed moderate levels of transmitted drug resistance. Main detected mutations included NNRTI-resistance mutations (K103N, Y181C) and M184V and to a lesser extent TAMs (thymidine analogue mutations). Pooled analysis indicated that the estimated prevalence of transmitted HIV drug resistance to NNRTIs increased between 2004 and 2010, particularly in the African region. The data suggested that greater coverage of ART was associated with a higher prevalence of TDR, particularly to NNRTIs (Fig. 4) (World Health Organization 2012). The PharmAccess African Studies to Evaluate Resistance Monitoring (PASER-M) cohort study among 2,436 antiretroviral-naïve individuals in 11 geographic areas in Kenya, Nigeria, South Africa, Uganda, Zambia, and Zimbabwe reported an overall baseline prevalence of drug resistance of 5.6 %. They estimated a 38 % increase of the average rate of resistance per year since ART rollout (Hamers et al. 2011).

In Asia, ART is also being rapidly scaled up, based on a similar public health approach as seen in sub-Saharan Africa. Several surveys have been done, but generally the studies have small sample sizes. Furthermore, generalizability is limited because the methodology is often unstandardized and based on convenience sampling that is often performed in urban populations or only in a particular risk group. Despite these caveats, most of the performed surveys report a low prevalence of TDR (Trotter et al. 2013; Yu et al. 2011). The TREAT Asia Studies to Evaluate Resistance Monitoring (TASER-M) program studied prevalence of transmitted drug resistance in 1,340 ART-naïve patients from 11 sites in Thailand, Malaysia, Hong Kong, Philippines, and Indonesia from 2007 to 2010 (Kiertiburanakul et al. 2013). With use of the WHO surveillance list for TDR, they reported a prevalence of 4.0 %. The TASER-S (Surveillance) program included 458 recently infected patients from four sites and reported a slightly higher prevalence of 6.1 % (Kiertiburanakul et al. 2013). A recent review of available studies in naïve patients from Asia that also used the WHO surveillance list for TDR reported an overall prevalence of 7.6 % (Stadeli and Richman 2013). Regarding the different drug classes, resistance mutations related to NRTIs (4.3 %) and NNRTIs (3.8 %) were observed most frequently. Only 0.3 % had resistance mutations associated with PIs. Compared to patients in Africa, Asian patients were more likely to harbor a virus with resistance mutations. In some Asian countries such as Thailand and Vietnam, ART has been available since the mid-1990s and included the use of suboptimal dual nucleoside regimens which may have resulted in higher levels of acquired drug resistance and subsequent transmitted drug resistance.

Recently a comprehensive global assessment of published studies and WHO surveys was performed on HIV-1 drug resistance in untreated patients, including 26,102 persons in 42 countries (Gupta et al. 2012). East Africa had the highest estimated rate of increase at 29 % per year since rollout, with estimated resistance prevalence at 8 years after rollout of 7.4 %. An annual increase of 14 % was estimated in Southern Africa. For West and Central Africa, Latin America, and Caribbean, no such increase was found. For Asia, no consistent trend could be observed due to the small amount of studies that were mainly done in Thailand, China, India, and Vietnam and due to the large differences among these countries.

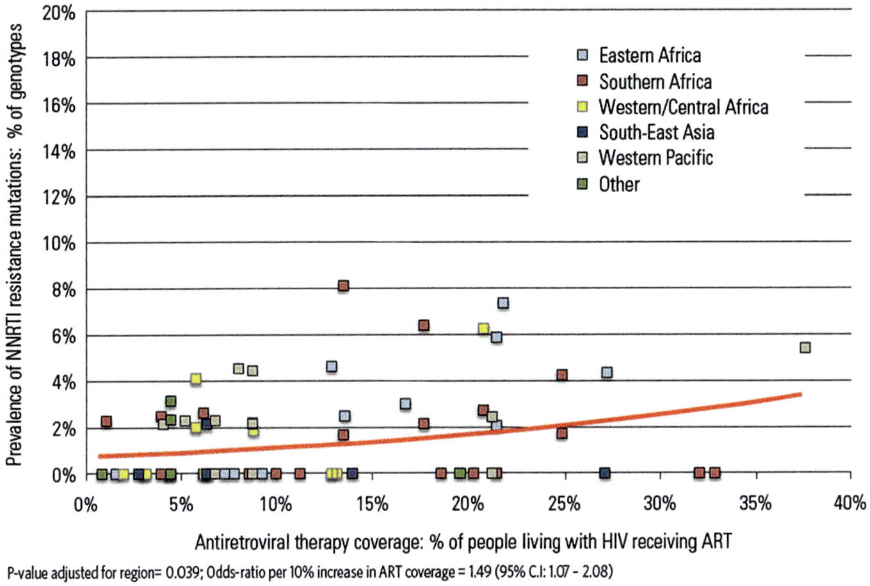

Fig. 4 Relationship between transmitted resistance mutations to NNRTI drugs and antiretroviral therapy coverage (Adapted from World Health Organization, *The HIV drug resistance report – 2012* (World Health Organization 2012))

Particularly NNRTI resistance increased substantially in east and southern Africa. However, a limitation of the meta-analysis was that the data included in the analyses were not likely to represent national prevalences, since most studies included urban populations, where ART coverage and pre-rollout ART use is likely to be higher than in rural areas.

In summary, cumulated data suggest a rise in TDR in east and southern Africa after ART scale-up. The rise is mostly driven by NNRTI resistance, which is of particular concern, as this drug class constitutes the foundation of current first-line ART regimens and prophylaxis for prevention of mother-to-child transmission. It highlights the need for virological monitoring of therapy failure and the importance of establishing surveillance of transmitted drug resistance. However, despite the rise in transmitted drug resistance, the current standard first- and second-line regimens are still shown to be effective in the majority of patients in resource-limited settings (Barth et al. 2010; Schoffelen et al. 2013; Siripassorn et al. 2010).

Molecular Epidemiology: Sources of Transmitted Drug Resistance

The availability of baseline resistance data of newly diagnosed HIV patients allows studying phylogenetic relationships. A large percentage of patients with recent HIV infection are part of transmission clusters, indicating that patients in early stage of infection play an important role in the spread of HIV (Brenner et al. 2007, 2008). Longitudinal studies among HIV serodiscordant couples in the Ugandan Rakai cohort also showed that the rate of HIV transmission was highest during early-stage infection (Wawer et al. 2005). In the early stage of infection, HIV RNA plasma levels are high, and the majority of patients is still unaware of their infection and therefore may not have yet adapted their risk behavior. A Swiss study showed that almost half of the transmitted drug resistance was linked to transmission clusters that included only newly diagnosed individuals (Yerly et al. 2009). For a long time, it had been assumed that transmitted drug resistance reflects direct infection from drug-experienced individuals, but these results demonstrated that newly diagnosed untreated individuals are also a source of onward transmission of drug resistance.

Onward transmission of resistance by treatment-naïve individuals may represent a limit to the decline in transmitted drug resistance. In Europe, a stable prevalence is observed, in particular for NRTI-resistance mutations. Thymidine analogue mutations (TAMs), such as M41L and T215Y/F, are usually selected in patients failing on regimens that include zidovudine or stavudine. Despite the decreased use of these compounds in first-line regimens, M41L and T215 revertants are among the most frequent observed mutations in case of transmitted drug resistance, most likely due to onward transmission by naïve patients. This phenomenon is also proposed as an explanation for the substantial level of transmitted drug resistance (15 %) in acutely infected patients in San Francisco, besides the increasing NNRTI resistance (Jain et al. 2010). Phylogenetic analysis of more than 2500 HIV-infected MSM in Montreal (Canada) revealed between 2002 and 2009 an episodic expansion of sub-epidemics with NNRTI-resistant virus among therapy-naïve individuals (Brenner et al. 2012).

Cluster analyses in the UK and the Netherlands have shown that drug-resistant viruses can circulate for a prolonged time among therapy-naïve patients, up to 8 years (Hue et al. 2009; Hofstra et al. 2013b). In the cluster observed in the Netherlands, it concerned a virus harboring a partly reverted resistance pattern. In clinical practice when such a reverted pattern is detected in naïve patients, the possibility that reversion occurred in these patients and initial infection was established by a fully resistant virus is usually taken into account. Concerns for more extensive resistance present in the quasispecies then result in the choice of more complex initial regimens with a higher genetic barrier, increased pill burden, more frequent toxicity, and elevated costs. However, the prolonged onward transmission of this particular strain made it more likely that reversion occurred in previous hosts in the transmission chain (Hofstra et al. 2013b). Mutation patterns that are frequently observed are single mutations or combinations of partly reverted TAMs. These patterns have little effect on replicative capacity which could be one of the reasons these patterns are transmitted by and circulating among therapy-naïve individuals. In this case, fear of hidden extensive resistance may not be necessary and one can initiate standard first-line therapy. The use of phylogeny to identify clusters may provide insight into the risk of more extensive resistance patterns in the quasispecies and prevent excessive use of antivirals.

Transmissibility of Resistant Virus

As was already noted in the early reports on transmitted drug resistance, there is a discrepancy in resistant profiles observed in drug-experienced patients failing treatment and those detected in treatment-naïve patients. This has been attributed to the well-known fitness costs of certain resistance mutations, which have not only been observed in vitro but also in vivo, reflected by a lower pre-therapy viral load in patients with the M184V mutation (Harrison et al. 2010). Plasma HIV RNA levels are one of the correlates of risk of transmission (Quinn et al. 2000). It has been hypothesized that drug-resistant variants may also have reduced transmission capacity.

Clinical studies evaluated this issue by comparing the percentage of acquired drug resistance among potential transmitters to the actual detected percentage of transmitted drug resistance among acutely HIV-infected individuals in the same region. Both studies observed lower transmission of resistance than could be expected based on the prevalence of acquired drug resistance and suggested that this could be due to a lower transmissibility of resistant variants (Leigh Brown et al. 2003; Yerly et al. 2004). However, a possible confounder is the risk behavior of the potential transmitters. Patients who failed on therapy may be more ill and therefore more likely to have reduced sexual activity and/or may have adapted their risk behavior to their HIV-positive status. Furthermore, these studies may underestimate the prevalence of transmitted drug resistance due to reversion of resistance mutations in untreated individuals. A study that used a more sensitive method to detect resistant variants showed that the M184V mutation is transmitted at higher rates than currently detected in clinical practice because its presence wanes over time (Wainberg et al. 2011).

Two recent studies did show diminished transmission efficiency relative to wild-type virus. In macaques, efficient systemic infection with SHIV162P3 mutants (M184V and K65R) after rectal and vaginal exposure required an increase in the virus inocula compared to wild-type SHIV162P3 (Cong et al. 2011). In a skin model, drug-resistant variants with a low replicative capacity (M184V/I/T) were less able to infect primary Langerhans cells compared to resistant viruses with a higher replicative capacity (K103N) or wild-type virus. Subsequent transmission to target cells was also decreased in these resistant variants (Pingen et al. 2014). This issue needs further study in the future.

Clinical Outcome of Transmitted Drug Resistance

In 2002 the first studies showed that patients infected with a virus with drug resistance mutations needed a longer period of time after initiation of treatment to achieve virological suppression while the time to virological failure was shorter, compared to patients infected with wild-type virus (Little et al. 2002; Grant et al. 2002). Virological failure was not only observed earlier, but also more frequently in case of transmitted drug resistance (Violin et al. 2004; Kuritzkes et al. 2008). Chronically infected patients with primary resistance from a German cohort that received a first-line regimen based on the results of resistance testing reported a similar efficacy of first-line HAART as patients infected with wild type, which suggested that resistance test guidance for selection of first-line regimen could improve therapy outcome (Oette et al. 2006). This was recently confirmed in a retrospective study that included over 10,000 patients who initiated combination therapy after 1998 (Wittkop et al. 2011). Of patients with TDR who received a regimen that was not fully active against the virus, 15.1 % experienced virological failure at 12 months. In contrast, patients infected with wild-type virus or patients with TDR who received a regimen that was still fully active against the virus experienced virological failure at much lower rates (4.2 % and 4.7 %, respectively). Patients with low-level or intermediate resistance to at least one drug had a 2.2-fold higher risk for virological failure, while patients with high-level resistance to at least one drug had a 6.3 times higher risk (Fig. 5). A recent study among more than 1,600 patients from 13 European centers who are receiving an efavirenz (NNRTI)-based regimen as first-line regimen also showed that intermediate baseline resistance to one drug significantly increases the risk of virological failure (Swartz et al. 2015).

It is clear that transmitted drug resistance influences therapy outcome, but whether it also impacts the natural course of the infection remains subject of debate. A faster CD4 cell decline in the first year of infection in patients with transmitted drug resistance was observed. However, a negative impact on the longer term was not demonstrated (Pillay et al. 2006). An alarming case report described a patient who was recently infected with a viral variant of HIV resistant to multiple classes of antiretroviral but who progressed to symptomatic AIDS in 4–20 months (Markowitz et al. 2005). The probable source patient and his partner experienced a relatively indolent clinical course, suggesting that possibly other factors than the virologic properties (such as genetic, immunological, or behavioral factors) may have contributed to the rapid clinical decline described in the case report (Blick et al. 2007). Comparison of patients infected with resistant virus vs. wild-type virus showed no significant difference in progression to AIDS in the first year (Wensing et al. 2005b).

Minority HIV Variants

The high mutation rate of HIV allows quick adaptation to new environments, where the viral variant with the highest fitness will dominate the quasispecies. When wild-type virus is the dominant variant, resistance mutations can still be present in minority variants. Genotypic testing in clinical practice is performed with population (Sanger) sequencing, which is limited to the detection of viral variants that constitute 10–20 % of the total virus population in a sample (Larder et al. 1993). To detect minority variants, more sensitive methods have been developed, utilizing two main approaches: point mutations assays and newer sequencing technologies.

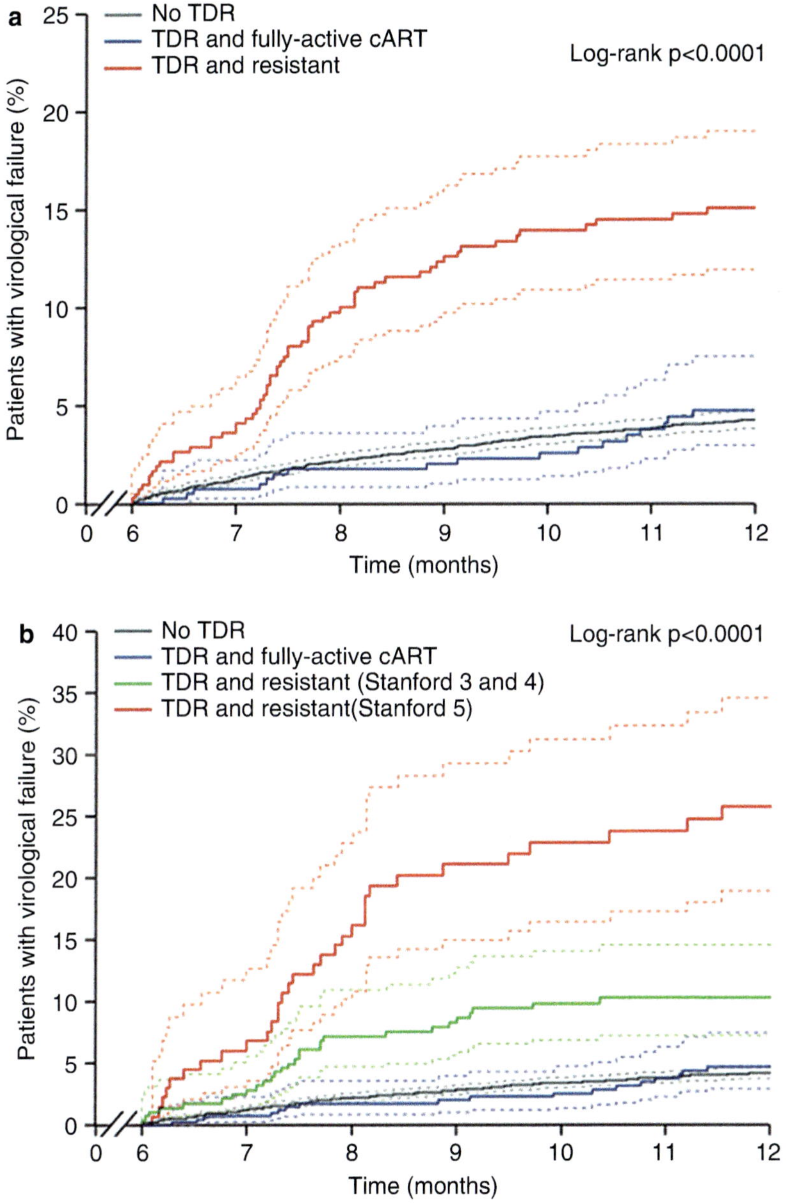

Fig. 5 Kaplan-Meier estimates of the proportion of patients with virological failure. (**a**) Risk of virological failure according to patient groups. (**b**) Risk of virological failure in patients with intermediate- and high-level resistance. *cART* combination antiretroviral therapy. *TDR* transmitted drug resistance. *Dotted lines* = 95 % CI (Adapted from Wittkop et al. (2011))

Point mutation assays such as allele-specific polymerase chain reaction (AS-PCR) are generally highly sensitive and specific for detecting a selected minority drug resistance mutation, but are limited to the detection of only a single point mutation at a time. In contrast, newer sequencing methods including single-genome sequencing (SGS) and ultra-deep pyrosequencing (UDPS) permit analyses of the entire sequence context but are more labor intensive and costly than point mutation assays. Allele-specific PCR can detect minorities at frequencies as low as 0.01 %, but may generate false positive results at the lower level of detection. Therefore, for each mutation one needs to assess the individual cutoff of detection. This is not necessary for the newer sequencing methods, which can detect viral variants at frequencies <1 %. For both approaches, the tested sample must have a large enough viral population size to ensure representative results on the minority variants present (Gianella and Richman 2010).

Using these more sensitive methods, minority resistant variants have been detected in acutely infected individuals that were not detected by population sequencing (Metzner et al. 2005; Toni et al. 2009). Possibly current surveillance studies with use of population sequencing are underestimating transmission of drug resistance. It had been shown that persisting minority resistant variants in NNRTI-experienced patients contributed to failure of an NNRTI regimen (Halvas et al. 2010). Whether the presence of minority resistant variants in therapy-naïve patients may affect the response to antiretroviral treatment is an essential question that remains subject of debate.

To date, several studies have been performed to determine the prevalence of baseline minority resistance mutations and their influence on rates of virological failure. Minority drug resistance mutations were detected in patients with wild-type virus by standard population sequencing (Paredes et al. 2010; Johnson et al. 2008). With the use of AS-PCR that could detect minority variants with K103N at levels as low as 0.003 % and Y181C at 0.03 %, one study detected minority variants in up to 40 % of patients (Paredes et al. 2010). Most studies showed that minority NNRTI- and NRTI-resistant variants significantly increased the risk of failure, particularly for NNRTI-based regimens, but not all could demonstrate such an effect. The studies have been performed on small cohorts, usually less than 100 patients. Therefore, a pooled analysis of the data of 10 studies was performed, including 1,263 patients, which showed that the presence of drug-resistant minority variants was associated with more than twice the risk of virological failure in patients receiving an initial NNRTI-based regimen, after controlling for adherence, race, baseline CD4 cell count, and baseline HIV RNA load (Li et al. 2011).

Not all patients with presence of drug-resistant minority variants experienced virological failure. It was shown that the presence of minority variants above 1 % conferred a higher risk of failure compared to minority variants present at less than 1 %. To explain this observation, the authors proposed a theory that minorities can arise from different sources: mutations present at frequencies >1 % may represent transmitted drug resistance that over time has been replaced by wild-type revertants, whereas mutations at lower frequencies could be the result of de novo mutations resulting from random error or laboratory artifacts (Li et al. 2011).

A previous study proposed to distinguish between proportion and magnitude of drug-resistant variants in the population. By multiplying the proportion of virus harboring resistance mutation K103N in RT and the viral load, Goodman et al. showed that the number of resistant copies correlated better with the rate of failure than the proportion of drug-resistant variants (Goodman et al. 2011). It has been frequently shown that viral load correlates with failure. In some clinical trials, particular regimens were less successful in patients with higher viral loads, which could be due to a higher load of resistant variants. The pooled analysis also showed an increasing risk of failure when the number of resistant copies increased (Li et al. 2011).

Resistance testing after the occurrence of virological failure in the patients of the pooled analysis showed that the presence of NNRTI-resistant minority variants was associated with an increased risk of NNRTI resistance detected at virological failure. However, the emerged resistance at failure frequently differed from those detected as minority variants at baseline. The researchers proposed several explanations for this unexpected finding: minority variants could predispose for the development of additional resistance mutations or more fit resistant variants have been selected before failure was detected. They also suggest the possibility that there could have been other undetected resistance mutations that eventually became the dominant species (Li et al. 2013).

The question is whether results of these sensitive assays can guide clinical decisions on treatment in the future. More research is necessary to establish a threshold and understand at what point a minority resistant variant may become clinically relevant.

Transmitted Drug Resistance to Other Classes

Maraviroc is an antagonist of CC chemokine receptor 5 (CCR5), one of the coreceptors used by the virus for cell binding and is the only antiretroviral drug aiming at a human instead of viral target. Resistance to maraviroc is not fully understood. There is yet no consensus on specific signature mutations that are associated with resistance of CCR5-tropic viruses to maraviroc. Resistance may also evolve from a tropism switch resulting in the use of the CXCR4 coreceptor, which also occurs without maraviroc pressure. As such no data can be presented on transmitted resistance to maraviroc.

Enfuvirtide is a fusion inhibitor that is not often used in clinical practice because it needs to be injected twice daily. In contrast to maraviroc, for enfuvirtide several signature mutations in the first heptad repeat (HR1) region of the gp41 envelope gene are described (Wensing et al. 2014). In 2007 the first two cases of transmitted drug resistance to enfuvirtide were reported in a cohort of 53 newly infected patients (Peuchant et al. 2007). Surveillance studies usually include only the *pol* region; therefore, no extensive baseline reports for transmitted resistance to enfuvirtide are available.

Integrase inhibitors (INIs) are a potent option for treatment of HIV and are becoming more in use in first-line treatment. Both raltegravir and elvitegravir are highly efficacious in first-line ART with small numbers of failure in clinical trials. However, both have a relatively low genetic barrier to resistance and cross-resistance between the two drugs precludes their sequential use. Dolutegravir does retain activity against most viruses that are resistant to raltegravir and elvitegravir (Geretti et al. 2012). With the increasing use in clinical practice, acquired resistance to INIs and subsequent transmitted drug resistance may emerge. The first two cases of transmitted drug resistance to INIs were reported in 2011 (Boyd et al. 2011; Young et al. 2011). Both cases were antiretroviral-naïve patients with multidrug resistance. In a cohort of 79 antiretroviral-naïve patients who were recently infected in a time when INIs were in use, no transmitted INI drug resistance was observed (Cossarini et al. 2011). It is too early to perform INI resistance testing routinely, but the two case reports show that INI resistance testing currently has additional value in patients that present with multiclass transmitted drug resistance. More surveys will be done in the future to determine at which point in time the prevalence of integrase mutations among treatment-naïve patients rises to a level that warrants routine baseline resistance testing for INI resistance.

Conclusion

Transmitted drug resistance remains an issue of concern. Due to onward transmission of drug resistance by therapy-naïve individuals that is observed in developed countries and the rise in acquired drug resistance and subsequent transmitted drug resistance after ART rollout in resource-limited settings, it is unlikely that the prevalence of transmitted drug resistance will decrease in the near future. In particular, the rising resistance to NNRTIs, a drug class that is frequently used as first line – in both developed countries and resource-limited settings – warrants continued surveillance. As this drug class has a low genetic barrier to development of resistance, possibly even minority resistant variants may have an impact on clinical outcome. Future research with the use of more sensitive assays is necessary to establish a threshold for clinically relevant resistant variants. In addition, future surveillance efforts will include *integrase* resistance testing, to monitor transmitted drug resistance to integrase inhibitors, a drug class that will be increasingly used in first-line therapy.

References

Barth RE et al (2010) Virological follow-up of adult patients in antiretroviral treatment programmes in sub-Saharan Africa: a systematic review. Lancet Infect Dis 10(3):155–166

Barth RE et al (2012) Accumulation of drug resistance and loss of therapeutic options precede commonly used criteria for treatment failure in HIV-1 subtype-C-infected patients. Antivir Ther 17(2):377–386

Bennett DE et al (2009) Drug resistance mutations for surveillance of transmitted HIV-1 drug-resistance: 2009 update. PLoS One 4(3):e4724

Blick G et al (2007) The probable source of both the primary multidrug-resistant (MDR) HIV-1 strain found in a patient with rapid progression to AIDS and a second recombinant MDR strain found in a chronically HIV-1-infected patient. J Infect Dis 195(9):1250–1259

Boden D et al (1999) HIV-1 drug resistance in newly infected individuals. JAMA 282 (12):1135–1141

Boyd SD et al (2011) Transmitted raltegravir resistance in an HIV-1 CRF_AG-infected patient. Antivir Ther 16(2):257–261

Brenner BG et al (2007) High rates of forward transmission events after acute/early HIV-1 infection. J Infect Dis 195(7):951–959

Brenner BG et al (2008) Transmission networks of drug resistance acquired in primary/early stage HIV infection. AIDS 22(18):2509–2515

Brenner BG et al (2012) Spread of sub-epidemics resistant to non-nucleoside analogues among treatment-naive MSM: Montreal. In: 19th conference on retroviruses and opportunistic infections, Seattle, p Paper # 73

Burchell AN et al (2012) Increase in transmitted HIV drug resistance among persons undergoing genotypic resistance testing in Ontario, Canada, 2002–09. J Antimicrob Chemother 67 (11):2755–2765

Castor D et al (2012) Transmitted drug resistance and phylogenetic relationships among acute and early HIV-1-infected individuals in New York City. J Acquir Immune Defic Syndr 61 (1):1–8

Castro H et al (2013) Persistence of HIV-1 transmitted drug resistance mutations. J Infect Dis 208:1459–1463

Collins JA et al (2004) Competitive fitness of nevirapine-resistant human immunodeficiency virus type 1 mutants. J Virol 78(2):603–611

Cong ME et al (2011) Generation and mucosal transmissibility of emtricitabine- and tenofovir-resistant SHIV162P3 mutants in macaques. Virology 412(2):435–440

Cossarini F et al (2011) Integrase and fusion inhibitors transmitted drug resistance in naive patients with recent diagnosis of HIV-1 infection. J Acquir Immune Defic Syndr 56(2):e51–e54

de Ronde A et al (1996) First case of new infection with zidovudine-resistant HIV-1 among prospectively studied intravenous drug users and homosexual men in Amsterdam, The Netherlands. AIDS 10(2):231–232

Eigen M (1993) Viral quasispecies. Sci Am 269(1):42–49

Erice A et al (1993) Brief report: primary infection with zidovudine-resistant human immunodeficiency virus type 1. N Engl J Med 328(16):1163–1165

Frentz D et al (2011) Transmission of HIV resistant to non-nucleoside RT inhibitors is rising in MSM in Europe. In: 13th European AIDS conference, Belgrade, p Abstract PS1/5

Geretti AM, Armenia D, Ceccherini-Silberstein F (2012) Emerging patterns and implications of HIV-1 integrase inhibitor resistance. Curr Opin Infect Dis 25(6):677–686

Gianella S, Richman DD (2010) Minority variants of drug-resistant HIV. J Infect Dis 202 (5):657–666

Goodman DD et al (2011) Low level of the K103N HIV-1 above a threshold is associated with virological failure in treatment-naive individuals undergoing efavirenz-containing therapy. AIDS 25(3):325–333

Grant RM et al (2002) Time trends in primary HIV-1 drug resistance among recently infected persons. JAMA 288(2):181–188

Gupta RK et al (2012) Global trends in antiretroviral resistance in treatment-naive individuals with HIV after rollout of antiretroviral treatment in resource-limited settings: a global collaborative study and meta-regression analysis. Lancet 380(9849):1250–1258

Halvas EK et al (2010) Low frequency nonnucleoside reverse-transcriptase inhibitor-resistant variants contribute to failure of efavirenz-containing regimens in treatment- experienced patients. J Infect Dis 201(5):672–680

Hamers RL et al (2011) HIV-1 drug resistance in antiretroviral-naive individuals in sub-Saharan Africa after rollout of antiretroviral therapy: a multicentre observational study. Lancet Infect Dis 11(10):750–759

Hamers RL et al (2013) Emerging HIV-1 drug resistance after roll-out of antiretroviral therapy in sub-Saharan Africa. Curr Opin HIV AIDS 8(1):19–26

Harrison L et al (2010) The effect of transmitted HIV-1 drug resistance on pre-therapy viral load. AIDS 24(12):1917–1922

Hecht FM et al (1998) Sexual transmission of an HIV-1 variant resistant to multiple reverse-transcriptase and protease inhibitors. N Engl J Med 339(5):307–311

Hirsch MS et al (1998) Antiretroviral drug resistance testing in adults with HIV infection: implications for clinical management. International AIDS Society – USA Panel. JAMA 279 (24):1984–1991

Hirsch MS et al (2003) Antiretroviral drug resistance testing in adults infected with human immunodeficiency virus type 1: 2003 recommendations of an International AIDS Society-USA Panel. Clin Infect Dis 37(1):113–128

Hirsch MS et al (2008) Antiretroviral drug resistance testing in adult HIV-1 infection: 2008 recommendations of an International AIDS Society-USA panel. Clin Infect Dis 47(2):266–285

Hofstra LM et al (2013a) Stable proportion but increasing number of HIV-1 diagnoses with transmitted drug resistance across Europe. In: 14th European AIDS conference, Brussels

Hofstra LM et al (2013b) Evolution and viral characteristics of a long-term circulating resistant HIV-1 strain in a cluster of treatment-naive patients. J Antimicrob Chemother 68(6):1246–1250

Hue S et al (2009) Demonstration of sustained drug-resistant human immunodeficiency virus type 1 lineages circulating among treatment-naive individuals. J Virol 83(6):2645–2654

Huigen M, Albert J, Lindstrom A (2006) Compensatory fixation explains long term persistence of the M41L in HIV-1 reverse transcriptase in a large transmission cluster. In: 15th international HIV drug resistance workshop: basic principles and clinical implications, Sitges

Jain V et al (2010) Transmitted drug resistance in persons with acute/early HIV-1 in San Francisco, 2002–2009. PLoS One 5(12):e15510

Jain V et al (2011) Differential persistence of transmitted HIV-1 drug resistance mutation classes. J Infect Dis 203(8):1174–1181

Johnson JA et al (2008) Minority HIV-1 drug resistance mutations are present in antiretroviral treatment-naive populations and associate with reduced treatment efficacy. PLoS Med 5(7):e158

Katzenstein DA, Holodniy M (1995) HIV viral load quantification, HIV resistance, and antiretroviral therapy. AIDS Clin Rev 96:277–303

Kiertiburanakul S et al (2013) Comparisons of primary HIV-1 drug resistance between recent and Chronic HIV-1 infection within a sub-regional cohort of Asian patients. PLoS One 8(6): e62057

Kim D et al (2013) Trend in transmitted HIV-1 ARV drug resistance-associated mutations: 10 HIV surveillance areas, US, 2007–2010. In: 20th conference on retroviruses and opportunistic infections, Atlanta, Paper #149

Kuritzkes DR et al (2008) Preexisting resistance to nonnucleoside reverse-transcriptase inhibitors predicts virologic failure of an efavirenz-based regimen in treatment-naive HIV-1-infected subjects. J Infect Dis 197(6):867–870

Larder BA et al (1993) Quantitative detection of HIV-1 drug resistance mutations by automated DNA sequencing. Nature 365(6447):671–673

Leigh Brown AJ et al (2003) Transmission fitness of drug-resistant human immunodeficiency virus and the prevalence of resistance in the antiretroviral-treated population. J Infect Dis 187 (4):683–686

Li JZ et al (2011) Low-frequency HIV-1 drug resistance mutations and risk of NNRTI-based antiretroviral treatment failure: a systematic review and pooled analysis. JAMA 305 (13):1327–1335

Li JZ et al (2013) Impact of minority nonnucleoside reverse transcriptase inhibitor resistance mutations on resistance genotype after virologic failure. J Infect Dis 207(6):893–897

Little SJ et al (2002) Antiretroviral-drug resistance among patients recently infected with HIV. N Engl J Med 347(6):385–394
Little SJ et al (2008) Persistence of transmitted drug resistance among subjects with primary human immunodeficiency virus infection. J Virol 82(11):5510–5518
Lorenzi P et al (1999) Impact of drug resistance mutations on virologic response to salvage therapy. Swiss HIV Cohort Study. AIDS 13(2):F17–F21
Markowitz M et al (2005) Infection with multidrug resistant, dual-tropic HIV-1 and rapid progression to AIDS: a case report. Lancet 365(9464):1031–1038
Mayers DL et al (1995) Prevalence and clinical course of persons seroconverting with AZT-resistant HIV-1 in Switzerland, Australia and the United States between 1988 and 1994. AIDS Res Hum Retroviruses 11(suppl 1):S162 (abstract)
Metzner KJ et al (2005) Detection of minor populations of drug-resistant HIV-1 in acute seroconverters. AIDS 19(16):1819–1825
Oette M et al (2006) Primary HIV drug resistance and efficacy of first-line antiretroviral therapy guided by resistance testing. J Acquir Immune Defic Syndr 41(5):573–581
Paredes R et al (2010) Pre-existing minority drug-resistant HIV-1 variants, adherence, and risk of antiretroviral treatment failure. J Infect Dis 201(5):662–671
Perelson AS et al (1996) HIV-1 dynamics in vivo: virion clearance rate, infected cell life-span, and viral generation time. Science 271(5255):1582–1586
Peuchant O et al (2007) Primary resistance to enfuvirtide (T20) in recently HIV-1 infected, antiretroviral-naive patients from the ANRS Aquitaine Cohort. Antivir Ther 12(4):559–562
Pillay D et al (2006) The impact of transmitted drug resistance on the natural history of HIV infection and response to first-line therapy. AIDS 20(1):21–28
Pingen M et al (2011) Evolutionary pathways of transmitted drug-resistant HIV-1. J Antimicrob Chemother 66(7):1467–1480
Pingen M et al (2014) Diminished transmission of drug resistant HIV-1 variants with reduced replication capacity in a human transmission model. Retrovirology 11(1):113
Quinn TC et al (2000) Viral load and heterosexual transmission of human immunodeficiency virus type 1. Rakai Project Study Group. N Engl J Med 342(13):921–929
Sawe F et al (2013) Superiority of routine viral load monitoring in rural Kenya: the Kericho Clinic-based ART Diagnostic Evaluation (CLADE) Trial. In: 20th conference on retroviruses and opportunistic infections, Atlanta
Schoffelen AF et al (2013) Sustained virological response on second-line antiretroviral therapy following virological failure in HIV-infected patients in rural South Africa. PLoS One 8(3): e58526
Schuurman R et al (1995) Rapid changes in human immunodeficiency virus type 1 RNA load and appearance of drug-resistant virus populations in persons treated with lamivudine (3TC). J Infect Dis 171(6):1411–1419
Siripassorn K et al (2010) Effectiveness of boosted protease inhibitor-based regimens in HIV type 1-infected patients who experienced virological failure with NNRTI-based antiretroviral therapy in a resource-limited setting. AIDS Res Hum Retroviruses 26(2):139–148
Stadeli KM, Richman DD (2013) Rates of emergence of HIV drug resistance in resource-limited settings: a systematic review. Antivir Ther 18(1):115–123
Swartz JE et al (2015) Efficacy of tenofovir and efavirenz in combination with lamivudine or emtricitabine in antiretroviral-naive patients in Europe. J Antimicrob Chemother pii:dkv033 [Epub ahead of print]
Toni TA et al (2009) Detection of human immunodeficiency virus (HIV) type 1 M184V and K103N minority variants in patients with primary HIV infection. Antimicrob Agents Chemother 53 (4):1670–1672
Trotter AB et al (2013) Systematic review of HIV drug resistance in Southeast Asia. AIDS Rev 15 (3):162–170
Vandamme AM et al (2004) Updated European recommendations for the clinical use of HIV drug resistance testing. Antivir Ther 9(6):829–848

Vercauteren J et al (2009) Transmission of drug-resistant HIV-1 is stabilizing in Europe. J Infect Dis 200(10):1503–1508
Violin M et al (2004) Risk of failure in patients with 215 HIV-1 revertants starting their first thymidine analog-containing highly active antiretroviral therapy. AIDS 18(2):227–235
Wainberg MA et al (2011) Transmission dynamics of the M184V drug resistance mutation in primary HIV infection. J Antimicrob Chemother 66(10):2346–2349
Wawer MJ et al (2005) Rates of HIV-1 transmission per coital act, by stage of HIV-1 infection, in Rakai, Uganda. J Infect Dis 191(9):1403–1409
Wensing AM, Boucher CA (2003) Worldwide transmission of drug-resistant HIV. AIDS Rev 5 (3):140–155
Wensing AM et al (2005a) Prevalence of drug-resistant HIV-1 variants in untreated individuals in Europe: implications for clinical management. J Infect Dis 192(6):958–966
Wensing AM et al (2005b) Comparative disease progression observed in newly diagnosed patients infected with drug resistant and susceptible HIV-1, the FORECAST-study: no signs for increased virulence. In 3rd IAS conference, Rio de Janeiro
Wensing AM et al (2014) 2014 Update of the drug resistance mutations in HIV-1. Top Antivir Med 22(3):642–50
Wittkop L et al (2011) Effect of transmitted drug resistance on virological and immunological response to initial combination antiretroviral therapy for HIV (EuroCoord-CHAIN joint project): a European multicohort study. Lancet Infect Dis 11(5):363–371
World Health Organization (2012) The HIV drug resistance report – 2012. World Health Organization, Geneva
World Health Organization (2013) Consolidated guidelines on the use of antiretroviral drugs for treating and preventing HIV infection – recommendations for a public health approach. World Health Organization, Geneva
World Health Organization, UNAIDS, UNICEF (2011) Global HIV/AIDS response: epidemic update and health sector progress towards universal access: progress report 2011. World Health Organization, Geneva
Yerly S et al (1999) Transmission of antiretroviral-drug-resistant HIV-1 variants. Lancet 354 (9180):729–733
Yerly S et al (2004) Infrequent transmission of HIV-1 drug-resistant variants. Antivir Ther 9 (3):375–384
Yerly S et al (2009) The impact of transmission clusters on primary drug resistance in newly diagnosed HIV-1 infection. AIDS 23(11):1415–1423
Young B et al (2011) Transmission of integrase strand-transfer inhibitor multidrug-resistant HIV-1: case report and response to raltegravir-containing antiretroviral therapy. Antivir Ther 16 (2):253–256
Yu D et al (2011) HIV drug resistance assessment in the Western Pacific region. A systematic review. AIDS Rev 13(4):214–226

HIV-1 Drug Resistance in Pre-exposure Prophylaxis Trials

Teri Liegler and Robert Grant

Contents

Abstract

When used with other proven strategies for prevention of HIV-1 acquisition, oral and topical preexposure prophylaxis (PrEP) has been shown to be effective in multiple randomized, placebo-controlled clinical trials throughout the world. Preexposure prophylaxis trials have included over 20,000 men and women at

T. Liegler (✉)
Department of Medicine, University of California, San Francisco, CA, USA
e-mail: teri.liegler@ucsf.edu

R. Grant
Department of Medicine, University of California, San Francisco, CA, USA

Gladstone Institute of Virology and Immunology, San Francisco, CA, USA

San Francisco AIDS Foundation, San Francisco, CA, USA
e-mail: robert.grant@ucsf.edu

M. Gotte et al. (eds.), *Handbook of Antimicrobial Resistance*,
DOI 10.1007/978-1-4939-0694-9_24

risk for HIV infection through sexual or intravenous exposure. A consistent finding is that drug exposure is essential for PrEP efficacy. In PrEP users with breakthrough infection, selection of drug-resistant virus is a possible outcome, presenting a unique sequence of events and outcomes compared with therapeutic use of antiretroviral drugs. Study findings have indicated that drug resistance selected by PrEP occurs rarely, except in cases where PrEP is initiated in very early infection, prior to seroconversion, and detectable only with nucleic acid tests. In this review, we discuss the factors associated with PrEP which may contribute to drug resistance and summarize the frequency and characteristics of HIV-1 drug resistance reported to date from global clinical trials. A theoretical framework of the causes and consequences of drug resistance in PrEP is considered as a basis of the real-life outcomes and challenges in implementing PrEP.

Keywords
Preexposure prophylaxis • PrEP • HIV-1 • Antiretrovirals • Drug resistance

Introduction

The concept of chemoprophylaxis, or using antimicrobial agents in uninfected humans to prevent infection, is a widely used and successful strategy for prevention of infection with endemic microbes such as malaria (Breman and Brandling-Bennett 2011). One of the great successes in HIV prevention is providing antiretroviral therapy (ART) perinatally to infected pregnant women to block mother-to-child transmission (MTCT) (Connor et al. 1994). Now with the availability of a large number of potent antiviral drugs, coupled with reduced toxicities and convenient dosing formulations (Gandhi and Gandhi 2014), the benefits of using oral or topical ART as preexposure prophylaxis (PrEP) may outweigh risks of prolonged drug exposure in healthy, uninfected people. As a result, using preexposure prophylaxis (PrEP) to prevent HIV infection in at-risk individuals has moved from the conceptual realm (Youle and Wainberg 2003a, b) to phase II/III safety and efficacy trials and now to initial implementation in demonstration projects and clinical practice.

However, as was revealed in early single-dose treatment strategies for MTCT prevention, suboptimal exposure to ART can result in PrEP failure and selection for drug-resistant variants in the infected infants (Arrive et al. 2007; Eshleman and Jackson 2002; Eshleman et al. 2001; Johnson et al. 2005; Micek et al. 2010). Due to the incidence and nature of drug resistance in this setting, concern over the use of PrEP for sexual transmission has been raised (Cohen and Baden 2012; Hurt et al. 2011; Liu et al. 2006). While the clinical impact and treatment options of viruses harboring drug-resistance mutations acquired by suboptimal ART initiated after established infection are well known and may be relevant to breakthrough infections during PrEP, the potential impact of PrEP-selected drug resistance at the population level is less clear. The benefits (infections averted) versus risks (drug resistance) with PrEP use have been modeled with significantly differing outcomes and interpretations based on input variables and assumptions (Abbas et al. 2011;

Baggaley et al. 2011; Dolling et al. 2012). In addition, in antiretroviral drug-experienced populations, the prevalence of circulating strains with drug resistance to PrEP agent(s) may impair the efficacy of PrEP. Now, with accumulating results from initial global randomized PrEP efficacy trials, the benefits and risks of PrEP use for HIV acquisition can undergo evidence-based assessment, allowing an in-depth understanding of the nature and frequency of PrEP-associated drug resistance, a critical step toward optimizing its use as a prevention strategy in all at-risk populations.

PrEP Efficacy for Prevention of HIV Sexual Transmission: Summary of Results from Randomized Controlled Trials

There are now multiple reports from randomized double-blind placebo-controlled clinical trials spanning four continents and over 20,000 individuals testing the safety and efficacy of oral and topical PrEP coupled with other proven prevention strategies [reviewed in (Baeten and Celum 2013; Celum and Baeten 2012)]. Topical PrEP as 1 % tenofovir (TVF) vaginal gel used pre- and postcoitally was first shown to be effective in preventing HIV transmission by sexual exposure in African women (Abdool Karim et al. 2010). Daily oral dosing of tenofovir disoproxil fumarate (TDF, the oral prodrug of TFV) used alone or co-formulated with emtricitabine (FTC) proved efficacious in preventing sexual transmission in men who have sex with men and transgender women (MSM/TGW) from South America, South Africa, Thailand, and the United States in the iPrEx study (Grant et al. 2010), in serodiscordant African male and female partners in the Partners PrEP study (Baeten et al. 2012), and in African men and women in the TDF2 study (Thigpen et al. 2012). Finally, the Bangkok tenofovir study demonstrated that daily oral TDF dosing was associated with a 48.9 % reduction in HIV infections in injecting drug users randomized to taking TDF compared with placebo (Choopanya et al. 2013). A consistent finding from these studies showing a reduction in HIV-1 acquisition ranging from 42 % to 73 % in participants randomized to the PrEP arms is that PrEP efficacy is directly associated with drug exposure. In nested, case-control studies within each of these trials, the overall relative infection risk reduction further increased to over 90 % in participants with measurable plasma or cellular drug levels.

Not all PrEP trials with similar designs have shown reduced infections in the active drug arms when compared to placebo. The FEM-PrEP study, which enrolled African women, was stopped early due to futility where a similar infection frequency occurred in participants randomized to oral FTC/TDF and placebo (Van Damme et al. 2012). And in the multi-arm VOICE trial, a statistically indistinguishable number of infections occurred in women randomized to either 1 % TFV vaginal gel, daily oral TDF or FTC/TDF, or placebo (Marrazzo et al. 2013). The basis of differences in efficacy outcomes between these two studies and those demonstrating protection against HIV acquisition is an active area on investigation. One key factor is product adherence, determined directly by antiretroviral drug level measurements in the blood plasma and cells. Overall, women randomized to the active arms in the

FEM-PrEP and VOICE trials had insufficient product use to measure efficacy. While it is evident that distinct PrEP modalities will need to be tailored to particular at-risk populations and their circumstances contributing to HIV-1 transmission and that tenofovir-based PrEP regimens can effectively block HIV acquisition when used regularly and in combination with other prevention methods, a setting of incomplete adherence coupled with exposure risk potentially increases the chances of infection and selection for PrEP-associated resistance.

Selection and Expansion of Drug-Resistant HIV in Response to Suboptimal Antiretroviral Therapy

There are now nearly three decades of experience with therapeutic antiretroviral agents designed to target multiple stages in the HIV-1 life cycle (Arts and Hazuda 2012). Regular use of combination therapy can provide durable virologic suppression within an individual to levels below that detected by standard clinical viral load assays and can have a favorable impact in lowering the community viral load or the aggregate level within a defined geographical region (Das et al. 2010; Montaner et al. 2010). But although the available arsenal of antiretroviral drugs shows continued improvement in potency, pharmacodynamics, formulation, and toxicities, the generation and selection of drug-resistant variants continue to be a barrier to durable suppression, especially in developing countries with limited regimen choice and lack of regular virologic monitoring (Hamers et al. 2013; Sigaloff et al. 2011).

In individuals with existing infection and ongoing viral replication, sustained use of non-suppressive therapy or intermittent use of suppressive therapy will quickly promote selection and expansion of drug-resistant variants. Even during subsequent virologic suppression following a regimen change, drug-resistant variants remain archived in target cells as proviral DNA, potentially limiting future therapeutic options. Distinct outcomes of ART use following established infection within an individual are shown schematically in Fig. 1a–c to highlight the dynamic makeup of quasispecies that may arise during treatment failure. The same ART used as PrEP can also select for drug-resistant variants when breakthrough infections occur or when PrEP is initiated with unrecognized infection (Fig. 1d–f), underscoring the importance of careful virologic monitoring before and during PrEP use. The outcomes schematized in Fig. 1 have been observed in many of the PrEP trials where regular serologic testing was performed.

The development of resistance to any particular drug is driven by the high error rate in HIV-1 reverse transcriptase. With a mutation frequency of approximately 4×10^{-5} per target base per replication cycle and a nearly 10 kb genome size, there is roughly one mutation produced per replication cycle (Mansky 1996; Mansky and Temin 1995). Coupled with an estimated 10^{10} virions produced per day (Ho et al. 1995; Wei et al. 1995; Perelson et al. 1996), the fixation of a new, randomly generated mutation under targeted selection can be rapid, as notably illustrated by M184V selection after suboptimal lamivudine monotherapy (Wainberg et al. 1995; Larder et al. 1995; Schuurman et al. 1995). While mutations conferring reduced

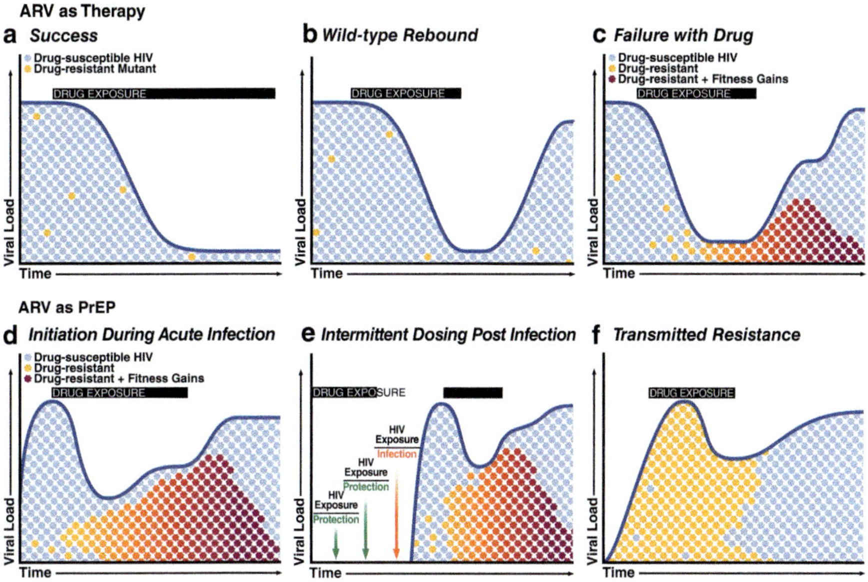

Fig. 1 Antiretroviral (ARV) drug exposure and the emergence of drug-resistant variants when used as therapy versus PrEP. The frequency of emergent drug-resistant variants and relative abundance within the viral quasispecies during distinct treatment modalities are influenced by factors such as the genetic barrier in establishing the codon(s) conferring resistance, the drug activity within a given target of viral replication, and the replication capacity in a particular environment (fitness). The *top panel* (**a**–**c**) is a schematic of possible outcomes in which ARVs are administered therapeutically, after incident infection. (a) Through random mutation, drug-resistant variants are generated sporadically in individuals with ongoing replication but remain at residual levels in settings of successful therapeutic ARV. (**b**) Treatment interruption leads to rapid virologic rebound of the more highly fit, wild-type species. (**c**) Drug-resistant variants may be selected in settings of non-suppressive therapy where continued exposure with ongoing replication may select for increasingly more fit viruses (*darker symbols*). If drug exposure is removed, residual archived wild-type virus will typically outgrow the drug-resistant species and predominate. The *lower panel* (**d**–**f**) shows possible outcomes when ARVs are inadvertently administered as PrEP in a setting of unrecognized infection. (**d**) When administered as PrEP in a setting of unrecognized infection, inadvertent postexposure initiation of ARV may be ineffective for durable suppression, selecting for minor variant drug-resistant species that may expand and evolve with fitness gains due to continued exposure. Following treatment interruption, archived wild-type virus outgrows. (**e**) Intermittent dosing with temporal lapses of protective drug exposure risks selection and outgrowth of drug-resistant variants during periods of continued ARV exposure. (**f**) Acquisition of transmitted or primary drug resistance to PrEP regimens will result in PrEP failure. Reversion by back mutation to wild-type, drug-susceptible virus can occur after discontinuation of PrEP, followed by eventual outgrowth of drug-susceptible variants if gains in fitness occur. Residual drug-resistant variants remain archived as proviruses in the cellular reservoir and may influence future treatment outcomes

susceptibility to ART often have impaired fitness in the absence of selection compared with wild-type, drug-susceptible strains, continued replication under selection can further select for additional compensatory mutations conferring fitness gains in the host's viral population (Condra et al. 1995; Cote et al. 2001; Gatanaga et al. 2002; Molla et al. 1996; Zhang et al. 1997), altered tropism, and virulence

(Coffin 1995; Kuritzkes 1996; Milich et al. 1993; Nijhuis et al. 2001) as shown in Fig. 1c. Following transmission of monophyletic or a limited number of polyphyletic founder viruses (Keele et al. 2008), the rapid expansion, high mutation and recombination frequencies (Onafuwa-Nuga and Telesnitsky 2009), multiple host, and therapeutic selection pressures can collectively promote the creation of complex viral quasispecies within an individual. Sensitive diagnostic assays that can quantify drug-resistant variants present at a minor proportion of the population within an individual have revealed mutations conferring drug resistance in ART-naïve individuals at residual levels ($\approx$1 %) within the viral quasispecies (Johnson et al. 2007, 2008; Liu et al. 2011; Metzner et al. 2011; Simen et al. 2009; Havlir et al. 1996). Preexisting low-level or minor variant drug resistance in treatment-naïve individuals can affect treatment outcomes, especially with particular NRTI- and NNRTI-selected mutations (Simen et al. 2009; Johnson et al. 2008; Havlir et al. 1996; Metzner et al. 2009; Li et al. 2011).

An alternative source of drug-resistant HIV-1 is that transmitted from a treatment-experienced partner, also known as primary resistance. Individual mutations conferring drug resistance can be detected in upwards of 20 % of the circulating strains in geographical areas that have access to ARV, changing with regional exposure levels and predominate treatment regimens over time (Chaix et al. 2009; Grant et al. 2002; Hamers et al. 2011; Jain et al. 2010; Little et al. 2002; Yerly et al. 2007; Wheeler et al. 2010). Such levels of circulating resistance within a population have driven national treatment guidelines to include baseline, pretreatment genotyping. How transmitted resistance might impact PrEP efficacy is an area of interest, especially where ARV included in PrEP regimens are also a component of first- and second-line therapies. Interestingly, numerous outcome predictions based on modeling the impact of the spread of drug resistance result in disparate scenarios [reviewed in (Baggaley et al. 2011)].

When assessing the role of PrEP agents in contributing to the selection and expansion of drug-resistant viruses, it is important to consider drug resistance in the context of drug exposure within the infection window to aid in differentiating transmitted from acquired (drug-selected) resistance. While transmitted resistance can be unequivocally confirmed by phylogenetic mapping of the source and index virus within the partnership, the presence of drug-resistance mutations associated with any particular PrEP regimen in the absence of drug exposure is highly likely to originate from transmitted strain(s) and not selected de novo by PrEP. As the frequency, nature, and origin (e.g., whether PrEP selected or transmitted) of drug-resistance findings accumulate from randomized clinical trials and demonstration projects, the impact of circulating resistance on PrEP efficacy can be directly assessed.

Detecting Drug Resistance in PrEP Studies

HIV-1 drug resistance in clinical practice is primarily measured and interpreted through two distinct but complementary approaches: (1) genotype testing, which includes direct sequencing of the HIV-1 drug target reading frames, usually *pol*, and

Table 1 Drug resistance assays used in phase II/III PrEP trials

	Genotype	Phenotype	Ultrasensitive
CAPRISA 004	In-house	None	AS-PCR
iPrEx	TRUGENE	PhenoSense	AS-PCR UDS[a]
Partners PrEP	ViroSeq, In-house	None	UDS
TDF2	In-house	None	AS-PCR
FEM-PrEP	TRUGENE	PhenoSense	AS-PCR UDS
Bangkok tenofovir study	TRUGENE	None	None

[a]*UDS* Ultradeep sequencing

(2) phenotypic susceptibility testing, which involves determining the concentration of a given compound necessary to inhibit viral growth in vitro [reviewed in (Tang and Shafer 2012)]. Both approaches measure the bulk population of viruses within an individual and, as a result, are insensitive to viral species carrying drug-resistance mutations below a given threshold (e.g., ≈20 % for population genotyping). As a research tool, multiple methods have been used to detect and quantify minor variant drug resistance within a population but below that detected by clinical tests, including allele-specific PCR-based assays that differentiate single-base changes conferring resistance, probe-based ligation assays, clonal sequencing, and highly parallel ultradeep sequencing [reviewed in (Gianella and Richman 2010)]. Ideally, genotype, phenotype, and ultrasensitive detection methods would be used together for monitoring drug resistance in PrEP failures as each approach can provide unique insights into the extent and nature of drug resistance. However, due to the high clinical diagnostic value, global accessibility, standardization of interpretation, and relatively low cost, drug-resistance genotyping is the primary diagnostic tool for drug-resistance monitoring in PrEP clinical trials (Table 1).

Designing PrEP Regimens to Minimize Drug Resistance

When designing effective regimens for PrEP, a number of factors are taken into consideration (Anderson et al. 2011; Derdelinckx et al. 2006; Fernandez-Montero et al. 2012; Garcia-Lerma et al. 2008; Amico 2012). Ideally, these include selecting compounds that target pre-integration events in the viral life cycle, demonstrate high antiviral activity and extended half-life in target tissues, exhibit synergies in activity and mutation impact if used in combination, and posses a high genetic barrier to resistance, which is the combined components that contribute to the generation of the specified resistance mutation and maintenance of the viral species in the population (Luber 2005). For these reasons, coupled with relatively favorable toxicity profiles, flexible formulations, efficacy in preventing transmission in nonhuman primate models under conditions that mimic sexual transmission in humans (Garcia-Lerma et al. 2008; Van Rompay et al. 2006; Subbarao et al. 2006; Radzio et al. 2012), and extensive history of therapeutic use, two nucleoside/nucleotide reverse transcriptase inhibitors (NRTI) have been used in the completed clinical trials to date.

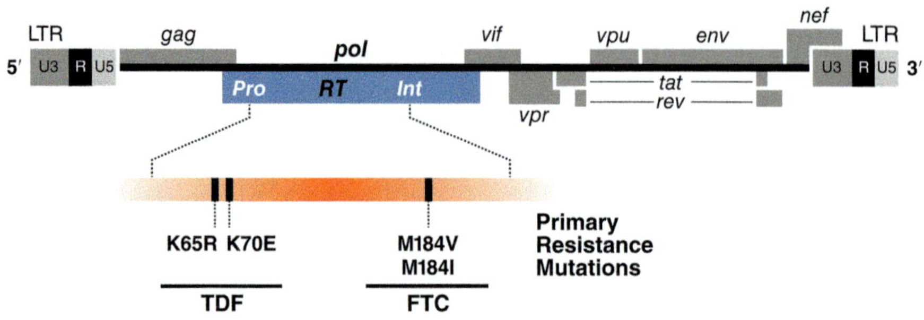

Fig. 2 Drug-resistance mutations in HIV-1 reverse transcriptase selected by FTC/TDF PrEP. Two primary drug-resistance mutations in HIV-1 reverse transcriptase are selected by each of tenofovir (TFV/TDF) and emtricitabine (FTC). TFV-associated codon changes are K65R (Lys to Arg) and K70E (Lys to Glu) and FTC-associated codon changes are M184I or V (Met to Ile or Val). Each mutation confers reduced susceptibility in vitro and in vivo. A single-base nucleotide change in RT codon A62V (Ala to Val) or S68G (Ser to Gly) does not directly confer changes in susceptibility to TFV but is a compensatory mutation associated with TFV exposure and partially restores viral replication capacity impairment conferred by K65R

Tenofovir (TFV), formulated as either a 1 % topical vaginal gel or as the orally available prodrug tenofovir disoproxil fumarate (TDF), has been administered as PrEP alone or together with emtricitabine (FTC). The co-formulated FTC/TDF oral pill TRUVADA™ is cleared by the US Food and Drug Administration for use as prevention in uninfected adults at high risk of HIV acquisition through sexual exposure. Both compounds act at pre-integration steps by terminating the nascent DNA chains in RNA-dependent and DNA-dependent DNA synthesis during the viral life cycle (Arts and Hazuda 2012).

The viral mutations associated with reduced susceptibility to TFV/TDF and related drugs are K65R and K70E (Margot et al. 2006a; Miller et al. 1999; Wainberg et al. 1999; Gallant et al. 2004) and to FTC are M184V and M184I (M184V/I) (Margot et al. 2006b), where the first amino acid listed for a given codon in RT represents the wild-type, drug-susceptible form and the second represents the mutant, drug-resistant form (Fig. 2). Additional RT mutations A62V and S68G associated with TDF exposure are considered compensatory mutations that improve viral replication capacity of poorly fit K65R mutants (Margot et al. 2006b; Svarovskaia et al. 2008). Although K65R and M184V/I are generated by a single-base substitution and thus may arise frequently in the course of HIV replication, viral species with these mutations demonstrate significantly reduced replication capacity and fitness in vitro and in vivo in the absence of selection (Yerly et al. 2007; Wheeler et al. 2010; Margot et al. 2006a; Petrella and Wainberg 2002; Miller et al. 2002; White et al. 2002; Frankel et al. 2007) thus conferring a relatively high barrier to resistance. Additionally, the presence of M184V causes increased sensitivity to TDF (Miller et al. 1999; Whitcomb et al. 2003; Deval et al. 2004), a synergy that is often taken advantage of in clinical practice (Wainberg and Gotte 2000). Finally, these ARVs provide a strong pharmacological barrier for sexual transmission. Emtricitabine concentrations are significantly higher in vaginal secretions compared to that measured in blood after single oral dosing, while TDF-DP (the active intracellular form) is up to 100× higher in the colorectal mucosa compared with vaginal and cervical tissues following a single dose (Anderson et al. 2011; Kwara et al. 2008; Patterson et al. 2011).

Genotypic, Phenotypic, and Minor Variant Drug Resistance in PrEP Trials

To date there are six completed phase III, randomized, placebo-controlled PrEP trials reporting drug-resistance results. The overall study design for monitoring HIV-1 infection status and drug resistance was similar across studies. HIV status at screening, entry, and post-randomization visits was assessed by serologic monitoring. Blood plasma, cells, or other tissue samples were typically collected and archived for retrospective measurements of HIV-1 nucleic acid and/or drug levels and, when collected at sufficient frequency, were used to establish the infection window and drug exposure levels. Upon receiving a positive rapid test result post-randomization, study drug was discontinued and confirmatory serotesting and/or RNA testing performed. In the iPrEx, Partners PrEP and TDF2 studies, participants with unrecognized, acute infection (RNA positive, seronegative) at entry were retrospectively identified. In confirmed seropositives, blood plasma collected at or proximal to the initial seropositive visit was tested for drug resistance by standard genotyping. In some studies, additional diagnostics were performed including drug-resistance phenotype and allele-specific PCR and/or deep sequencing for ultrasensitive detection of minor variant drug resistance (Table 1). In the iPrEx and FEM-PrEP studies, longitudinal sampling and testing was performed to monitor drug resistance over time in participants with FTC/TDF-associated resistance at seroconversion and randomized to the active drug arm (Grant et al. in press; Liegler et al. 2014).

The drug-resistance mutations and frequencies reported from the CAPRISA 004 (Abdool Karim et al. 2010; Wei et al. 2014), the iPrEx (Grant et al. 2010; Liegler et al. 2014), Partners PrEP (Baeten et al. 2012; Lehman et al. in press), TDF2 (Thigpen et al. 2012), FEM-PrEP (Van Damme et al. 2012; Grant et al. in press), and the Bangkok tenofovir (Choopanya et al. 2013) trials are summarized in Table 2, categorized by participants' timing of infection (pre-randomization vs incident) and randomization arm. Overall, in participants with incident (on-study post-randomization) infection, the frequency of TFV/TDF- or FTC-associated drug resistance was low, including those randomized to the PrEP arms with measurable drug levels near the infection window. Of the 142 seroconverters with incident infections and in the PrEP arms of the CAPRISA 004, iPrEx, Partners PrEP, TDF2, and Bangkok tenofovir studies, none showed genotypic or phenotypic drug resistance associated with the PrEP regimens used at or near the seroconversion visit. In contrast, four of 33 (12 %) women on the oral FTC/TDF arm in the FEM-PrEP study showed genotypic and phenotypic resistance to FTC (M184V/I) at the seroconversion visit (Van Damme et al. 2012; Grant et al. in press). Tenofovir resistance was not observed, and two showed phenotypic hypersusceptibility to this drug. Two of

Table 2 Genotypic drug-resistance testing results reported from PrEP trials

			Infected at entry				Incident infection			
			Study drug		Placebo		Study drug		Placebo	
Study	Subjects randomized	Agent	Resist/ Tot Tested	PrEP-associated mutations	Resist/ Tot Tested	PrEP-associated mutations	Resist/ Tot Tested	PrEP-associated mutations	Resist/ Tot Tested	PrEP-associated mutations
CAPRISA 004	1,085 women	1 % TFV gel coitally dependent use	0/1	none	0/9[a]	none	0/38	none	0/60	none
iPrEx	2,499 MSM and transgender women	FTC/TDF daily oral use	2/2	M184V selected[b] M184I unknown[c]	1/8	M184V transmitted	0/48	none	0/83	none
Partners PrEP	4,758 male/ female couples	TDF daily oral use	1/5	K65R selected[d]	0/6	none	0/15	none	0/51	none
		FTC/TDF daily oral use	1/3	M184V selected[e]			0/12	none		
TDF2	1,219 men and women	FTC/TDF daily oral use	1/1	K65R M184V A62V selected[f]	0/2	none	0/9	none	0/24	none
FEM-PrEP	2,120 women	FTC/TDF daily oral use	0/1	none	0/1	none	4/33	1 ea M184I selected[g] 3 ea M184V 2 transmitted 1 selected[h]	1/35	M184V transmitted
Bangkok tenofovir study	2,413 men and women (IVDU)	TDF daily oral use	none	none	0/2	none	0/15	none	0/32	none

[a]Two participants randomized to placebo were deemed ineligible for study.
[b]Mutation not found at enrollment. FTC-selected resistance
[c]Unable to genotype sample (VL = 48 cps/mL). Presence of mutation at enrollment unknown
[d]Mutation not found at enrollment. TDF-selected resistance
[e]Mutation not found at enrollment. FTC-selected resistance
[f]Mutations not found at enrollment. FTC- and TDF-selected resistance
[g]FTC detected in plasma during infection window
[h]FTC detected in plasma during infection window

these participants, 1 with M184I and 1 with M184V, had moderate- and high-study drug levels at seroconversion, respectively, implicating selection by the PrEP regimen. However, seroconversion occurred within 4 (M184V) and 8 (M184I) weeks of study entry, leaving open the possibility that infection was incubating prior to PrEP initiation – a situation with increased frequencies of emergent drug resistance.

In PrEP studies reporting ultrasensitive testing for minor variant drug resistance in seroconverters performed by AS-PCR and/or deep sequencing, background mutation frequencies (that observed in WT viruses in the absence of drug selection) were established for each individual assay and were typically $\leq$1 %. While minor variant drug resistance was observed above background levels from seroconverters in both placebo and active drug arms, examples seen in subjects randomized to the PrEP arms and therefore potentially PrEP selected are highlighted here.

In CAPRISA 004 (Wei et al. 2014) and TDF2 (Thigpen et al. 2012), AS-PCR measurements in blood plasma and vaginal swabs (CAPRISA 004) near the seroconversion visit showed no evidence of minor variant resistance to TFV. Seven of 27 (26 %) women in the CAPRISA 004 TFV gel arm had measurable TFV in vaginal fluids. However the majority had insignificant or undetectable TFV levels indicating the absence of drug selection pressure.

In the iPrEx and FEM-PrEP studies, minor variant DR in blood plasma from participants randomized to the FTC/TDF arms was observed, however infrequent and at very low proportions within the population measured by AS-PCR and 454 deep sequencing (Grant et al. in press; Liegler et al. 2011). In iPrEx, one seroconverter's virus had M184I detected at 0.53 % of the plasma viral population by AS-PCR but below background by 454 sequencing This subject had detectable but low drug levels in blood plasma and cells, opening the possibility of selection by PrEP but without significant outgrowth within the population. Similarly, one FEM-PrEP seroconverter showed M184I at 0.66 % of the population but at background levels by 454 sequencing. Study drug was not detected in this woman near the seroconversion window, suggesting spurious detection of drug-resistance mutations near the background cutoff level, rather than PrEP-selected resistance.

Blood plasma samples at the seroconversion and proximal follow-up visits from subjects in the Partners PrEP study (oral FTC/TDF, TDF alone, placebo) were analyzed for minor variant drug resistance by 454 deep sequencing (Lehman et al. in press). Of those in the oral FTC/TDF arm, a virus from 1 subject showed M184V at 16 % of the viral population (SC visit), decreasing to 1.7 % 4 weeks later, without detectable study drug. Viruses from two other participants with detectable drug showed minor variant resistance mutations: 1 with M184V at 1.9 % from the post-seroconversion visit and another with M184V (at 7.7 %), M184I (at 5.4 %), and K65R (at 1.2 %) in the seroconversion visit sample. This rare example of K65R in incident infections may reflect the significantly impaired fitness or replication capacity conferred by K65R, especially when in combination with M184V (Miller et al. 1999, 2002; Margot et al. 2006b; Petrella and Wainberg 2002; White et al. 2002; Frankel et al. 2007), and/or insufficient drug exposure, as PrEP was discontinued at the first evidence of seroconversion. In the oral TDF arm, 1 of 30 participants showed M184I at a low level (2.5 %), a mutation that is not selected by TDF. This mutation was detected as a minor variant in the placebo arm of Partners PrEP, FEM-PrEP, and iPrEx participants, possibly maintained at low levels by APOBEC3G-induced G-to-A hypermutation (Neogi et al. 2013).

Development of Elevated Drug-Resistance Frequencies When Initiating PrEP During Acute, Seronegative Infection

A striking finding from these studies is the relatively high frequency of PrEP-associated drug-resistance mutations seen in subjects who inadvertently initiated PrEP with unrecognized (RNA positive, seronegative) infection at randomization when compared to that seen in study participants with incident infections. Of the 13 participants with unknown acute infection initiating PrEP at randomization, five in the combined iPrEx, Partners PrEP, and TDF2 studies showed genotypic resistance to FTC (M184V) or TDF (K65R) at their initial seroconversion visit. In four of these participants, the virus at enrollment did not carry these resistance mutations, favoring selection by PrEP regimens during the initial 4 weeks of use. The additional subject from the iPrEx study with M184I had a low viral load at entry that was insufficient for a genotype (48 copies/mL), so it cannot be unequivocally determined whether the mutation conferring resistance to FTC was transmitted or selected. Of note, one subject from the TDF2 study developed multidrug resistance in a stepwise manner over time where M184V was detected at the first visit after study entry, followed by additional TDF-associated mutations K65R and A62V at the second visit 6 months later. Although enrollment of participants with unrecognized acute infection who went on to develop PrEP-selected resistance was rare among all in PrEP studies, the relative frequency of generating resistance in this subset of participants was high (5/13, 38 %) and possibly avoidable with HIV-1 RNA testing prior to PrEP initiation and delaying PrEP in those with symptoms consistent with acute viral infections.

In the absence of continued selection by PrEP, the FTC-associated resistance in blood plasma virions declines to residual levels over time, through outgrowth of the more highly fit WT variant generated through back mutation, or presents at very low levels under PrEP selection. Participants in both the iPrEx and FEM-PrEP trials with FTC resistance mutations M184V/I were followed longitudinally after stopping PrEP for up to nearly 18 months, and blood plasma samples were assayed for the relative proportion of coexisting drug-resistant and susceptible variants by sensitive allele-specific PCR and deep sequencing assays (Grant et al. in press; Liegler et al. 2012, 2014) and unpublished data). In all cases analyzed from both the placebo and control arms ($n = 7$), the drug-resistant variants proportionally decreased from 95 % to 100 % at seroconversion to residual levels (<0.5 %) in the blood plasma over time. Although most demonstrated a more prolonged time course for complete reversion (median 9 months), one participant showed complete reversion and overgrowth at the RT codon 184 from Ile to Met within 4 weeks of discontinuing study drug. These results are consistent with the time course of transmitted M184V reversion over time in ARV-naïve subjects (Liegler et al. 2011; Jain et al. 2011) and highlight the value of baseline resistance testing as early in infection as possible.

Distinct Patterns of Drug Resistance in PrEP: What Is Driving It?

The frequencies and nature of PrEP-associated drug resistance fall into distinct patterns that are likely outcomes of multiple diverse factors including the temporal sequela of exposure to drug and infectious virus, the pharmacodynamics of the individual compounds and formulations in diverse anatomical target sites under changing physiologic states, and the genetic barrier to resistance specific for each PrEP regimen and other factors. The interplay between the drug activity, viral resistance barriers, and how these factors might affect the relative risk of infection and frequency of resistance is schematized in Fig. 3. The distinct scenarios diagramed in panels A to D reflect various outcomes noted with use of chemoprophylaxis and HIV infection. Panel A represents effective PrEP where infection occurs only with very low drug exposure and where the overall genetic barrier to resistance is sufficiently high to prevent its emergence. This scenario reflects WT

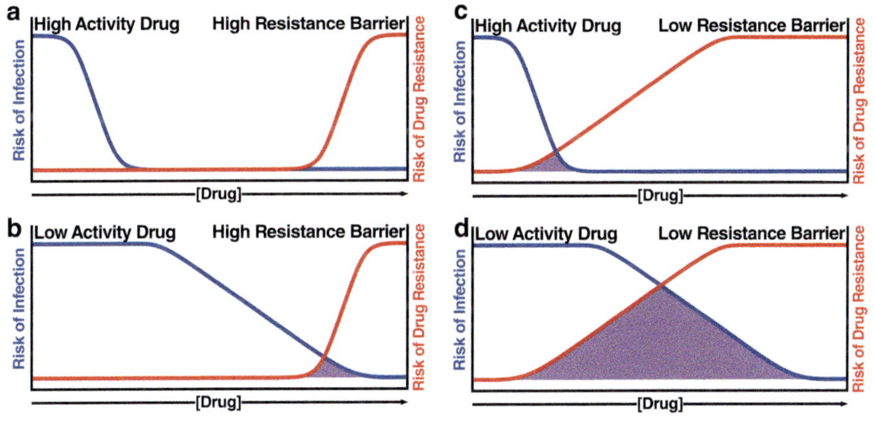

Fig. 3 Schematic of the interplay between pharmacologic and virologic factors that influence the risk of infection and drug resistance in a PrEP setting. Panels **a to d** represent theoretical schematics of the relative frequency of generating drug-resistant HIV-1 (*shaded area* at curve intersections) in settings of breakthrough infection during PrEP use. The relative risk of infection (*blue line*) is plotted against the relative risk of emergent drug resistance (*red line*) with increasing drug concentration at the anatomical and subcellular target of entry. (**a**) In a setting of high drug activity and a high barrier to resistance, the infection window occurs with insufficient drug levels to select for resistance. (**b–c**) Drug resistance can occur, although infrequently with either low drug activity or a low barrier to resistance where drug levels are suboptimal, allowing viral replication, but sufficiently high to select for drug resistance. (**d**). Increased frequency of drug resistance may occur in a setting of both low drug activity and low resistance barrier, such as that resulting from single-dose nevirapine treatment given to pregnant women to prior to delivery to prevent mother-to-child transmission

infection seen in the majority of seroconverters in PrEP studies with low or undetectable drug levels. Panels B and C may reflect the infrequent cases of resistance seen in PrEP where local concentrations of the drug may be insufficient to block infection and/or create a sufficient barrier to resistance. Distinct tissue-specific pharmacodynamics for FTC and TFV may uncouple the combined synergy in target tissues such as the cervicovaginal or colorectal mucosa (Thompson et al. 2013), leading to the observed predominance of FTC-selected mutations M184V/I in FTC/TDF oral PrEP. Finally, panel D represents settings where drug resistance is high, such as that observed with limited dosing monotherapy for prevention of MTCT. A deeper understanding of the factors that influence ARV activity and emergence of resistance in target tissues of viral entry and dissemination is critical for designing more effective PrEP regimens, formulations, and dosing strategies.

Progress Toward Next-Generation PrEP

Favorable results from initial randomized placebo-controlled PrEP efficacy trials and the US Food and Drug Administration's first label approval for an antiretroviral compound to be used as chemoprophylaxis for prevention of sexual HIV-1 transmission have led to demonstration projects worldwide where PrEP efficacy is tested in open-label, clinical settings. Ongoing demonstration projects include daily oral FTC/TDF PrEP [reviewed in (Baeten et al. 2013)], allowing direct comparisons to the PrEP efficacy trials. Comprehensive monitoring for drug resistance and drug exposure in seroconverters from these studies should yield additional insights into the overall impact of PrEP use and drug resistance. There is, however, room for overall improvement in strategies for optimizing PrEP and monitoring virologic, behavioral, toxicity, and other outcomes.

Additional compounds and formulations with improved penetration in target tissues, innovative dosing and delivery strategies, and additional viral targets are needed to further increase PrEP efficacy with expanded use while maintaining low toxicity and high genetic resistance barriers [reviewed in (Abraham and Gulick 2012)]. The ÉCLAIR study is a phase IIa safety and tolerability study evaluating the injectable long-acting investigational integrase inhibitor GSK-744 LA in uninfected men. Promising results were reported using a long-lasting nanoparticle formulation of the HIV-1 integrase inhibitor dolutegravir, with successful protection against rectal SHIV challenges (Andrews et al. 2013). Other long-lasting nanoparticle ARV formulations intended for periodic injections and targeting multiple HIV-1 pol enzymes are in various stages of investigation in small animal models measuring pharmacokinetic profiles in target tissues and cells (Puligujja et al. 2013; Martin et al. 2013).

There are multiple ongoing trials testing oral tenofovir-based PrEP dosing strategies and drug combinations to reduce pill burden and minimize overall drug exposure but maintain effective exposure for situational risk. Intermittent PrEP (pre- and postexposure) use has been shown to be efficacious in reducing SHIV infection through rectal exposure in macaques (Garcia-Lerma et al. 2010). In this study of multiple dosing strategies, none of the breakthrough infections showed evidence of drug resistance. The ANRS IPERGAY study includes MSM and "on demand" oral FTC/TDF, taken at the time of sexual exposure. The HIV Prevention Trials Network (HPTN) 067 study ADAPT, enrolling MSM/TGW and women who have sex with men (WSM), is a behavioral study with a 1:1:1 randomization of three arms using oral FTC/TDF with either daily dosing, time-driven dosing, or event-driven dosing. The NEXT-PrEP (HPTN 069/ACTG 5305) study is a four-arm phase II safety and tolerability trial investigating combinations of oral daily FTC, TDF, and the HIV-1 entry inhibitor maraviroc (MVC). Drug concentration measurements in all study participants and drug resistance testing in seroconverters in these various studies will aid in determining the oral dosing formulation and timing needed to prevent infection while minimizing exposure for reduced toxicity. This relationship was estimated using drug level measurements in blood and levels of protection from HIV acquisition in the iPrEx trial combined with defined intermittent and daily dosing strategies in the STRAND study (Anderson et al. 2012). While this serves as an important basis for determining the most effective and least harmful dosing strategy, further evaluations within these and other trials are necessary to further optimize the next-generation PrEP for diverse user needs.

Conclusions

The proven efficacy of PrEP in preventing HIV acquisition in clinical trial settings is one of the celebrated successes in HIV prevention research and brings cautious optimism for continued success with more widespread use. One clear message from PrEP trials is that successful PrEP requires drug uptake. The risk of infection increases with suboptimal PrEP use, as does the potential drug resistance. Despite a range of efficacies and adherence levels reported, drug resistance selected by PrEP was largely seen in subjects initiating PrEP during acute, unrecognized infection. Monitoring for acute viral symptomatology and the presence of HIV nucleic acids may be useful diagnostic tools at PrEP initiation. Additionally, using combination regimens and drug formulations with increased potency at PrEP initiation may minimize this occurrence. In incident infections, the occurrence of drug resistance, even as minor variants, was infrequent in participants with measurable drug levels indicating exposure. However, there are limitations in interpreting these findings – in all PrEP trials, study drug was discontinued at the first evidence of infection, thus limiting drug exposure that may generate resistance with longer duration. Guidelines for PrEP use in clinical practice indicate monitoring for infection with PrEP at a minimum of every 12 weeks (Centers for Disease Control and Prevention 2011, 2012), less frequent than the monthly monitoring in clinical trials.

Continued rigorous assessment of drug resistance in breakthrough infections while using PrEP is necessary with expanded use in clinical settings and as other compounds, formulations, dosing strategies, and novel drugs are tested and implemented.

References

Abbas UL, Hood G, Wetzel AW, Mellors JW (2011) Factors influencing the emergence and spread of HIV drug resistance arising from rollout of antiretroviral pre-exposure prophylaxis (PrEP). PLoS One 6:e18165

Abdool Karim Q et al (2010) Effectiveness and safety of tenofovir gel, an antiretroviral microbicide, for the prevention of HIV infection in women. Science 329:1168

Abraham BK, Gulick R (2012) Next-generation oral preexposure prophylaxis: beyond tenofovir. Curr Opin HIV AIDS 7:600

Amico KR (2012) Adherence to preexposure chemoprophylaxis: the behavioral bridge from efficacy to effectiveness. Curr Opin HIV AIDS 7:542

Anderson PL et al (2011) Pharmacological considerations for tenofovir and emtricitabine to prevent HIV infection. J Antimicrob Chemother 66:240

Anderson PL et al (2012) Emtricitabine-tenofovir concentrations and pre-exposure prophylaxis efficacy in men who have sex with men. Sci Transl Med 4:151ra125

Andrews CGA, Russell-Lodrigue K, Moss L, Mohri H, Spreen W, ChengMayer HZ, Markowitz M, Ho D (2013) Paper presented at the 20th conference on retroviruses and opportunistic infections, Atlanta

Arrive E et al (2007) Prevalence of resistance to nevirapine in mothers and children after single-dose exposure to prevent vertical transmission of HIV-1: a meta-analysis. Int J Epidemiol 36:1009

Arts EJ, Hazuda DJ (2012) HIV-1 antiretroviral drug therapy. Cold Spring Harbor Perspect Med 2: a007161

Baeten J, Celum C (2013) Systemic and topical drugs for the prevention of HIV infection: antiretroviral pre-exposure prophylaxis. Annu Rev Med 64:219

Baeten JM et al (2012) Antiretroviral prophylaxis for HIV prevention in heterosexual men and women. N Engl J Med 367:399

Baeten JM, Haberer JE, Liu AY, Sista N (2013) Preexposure prophylaxis for HIV prevention: where have we been and where are we going? J Acquir Immune Def Syndr 63(Suppl 2):S122

Baggaley RF, Powers KA, Boily MC (2011) What do mathematical models tell us about the emergence and spread of drug-resistant HIV? Curr Opin HIV AIDS 6:131

Breman JG, Brandling-Bennett AD (2011) The challenge of malaria eradication in the twenty-first century: research linked to operations is the key. Vaccine 29(Suppl 4):D97

Centers for Disease Control and Prevention (2011) MMWR 60:65–68

Centers for Disease Control and Prevention (2012) MMWR 61:586–589

Celum C, Baeten JM (2012) Tenofovir-based pre-exposure prophylaxis for HIV prevention: evolving evidence. Curr Opin Infect Dis 25:51

Chaix ML et al (2009) Stable frequency of HIV-1 transmitted drug resistance in patients at the time of primary infection over 1996–2006 in France. Aids 23:717

Choopanya K et al (2013) Antiretroviral prophylaxis for HIV infection in injecting drug users in Bangkok, Thailand (the Bangkok Tenofovir Study): a randomised, double-blind, placebo-controlled phase 3 trial. Lancet 381:2083

Coffin JM (1995) HIV population dynamics in vivo: implications for genetic variation, pathogenesis, and therapy. Science 267:483

Cohen MS, Baden LR (2012) Preexposure prophylaxis for HIV–where do we go from here? N Engl J Med 367:459

Condra JH et al (1995) In vivo emergence of HIV-1 variants resistant to multiple protease inhibitors. Nature 374:569

Connor EM et al (1994) Reduction of maternal-infant transmission of human immunodeficiency virus type 1 with zidovudine treatment. Pediatric AIDS Clinical Trials Group Protocol 076 Study Group. N Engl J Med 331:1173

Cote HC, Brumme ZL, Harrigan PR (2001) Human immunodeficiency virus type 1 protease cleavage site mutations associated with protease inhibitor cross-resistance selected by indinavir, ritonavir, and/or saquinavir. J Virol 75:589
Das M et al (2010) Decreases in community viral load are accompanied by reductions in new HIV infections in San Francisco. PLoS One 5:e11068
Derdelinckx I et al (2006) Criteria for drugs used in pre-exposure prophylaxis trials against HIV infection. PLoS Med 3:e454
Deval J et al (2004) Mechanistic basis for reduced viral and enzymatic fitness of HIV-1 reverse transcriptase containing both K65R and M184V mutations. J Biol Chem 279:509
Dolling D et al (2012) Evaluating the extent of potential resistance to pre-exposure prophylaxis within the UK HIV-1-infectious population of men who have sex with men. HIV Med 13:309
Eshleman SH, Jackson JB (2002) Nevirapine resistance after single dose prophylaxis. AIDS Rev 4:59
Eshleman SH et al (2001) Selection and fading of resistance mutations in women and infants receiving nevirapine to prevent HIV-1 vertical transmission (HIVNET 012). Aids 15:1951
Fernandez-Montero JV, Barreiro P, Del Romero J, Soriano V (2012) Antiretroviral drugs for pre-exposure prophylaxis of HIV infection. AIDS Rev 14:54
Frankel FA, Invernizzi CF, Oliveira M, Wainberg MA (2007) Diminished efficiency of HIV-1 reverse transcriptase containing the K65R and M184V drug resistance mutations. Aids 21:665
Gallant JE et al (2004) Efficacy and safety of tenofovir DF vs stavudine in combination therapy in antiretroviral-naive patients: a 3-year randomized trial. JAMA 292:191
Gandhi M, Gandhi RT (2014) Single-pill combination regimens for treatment of HIV-1 infection. N Engl J Med 371:248
Garcia-Lerma JG et al (2008) Prevention of rectal SHIV transmission in macaques by daily or intermittent prophylaxis with emtricitabine and tenofovir. PLoS Med 5:e28
Garcia-Lerma JG et al (2010) Intermittent prophylaxis with oral truvada protects macaques from rectal SHIV infection. Sci Transl Med 2:14ra4
Gatanaga H et al (2002) Amino acid substitutions in Gag protein at non-cleavage sites are indispensable for the development of a high multitude of HIV-1 resistance against protease inhibitors. J Biol Chem 277:5952
Gianella S, Richman DD (2010) Minority variants of drug-resistant HIV. J Infect Dis 202:657
Grant RM et al (2002) Time trends in primary HIV-1 drug resistance among recently infected persons. JAMA 288:181
Grant RM et al (2010) Preexposure chemoprophylaxis for HIV prevention in men who have sex with men. N Engl J Med 363:2587
Grant RM et al (in press) Drug resistance and plasma viral RNA level after ineffective use of oral pre-exposure prophylaxis in women. Aids
Hamers RL et al (2011) HIV-1 drug resistance in antiretroviral-naive individuals in sub-Saharan Africa after rollout of antiretroviral therapy: a multicentre observational study. Lancet Infect Dis 11:750
Hamers RL, Sigaloff KC, Kityo C, Mugyenyi P, de Wit TF (2013) Emerging HIV-1 drug resistance after roll-out of antiretroviral therapy in sub-Saharan Africa. Curr Opin HIV AIDS 8:19
Havlir DV, Eastman S, Gamst A, Richman DD (1996) Nevirapine-resistant human immunodeficiency virus: kinetics of replication and estimated prevalence in untreated patients. J Virol 70:7894
Ho DD et al (1995) Rapid turnover of plasma virions and CD4 lymphocytes in HIV-1 infection. Nature 373:123
Hurt CB, Eron JJ Jr, Cohen MS (2011) Pre-exposure prophylaxis and antiretroviral resistance: HIV prevention at a cost? Clin Infect Dis 53:1265
Jain V et al (2010) Transmitted drug resistance in persons with acute/early HIV-1 in San Francisco, 2002–2009. PLoS One 5:e15510

Jain V et al (2011) Differential persistence of transmitted HIV-1 drug resistance mutation classes. J Infect Dis 203:1174
Johnson JA et al (2005) Emergence of drug-resistant HIV-1 after intrapartum administration of single-dose nevirapine is substantially underestimated. J Infect Dis 192:16
Johnson JA et al (2007) Simple PCR assays improve the sensitivity of HIV-1 subtype B drug resistance testing and allow linking of resistance mutations. PLoS One 2:e638
Johnson JA et al (2008) Minority HIV-1 drug resistance mutations are present in antiretroviral treatment-naive populations and associate with reduced treatment efficacy. PLoS Med 5:e158
Keele BF et al (2008) Identification and characterization of transmitted and early founder virus envelopes in primary HIV-1 infection. Proc Natl Acad Sci U S A 105:7552
Kuritzkes DR (1996) Clinical significance of drug resistance in HIV-1 infection. Aids 10(Suppl 5): S27
Kwara A et al (2008) Antiretroviral drug concentrations and HIV RNA in the genital tract of HIV-infected women receiving long-term highly active antiretroviral therapy. Clin Infect Dis 46:719
Larder BA, Kemp SD, Harrigan PR (1995) Potential mechanism for sustained antiretroviral efficacy of AZT-3TC combination therapy. Science 269:696
Lehman DA et al (in press) Risk of drug resistance among persons acquiring HIV within a randomized clinical trial of single or dual-agent pre-exposure prophylaxis. J Infect Dis
Li JZ et al (2011) Low-frequency HIV-1 drug resistance mutations and risk of NNRTI-based antiretroviral treatment failure: a systematic review and pooled analysis. JAMA 305:1327
Liegler T, Abdel-Mohsen M, Jain V, Schmidt T, Spotts G, Hartogensis W, Grant R, Hecht F (2011) Paper presented at the 18th conference on retroviruses and opportunistic infections, Boston
Liegler T et al (2012) Drug resistance among HIV-1 seroconverters in the FEM-PrEP Study. Antiviral therapy 17(Suppl 1):37
Liegler T et al (2014) HIV-1 drug resistance in the iPrEx preexposure prophylaxis trial. J Infect Dis 210:1217
Little SJ et al (2002) Antiretroviral-drug resistance among patients recently infected with HIV. New Engl J Med 347:385
Liu AY, Grant RM, Buchbinder SP (2006) Preexposure prophylaxis for HIV: unproven promise and potential pitfalls. JAMA 296:863
Liu J et al (2011) Analysis of low-frequency mutations associated with drug resistance to raltegravir before antiretroviral treatment. Antimicrob Agents Chemother 55:1114
Luber AD (2005) Genetic barriers to resistance and impact on clinical response. Med Gen Med 7:69
Mansky LM (1996) Forward mutation rate of human immunodeficiency virus type 1 in a T lymphoid cell line. AIDS Res Hum Retroviruses 12:307
Mansky LM, Temin HM (1995) Lower in vivo mutation rate of human immunodeficiency virus type 1 than that predicted from the fidelity of purified reverse transcriptase. J Virol 69:5087
Margot NA, Lu B, Cheng A, Miller MD (2006a) Resistance development over 144 weeks in treatment-naive patients receiving tenofovir disoproxil fumarate or stavudine with lamivudine and efavirenz in Study 903. HIV Med 7:442
Margot NA, Waters JM, Miller MD (2006b) In vitro human immunodeficiency virus type 1 resistance selections with combinations of tenofovir and emtricitabine or abacavir and lamivudine. Antimicrob Agents Chemother 50:4087
Marrazzo J et al (2013) Paper presented at the 20th Conference on Retroviruses and Opportunistic Infections, Atlanta
Martin PLN, McDonald T, Giardiello M, Roberts P, Curley P, Smith D, Siccardi M, Rannard S, Owen A (2013) Paper presented at the 20th conference on retroviruses and opportunistic Infections, Atlanta
Metzner KJ et al (2009) Minority quasispecies of drug-resistant HIV-1 that lead to early therapy failure in treatment-naive and -adherent patients. Clin Infect Dis 48:239

Metzner KJ et al (2011) Prevalence of key resistance mutations K65R, K103N, and M184V as minority HIV-1 variants in chronically HIV-1 infected, treatment-naive patients. J Clin Virol 50:156
Micek MA et al (2010) Nevirapine resistance by timing of HIV type 1 infection in infants treated with single-dose nevirapine. Clin Infect Dis 50:1405
Milich L, Margolin B, Swanstrom R (1993) V3 loop of the human immunodeficiency virus type 1 Env protein: interpreting sequence variability. J Virol 67:5623
Miller MD, Anton KE, Mulato AS, Lamy PD, Cherrington JM (1999) Human immunodeficiency virus type 1 expressing the lamivudine-associated M184V mutation in reverse transcriptase shows increased susceptibility to adefovir and decreased replication capability in vitro. J Infect Dis 179:92
Miller V, Stark T, Loeliger AE, Lange JM (2002) The impact of the M184V substitution in HIV-1 reverse transcriptase on treatment response. HIV Med 3:135
Molla A et al (1996) Ordered accumulation of mutations in HIV protease confers resistance to ritonavir. Nat Med 2:760
Montaner JS et al (2010) Association of highly active antiretroviral therapy coverage, population viral load, and yearly new HIV diagnoses in British Columbia, Canada: a population-based study. Lancet 376:532
Neogi U et al (2013) Human APOBEC3G-mediated hypermutation is associated with antiretroviral therapy failure in HIV-1 subtype C-infected individuals. J Int AIDS Soc 16:18472
Nijhuis M, Deeks S, Boucher C (2001) Implications of antiretroviral resistance on viral fitness. Curr Opin Infect Dis 14:23
Onafuwa-Nuga A, Telesnitsky A (2009) The remarkable frequency of human immunodeficiency virus type 1 genetic recombination. Microbiol Mol Biol Rev 73:451
Patterson KB et al (2011) Penetration of tenofovir and emtricitabine in mucosal tissues: implications for prevention of HIV-1 transmission. Sci Transl Med 3:112re4
Perelson AS, Neumann AU, Markowitz M, Leonard JM, Ho DD (1996) HIV-1 dynamics in vivo: virion clearance rate, infected cell life-span, and viral generation time. Science 271:1582
Petrella M, Wainberg MA (2002) Might the M184V substitution in HIV-1 RT confer clinical benefit? AIDS Rev 4:224
Puligujja PGH, Kendrick L, Smith N, Balkundi S, Roy R, Veerubhotla R, McMillan J, Liu X (2013) Paper presented at the 20th conference on retroviruses and opportunistic infections, Atlanta
Radzio J et al (2012) Prevention of vaginal SHIV transmission in macaques by a coitally-dependent Truvada regimen. PLoS One 7:e50632
Schuurman R et al (1995) Rapid changes in human immunodeficiency virus type 1 RNA load and appearance of drug-resistant virus populations in persons treated with lamivudine (3TC). J Infect Dis 171:1411
Sigaloff KC, Calis JC, Geelen SP, van Vugt M, de Wit TF (2011) HIV-1-resistance-associated mutations after failure of first-line antiretroviral treatment among children in resource-poor regions: a systematic review. Lancet Infect Dis 11:769
Simen BB et al (2009) Low-abundance drug-resistant viral variants in chronically HIV-infected, antiretroviral treatment-naive patients significantly impact treatment outcomes. J Infect Dis 199:693
Subbarao S et al (2006) Chemoprophylaxis with tenofovir disoproxil fumarate provided partial protection against infection with simian human immunodeficiency virus in macaques given multiple virus challenges. J Infect Dis 194:904
Svarovskaia ES et al (2008) The A62V and S68G mutations in HIV-1 reverse transcriptase partially restore the replication defect associated with the K65R mutation. J Acquir Immune Defic Syndr 48:428
Tang MW, Shafer RW (2012) HIV-1 antiretroviral resistance: scientific principles and clinical applications. Drugs 72:e1

Thigpen MC et al (2012) Antiretroviral preexposure prophylaxis for heterosexual HIV transmission in Botswana. N Engl J Med 367:423
Thompson CG, Cohen MS, Kashuba AD (2013) Antiretroviral pharmacology in mucosal tissues. J Acquir Immune Defic Syndr 63(Suppl 2):S240
Van Damme L et al (2012) Preexposure prophylaxis for HIV infection among African women. N Engl J Med 367:411
Van Rompay KK et al (2006) Evaluation of oral tenofovir disoproxil fumarate and topical tenofovir GS-7340 to protect infant macaques against repeated oral challenges with virulent simian immunodeficiency virus. J Acquir Immune Defic Syndr 43:6
Wainberg MA, Gotte M (2000) Should the M184V mutation in RT be maintained as a component of HIV treatment strategies? Aids 14:S33
Wainberg MA et al (1995) Development of HIV-1 resistance to (−)2'-deoxy-3'-thiacytidine in patients with AIDS or advanced AIDS-related complex. Aids 9:351
Wainberg MA et al (1999) In vitro selection and characterization of HIV-1 with reduced susceptibility to PMPA. Antivir Ther 4:87
Wei X et al (1995) Viral dynamics in human immunodeficiency virus type 1 infection. Nature 373:117
Wei X et al (2014) Sensitive tenofovir resistance screening of HIV-1 from the genital and blood compartments of women with breakthrough infections in the CAPRISA 004 tenofovir gel trial. J Infect Dis 209:1916
Wheeler WH et al (2010) Prevalence of transmitted drug resistance associated mutations and HIV-1 subtypes in new HIV-1 diagnoses, US-2006. Aids 24:1203
Whitcomb JM, Parkin NT, Chappey C, Hellmann NS, Petropoulos CJ (2003) Broad nucleoside reverse-transcriptase inhibitor cross-resistance in human immunodeficiency virus type 1 clinical isolates. J Infect Dis 188:992
White KL et al (2002) Molecular mechanisms of resistance to human immunodeficiency virus type 1 with reverse transcriptase mutations K65R and K65R + M184V and their effects on enzyme function and viral replication capacity. Antimicrob Agents Chemother 46:3437
Yerly S et al (2007) Transmission of HIV-1 drug resistance in Switzerland: a 10-year molecular epidemiology survey. Aids 21:2223
Youle M, Wainberg MA (2003a) Pre-exposure chemoprophylaxis (PREP) as an HIV prevention strategy. J Int Assoc Physicians AIDS Care 2:102
Youle M, Wainberg MA (2003b) Could chemoprophylaxis be used as an HIV prevention strategy while we wait for an effective vaccine? Aids 17:937
Zhang YM et al (1997) Drug resistance during indinavir therapy is caused by mutations in the protease gene and in its Gag substrate cleavage sites. J Virol 71:6662

HIV-1 Entry Inhibitor Resistance

Victor G. Kramer and Mark A. Wainberg

Contents

Abstract

Purpose of review: This review discusses resistance to HIV entry inhibitors with a focus on currently approved drugs and future uses.

Recent findings: The HIV entry inhibitor class is unique among HIV antiretrovirals as it encompasses drugs that target the different stages of the HIV entry cascade. There are currently 2 FDA-approved drugs in this class, the chemokine receptor-5 (CCR5) antagonist maraviroc (MVC) and the fusion inhibitor enfuvirtide (T-20). Attachment inhibitors are still under development, with

V.G. Kramer (✉)
Department of Experimental Medicine, McGill University, Montreal, QC, Canada
e-mail: victor.kramer@mail.mcgill.ca

M.A. Wainberg
Department of Microbiology and Immunology, McGill University, Montreal, QC, Canada
e-mail: mark.wainberg@mcgill.ca

M. Gotte et al. (eds.), *Handbook of Antimicrobial Resistance*,
DOI 10.1007/978-1-4939-0694-9_25

multiple candidates in various states of development. Coreceptor antagonists are the most widely studied because patients who lack CCR5 are protected from HIV infection. CXCR4-antagonist development has proceeded more cautiously, due to limited antiviral effect in clinical trials. Fusion inhibitor development is advancing slowly, with the majority of research focusing on orally available small-molecule inhibitors. Resistance to these subclasses manifests in a complex manner and does not conform to the resistance paradigm of other antiretroviral classes.

Summary: This review will describe this heterogeneous class of antiretrovirals and the unique challenges and opportunities that they present in the pursuit of improving options for treatment.

Keywords

HIV • entry inhibitors • resistance • antiretrovirals • tropism

Key Points

1. Entry inhibitors are effective antiviral agents against HIV.
2. Two entry inhibitors are currently approved for treatment.
3. Entry inhibitors in development target alternative steps of the entry cascade that include CD4 and CXCR4.
4. Resistance to current entry inhibitors represents a unique challenge unseen with other antiretroviral classes.
5. The limitations of entry inhibitors are still being investigated and have implications for treatment that extend beyond antiviral activity.

Introduction

The development of highly active antiretroviral therapy (HAART) for HIV has led to a marked decrease in morbidity and mortality. Drug candidates for HAART regimens come from the following classes: reverse transcriptase inhibitors, protease inhibitors, integrase strand-transfer inhibitors, and entry inhibitors. A typical regimen includes two reverse transcriptase inhibitors and either a non-nucleoside reverse transcription inhibitor or a protease inhibitor. A number of concerns arise as a result of lifelong HAART, including development of drug resistance, long-term toxicity, and unfavorable drug-drug reactions. It is therefore vital to continue to develop and refine new drug classes in an effort to broaden the treatment options that are available. This review focuses on currently approved and candidate entry inhibitors and the development of resistance to said inhibitors.

HIV enters host target cells through a complex, stepwise process that begins with virus envelope subunit gp120 binding to the CD4 receptor on the cell surface (reviewed in Kuritzkes 2009, Tilton and Doms 2010). The gp41 and gp120 subunits are the result of furin cleavage of gp160, which is the major product of the HIV *env* gene, in the Golgi apparatus (Moulard and Decroly 2000). After cleavage, noncovalently associated trimers that are the result of their cleavage are transported to the cell membrane where new virions incorporate them onto their surfaces via budding (Freed and Martin 1995). CD4 D1 domain binding to a conserved site on gp120 causes the latter to undergo a conformational shift that allows it to bind to one of two chemokine coreceptors at the cell surface, CCR5 or CXCR4. These chemokine coreceptors are G-protein coupled receptors that possess an extracellular N-terminus, intracellular C-terminus, and 6 loops – equally divided into intracellular and extracellular loops. These receptors are responsible for lymphocyte chemotaxis and activation and are expressed on T cells, monocytes, macrophages, and dendritic cells. The conformational shift involves V1/V2 loop changes as well as exposure of the V3 loop (Chen et al. 2005; Kwong et al. 1998; Huang et al. 2005). The specific coreceptor that gp120 interacts with is determined by the amino acid composition of the V3 loop (De Jong et al. 1992; Shioda et al. 1991, 1992). Viruses that interact with CXCR4 are positively charged at amino acids 11, 24, and 25 on the V3 loop. Once gp120 binds to a coreceptor, it induces further conformational change that allows the gp41 fusion peptide to insert itself into the cell membrane. This precipitates the formation of a six-helix bundle comprised of six heptad repeat domains, three of which are termed HR1 and three others that are termed HR2 (Delwart et al. 1990; Chambers et al. 1990; Gallaher et al. 1989). The bundle is formed when the C-terminal HR2 region binds to the N-terminal HR1 region in an opposing orientation. The formation of this bundle brings the virus and cell membrane into close proximity and culminates in fusion, allowing the viral capsid to enter the cytoplasm and begin reverse transcription (Figs. 1 and 2).

Each step of the entry cascade has potential targets for inhibition. Thus, unlike other antiretroviral classes, the entry inhibitor class consists of a number of agents with diverse antiviral mechanisms that act at disparate points in the viral entry cascade. These steps include: CD4 binding, coreceptor binding, and membrane fusion. The first step in the cascade, CD4 binding, is not targeted by any currently approved agent. Although previous candidates were shown to inhibit HIV entry in tissue culture, this was not reflected in patients (Daar et al. 1990; Schooley et al. 1990). The blockage of the CD4 receptor carries an inherent risk of immunological disruption, as this receptor is essential in processes involving antigen recognition. Soluble CD4 (sCD4) was developed as a promising early candidate following identification of the role of CD4 in entry. Despite promising results in vitro, sCD4 was ineffective in patients in clinical trials, and subinhibitory concentrations of sCD4 were found to enhance infection (Sullivan et al. 1998). Candidate compounds still under development in this subclass include BMS-663068 (Nettles et al. 2012), a drug that binds to gp120 and prevents attachment to CD4. Earlier generations of this drug (BMS-488043) required high doses for antiviral activity (Hanna et al. 2011). BMS-663068 has now been shown to lower HIV-1 viral load by at least 1 $\log_{10}$ during 8 days of monotherapy (Nettles et al. 2012). These compounds induce a conformational change in gp120 that render it unable to bind to CD4 (Ho et al. 2006).

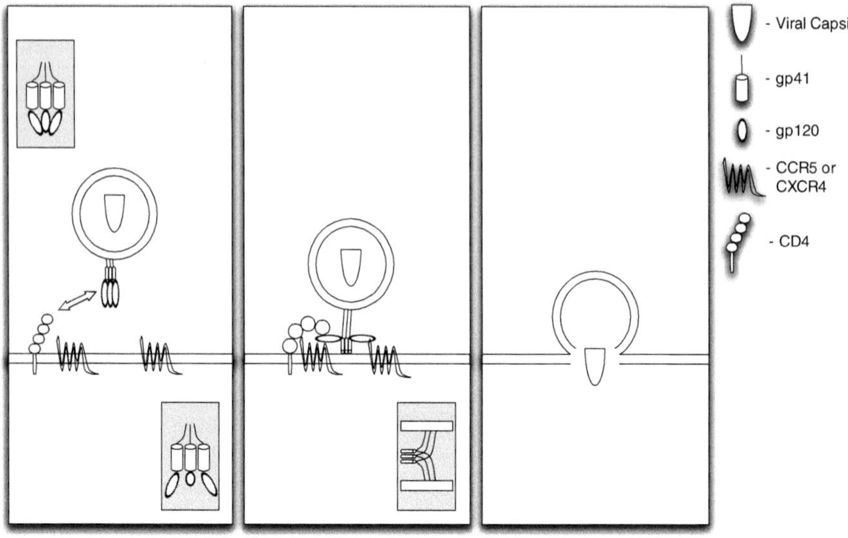

Fig. 1 Diagram of HIV-1 entry. *Left panel*: gp120/gp41 trimer on the virus surface attaches to CD4 on the surface of the cell membrane. *Left panel, insert; top left*: Native gp120/gp41 trimer, unbound to CD4. *Left panel, insert; bottom right*: gp120 conformation bound to CD4. *Middle panel*: Interaction between gp120 and coreceptor, post-CD4 attachment. gp120 binds to the N-terminus and extracellular loop 2 of the coreceptor. This allows the gp41 fusion peptide to insert into the cell membrane. *Middle panel, insert; bottom right*: Formation of the six-helix bundle following interaction of the HR1 and HR2 domains of gp41, post-fusion peptide insertion. This brings together viral and cellular membranes for fusion. *Right panel*: Fusion of viral and cellular membranes creates a pore that viral capsid uses to enter the target cell

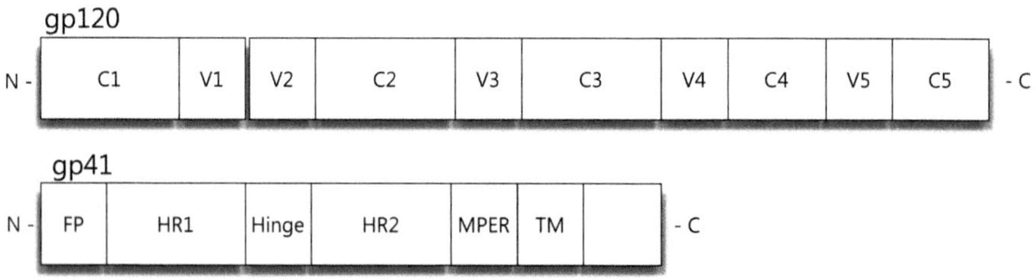

Fig. 2 Schematic representation of HIV gp120 and gp41 envelope proteins on the virion surface. *Top*: gp120 contains five conserved domains (C1–C5) and five variable domains (V1–V5). *Bottom*: gp41 contains a fusion peptide (FP), heptad repeat region 1 (HR1), heptad repeat region 2 (HR2), and the hinge region between both the membrane proximal external region (MPER) and the transmembrane anchor (TM)

A post-attachment inhibitor, the monoclonal antibody ibalizumab, has been developed that targets the D2 domain of the CD4 receptor (Burkly et al. 1992). It blocks gp120 conformational change following the gp120-CD4 interaction. Used as a single dose, it has shown antiviral activity with HIV viral load reductions up to

1.5 $\log_{10}$ when given together with optimized background therapy (OBT) (Kuritzkes et al. 2004). Phase IIb trials demonstrated that weekly or biweekly doses led to viral load reductions of up to 1.7 $\log_{10}$ together with OBT (Jacobson et al. 2009). Ibalizumab is currently in phase I subcutaneous administration dose-escalation trials for subcutaneous administration in HIV-negative individuals (www.clinicaltrials.gov, NCT01292174). CD4 inhibitors are currently the only subclass of entry inhibition without drugs for HIV therapy.

CCR5 coreceptor inhibitors are the best researched entry inhibitor subclass. This is due to a variety of factors such as (1) the existence of individuals who do not express CCR5 due to a homozygous gene variant (CCR5 delta32/delta32). These individuals possess a high level of resistance to HIV-1 R5-tropic infection (Dean et al. 1996; Liu et al. 1996; Samson et al. 1996). Heterozygotes for this deletion experienced slower disease progression (Dean et al. 1996; Samson et al. 1996; Huang et al. 1996; Michael et al. 1997; Rappaport et al. 1997). (2) A lack of CCR5 has not led to major detrimental effects. Interestingly, CCR5 homozygotes show increased susceptibility to West Nile virus and tick-borne encephalitis infections (Kindberg et al. 2008; Lim et al. 2008). (3) Recent reports described several potential benefits of CCR5 antagonists that extend beyond antiviral effect such as a reduction in inflammation (Funderburg et al. 2010; Schroder et al. 2007), although not on progression of rheumatoid arthritis (Fleishaker et al. 2012). CCR5 blockade has also led to an increase in levels of CD4 T cells, though it is unknown whether these regenerated T cells are extant cells that have gone uninfected or a *de novo* population of other replicative cells (Funderburg et al. 2010). Finally, one HIV-positive patient who had his viremia controlled by HAART subsequently developed acute myeloid leukemia and received a hematopoietic stem cell transplant from a homozygous CCR5 delta32/delta32 donor (Hütter et al. 2009). HAART was stopped before transplantation and, after 5 years, his viremia has not returned (Allers et al. 2011; Symons et al. 2012). This has been attributed to the fact that the donor was a homozygous CCR5 delta32/delta32 donor. The success of this patient as proof of concept of HIV cure, notwithstanding the impracticality of hematopoietic stem cell transplant solely for HIV treatment, is among the reasons that CCR5-blockade research is so important.

CXCR4 is the alternative coreceptor that a virus may use to enter cells in conjunction with CD4. It is unknown what the long-term effects of CXCR4 blockade are, though there are concerns that it may have serious ramifications due to the fact that cases of CXCR4-receptor augmentation in humans often result in serious immunodeficiency (WHIM syndrome) (Hernandez et al. 2003; Liu et al. 2012) and CXCR4 knockout in mice led to abnormalities in embryonic development (Tachibana et al. 1998; Zou et al. 1998; Ma et al. 1998; Nagasawa et al. 1996). CXCR4 functions as a receptor of SDF-1 and does not appear to be as redundant, as CCR5. But, homozygotes possessing mutant ligand SDF1-3′A also displayed delayed progression to AIDS (Winkler et al. 1998). Promising CXCR4 inhibitors such as AMD3100 have demonstrated antiviral activity in vitro but did not exhibit the same antiviral efficacy in vivo (Hendrix et al. 2004; Donzella et al. 1998). This may be attributed to the fact that X4-tropic strains of HIV are rarely found on their

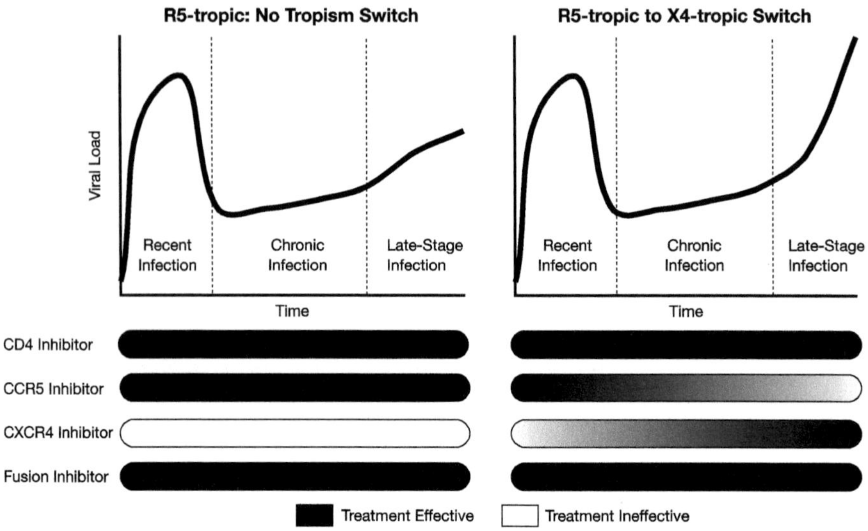

Fig. 3 Relative viral load through three stages of HIV-1 disease course and corresponding efficacy of entry inhibitor subclasses. *Left*: Patients infected with a CCR5-tropic virus that does not undergo tropism switch. CD4, CCR5, and fusion inhibitors are effective for treatment; CXCR4 inhibitors are not. *Right*: Patients infected with a CCR5-tropic virus that switches tropism to CXCR4, characterized by a pronounced increase in viral load at late-stage disease. CD4 and fusion inhibitors are effective throughout disease course. The efficacy of CCR5 inhibitors decreases with a concomitant rise in CXCR4 tropism during chronic and late-stage infection; CXCR4 inhibitors are more effective during these stages

own in vivo; they generally appear in the presence of R5-tropic virus, even in late-stage disease (Moyle et al. 2005; Wilkin et al. 2007; Brumme et al. 2005; Regoes et al. 2005) (Fig. 3). Although CXCR4 blockade may completely inhibit the X4-tropic component of the viral quasispecies, R5-tropic replication may continue unabated in the presence of CXCR4 antagonists. AMD3100, initially developed as an HIV antiretroviral, is no longer being developed for HIV therapy but is now being used as a hematopoietic stem cell mobilizer (plerixafor) in order to increase stem cell harvests before transplantation. Additionally, AMD3100 is now undergoing clinical trials for treatment of WHIM syndrome as it ablates hyper-CXCR4 signaling following binding to SDF-1 (Liu et al. 2012; McDermott et al. 2011a, b).

Entry Inhibitors Currently Approved for Treatment

Maraviroc

Maraviroc is a CCR5 entry inhibitor that prevents R5-tropic virus from infecting a target cell. It is currently the only CCR5 inhibitor approved for HIV-1 treatment by the US Food and Drug Administration and other regulatory agencies for both first-line and second-line therapies (USFDA 2009). It is not yet licensed for first-line therapy in Europe (Society EAC. Guidelines 2011). Since a majority of new transmissions are R5-tropic (Pope and Haase 2003), it is reasonable that MVC could have its greatest benefit early in treatment (Fig. 3). X4-tropic variants are more likely to develop over time, rendering the use of maraviroc inappropriate (Brumme et al. 2005; Regoes et al. 2005; Schuitemaker et al. 1992; Saag et al. 2009).

MVC is unique among currently approved antiretrovirals in that it exerts its antiviral properties by binding to a cellular target rather than a viral one. It binds at a hydrophobic transmembrane pocket on extracellular loop 2 (ECL2) that is distinct from the gp120 binding site and induces a conformational change that renders the receptor unusable for entry (Dorr et al. 2005; Garcia-Perez et al. 2011). This allosteric inhibition prevents CCR5 ligand (MIP-1a, MIP-1b, and RANTES) signaling, although there does not appear to be any sequelae associated with such interference (Dorr et al. 2005).

MVC, as a cellular inhibitor, may have effects beyond its ostensible antiviral activity. The results of the MOTIVATE-1 and MOTIVATE-2 trials showed that treatment-experienced patients who received MVC with OBT had increased CD4+ T-cell counts versus placebo groups (Fatkenheuer et al. 2008; Gulick et al. 2008). This increase in CD4+ T-cell count was observed in both patients with solely R5-tropic virus and also in patients harboring X4 and dual/mixed population virus at failure. It is possible that the increase in CD4+ T cells results from anti-inflammatory effects that are a natural consequence of CCR5-blockade, since naive cells may no longer be recruited to sites of inflammation. The precise mechanisms responsible for the increased CD4+ cell count are still under investigation.

MVC appears to limit graft versus host disease (GVHD) in patients receiving allogeneic stem cell transplants. Phase I and II trials revealed decreased incidence of GVHD in patients taking a 33-day course of combination maraviroc, tacrolimus, and methotrexate (23.6 %, grade II to IV disease; 5.9 %, grade III or IV) compared to patients taking only tacrolimus and methotrexate (38.5 %, grade II to IV disease; 21.9 %, grade III or IV) (Reshef et al. 2012). This is attributed to MVC-mediated inhibition of CCR5 internalization and lymphocyte recruitment.

CCR5 was recently implicated as the receptor required for *Staphylococcus aureus*-produced leukotoxin ED toxicity (Alonzo et al. 2013). Leukotoxin ED is one of four pore-forming toxins produced by the bacteria and is responsible for targeted killing of macrophages, dendritic cells, and effector memory T cells and can serve as an immune evasion strategy by this bacterial pathogen. MVC, along with natural ligands and a monoclonal antibody to ECL-2, reduced the interaction between leukotoxin and CCR5, whereas antibody 3A9, specific for the CCR5 N-terminus, did not affect the interaction. Although MVC treatment had no effect on leukotoxin ED-mediated killing of neutrophils and monocytes, CCR5 antagonists may potentially represent complementary therapeutic strategies in the treatment of *S. aureus* infections.

CCR5 delta32/delta32 homozygotes appear to have more favorable outcomes in rheumatoid arthritis (Prahalad 2006; Wheeler et al. 2007). Indeed, it had been hypothesized that CCR5 blockade might mediate rheumatoid arthritis and maraviroc was originally developed with antiarthritic use in mind. However, maraviroc did not demonstrate any beneficial effects when used to treat rheumatoid arthritis in conjunction with methotrexate (Fleishaker et al. 2012).

Enfuvirtide (T-20)

Fusion inhibitors exert their antiviral effect during the last stage of viral entry through inhibition of virus and cell membrane fusion. Enfuvirtide (T-20) is the only approved representative of the fusion inhibitor subclass of HIV entry inhibitors. It was the first entry inhibitor approved for therapy and is indicated for inclusion in salvage regimens in treatment-experienced patients despite requiring subcutaneous administration. Two randomized phase III trials (TOROs 1 and 2) showed reduced viral loads to <400 copies/ml in a greater percentage of patients than a placebo arm after 48 weeks (Lalezari et al. 2003a; Lazzarin et al. 2003; Nelson et al. 2005). A 96-week follow-up demonstrated viral loads below 400 copies/ml in 26.5 % of patients, with 17.5 % achieving viral loads <50 copies/ml (Reynes et al. 2007).

T-20 is a 36-amino-acid synthetic peptide that mimics the HR2 region of gp41. T-20 prevents formation of the six-helix bundle required to bring viral and cell membranes into close proximity by competitively binding to HR1 (Wild et al. 1993). It has demonstrated antiviral efficacy across all viral subtypes and tropisms in vitro and in vivo (Kilby et al. 1998, 2002; Lalezari et al. 2003b; Derdeyn et al. 2000). As such, it has a broader antiviral range than coreceptor inhibitors. However, the need for twice-daily subcutaneous injection as a consequence of a short plasma half-life (~4 h) has meant that the use of T-20 is limited (Zhang et al. 2002; Makinson and Reynes 2009).

Other Entry Inhibitors in Development

CCR5 Inhibitors

The recent case of the Berlin patient has renewed interest in development of entry inhibitors as a potent antiretroviral class. CCR5 entry inhibitors currently in development include an anti-CCR5 antibody PRO-140, which binds to an extracellular region of ECL2 on CCR5 (Olson et al. 1999). PRO-140 has yielded declines in viral load of up to 1.83 $\log_{10}$ in single-dose studies (Jacobson et al. 2008). It has also shown favorable results in dose-escalation studies, in which 0.99 to 1.65 $\log_{10}$ viral load reductions were witnessed after weekly (162 mg, 324 mg) or biweekly (324 mg) subcutaneous administration (Jacobson et al. 2010). There was no detectable rebound in viremia between doses. Phase IIb studies using PRO-140 as an adjunct to oral antiretroviral treatment in treatment-experienced patients are ongoing (www.clinicaltrials.gov; NCT01272258).

Cenicriviroc (CVC) (TBR-652) is a small-molecule CCR5 inhibitor that has shown promise in phase IIb dose-finding studies. It demonstrated a favorable tolerability profile and potent antiviral efficacy with a reduction of up to 1.8 $\log_{10}$ viral load copies in a phase IIb study (Lalezari et al. 2011; Marier et al. 2011). Treatment-experienced patients who received 10-day monotherapy with escalating doses of drug displayed dose-dependent reductions in viral load. The plasma half-life of CVC is 35–40 h and is not influenced by cytochrome P450. As such, it is suitable for once-daily dosing. Interestingly, CVC may also possess anti-inflammatory effects by virtue of its ability to antagonize CCR2 (Baba et al. 2005). Levels of the CCR2 ligand macrophage chemoattractant protein 1 (MCP-1) were increased in patients receiving CVC monotherapy, also suggesting CCR2 antagonism (Lalezari et al. 2011). The MCP-1/CCR2 pathway has been implicated in a number of inflammatory diseases, and CVC that can simultaneously antagonize CCR2 and CCR5 bears further investigation in HIV-1-infected patients. Phase IIb studies of CVC plus two nucleoside reverse transcriptase inhibitors (NRTIs) versus efavirenz plus two NRTIs in treatment-naïve patients are ongoing (www.clinicaltrials.gov; NCT01338883).

Fusion Inhibitors

Fusion inhibitor development has proceeded with the goal of achieving oral availability or at least a reduction in the numbers of injections required for dosing. As mentioned, enfuvirtide (T-20) must be injected subcutaneously twice daily, leading to painful treatment-site reactions. The pursuit of oral bioavailability has led to successive generations of inhibitors; the third-generation compounds T-2635 (Eggink et al. 2011) and sifuvirtide (He et al. 2008) show potent antiviral efficacy in vitro and have a longer half-life than T-20 as a result of stabilization between HR1 and HR2 mimetics (reviewed in Eggink et al. 2010). This stability was a product of ion pair interactions that increased α-helix stability in these monomeric peptides that, in turn, stabilized the six-helix bundle. As a result, sifuvirtide has a higher potency and longer half-life than T-20 (26 h). Prolongation of half-life is also being pursued for T-20 with novel strategies that include the use of antibodies attached to T-20. The serum half-life of this conjugate was 72 h in mice and antiviral potency was increased (Chang et al. 2012).

CXCR4 Inhibitors

AMD070 is a derivative of the CXCR4 inhibitor AMD3100. It has antiviral potency in vivo and in vitro and has completed dose-escalation phase I studies (Moyle et al. 2009; Stone et al. 2007); oral bioavailability is currently being improved (Skerlj et al. 2010, 2011). Phase IIa and IIb safety and antiviral activity trials have been completed and results are expected soon (www.clinicaltrials.gov; NCT00089466, NCT00063804).

Resistance to Current Entry Inhibitors

There are concerns and limitations unique to entry inhibitors since resistance to entry inhibitors, particularly chemokine receptors, is unlike resistance to other antiretroviral agents. Entry inhibitors act either directly or indirectly against the viral envelope, one of HIV's most mutable proteins. Therefore, in addition to development of resistance, baseline sensitivities of patient viruses must also be taken into consideration (Tilton et al. 2010; Yu et al. 2011; Covens et al. 2009; Leung et al. 2010; Araujo et al. 2012).

Susceptibility to entry inhibitors can vary widely among different patient isolates, up to 1000-fold in cases. This difference is the result of envelope diversity at baseline. The envelope diversity of HIV results from a number of factors, including level of glycosylation, structural plasticity, continuous immune pressure, incomplete processing, and availability of target cells.

Resistance to each entry inhibitor subclass is unique and develops differently for each inhibitor. Resistance to the BMS attachment inhibitor compounds has involved mutations in gp41 and gp120, particularly in the CD4 binding site. Resistance to BMS-378806 which was discontinued following phase II clinical studies developed in vitro in gp41 (I595F, K655E) (Lin et al. 2003; Zhou et al. 2010). This was in addition to mutations in the CD4 binding site. However, the presence of these mutations did not correlate completely with in vivo resistance, revealing the complexities involved. One mutation that appeared in patients and in in vitro selections was M426L in the CD4 binding site (Zhou et al. 2011). This mutation also conferred resistance to BMS-626529 (Charpentier et al. 2012; Soulie et al. 2013). Although the appearance of M426L was common to both these drugs, two distinct mechanisms of resistance may be at work, as BMS-378806 is thought to prevent gp120-induced gp41 exposure, while BMS-626529 prevents gp120-CD4 interactions through induced gp120 conformational change. The M426L polymorphism was observed primarily in attachment-inhibitor-naïve patients harboring subtypes D and CRF_02 and did not frequently appear in subtype B. Virus tropism was evenly distributed among patient viruses harboring this polymorphism. Synergy between this inhibitor and all other antiretroviral classes was observed in vitro (Zhou et al. 2011). Resistance to ibalizumab has shown dependence on the loss of potential N-linked glycosylation sites in the V5 loop of gp120, although the molecular mechanism of resistance is still undefined (Pace et al. 2013; Toma et al. 2011).

Ibalizumab-resistant viruses demonstrated higher levels of infectivity versus wild type and sensitivity to soluble CD4. However, the resistant viruses did not regain wild-type infectivity in the presence of fully inhibitory concentrations of antibody (Toma et al. 2011). This implies that a possible mechanism of resistance may involve the ability of an ibalizumab-resistant virus to use antibody-bound CD4 in entry as a result of increased efficiency of CD4 usage, an enhancement of CD4-induced conformational change, or a combination of the two.

In regard to coreceptor inhibitors, resistance can occur in one of two ways. The first mechanism of resistance is a tropism switch that is defined as the emergence of X4-tropic strains from a predominantly R5-tropic virus population. In natural infections, tropism switches occur in ~50 % of patients and are usually accompanied by disease progression and a steep decline in CD4 T cells (Scarlatti et al. 1997; Connor et al. 1997; Berger et al. 1999). Whether this tropism switch is the cause or consequence of advanced disease progression is still the subject of debate. In consideration of conflicting reports showing antiviral activity against dual/mixed (D/M) tropic viruses (Saag et al. 2009; Ceccherini-Silberstein et al. 2011; Perez-Olmeda et al. 2012; Symons et al. 2011), maraviroc and other CCR5 inhibitors can only be administered following a tropism test that indicates a purely R5-tropic virus population. Whether the emergence of detectable X4-tropic strains represents R5-tropic envelope evolution or an outgrowth of preexisting X4-tropic strains is a question that requires further investigation (Savkovic et al. 2012; Pastore et al. 2004; Fiser et al. 2010; Trkola et al. 2002). In vitro selection studies performed in PBMCs have demonstrated that tropism switch does not occur and that the inhibitor-resistant strains can still use CCR5 for entry. This was shown regardless of which entry inhibitor or CCR5-tropic virus was used.

In the MOTIVATE trials, 50 % of patients who failed MVC-containing regimens harbored X4/dual-tropic virus as opposed to the control group, for which only 6 % of patients failing treatment exhibited altered tropism (Fatkenheuer et al. 2008; Gulick et al. 2008). The emergence of X4-tropic virus was also observed in the MERIT trial in which a tropism test was used to screen out patients possessing X4 or dual-tropic virus at baseline. 31 % of patients who failed MVC-containing regimens harbored X4-tropic virus and 14 % harbored CCR5-tropic virus resistant to MVC (Cooper et al. 2010). A number of patients in clinical trials that failed on MVC treatment were found to harbor CXCR4-tropic virus at baseline. In a study of patients failing MVC treatment, 30 % of patients who experienced virologic failure harbored CXCR4. Of these, patients who exhibited X4-tropic virus at baseline displayed an outgrowth of these viruses (Recordon-Pinson et al. 2013). In MVC-treated patients in whom CXCR4 virus appeared, cessation of CCR5-inhibitor therapy resulted in a return of CCR5-tropic virus predominance suggesting that CCR5 variants may be more replication fit than CXCR4 variants (Gulick et al. 2007; Lalezari et al. 2005; Westby et al. 2006). It remains to be seen whether subtype-specific differences play a role in the development of this resistance pathway, as particular subtypes such as subtype C are far less prone to tropism switch during the course of infection (Cecilia et al. 2000; Coetzer et al. 2011).

Resistance to CCR5 coreceptor inhibitors can also occur if the virus is able to use drug-bound CCR5 for entry. This has notably been demonstrated in vitro. Different CCR5 antagonists have shown different resistance profiles in vitro, complicating the characterization of R5 resistance in general. Variations in envelope between different isolates, as well as the particular CCR5 antagonist used, have led to different manifestations of resistance with little overlap. MVC-resistant virus has been shown to use drug-bound receptor through a noncompetitive mechanism where an increase in drug concentration has no effect on entry. This has also been shown for attachment inhibitors (Nowicka-Sans et al. 2012). Evidence of a competitive mechanism has also been shown in vitro (Ratcliff et al. 2013), whereby an increase in IC50 has characterized a resistant virus that is still inhibited by high amounts of MVC.

Furthermore, coreceptor inhibitor mutations that appear in one HIV strain may not necessarily confer resistance when introduced into another (Henrich et al. 2010; Kuhmann et al. 2004; Marozsan et al. 2005; McNicholas et al. 2010, 2011; Tsibris et al. 2008).

Viral efficiency in utilizing CD4 and CCR5 appears to play a role in development of resistance (Fig. 4). A recent study compared the MVC-resistant viruses of two different patients. One of these was characterized as having strong resistance as evidenced by a low maximal percent inhibition (Roche et al. 2013). The other had weak resistance characterized by a high maximal percent inhibition. These viruses exhibited disparate Env mutations, but both showed a high reliance on sulfated tyrosine residues on the CCR5 N-terminus. The virus characterized by weak resistance could not efficiently engage maraviroc-bound receptors; the strongly resistant virus could efficiently use the maraviroc-bound receptor. Strains that utilize CCR5 efficiently appear to be more prone to developing resistance to CCR5 antagonists (Roche et al. 2011a), and resistance to CCR5 inhibitors may be related to baseline viral use of drug-bound coreceptor (Roche et al. 2011b). Interestingly, viral entry in the presence of CCR5-inhibitor vicriviroc may partially depend on the presence of the drug (Putcharoen et al. 2012). This is in contrast to what had been shown for aplaviroc, a CCR5 inhibitor that is no longer being clinically pursued (Pfaff et al. 2010).

Viral strains resistant to CVC have been generated that harbor changes in the V3 loop. Cenicriviroc selected T306K and Q309E in tissue culture in addition to changes in C2 (K221N), C4 (M424T), and gp41 (V766A, I769) (Baba et al. 2007). It is important to note that no one amino acid was considered sufficient for resistance to cenicriviroc. Rather, the accumulation of amino acid changes at various locations was required. Resistant viruses to other small-molecule CCR5 inhibitors have followed a similar pattern whereby the V3 loop mutations occurred most frequently though but were not the only Env mutations that were observed.

Pure X4-tropic viral populations in patients are rare, and it is unknown whether an X4 blockade might lead to resistance. One study showed that treatment of PBMCs with AMD3100 would lead to the emergence of R5 tropism in clinical isolates (Harrison et al. 2008; Armand-Ugon et al. 2003; Este et al. 1999). However, the clonal X4 virus NL4-3 did not exhibit a tropism switch when used in in vitro selections with the CXCR4 inhibitors SDF-1α and T134 (Kanbara et al. 2001; Schols et al. 1998). It is unclear what consequences may arise from resistance to CXCR4 blockade and what the impact on late-stage HIV pathogenesis might be.

Resistance to T-20 is more straightforward and does involve mutations within the HR1 region of gp41 that allows preferential binding to occur to HR2 instead of enfuvirtide (Marcelin et al. 2004; Carmona et al. 2005). These mutations localize between amino acids 36 and 45 in the N-terminal region. Common mutations include G36D, V38M, N42D, and N43D/Q. Combinations of these and other mutations in HR1 can select for high-level resistance to T-20. There is no cross-resistance between T-20 and other antiretrovirals (Greenberg and Cammack 2004).

These resistance mutations decrease the efficiency of the fusion process, causing T-20-resistant strains to be more sensitive to neutralizing antibodies

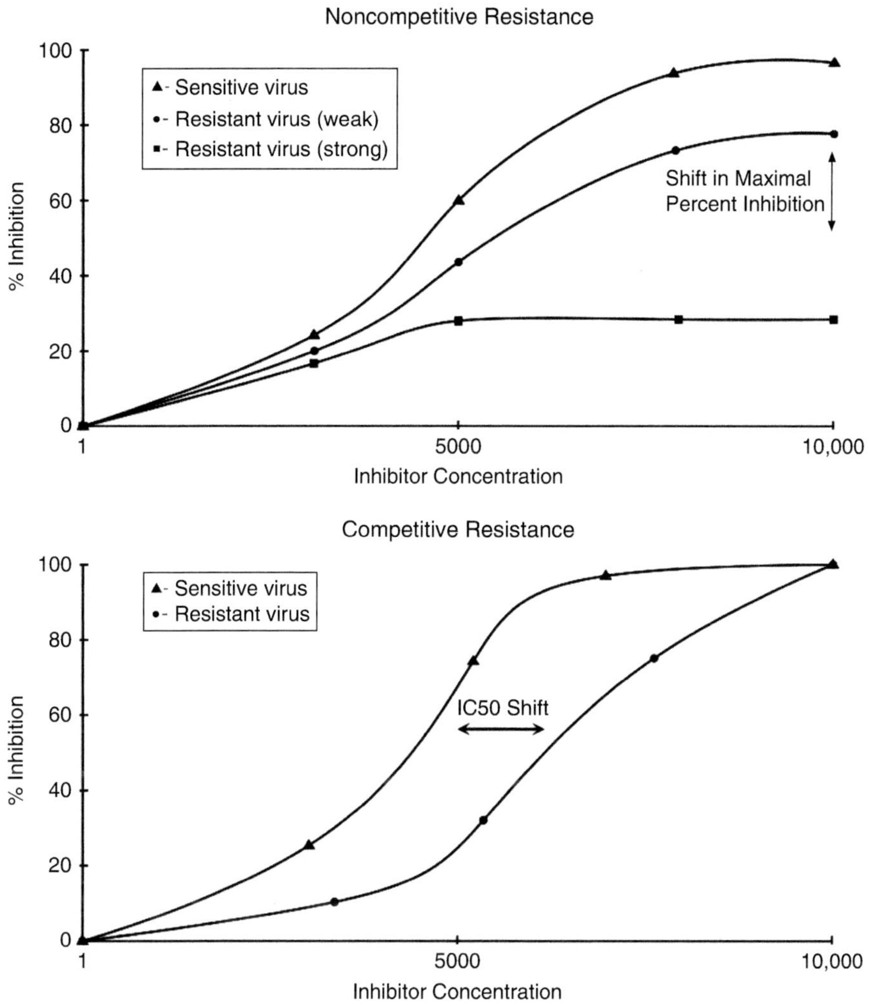

Fig. 4 Representations of noncompetitive and competitive resistance to entry inhibitors. *Top*: Noncompetitive entry inhibition allows for resistant virus to utilize drug-bound receptor. The virus does not compete with drug in receptor binding. The difference between sensitive, weakly, and strongly resistant viruses can be compared by maximal percent inhibition, defined as the percent inhibition of infection in overwhelmingly inhibitory concentrations of drug. The difference between weakly and strongly resistant viruses is a result of their efficiency in drug-bound receptor utilization. *Bottom*: Competitive entry inhibition occurs when the virus competes with drug for binding to the receptor. The difference between sensitive and resistant viruses is represented by a fold change in IC50 values. Resistant virus outcompetes the drug for binding to the receptor, but increasing amounts of drug will produce full inhibition of entry

(Reeves et al. 2005). The notion that a less efficient process of entry allows more time for a virion to be bound by neutralizing antibodies (Platt et al. 2012) may be one of the mechanisms involved and may also play a role in antiviral synergy among different entry inhibitors. The accumulation of varying mutations to different entry inhibitors may lead to a severe fitness cost to the virus. N125D in HR2 can compensate for the loss of fitness as a result of the resistance mutations Q40H and Q56R. S138A is another compensatory mutation that can restore entry efficiency following selection of N43D (Izumi et al. 2009; Ray et al. 2009; Xu et al. 2005). Two mechanisms may account for restoration of entry efficiency. First, compensatory mutations in HR2 can restore its affinity for HR1 (Baldwin and Berkhout 2008). Second, mutations in both gp41 and stem loop 3 of the Rev-responsive element can result in an E57A mutation that is associated with an increase in viremia in patients harboring T-20-resistant viruses (Svicher et al. 2008) that is in contrast to results of other studies in which CD4 increases were observed in patients harboring T-20-resistant isolates (Deeks et al. 2007; Melby et al. 2007; Soria et al. 2008).

Limitations of Current Entry Inhibitors

The results of recent clinical trials involving maraviroc as part of an antiretroviral regimen for treatment-naïve patients showed that a greater percentage of patients in the maraviroc treatment group harbored viral loads between 50 and 400 copies/ml compared with patients taking either an RT inhibitor or an integrated strand-transfer inhibitor (INSTI) together with optimized background therapy (Cooper et al. 2010; Sierra-Madero et al. 2010; Mills et al. 2012). With more laboratories switching to viral load assays with a limit of 20 copies/ml, the entry inhibitor class may not appear to be as potent as other classes. Furthermore, antiretrovirals of various classes may have differing effects on the overall rate of viral load decline. Integrase inhibitors, for example, led to a much steeper decline in viral load than reverse transcriptase and protease inhibitors, by virtue of their method of action (Donahue et al. 2010; Markowitz et al. 2007; Grinsztejn et al. 2007; Sedaghat et al. 2008). Clinical trials have empirically shown that entry inhibitors do not exhibit a faster rate of decline on viral loads compared to other classes (Mills et al. 2012). This may be attributed to a number of factors: (1) inherent antiretroviral activity (Sedaghat et al. 2008), (2) increased CD4 trafficking (Gulick et al. 2008), or (3) redistribution of repelled virus (Kramer et al. 2012). The clinical implications of a slightly elevated viral load (>50 copies/ml) as a result of entry inhibitor suppression bear further investigation.

Conclusions

Targeting HIV entry has yielded an antiretroviral drug class with two representatives approved for treatment. The complexity of the entry process has given rise to a number of candidates, each with novel antiviral mechanisms, which are currently progressing in the clinic. The diversity of the class demands consideration of a number of issues: antiviral efficacy, treatment indications, development of resistance, and the importance of viral tropism. The need for further study to precisely designate the role of this class in HIV treatment is warranted by the potential that this class represents in both early treatment/prophylaxis and functional cure.

References

Allers K, Hütter G, Hofmann J et al (2011) Evidence for the cure of HIV infection by Ccr5{delta}32/{δ}32 stem cell transplantation. Blood 117:2791–2799

Alonzo F 3rd, Kozhaya L, Rawlings SA et al (2013) Ccr5 is a receptor for *Staphylococcus aureus* leukotoxin Ed. Nature 493(7430):51–55, Epub 14 Dec 2012

Araujo LA, Junqueira DM, de Medeiros RM et al (2012) Naturally occurring resistance mutations to HIV-1 entry inhibitors in subtypes B, C, and Crf31_Bc. J Clin Virol 54(1):6–10, Epub 18 Feb 2012

Armand-Ugon M, Quinones-Mateu ME, Gutierez A et al (2003) Reduced fitness of HIV-1 resistant to Cxcr4 antagonists. Antivir Ther 8(1):1–8, Epub 26 Apr 2003

Baba M, Takashima K, Miyake H et al (2005) Tak-652 inhibits Ccr5-mediated human immunodeficiency virus type 1 infection in vitro and has favorable pharmacokinetics in humans. Antimicrob Agents Chemother 49(11):4584–4591, Epub 28 Oct 2005

Baba M, Miyake H, Wang X et al (2007) Isolation and characterization of human immunodeficiency virus type 1 resistant to the small-molecule Ccr5 antagonist Tak-652. Antimicrob Agents Chemother 51(2):707–715, Epub 23 Nov 2006

Baldwin C, Berkhout B (2008) Mechanistic studies of a T20-dependent human immunodeficiency virus type 1 variant. J Virol 82(15):7735–7740, Epub 16 May 2008

Berger EA, Murphy PM, Farber JM (1999) Chemokine receptors as HIV-1 coreceptors: roles in viral entry, tropism, and disease. Annu Rev Immunol 17:657–700, Epub 08 Jun 1999

Brumme ZL, Goodrich J, Mayer HB et al (2005) Molecular and clinical epidemiology of Cxcr4-using HIV-1 in a large population of antiretroviral-naive individuals. J Infect Dis 192(3):466–474, Epub 05 July 2005

Burkly LC, Olson D, Shapiro R et al (1992) Inhibition of HIV infection by a novel Cd4 domain 2-specific monoclonal antibody. Dissecting the basis for its inhibitory effect on HIV-induced cell fusion. J Immunol 149(5):1779–1787, Epub 01 Sept 1992

Carmona R, Perez-Alvarez L, Munoz M et al (2005) Natural resistance-associated mutations to enfuvirtide (T20) and polymorphisms in the Gp41 region of different HIV-1 genetic forms from T20 naive patients. J Clin Virol 32(3):248–253, Epub 22 Feb 2005

Ceccherini-Silberstein F, Alteri C, Surdo M et al (eds) (2011) HIV-1 dual/mixed-tropic viruses can be inhibited in vitro as in vivo by Maraviroc: a refined analysis from patients enrolled in the phase-Iib study-A4001029. In: IAS 2011, Rome

Cecilia D, Kulkarni SS, Tripathy SP et al (2000) Absence of coreceptor switch with disease progression in human immunodeficiency virus infections in India. Virology 271(2):253–258, Epub 22 Jun 2000

Chambers P, Pringle CR, Easton AJ (1990) Heptad repeat sequences are located adjacent to hydrophobic regions in several types of virus fusion glycoproteins. J Gen Virol 71(Pt 12):3075–3080, Epub 01 Dec 1990

Chang CH, Hinkula J, Loo M et al (2012) A novel class of anti-HIV agents with multiple copies of enfuvirtide enhances inhibition of viral replication and cellular transmission in vitro. PLoS One 7(7):e41235, Epub 31 July 2012

Charpentier C, Larrouy L, Visseaux B et al (2012) Prevalence of subtype-related polymorphisms associated with in vitro resistance to attachment inhibitor Bms-626529 in HIV-1 'Non-B '-infected patients. J Antimicrob Chemother 67(6):1459–1461, Epub 03 Mar 2012

Chen B, Vogan EM, Gong H et al (2005) Structure of an unliganded simian immunodeficiency virus Gp120 core. Nature 433(7028):834–841, Epub 25 Feb 2005
Coetzer M, Nedellec R, Cilliers T et al (2011) Extreme genetic divergence is required for coreceptor switching in HIV-1 subtype C. J Acquir Immune Defic Syndr 56(1):9–15, Epub 06 Oct 2010
Connor RI, Sheridan KE, Ceradini D et al (1997) Change in coreceptor use correlates with disease progression in HIV-1–infected individuals. J Exp Med 185(4):621–628, Epub 17 Feb 1997
Cooper DA, Heera J, Goodrich J et al (2010) Maraviroc versus efavirenz, both in combination with zidovudine-lamivudine, for the treatment of antiretroviral-naive subjects with Ccr5-tropic HIV-1 infection. J Infect Dis 201(6):803–813
Covens K, Kabeya K, Schrooten Y et al (2009) Evolution of genotypic resistance to enfuvirtide in HIV-1 isolates from different group M subtypes. J Clin Virol 44(4):325–328, Epub 25 Feb 2009
Daar ES, Li XL, Moudgil T et al (1990) High concentrations of recombinant soluble Cd4 Are required to neutralize primary human immunodeficiency virus type 1 isolates. Proc Natl Acad Sci U S A 87(17):6574–6578, Epub 01 Sept 1990
De Jong JJ, De Ronde A, Keulen W et al (1992) Minimal requirements for the human immunodeficiency virus type 1 V3 domain to support the syncytium-inducing phenotype: analysis by single amino acid substitution. J Virol 66(11):6777–6780, Epub 01 Nov 1992
Dean M, Carrington M, Winkler C et al (1996) Genetic restriction of HIV-1 infection and progression to AIDS by a deletion allele of the Ckr5 structural gene. Hemophilia growth and development study, multicenter AIDS cohort study, multicenter hemophilia cohort study, San Francisco city cohort, alive study. Science 273(5283):1856–1862, Epub 27 Sept 1996
Deeks SG, Lu J, Hoh J et al (2007) Interruption of enfuvirtide in HIV-1 infected adults with incomplete viral suppression on an enfuvirtide-based regimen. J Infect Dis 195(3):387–391, Epub 06 Jan 2007
Delwart EL, Mosialos G, Gilmore T (1990) Retroviral envelope glycoproteins contain a "leucine zipper"-like repeat. AIDS Res Hum Retroviruses 6(6):703–706, Epub 01 Jun 1990
Derdeyn CA, Decker JM, Sfakianos JN et al (2000) Sensitivity of human immunodeficiency virus type 1 to the fusion inhibitor T-20 is modulated by coreceptor specificity defined by the V3 loop of Gp120. J Virol 74(18):8358–8367, Epub 23 Aug 2000
Donahue DA, Sloan RD, Kuhl BD et al (2010) Stage-dependent inhibition of HIV-1 replication by antiretroviral drugs in cell culture. Antimicrob Agents Chemother 54(3):1047–1054
Donzella GA, Schols D, Lin SW et al (1998) Amd3100, a small molecule inhibitor of HIV-1 entry via the Cxcr4 Co-receptor. Nat Med 4(1):72–77, Epub 14 Jan 1998
Dorr P, Westby M, Dobbs S et al (2005) Maraviroc (Uk-427,857), a potent, orally bioavailable, and selective small-molecule inhibitor of chemokine receptor Ccr5 with broad-spectrum anti-human immunodeficiency virus type 1 activity. Antimicrob Agents Chemother 49(11):4721–4732
Eggink D, Berkhout B, Sanders RW (2010) Inhibition of HIV-1 by fusion inhibitors. Curr Pharm Des 16(33):3716–3728, Epub 07 Dec 2010
Eggink D, Bontjer I, Langedijk JP et al (2011) Resistance of human immunodeficiency virus type 1 to a third-generation fusion inhibitor requires multiple mutations in Gp41 and is accompanied by a dramatic loss of Gp41 function. J Virol 85(20):10785–10797, Epub 13 Aug 2011
Este JA, Cabrera C, Blanco J et al (1999) Shift of clinical human immunodeficiency virus type 1 isolates from X4 to R5 and prevention of emergence of the syncytium-inducing phenotype by blockade of Cxcr4. J Virol 73(7):5577–5585, Epub 11 Jun 1999
European AIDS Clinical Society (2011) European AIDS Clinical Society (EACS): Treatment Guidelines Version 6.0
Fatkenheuer G, Nelson M, Lazzarin A et al (2008) Subgroup analyses of maraviroc in previously treated R5 HIV-1 infection. N Engl J Med 359(14):1442–1455, Epub 04 Oct 2008
Fiser A-L, Vincent T, Brieu N et al (2010) High Cd4+ T-cell surface Cxcr4 density as a risk factor for R5 to X4 switch in the course of HIV-1 infection. J Acquir Immune Defic Syndr 55(5):529–535
Fleishaker DL, Garcia Meijide JA, Petrov A et al (2012) Maraviroc, a chemokine receptor-5 antagonist, fails to demonstrate efficacy in the treatment of patients with rheumatoid arthritis

in a randomized, double-blind placebo-controlled trial. Arthritis Res Ther 14(1):R11, Epub 19 Jan 2012
Freed EO, Martin MA (1995) The role of human immunodeficiency virus type 1 envelope glycoproteins in virus infection. J Biol Chem 270(41):23883–23886, Epub 13 Oct 1995
Funderburg N, Kalinowska M, Eason J et al (2010) Effects of maraviroc and efavirenz on markers of immune activation and inflammation and associations with Cd4 cell rises in HIV-infected patients. PLoS One 5:10
Gallaher WR, Ball JM, Garry RF et al (1989) A general model for the transmembrane proteins of HIV and other retroviruses. AIDS Res Hum Retroviruses 5(4):431–440, Epub 01 Aug 1989
Garcia-Perez J, Rueda P, Alcami J et al (2011) Allosteric model of maraviroc binding to Cc chemokine receptor 5 (Ccr5). J Biol Chem 286(38):33409–33421, Epub 22 July 2011
Greenberg ML, Cammack N (2004) Resistance to enfuvirtide, the first HIV fusion inhibitor. J Antimicrob Chemother 54(2):333–340, Epub 03 July 2004
Grinsztejn B, Nguyen BY, Katlama C et al (2007) Safety and efficacy of the HIV-1 integrase inhibitor raltegravir (Mk-0518) in treatment-experienced patients with multidrug-resistant virus: a phase Ii randomised controlled trial. Lancet 369(9569):1261–1269, Epub 17 Apr 2007
Gulick RM, Su Z, Flexner C et al (2007) Phase 2 study of the safety and efficacy of vicriviroc, a Ccr5 inhibitor, in HIV-1-infected, treatment-experienced patients: AIDS clinical trials group 5211. J Infect Dis 196(2):304–312, Epub 16 Jun 2007
Gulick RM, Lalezari J, Goodrich J et al (2008) Maraviroc for previously treated patients with R5 HIV-1 infection. N Engl J Med 359(14):1429–1441, Epub 04 Oct 2008
Hanna GJ, Lalezari J, Hellinger JA et al (2011) Antiviral activity, pharmacokinetics, and safety of Bms-488043, a novel oral small-molecule HIV-1 attachment inhibitor, in HIV-1-infected subjects. Antimicrob Agents Chemother 55(2):722–728, Epub 17 Nov 2010
Harrison JE, Lynch JB, Sierra LJ et al (2008) Baseline resistance of primary human immunodeficiency virus type 1 strains to the Cxcr4 inhibitor Amd3100. J Virol 82(23):11695–11704, Epub 19 Sept 2008
He Y, Xiao Y, Song H et al (2008) Design and evaluation of sifuvirtide, a novel HIV-1 fusion inhibitor. J Biol Chem 283(17):11126–11134, Epub 28 Feb 2008
Hendrix CW, Collier AC, Lederman MM et al (2004) Safety, pharmacokinetics, and antiviral activity of Amd3100, a selective Cxcr4 receptor inhibitor, in HIV-1 infection. J Acquir Immune Defic Syndr 37(2):1253–1262, Epub 24 Sept 2004
Henrich TJ, Tsibris AM, Lewine NR et al (2010) Evolution of Ccr5 antagonist resistance in an HIV-1 subtype C clinical isolate. J Acquir Immune Defic Syndr 55(4):420–427, Epub 22 Sept 2010
Hernandez PA, Gorlin RJ, Lukens JN et al (2003) Mutations in the chemokine receptor gene Cxcr4 are associated with whim syndrome, a combined immunodeficiency disease. Nat Genet 34(1):70–74, Epub 15 Apr 2003
Ho HT, Fan L, Nowicka-Sans B et al (2006) Envelope conformational changes induced by human immunodeficiency virus type 1 attachment inhibitors prevent Cd4 binding and downstream entry events. J Virol 80(8):4017–4025, Epub 31 Mar 2006
Huang Y, Paxton WA, Wolinsky SM et al (1996) The role of a mutant Ccr5 allele in HIV-1 transmission and disease progression. Nat Med 2(11):1240–1243, Epub 01 Nov 1996
Huang CC, Tang M, Zhang MY et al (2005) Structure of a V3-containing HIV-1 Gp120 core. Science 310(5750):1025–1028, Epub 15 Nov 2005
Hütter G, Allers K, Schneider T (2009) The additional use of viral entry inhibitors during autologous hematopoietic stem cell transplantation in patients with non-Hodgkin S Lymphoma and HIV-1 infection. Biol Blood Marrow Transplant 17(4):586–587
Izumi K, Kodama E, Shimura K et al (2009) Design of peptide-based inhibitors for human immunodeficiency virus type 1 strains resistant to T-20. J Biol Chem 284(8):4914–4920, Epub 17 Dec 2008
Jacobson JM, Saag MS, Thompson MA et al (2008) Antiviral activity of single-dose Pro 140, a Ccr5 monoclonal antibody, in HIV-infected adults. J Infect Dis 198(9):1345–1352, Epub 06 Sept 2008

Jacobson JM, Kuritzkes DR, Godofsky E et al (2009) Safety, pharmacokinetics, and antiretroviral activity of multiple doses of ibalizumab (formerly Tnx-355), an anti-Cd4 monoclonal antibody, in human immunodeficiency virus type 1-infected adults. Antimicrob Agents Chemother 53 (2):450–457, Epub 19 Nov 2008

Jacobson JM, Thompson MA, Lalezari JP et al (2010) Anti-HIV-1 activity of weekly or biweekly treatment with subcutaneous Pro 140, a Ccr5 monoclonal antibody. J Infect Dis 201 (10):1481–1487, Epub 10 Apr 2010

Kanbara K, Sato S, Tanuma J et al (2001) Biological and genetic characterization of a human immunodeficiency virus strain resistant to Cxcr4 antagonist T134. AIDS Res Hum Retroviruses 17(7):615–622, Epub 26 May 2001

Kilby JM, Hopkins S, Venetta TM et al (1998) Potent suppression of HIV-1 replication in humans by T-20, a peptide inhibitor of Gp41-mediated virus entry. Nat Med 4(11):1302–1307, Epub 11 Nov 1998

Kilby JM, Lalezari JP, Eron JJ et al (2002) The safety, plasma pharmacokinetics, and antiviral activity of subcutaneous enfuvirtide (T-20), a peptide inhibitor of Gp41-mediated virus fusion, in HIV-infected adults. AIDS Res Hum Retroviruses 18(10):685–693, Epub 09 Aug 2002

Kindberg E, Mickiene A, Ax C et al (2008) A deletion in the chemokine receptor 5 (Ccr5) gene is associated with tickborne encephalitis. J Infect Dis 197(2):266–269, Epub 09 Jan 2008

Kramer VG, Schader SM, Oliveira M et al (2012) Maraviroc and other HIV-1 entry inhibitors exhibit a class-specific redistribution effect that results in increased extracellular viral load. Antimicrob Agents Chemother 56(8):4154–4160, Epub 23 May 2012

Kuhmann SE, Pugach P, Kunstman KJ et al (2004) Genetic and phenotypic analyses of human immunodeficiency virus type 1 escape from a small-molecule Ccr5 inhibitor. J Virol 78 (6):2790–2807, Epub 03 Mar 2004

Kuritzkes DR (2009) HIV-1 entry inhibitors: an overview. Curr Opin HIV AIDS 4(2):82–87, Epub 03 Apr 2009

Kuritzkes DR, Jacobson J, Powderly WG et al (2004) Antiretroviral activity of the anti-Cd4 monoclonal antibody Tnx-355 in patients infected with HIV type 1. J Infect Dis 189 (2):286–291, Epub 15 Jan 2004

Kwong PD, Wyatt R, Robinson J et al (1998) Structure of an HIV Gp120 envelope glycoprotein in complex with the Cd4 receptor and a neutralizing human antibody. Nature 393(6686):648–659, Epub 26 Jun 1998

Lalezari JP, Henry K, O'Hearn M et al (2003a) Enfuvirtide, an HIV-1 fusion inhibitor, for drug-resistant HIV infection in north and south America. N Engl J Med 348(22):2175–2185

Lalezari JP, Eron JJ, Carlson M et al (2003b) A phase Ii clinical study of the long-term safety and antiviral activity of enfuvirtide-based antiretroviral therapy. AIDS 17(5):691–698, Epub 21 Mar 2003

Lalezari J, Thompson M, Kumar P et al (2005) Antiviral activity and safety of 873140, a novel Ccr5 antagonist, during short-term monotherapy in HIV-infected adults. AIDS 19(14):1443–1448, Epub 02 Sept 2005

Lalezari J, Gathe J, Brinson C et al (2011) Safety, efficacy, and pharmacokinetics of Tbr-652, a Ccr5/Ccr2 antagonist, in HIV-1-infected, treatment-experienced, Ccr5 antagonist-naive subjects. J Acquir Immune Defic Syndr 57(2):118–125, Epub 15 Feb 2011

Lazzarin A, Clotet B, Cooper D et al (2003) Efficacy of enfuvirtide in patients infected with drug-resistant HIV-1 in Europe and Australia. N Engl J Med 348(22):2186–2195, Epub 30 May 2003

Leung PH, Chen JH, Wong KH et al (2010) High prevalence of primary enfuvirtide (Enf) resistance-associated mutations in HIV-1-infected patients in Hong Kong. J Clin Virol 47 (3):273–275, Epub 02 Feb 2010

Lim JK, Louie CY, Glaser C et al (2008) Genetic deficiency of chemokine receptor Ccr5 is a strong risk factor for symptomatic west Nile virus infection: a meta-analysis of 4 cohorts in the Us epidemic. J Infect Dis 197(2):262–265, Epub 09 Jan 2008

Lin PF, Blair W, Wang T et al (2003) A small molecule HIV-1 inhibitor that targets the HIV-1 envelope and inhibits Cd4 receptor binding. Proc Natl Acad Sci U S A 100(19):11013–11018, Epub 22 Aug 2003

Liu R, Paxton WA, Choe S et al (1996) Homozygous defect in HIV-1 coreceptor accounts for resistance of some multiply-exposed individuals to HIV-1 infection. Cell 86(3):367–377, Epub 09 Aug 1996

Liu Q, Chen H, Ojode T et al (2012) Whim syndrome caused by a single amino acid substitution in the carboxy-tail of chemokine receptor Cxcr4. Blood 120(1):181–189, Epub 19 May 2012

Ma Q, Jones D, Borghesani PR et al (1998) Impaired B-lymphopoiesis, myelopoiesis, and derailed cerebellar neuron migration in Cxcr4- and Sdf-1-deficient mice. Proc Natl Acad Sci U S A 95 (16):9448–9453, Epub 05 Aug 1998

Makinson A, Reynes J (2009) The fusion inhibitor enfuvirtide in recent antiretroviral strategies. Curr Opin HIV AIDS 4(2):150–158, Epub 03 Apr 2009

Marcelin AG, Reynes J, Yerly S et al (2004) Characterization of genotypic determinants in Hr-1 and Hr-2 Gp41 domains in individuals with persistent HIV viraemia under T-20. AIDS 18 (9):1340–1342, Epub 15 Sept 2004

Marier JF, Trinh M, Pheng LH et al (2011) Pharmacokinetics and pharmacodynamics of Tbr-652, a novel Ccr5 antagonist, in HIV-1-infected, antiretroviral treatment-experienced, Ccr5 antagonist-naive patients. Antimicrob Agents Chemother 55(6):2768–2774, Epub 14 Apr 2011

Markowitz M, Nguyen BY, Gotuzzo E et al (2007) Rapid and durable antiretroviral effect of the HIV-1 integrase inhibitor raltegravir as part of combination therapy in treatment-naive patients with HIV-1 infection: results of a 48-week controlled study. J Acquir Immune Defic Syndr 46 (2):125–133, Epub 28 Aug 2007

Marozsan AJ, Kuhmann SE, Morgan T et al (2005) Generation and properties of a human immunodeficiency virus type 1 isolate resistant to the small molecule Ccr5 inhibitor, Sch-417690 (Sch-D). Virology 338(1):182–199, Epub 07 Jun 2005

McDermott DH, Liu Q, Ulrick J et al (2011a) The Cxcr4 antagonist plerixafor corrects panleukopenia in patients with whim syndrome. Blood 118(18):4957–4962, Epub 06 Sept 2011

McDermott DH, Lopez J, Deng F et al (2011b) Amd3100 is a potent antagonist at Cxcr4(R334x), a hyperfunctional mutant chemokine receptor and cause of whim syndrome. J Cell Mol Med 15 (10):2071–2081, Epub 13 Nov 2010

McNicholas P, Wei Y, Whitcomb J et al (2010) Characterization of emergent HIV resistance in treatment-naive subjects enrolled in a vicriviroc phase 2 trial. J Infect Dis 201(10):1470–1480, Epub 09 Apr 2010

McNicholas PM, Mann PA, Wojcik L et al (2011) Mapping and characterization of vicriviroc resistance mutations from HIV-1 isolated from treatment-experienced subjects enrolled in a phase Ii study (victor-E1). J Acquir Immune Defic Syndr 56(3):222–229, Epub 07 Jan 2011

Melby TE, Despirito M, Demasi RA et al (2007) Association between specific enfuvirtide resistance mutations and Cd4 cell response during enfuvirtide-based therapy. AIDS 21(18):2537–2539, Epub 21 Nov 2007

Michael NL, Louie LG, Rohrbaugh AL et al (1997) The role of Ccr5 and Ccr2 polymorphisms in HIV-1 transmission and disease progression. Nat Med 3(10):1160–1162, Epub 23 Oct 1997

Mills A, Mildvan D, Podzamczer D et al (eds) (2012) Once-daily Maraviroc in combination with Ritonavir-boosted Atazanavir in treatment-NaïVe patients infected with Ccr5-tropic HIV-1 (Study A4001078): 96-Week results. In: IAS 2012, Washington, DC

Moulard M, Decroly E (2000) Maturation of HIV envelope glycoprotein precursors by cellular endoproteases. Biochim Biophys Acta 1469(3):121–132, Epub 07 Nov 2000

Moyle GJ, Wildfire A, Mandalia S et al (2005) Epidemiology and predictive factors for chemokine receptor use in HIV-1 infection. J Infect Dis 191(6):866–872, Epub 18 Feb 2005

Moyle G, DeJesus E, Boffito M et al (2009) Proof of activity with Amd11070, an orally bioavailable inhibitor of Cxcr4-tropic HIV type 1. Clin Infect Dis 48(6):798–805, Epub 06 Feb 2009

Nagasawa T, Hirota S, Tachibana K et al (1996) Defects of B-cell lymphopoiesis and bone-marrow myelopoiesis in mice lacking the Cxc chemokine pbsf/Sdf-1. Nature 382(6592):635–638, Epub 15 Aug 1996

Nelson M, Arasteh K, Clotet B et al (2005) Durable efficacy of enfuvirtide over 48 weeks in heavily treatment-experienced HIV-1-infected patients in the T-20 versus optimized background regimen only 1 and 2 clinical trials. J Acquir Immune Defic Syndr 40(4):404–412, Epub 11 Nov 2005

Nettles RE, Schurmann D, Zhu L et al (2012) Pharmacodynamics, safety, and pharmacokinetics of Bms-663068, an oral HIV-1 attachment inhibitor in HIV-1-infected subjects. J Infect Dis 206(7):1002–1011, Epub 17 Aug 2012

Nowicka-Sans B, Gong YF, McAuliffe B et al (2012) In vitro antiviral characteristics of HIV-1 attachment inhibitor Bms-626529, the active component of the prodrug Bms-663068. Antimicrob Agents Chemother 56(7):3498–3507, Epub 02 May 2012

Olson WC, Rabut GE, Nagashima KA et al (1999) Differential inhibition of human immunodeficiency virus type 1 fusion, Gp120 binding, and Cc-chemokine activity by monoclonal antibodies to Ccr5. J Virol 73(5):4145–4155, Epub 10 Apr 1999

Pace CS, Fordyce MW, Franco D et al (2013) Anti-Cd4 monoclonal antibody ibalizumab exhibits breadth and potency against HIV-1, with natural resistance mediated by the loss of a V5 glycan in envelope. J Acquir Immune Defic Syndr 62(1):1–9, Epub 02 Oct 2012

Pastore C, Ramos A, Mosier DE (2004) Intrinsic obstacles to human immunodeficiency virus type 1 coreceptor switching. J Virol 78(14):7565–7574, Epub 29 Jun 2004

Perez-Olmeda M, Cascajero A, Rastrojo A et al. (eds) (2012) Dynamic of HIV-1 quasi-species during a short exposure to Maraviroc in NaïVe patients using 454 ultra-deep sequencing. In: 19th conference on retroviruses and opportunistic infections, 2012, Seattle

Pfaff JM, Wilen CB, Harrison JE et al (2010) HIV-1 resistance to Ccr5 antagonists associated with highly efficient use of Ccr5 and altered tropism on primary Cd4+ T cells. J Virol 1–34

Platt EJ, Gomes MM, Kabat D (2012) Kinetic mechanism for HIV-1 neutralization by antibody 2g12 entails reversible glycan binding that slows cell entry. Proc Natl Acad Sci U S A 109(20):7829–7834, Epub 02 May 2012

Pope M, Haase AT (2003) Transmission, acute HIV-1 infection and the quest for strategies to prevent infection. Nat Med 9(7):847–852, Epub 02 July 2003

Prahalad S (2006) Negative association between the chemokine receptor Ccr5-Delta32 polymorphism and rheumatoid arthritis: a meta-analysis. Genes Immun 7(3):264–268, Epub 17 Mar 2006

Putcharoen O, Lee SH, Henrich TJ et al (2012) HIV-1 clinical isolates resistant to Ccr5 antagonists exhibit delayed entry kinetics that are corrected in the presence of drug. J Virol 86(2):1119–1128, Epub 18 Nov 2011

Rappaport J, Cho YY, Hendel H et al (1997) 32 Bp Ccr-5 gene deletion and resistance to fast progression in HIV-1 infected heterozygotes. Lancet 349(9056):922–923, Epub 29 Mar 1997

Ratcliff AN, Shi W, Arts EJ (2013) HIV-1 resistance to maraviroc conferred by a Cd4 binding site mutation in the envelope glycoprotein Gp120. J Virol 87(2):923–934, Epub 09 Nov 2012

Ray N, Blackburn LA, Doms RW (2009) Hr-2 mutations in human immunodeficiency virus type 1 Gp41 restore fusion kinetics delayed by Hr-1 mutations that cause clinical resistance to enfuvirtide. J Virol 83(7):2989–2995, Epub 21 Jan 2009

Recordon-Pinson P, Raymond S, Bellecave P et al (2013) HIV-1 dynamics and coreceptor usage in maraviroc-treated patients with ongoing replication. Antimicrob Agents Chemother 57(2):930–935, Epub 05 Dec 2012

Reeves JD, Lee FH, Miamidian JL et al (2005) Enfuvirtide resistance mutations: impact on human immunodeficiency virus envelope function, entry inhibitor sensitivity, and virus neutralization. J Virol 79(8):4991–4999, Epub 30 Mar 2005

Regoes RR, Bonhoeffer S (2005) The HIV coreceptor switch: a population dynamical perspective. Trends Microbiol 13(6):269–277

Reshef R, Luger SM, Hexner EO et al (2012) Blockade of lymphocyte chemotaxis in visceral graft-versus-host disease. N Engl J Med 367(2):135–145, Epub 13 July 2012

Reynes J, Arasteh K, Clotet B et al (2007) Toro: ninety-six-week virologic and immunologic response and safety evaluation of enfuvirtide with an optimized background of antiretrovirals. AIDS Patient Care STDS 21(8):533–543, Epub 23 Aug 2007

Roche M, Jakobsen M, Sterjovski J et al (2011a) HIV-1 escape from the Ccr5 antagonist maraviroc associated with an altered and less efficient mechanism of Gp120-Ccr5 engagement that attenuates macrophage-tropism. J Virol 85(9):4330–4342. doi:10.1128/JVI.00106-11v1

Roche M, Jakobsen MR, Ellett A et al (2011b) HIV-1 predisposed to acquiring resistance to maraviroc (Mvc) and other Ccr5 antagonists in vitro has an inherent, low-level ability to utilize Mvc-bound Ccr5 for entry. Retrovirology 8:89, Epub 08 Nov 2011

Roche M, Salimi H, Duncan R et al (2013) A common mechanism of clinical HIV-1 resistance to the Ccr5 antagonist maraviroc despite divergent resistance levels and lack of common Gp120 resistance mutations. Retrovirology 10(1):43, Epub 23 Apr 2013

Saag M, Goodrich J, Fatkenheuer G et al (2009) A double-blind, placebo-controlled trial of maraviroc in treatment-experienced patients infected with non-R5 HIV-1. J Infect Dis 199(11):1638–1647, Epub 13 May 2009

Samson M, Libert F, Doranz BJ et al (1996) Resistance to HIV-1 infection in Caucasian individuals bearing mutant alleles of the Ccr-5 chemokine receptor gene. Nature 382(6593):722–725, Epub 22 Aug 1996

Savkovic B, Symonds G, Murray JM (2012) Stochastic model of in-vivo X4 emergence during HIV infection: implications for the Ccr5 inhibitor maraviroc. PLoS One 7(7):e38755, Epub 07 Aug 2012

Scarlatti G, Tresoldi E, Bjorndal A et al (1997) In vivo evolution of HIV-1 Co-receptor usage and sensitivity to chemokine-mediated suppression. Nat Med 3(11):1259–1265, Epub 14 Nov 1997

Schols D, Este JA, Cabrera C et al (1998) T-cell-line-tropic human immunodeficiency virus type 1 that is made resistant to stromal cell-derived factor 1alpha contains mutations in the envelope Gp120 but does not show a switch in coreceptor use. J Virol 72(5):4032–4037, Epub 29 Apr 1998

Schooley RT, Merigan TC, Gaut P et al (1990) Recombinant soluble Cd4 therapy in patients with the acquired immunodeficiency syndrome (AIDS) and AIDS-related complex. A phase I-Ii escalating dosage trial. Ann Intern Med 112(4):247–253, Epub 15 Feb 1990

Schroder C, Pierson RN 3rd, Nguyen BN et al (2007) Ccr5 blockade modulates inflammation and alloimmunity in primates. J Immunol 179(4):2289–2299, Epub 07 Aug 2007

Schuitemaker H, Koot M, Kootstra NA et al (1992) Biological phenotype of human immunodeficiency virus type 1 clones at different stages of infection: progression of disease is associated with a shift from monocytotropic to T-cell-tropic virus population. J Virol 66(3):1354–1360, Epub 01 Mar 1992

Sedaghat AR, Dinoso JB, Shen L et al (2008) Decay dynamics of HIV-1 depend on the inhibited stages of the viral life cycle. Proc Natl Acad Sci U S A 105(12):4832–4837, Epub 26 Mar 2008

Shioda T, Levy JA, Cheng-Mayer C (1991) Macrophage and T cell-line tropisms of HIV-1 are determined by specific regions of the envelope Gp120 gene. Nature 349(6305):167–169, Epub 10 Jan 1991

Shioda T, Levy JA, Cheng-Mayer C (1992) Small amino acid changes in the V3 hypervariable region of Gp120 can affect the T-cell-line and macrophage tropism of human immunodeficiency virus type 1. Proc Natl Acad Sci U S A 89(20):9434–9438, Epub 15 Oct 1992

Sierra-Madero J, Di Perri G, Wood R et al (2010) Efficacy and safety of maraviroc versus efavirenz, both with zidovudine/lamivudine: 96-week results from the merit study. HIV Clin Trials 11 (3):125–132, Epub 26 Aug 2010

Skerlj RT, Bridger GJ, Kaller A et al (2010) Discovery of novel small molecule orally bioavailable C-X-C chemokine receptor 4 antagonists that are potent inhibitors of T-tropic (X4) HIV-1 replication. J Med Chem 53(8):3376–3388, Epub 20 Mar 2010

Skerlj R, Bridger G, McEachern E et al (2011) Design of novel Cxcr4 antagonists that Are potent inhibitors of T-tropic (X4) HIV-1 replication. Bioorg Med Chem Lett 21(5):1414–1418, Epub 08 Feb 2011

Soria A, Cavarelli M, Sala S et al (2008) Unexpected dramatic increase in Cd4+ cell count in a patient with AIDS after enfuvirtide treatment despite persistent viremia and resistance mutations. J Med Virol 80(6):937–941, Epub 23 Apr 2008

Soulie C, Lambert-Niclot S, Fofana DB et al (2013) Frequency of amino acid changes associated with resistance to attachment inhibitor Bms-626529 in R5- and X4-tropic HIV-1 subtype B. J Antimicrob Chemother 68(6):1243–1245, Epub 12 Feb 2013

Stone ND, Dunaway SB, Flexner C et al (2007) Multiple-dose escalation study of the safety, pharmacokinetics, and biologic activity of oral Amd070, a selective Cxcr4 receptor inhibitor, in human subjects. Antimicrob Agents Chemother 51(7):2351–2358, Epub 25 Apr 2007

Sullivan N, Sun Y, Binley J et al (1998) Determinants of human immunodeficiency virus type 1 envelope glycoprotein activation by soluble Cd4 and monoclonal antibodies. J Virol 72(8):6332–6338, Epub 11 July 1998

Svicher V, Aquaro S, D'Arrigo R et al (2008) Specific enfuvirtide-associated mutational pathways in HIV-1 Gp41 are significantly correlated with an increase in Cd4(+) cell count, despite virological failure. J Infect Dis 197(10):1408–1418, Epub 19 Apr 2008

Symons J, van Lelyveld SFL, Hoepelman AIM et al (2011) Maraviroc is able to inhibit dual-R5 viruses in a dual/mixed HIV-1-infected patient. J Antimicrob Chemother 66(4):890–895

Symons J, Deeks S, Hutter G et al (eds) (2012) The cure of the 'Berlin patient': why did pre-existing X4-variants not emergence after allogeneic Ccr5-Δ32 Sct? In: AIDS 2012, Washington, DC

Tachibana K, Hirota S, Iizasa H et al (1998) The chemokine receptor Cxcr4 is essential for vascularization of the gastrointestinal tract. Nature 393(6685):591–594, Epub 20 Jun 1998

Tilton JC, Doms RW (2010) Entry inhibitors in the treatment of HIV-1 infection. Antiviral Res 85(1):91–100, Epub 18 Aug 2009

Tilton JC, Amrine-Madsen H, Miamidian JL et al (2010) HIV type 1 from a patient with baseline resistance to Ccr5 antagonists uses drug-bound receptor for entry. AIDS Res Hum Retroviruses 26(1):13–24, Epub 09 Jan 2010

Toma J, Weinheimer SP, Stawiski E et al (2011) Loss of asparagine-linked glycosylation sites in variable region 5 of human immunodeficiency virus type 1 envelope is associated with resistance to Cd4 antibody ibalizumab. J Virol 85(8):3872–3880, Epub 04 Feb 2011

Trkola A, Kuhmann SE, Strizki JM et al (2002) HIV-1 escape from a small molecule, Ccr5-specific entry inhibitor does not involve Cxcr4 use. Proc Natl Acad Sci U S A 99(1):395–400, Epub 10 Jan 2002

Tsibris AM, Sagar M, Gulick RM et al (2008) In vivo emergence of vicriviroc resistance in a human immunodeficiency virus type 1 subtype C-infected subject. J Virol 82(16):8210–8214, Epub 23 May 2008

USFDA (2009) Food and Drug Administration: Expanded indication for Selzentry (maraviroc)

Westby M, Lewis M, Whitcomb J et al (2006) Emergence of Cxcr4-using human immunodeficiency virus type 1 (HIV-1) variants in a minority of HIV-1-infected patients following treatment with the Ccr5 antagonist maraviroc is from a pretreatment Cxcr4-using virus reservoir. J Virol 80 (10):4909–4920, Epub 28 Apr 2006

Wheeler J, McHale M, Jackson V et al (2007) Assessing theoretical risk and benefit suggested by genetic association studies of Ccr5: experience in a drug development programme for maraviroc. Antivir Ther 12(2):233–245, Epub 17 May 2007

Wild C, Greenwell T, Matthews T (1993) A synthetic peptide from HIV-1 Gp41 is a potent inhibitor of virus-mediated cell-cell fusion. AIDS Res Hum Retroviruses 9(11):1051–1053, Epub 01 Nov 1993

Wilkin TJ, Su Z, Kuritzkes DR et al (2007) HIV type 1 chemokine coreceptor use among antiretroviral-experienced patients screened for a clinical trial of a Ccr5 inhibitor: AIDS clinical trial group A5211. Clin Infect Dis 44(4):591–595, Epub 24 Jan 2007

Winkler C, Modi W, Smith MW et al (1998) Genetic restriction of AIDS pathogenesis by an Sdf-1 chemokine gene variant. Alive study, hemophilia growth and development study (hgds), multicenter AIDS cohort study (Macs), multicenter hemophilia cohort study (mhcs), San Francisco city cohort (sfcc). Science 279(5349):389–393, Epub 07 Feb 1998

Xu L, Pozniak A, Wildfire A et al (2005) Emergence and evolution of enfuvirtide resistance following long-term therapy involves heptad repeat 2 mutations within Gp41. Antimicrob Agents Chemother 49(3):1113–1119, Epub 25 Feb 2005

Yu X, Yuan L, Huang Y et al (2011) Susceptibility of HIV-1 subtypes B′, Crf07_Bc and Crf01_Ae that are predominantly circulating in china to HIV-1 entry inhibitors. PLoS One 6(3):e17605

Zhang X, Nieforth K, Lang JM et al (2002) Pharmacokinetics of plasma enfuvirtide after subcutaneous administration to patients with human immunodeficiency virus: inverse Gaussian density absorption and 2-compartment disposition. Clin Pharmacol Ther 72(1):10–19, Epub 02 Aug 2002

Zhou N, Fan L, Ho HT et al (2010) Increased sensitivity of HIV variants selected by attachment inhibitors to broadly neutralizing antibodies. Virology 402(2):256–261, Epub 20 Apr 2010

Zhou N, Nowicka-Sans B, Zhang S et al (2011) In vivo patterns of resistance to the HIV attachment inhibitor Bms-488043. Antimicrob Agents Chemother 55(2):729–737, Epub 17 Nov 2010

Zou YR, Kottmann AH, Kuroda M et al (1998) Function of the chemokine receptor Cxcr4 in haematopoiesis and in cerebellar development. Nature 393(6685):595–599, Epub 20 Jun 1998

HIV-1 Resistance to Reverse Transcriptase Inhibitors

Grant Schauer and Nicolas Sluis-Cremer

Contents

G. Schauer
Department of Cell Biology, Rockefeller University, New York, NY, USA
e-mail: gschauer@rockefeller.edu

N. Sluis-Cremer (✉)
Department of Medicine, Division of Infectious Diseases, University of Pittsburgh School of Medicine, Pittsburgh PA, USA
e-mail: nps2@pitt.edu

M. Gotte et al. (eds.), *Handbook of Antimicrobial Resistance*,
DOI 10.1007/978-1-4939-0694-9_26

Abstract

Purpose of Review: This review discusses the mutations and mechanisms associated with HIV-1 resistance to nucleoside reverse transcriptase (RT) inhibitors (NRTIs) and nonnucleoside RT inhibitors (NNRTIs).

Recent Findings: First-line antiretroviral therapy (ART) for the treatment of HIV-1 infection typically includes two NRTIs in combination with an NNRTI or a protease inhibitor. NRTIs and NNRTIs are also routinely used in second-line and salvage ART therapies. HIV-1 resistance to all of the FDA-approved NRTIs and NNRTIs has been documented. An understanding of the mutations associated with RT inhibitor (RTI) resistance, the antagonistic or complementary interactions between RTI-resistance mutations, and the mechanisms of HIV-1 resistance to RTIs is of critical importance for the development and formulation of effective ART therapies. Of concern, there has been a significant increase in circulating and transmitted NNRTI drug resistance in resource-limited settings due to the extensive use of NNRTIs in prevention and treatment strategies for HIV-1 infection. Despite this increase in NNRTI drug resistance, the diarylpyrimidine NNRTIs, dapivirine, etravirine, and rilpivirine, will be increasingly used in resource-limited settings. As such, there is a continued need to monitor and understand NNRTI resistance, particularly in sub-Saharan Africa where non-subtype B HIV-1 predominates.

Summary: This review describes HIV-1 resistance to NRTIs and NNRTIs.

Keywords

HIV • Reverse transcriptase • Nannucleosicle • Efavirens • Neviapine • Rilpivirine • Etravirine

Key Points

1. NRTIs and NNRTIs form the backbone of most first-line ART.
2. Thirteen RTIs (eight NRTIs and five NNRTIs) have been approved for treatment, although only ten of these are routinely used.
3. RTI therapy selects for viruses that have mutations in HIV-1 RT.
4. NRTI-associated resistance mutations can be broadly categorized into two groups depending on whether they confer resistance via a discrimination of excision phenotype.

5. HIV-1 resistance to NNRTIs correlates directly with mutations of one or more RT residues in the NNRTI-binding pocket.
6. Interactions between different NRTI and NNRTI-resistance mutations can be complementary or antagonistic.
7. There has been a significant increase in NNRTI drug resistance in resource-limited settings that could impact future prevention and treatment strategies.

Introduction

HIV-1 reverse transcriptase (RT) catalyzes the conversion of the viral single-stranded (+)RNA into double-stranded DNA. The enzyme is multifunctional and possesses both a DNA polymerase activity that can use either RNA or DNA as a template and a ribonuclease H (RNase H) activity that degrades the RNA strand in RNA/DNA duplexes. HIV-1 RT is composed of a 560-residue 66 kDa subunit (p66) and a p66-derived 440-residue 51 kDa (p51) subunit. The p66 subunit contains three domains, namely, DNA polymerase (residues 1–318), connection (residues 319–426), and RNase H (residues 427–560) (Kohlstaedt et al. 1992). In comparison, p51 comprises only the polymerase and connection domains. Each p66/p51 RT molecule has one binding cleft for the template/primer (T/P) nucleic acid substrate, one DNA polymerization active site, and one RNase H active site. Both the polymerase and RNase H active sites reside in p66; although p51 is identical in amino acid sequence to p66, the polymerase active site in this subunit is not functional (Kohlstaedt et al. 1992; Wang et al. 1994).

RT Inhibitors (RTIs)

The US Food and Drug Administration (FDA) has approved 13 RTIs for the treatment of HIV-1 infection, although only 11 of these are currently used (see below). These inhibitors, all of which bind at or near to the DNA polymerase active site of the enzyme, can be classified into two distinct groups: (1) the nucleoside and nucleotide RT inhibitors (NRTIs) and (2) the nonnucleoside RT inhibitors (NNRTIs).

The NRTIs are analogs of naturally occurring dNTPs that lack a 3′-hydroxyl group on the ribose sugar/pseudosugar. They were the first drugs used to treat HIV-1 infection, and they remain integral components of nearly all antiretroviral (ART) regimens. To exhibit antiviral activity, NRTIs must be metabolically converted by host-cell kinases to their corresponding triphosphate forms (NRTI-TP). The NRTI-TP inhibit HIV-1 RT DNA synthesis by acting as chain terminators of DNA synthesis (Goody et al. 1991). Eight NRTIs have been approved for clinical use, namely, 3′-azido-3′-deoxythymidine (zidovudine, AZT); 2′,3′-dideoxyinosine (didanosine, ddI); 2′,3′-dideoxycytidine (zalcitabine, ddC); (−)-β-2′,3′-dideoxy-3′-thiacytidine (lamivudine, 3TC); 2′-deoxy-2′,3′-didehydrothymidine (stavudine, d4T); (1*S*,4*R*)-4-[2-amino-6-(cyclopropyl-amino)-9H-purin-9-yl]-2-cyclopentene-1-

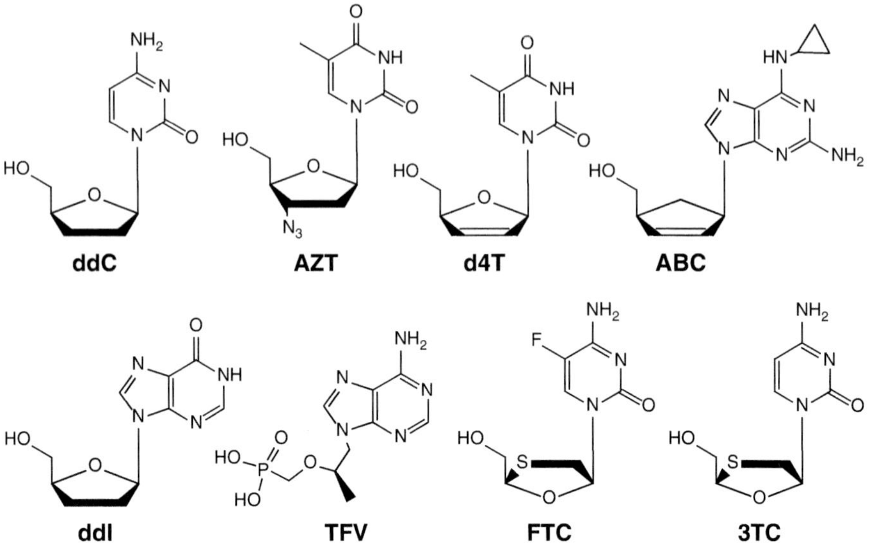

Fig. 1 Chemical structures of FDA-approved NRTIs

methanol succinate (abacavir, ABC); (*R*)-9-(2-phosphonylmethoxypropyl) adenine (TFV, tenofovir); and 5-fluoro-1-[(2*R*,5*S*)-2-(hydroxymethyl)-1,3-oxathiolan-5-yl]cytosine (emtricitabine, FTC) (Fig. 1). ddC is less potent than the other NRTIs, has inconvenient dosing schedules, and is associated with serious adverse events. For these reasons, it is now rarely used to treat HIV-1 infection. Similarly, the World Health Organization advocated that d4T should be phased out of use because of its long-term, irreversible side effects. However, d4T is still used in first-line therapy in developing countries due to its low cost and widespread availability.

The NNRTIs are a group of amphiphilic compounds that bind to a hydrophobic pocket in HIV-1 RT that is proximal to but distinct from the polymerase active site (Kohlstaedt et al. 1992; Sluis-Cremer et al. 2004). NNRTI are allosteric inhibitors of HIV-1 RT DNA polymerization reactions (Sluis-Cremer et al. 2004). FDA-approved NNRTIs include 11-cyclopropyl-4-methyl-5,11-dihydro-6*H*-dipyrido[3,2-*b*:2′,3′-*e*][1,4] diazepin-6-one (nevirapine; NVP); *N*-[2-({4-[3-(propan-2-ylamino)pyridin-2-yl] piperazin-1-yl}carbonyl)-1*H*-indol-5-yl]methanesulfonamide (delavirdine; DEL); (4*S*)-6-chloro-4-(2-cyclopropylethynyl)-4-(trifluoromethyl)-2,4-dihydro-1*H*-3,1-benzoxazin-2-one (efavirenz; EFV), 4-[6-Amino-5-bromo-2-[(4-cyanophenyl)amino] pyrimidin-4-yl]oxy-3,5-dimethylbenzonitrile (etravirine; ETV); and 4-{[4-({4-[(*E*)-2-cyanovinyl]-2,6-dimethylphenyl}amino)pyrimidin-2-yl]amino}benzonitrile (rilpivirine; RIL). The efficacy of delavirdine is lower than that of the other NNRTIs, especially EFV, and it also has an inconvenient dosing schedule. These factors have led the US Department of Health and Human Services (DHHS) to recommend against its use as part of initial therapy (Fig. 2).

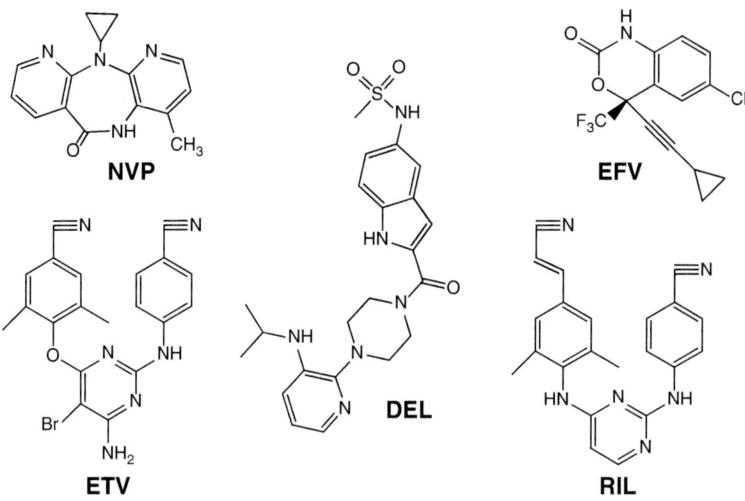

Fig. 2 Chemical structures of FDA-approved NNRTIs

HIV-1 Drug Resistance

Although combination therapies that contain two or more RTI have profoundly reduced morbidity and mortality from HIV-1 infection, their long-term efficacy is limited by the selection of drug-resistant variants of HIV-1. Antiviral drug resistance is defined by the presence of viral mutations that reduce drug susceptibility compared with the drug susceptibility of wild-type (WT) viruses. HIV-1 drug resistance within an individual arises from the genetic variability of the virus population and selection of subpopulations of resistant variants with therapy (Chen et al. 2004). HIV-1 genetic variability arises from the inability of HIV-1 RT to proofread nucleotide sequences during replication, the high rate of HIV-1 replication, the accumulation of proviral variants during the course of HIV-1 infection, and the genetic recombination when viruses of different sequence infect the same cell (Sluis-Cremer et al. 2004; Chen et al. 2004). As a consequence of these mechanisms, innumerable genetically distinct variants (termed quasispecies) evolve within an individual in the years following infection. Whether or not drug resistance develops depends on the extent to which virus replication continues during therapy, the ease of acquisition of a particular mutation (or set of mutations), and the effect of drug-resistance mutations on drug susceptibility and viral fitness (Chen et al. 2004). In general, RTI therapy selects for viruses that have mutations in RT. From a clinical perspective, the development of drug-resistant HIV-1 limits future treatment options by effectively decreasing the number of available drugs that remain active against the resistant virus. As a consequence, more complicated drug regimens are required that involve intense dosing schedules and greater risk of severe side effects due to drug toxicity. These factors often contribute to incomplete adherence to the drug regimen and lower therapeutic efficacy.

HIV-1 Resistance to NRTIs

NRTI-associated resistance mutations can be broadly categorized into two groups depending on their phenotypic mechanism of resistance (Sluis-Cremer et al. 2000a; Selmi et al. 2003; Deval et al. 2004a). The mutations K65R, K70E, L74V, Q151M (in complex with A62V, V75I, F77L, and F116Y), and M184V increase the selectivity of RT for incorporation of natural dNTP substrate versus the NRTI-TP (Selmi et al. 2001; Deval et al. 2002, 2004b, c; Feng and Anderson 1998; Sluis-Cremer et al. 2007). This resistance mechanism has been termed NRTI-TP discrimination. In comparison, the mutations M41L, D67N, K70R, L210W, T215F/Y, and K219Q/E are typically referred to as thymidine analog mutations (TAMs). These mutations augment the ability of HIV-1 RT to excise a chain-terminating NRTI monophosphate (NRTI-MP) from a prematurely terminated DNA chain (Arion et al. 1998; Meyer et al. 1998). This resistance mechanism has been termed NRTI-MP excision. Each of these mechanisms is described in more detail below. The locations of the mutations associated with the NRTI-TP discrimination and NRTI-MP excision phenotypes relative to the DNA polymerase active site of HIV-1 RT are shown in Fig. 3.

Drug-Resistance Mutations that Increase NRTI-TP Discrimination

This mechanism involves the acquisition of one or more resistance mutations in RT that improve the enzyme's ability to discriminate between the natural dNTP substrate and the NRTI-TP. Resistance by this mechanism is typically associated with decreased catalytic efficiency of NRTI-TP incorporation. NRTI-TP (and dNTP) catalytic efficiency is driven by two kinetic parameters: (i) the affinity of the nucleotide for the RT polymerase active site (K_d) and (ii) the maximum rate of nucleotide incorporation (k_{pol}), both of which can be determined using pre-steady-state kinetic analyses (Reardon 1992). In general, NRTI-TP discrimination is achieved by the resistance mutation affecting only one of these kinetic parameters, as described below.

K65R

The K65R mutation in HIV-1 RT decreases susceptibility to all FDA-approved NRTI, with the exception of AZT (Parikh et al. 2005). Residue K65 resides in the β3-β4 loop in the "fingers" subdomain of the 66 kDa subunit of HIV-1 RT, and in the crystal structure of the ternary HIV-1 RT-template/primer (T/P)-dNTP complex, the ε-amino group of K65 interacts with the γ-phosphate of the bound dNTP substrate (Huang et al. 1998). Pre-steady-state kinetic analyses have demonstrated that K65R

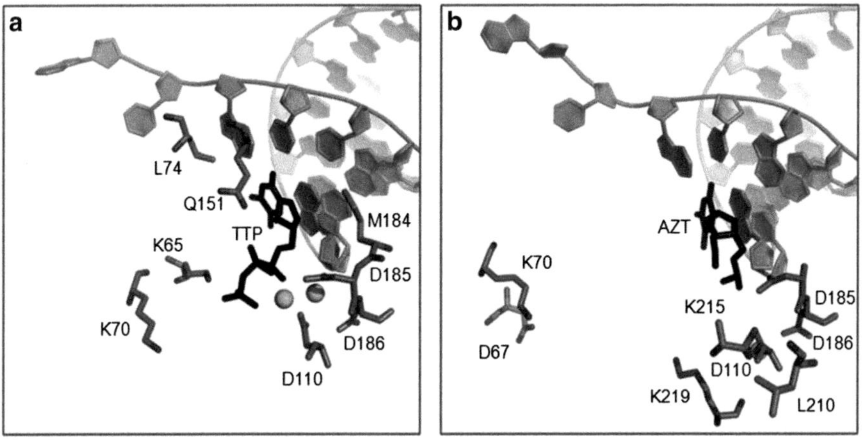

Fig. 3 Location of amino acid residues associated with the NRTI-TP discrimination (**a**) and NRTI-MP excision (**b**) resistance phenotypes

confers resistance to ddATP (active metabolite of ddI), 3TCTP, carbovir-TP (CBVTP, active metabolite of ABC), and TFV-diphosphate (DP) by selectively reducing k_{pol} without affecting K_d (Selmi et al. 2001; Deval et al. 2004b; Sluis-Cremer et al. 2007). However, for ddCTP, the resistance involves both reduction in k_{pol} and increase in K_d (Selmi et al. 2001). Structural studies suggest that the K65R mutation in HIV-1 RT distorts optimal positioning of the NRTI-TP in the active site, which decreases the catalytic efficiency of incorporation (Selmi et al. 2001; Sluis-Cremer et al. 2000b; Das et al. 2009).

K70E

The K70E mutation was initially selected in vitro with the NRTI adefovir (Cherrington et al. 1996). However, it has become more prevalent in clinical samples since the introduction of tenofovir and was recently reported in 10 % of antiretroviral-naïve subjects receiving the triple NRTI combination of tenofovir, ABC, and 3TC (Kagan et al. 2007). We demonstrated that K70E confers resistance to TFV-DP, CBVTP, and 3TCTP through a discrimination mechanism involving reduction in k_{pol} with little effect on K_d (Sluis-Cremer et al. 2007).

L74V

The L74V mutation was originally identified as causing ddI resistance but has also been associated with ABC resistance (Winters et al. 1994; Miller et al. 2000). Pre-steady-state kinetic experiments have demonstrated that the L74V mutation confers resistance to ddATP by decreasing k_{pol} without impacting K_d. Molecular modeling suggests that the L74V mutation leads to the loss of a stabilizing interaction between the nucleotide base of the incoming nucleotide and the side chain of L74 (Deval et al. 2004c). This may induce a rotation of the base (7° for ddATP compared with dATP), which indirectly affects the positioning of the phosphates and catalytic efficiency (Deval et al. 2004c).

Q151M Complex

The Q151M complex consists of a cluster of mutations in HIV-1 RT that includes the Q151M mutation plus four additional mutations: A62V, V75I, F77L, and F116Y (Ueno et al. 1995; Matsumi et al. 2003). The Q151M mutation generally occurs first before the acquisition of the other mutations (Ueno et al. 1995; Matsumi et al. 2003). Although rare (~1 % prevalence among resistance databases), the Q151M complex is most often selected by regimens containing d4T and ddI (Balotta et al. 2000). The mechanism of resistance mediated by Q151M and the Q151M complex is a selective reduction in the catalytic rate constant (k_{pol}) for incorporation of NRTI-TP (Deval et al. 2002).

M184I/V

The M184I/V mutation in HIV-1 RT causes high-level (>100-fold) resistance to 3TC and FTC resistance (Schinazi et al. 1993; Faraj et al. 1994). However, this mutation also confers resistance to ABC, ddC, and ddI (Winters et al. 1997; Miller et al. 2000; Hammond et al. 2005). Pre-steady-state kinetic analyses have demonstrated that M184V exerts a profound effect on the K_d for 3TCTP, without impacting k_{pol} (Deval et al. 2004b; Feng and Anderson 1998). M184 forms part of the highly conserved YMDD motif, and crystal structures of 3TC-resistant M184I RT, obtained in the presence or absence of a nucleic acid substrate, suggest that steric hindrance between the oxathiolane ring of 3TCTP and the side chain of the β-branched amino acids (Val or Ile) at position 184 reduces inhibitor binding thus increasing K_d (Gao et al. 2000).

Drug-Resistance Mutations Affecting NRTI-MP Excision

For the excision mechanism of NRTI resistance, the mutant HIV-1 RT does not discriminate between the natural dNTP substrate and the NRTI-TP at the nucleotide incorporation step (Kerr and Anderson 1997). Instead, RT containing excision-enhancing mutations shows an increased capacity to unblock NRTI-MP terminated primers in the presence of physiological concentrations of ATP (Meyer et al. 1998). Resistance mutations associated with the excision mechanism include thymidine analog mutations (TAMs) and T69S insertion mutations. These mutations are described below.

TAMs

AZT resistance is associated with multiple mutations in RT including M41L, D67N, K70R, L210W, T215F/Y, and K219E/Q (Larder and Kemp 1998; Kellam et al. 1992; Harrigan et al. 1996; Hooker et al. 1996). Because each of these mutations has also been selected with d4T therapy, they have been termed thymidine-analog mutations or TAMs (Ross et al. 2001). The presence of four or more TAMs in HIV-1 RT typically results in >100-fold resistance to AZT, fivefold to sevenfold reduced susceptibility to ABC, and twofold to fivefold reduced susceptibility to d4T, ddI, and TFV (Whitcomb et al. 2003). TAMs also reduce susceptibility to 3TC, but via a discrimination mechanism rather than an excision mechanism (Parikh et al. 2006, 2007). The efficiency of the NRTI-MP excision reaction by RT containing TAMs depends on the chain-terminating NRTI-MP residing in the nucleotide-binding site (N-site) of the RT active site. Under physiological conditions, the binding of the next-correct dNTP can drive the terminating nucleotide into the primer-binding site (P-site) resulting in the formation of a dead-end complex (DEC) (Meyer et al. 1998). Biochemical studies have proposed several mechanisms by which TAMs can increase the efficiency of RT to excise NRTI-MP from chain-terminated primers. These mechanisms include (i) an increase in the binding affinity of ATP for RT (Meyer et al. 1998), (ii) an increase in the kinetic rate of ATP-mediated NRTI-MP excision (Ray et al. 2003), (iii) a decrease in sensitivity of RT to DEC formation (Meyer et al. 1998), and (iv) a shift in the translocation equilibrium of the primer terminus between the N- and P-sites such that the N-site is favored (Marchand and Gotte 2003). While it has been suggested that the 3′-azido group of the AZTMP-terminated primer is the primary structural determinant for the excision phenotype, we recently showed that the potency of 3′-azido-2′,3′-dideoxyadenosine (3′-azido-ddA) and 3′-azido-2′,3-′-dideoxyguanosine (3′-azdio-ddG) is retained against AZT-resistant virus (Sluis-Cremer et al. 2005). This indicates that the nucleoside base has an important influence on the efficiency of excision resulting from TAMs.

T69S Insertions

HIV-1 RT containing dipeptide insertions (typically Ser-Ser, Ser-Gly, or Ser-Ala) between codons 69 and 70, together with the amino acid substitutions T69S, T215Y, and other TAMs, has been identified in heavily NRTI-experienced patients, albeit at low prevalence (0.5–2.7 %) (Winters and Merigan 2005). In phenotypic assays, viral isolates containing insertion mutations in RT demonstrate high-level resistance to AZT and moderate levels of resistance to other NRTI, such as d4T, ddC, ddI, ABC, and tenofovir. In combination with TAMs (in particular T215Y), the dipeptide insertions in HIV-1 RT confer enhanced ATP-dependent phosphorolytic activity that facilitates removal of terminating AZTMP, d4TMP, ddAMP, or tenofovir, even when relatively high levels of dNTPs are present in the reaction (Meyer et al. 2003; Boyer et al. 2002; Mas et al. 2000).

HIV-1 Resistance to NNRTIs

Typically, HIV-1 resistance to NNRTIs correlates directly with mutations of one or more RT residues in the NNRTI-binding pocket. Mutations associated with resistance to NVP and EFV include L100I, K101E/P, K103N/S, V106A/M, Y181C/I/V, Y188C/L/H, G190A/E/S, and M230L (Stanford University HIV Drug Resistance Database: http://hivdb.stanford.edu/). Although ETV and RIL have been reported to have higher in vitro genetic barriers to resistance than EFV or NVP (Andries et al. 2004; Azijn et al. 2010), 17 mutations in HIV-1 RT have been associated with decreased virologic response to ETV (V90I, A98G, L100I, K101E/H/P, V106I, E138A, V179D/F/T, Y181C/I/V, G190A/S, and M230L) (Vingerhoets et al. 2010) and 15 mutations with decreased virologic response to RIL (K101E/P, E138A/G/K/Q/R, V179L, Y181C/I/V, H221Y, F227C, and M230I/L) (Anta et al. 2013). The locations of the mutations associated with NVP, EFV, RIL, and ETV resistance are shown in Fig. 4. In general, these NNRTI-resistance mutations can affect inhibitor binding in a number of ways. (1) They can remove one or more favorable interactions between the inhibitor and NNRTI-binding pocket. For example, the Y181C mutation eliminates π-stacking interactions between this residue and the aromatic ring of the NNRTI pharmacophore (Ren et al. 2001). (2) They can introduce steric barriers to NNRTI binding. For example, the G190E mutation introduces a bulky side chain which may prevent NNRTI binding by sterically interfering with functional groups, such as the cyclopropyl ring of NVP (Huang et al. 2003; Yap et al. 2007). (3) The mutations may introduce or eliminate inter-residue contacts in the NNRTI-binding pocket, which interfere with the ability of other residues in the pocket to fold down over the NNRTI (Sluis-Cremer et al. 2004).

RTI-Resistance Mutations in the Connection Domain of HIV-1 RT

While genotypic analysis of HIV-1 isolates in infected patients is usually restricted to residues 1–250 of the RT, recent reports indicate that several residues in the connection domain of RT can also modulate NRTI and NNRTI resistance. Mutations in the connection domain of RT with potential clinical relevance include N348I, A360V, and A367S.

N348I

The N348I mutation in HIV-1 RT confers both NRTI (AZT) and NNRTI resistance (Yap et al. 2007; Hachiya et al. 2008; von Wyl et al. 2010; Sluis-Cremer et al. 2010). N348I can appear early in therapy and is found to be highly associated with TAMs, M184V/I, and the NNRTI-resistance mutations K103N, Y181C/I, and G190A/S (Yap et al. 2007). N348I was also found to be significantly associated with therapies that contained AZT and NVP (Yap et al. 2007). Yap et al. showed that N348I reduces the rate of RNA template degradation by RT in either a wild-type background or in

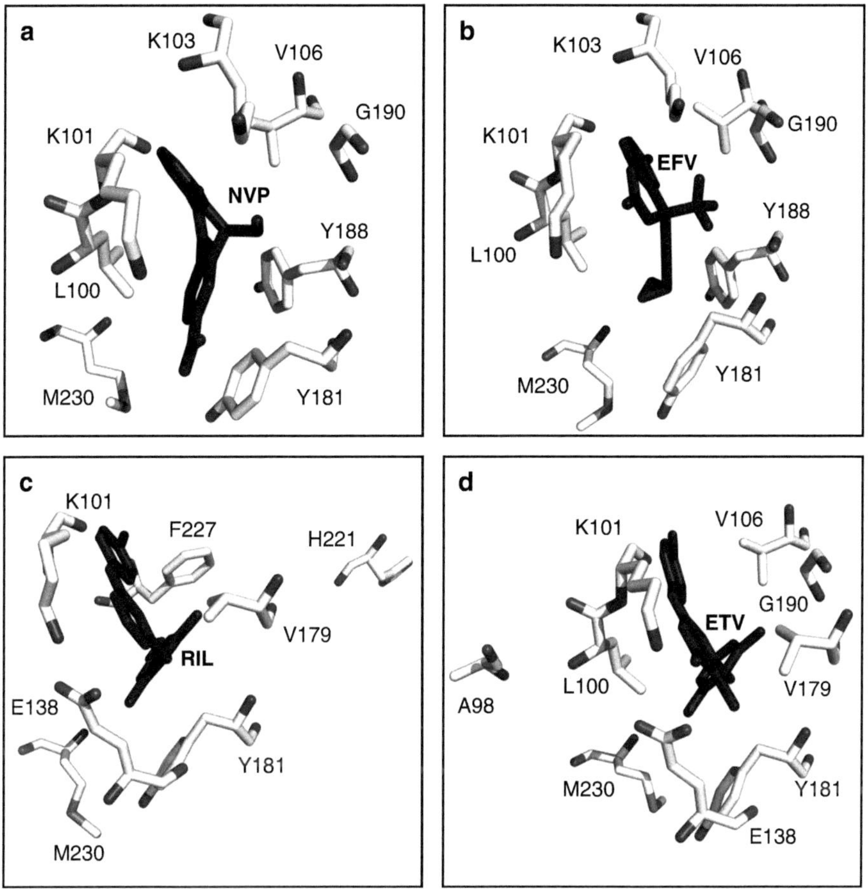

Fig. 4 Location of amino acid residues associated with NVP (**a**), EFV (**b**), RIL (**c**), and ETV (**d**) resistance

the presence of TAMs (Yap et al. 2007). This property would facilitate the excision of AZT-MP by giving RT more time to excise the blocking nucleoside analog from the terminated primer. However, it has been shown that N348I could also modulate the excision activity of the RT by an RNase H-independent mechanism, since this mutation could increase the processivity of HIV-1 RT in the absence or in the presence of TAMs (Ehteshami et al. 2008; Schuckmann et al. 2010). In regard to NNRTI resistance, three different mechanisms have been proposed to explain the resistant phenotype conferred by N348I. These include: (i) N348I directly decreases NNRTI binding affinity to RT (Schuckmann et al. 2010), (ii) N348I decreases RT RNase H activity (Radzio and Sluis-Cremer 2011; Nikolenko et al. 2010), and (iii) N348I impacts the orientation of RT relative to the T/P substrate, a property that appears to be critical for polypurine tract removal during plus strand DNA synthesis (Biondi et al. 2010).

A360V

The A360V in the connection domain of HIV-1 RT is also highly associated with TAMs (Ehteshami et al. 2008). Importantly, Brehm et al. showed that the A360V mutation was selected in HIV-infected individuals who received AZT monotherapy and contributed to AZT resistance (Brehm et al. 2012). Like N348I, the A360V mutation reduces the rate of RNA template degradation by WT and TAM containing RT, therefore providing more time for the enzyme to excise AZT-MP from the terminated primer (Brehm et al. 2012).

A376S

Paredes et al. reported that preexisting A376S was associated with an increased risk of virologic failure to NVP (relative hazard (RH) = 10.4; 95 % confidence interval (CI), 2.0–54.7), but did not affect EFV outcome the same way (RH = 0.5; 95 % CI, 0.1–2.2) ($p = 0.013$) (Paredes et al. 2011). A376S confers selective low-level NVP resistance in vitro (Paredes et al. 2011). Interestingly, Gupta et al. reported that virologic responses to an ETV-containing regimen were slightly diminished when A376S was present (Gupta et al. 2011).

Interactions Between RTI-Resistance Mutations

Antagonistic Interactions

Several NRTI (e.g., K65R, K70E, L74V, and M184V) and NNRTI mutations (e.g., Y181C) reverse HIV-1 resistance to AZT when added to a genetic background containing TAMs (Sluis-Cremer et al. 2007; Parikh et al. 2006; Miranda et al. 2005; Gotte et al. 2000; Larder 1992). It has also been shown that TAMs can antagonize the phenotypic effects of K65R, decreasing resistance to TFV, ABC, ddI, and d4T (Parikh et al. 2006). Biochemical studies have demonstrated that K65R, L74V, and M184V significantly reduce the ability of RT containing TAMs to excise NRTI-MP (Sluis-Cremer et al. 2007; Parikh et al. 2007; Miranda et al. 2005; Gotte et al. 2000). By contrast, TAMs decrease the extent to which RT containing K65R can discriminate against D-nucleotide analogs, but not L-nucleotide analogs (such as 3TC-TP), by partially restoring the maximum rate of NRTI-TP incorporation (Parikh et al. 2007). Despite this antagonism, multidrug-resistant HIV-1 can still develop, although the current literature suggests that this may require the accumulation of several additional mutations. For example, substitutions at RT codons 44, 118, 207, 208, 333, and 348 have been associated with increased AZT resistance in viruses that carry both TAMs and M184V (von Wyl et al. 2010; Girouard et al. 2003; Zelina et al. 2008; Radzio et al. 2010).

Complementary Interactions

In the phase III ECHO and THRIVE clinical trials which compared the efficacy of RIL versus EFV in treatment-naïve HIV-1-infected individuals, the most frequent mutation combination that emerged in the RIL virologic failures was E138K + M184I (Rimsky et al. 2013; Molina et al. 2013; Cohen et al. 2013). Typically, the M184I mutation emerges first during FTC or 3TC containing ART regimens but is rapidly replaced by the M184V mutation because viruses carrying M184V are fitter than the M184I mutants. In this case, it was found that the E138K mutation compensated for the poor replicative capacity of M184I (Hu and Kuritzkes 2011; Xu et al. 2011). Indeed, the replicative capacity of E138K/M184I HIV-1 was comparable to that of the WT virus in the absence of drug and was found to be significantly greater than that of the E138K and E138K/M184V mutants in the presence of ETV (Hu and Kuritzkes 2011). Kinetic analyses have demonstrated that E138K compensates for a deficit in dNTP usage that is inherent to the M184I HIV-1 RT (Xu et al. 2011).

Subtype Differences in HIV-1 Resistance to RTIs

The majority of research into HIV-1 drug resistance has focused on subtype B viruses, yet non-subtype B strains are responsible for 90 % of global infections. Importantly, there is increasing evidence of subtype differences in RTI drug resistance, as described below.

V106M

Subtype C viruses harbor GTG (valine) at codon 106 in HIV-1 RT, whereas subtype B harbors GTA (valine). The GTG polymorphism facilitates the emergence of subtype C virus with the V106M mutation (GTG to ATG) that confers resistance to all NNRTIs (Brenner et al. 2003).

E138A

Recent data from our group shows that a glutamic acid to alanine substitution at codon 138 in RT occurs significantly more frequently in subtype C than B sequences in both treatment-naïve and RT inhibitor-experienced HIV-1-infected individuals (Sluis-Cremer et al. 2013). E138A has been clinically associated with virologic failure of regimens that contain ETV or RIL.

Silent Mutations at Codons 64, 65, and 66 in Subtype C HIV-1 RT

Subtype C viruses harbor AAA (lysine), AAG (lysine), and AAG (lysine) at codons 64, 65, and 66 or HIV-1 RT, respectively. In contrast, all other HIV-1 subtypes harbor

AAG (lysine), AAA (lysine), and AAA (lysine) at the same codons. There is recent clinical evidence demonstrating frequent and early emergence of K65R on TNF-based first-line ART regimens in South Africa (Sunpath et al. 2012; Theys et al. 2013). In this regard, Mark Wainberg's group has shown that the difference in selection of K65R between subtypes B and C is related to the template nucleotide sequence and preferential pausing of reverse transcription at the homopolymeric stretch of adenine bases at codons 64, 65, and 66 of RT (Coutsinos et al. 2010; Invernizzi et al. 2009).

The Threat of Transmitted NNRTI Resistance in Resource-Limited Settings

The past decade has seen an enormous global scale-up of ART. In 2011, more than eight million people were receiving ART in low- and middle-income countries, which was 26 times higher than the number in 2003 (Together we will end AIDS). Although this widespread distribution of ART has dramatically reduced HIV/AIDs-related mortality, current data suggests that up to 24 % of individuals receiving first-line ART in sub-Saharan Africa experience virologic failure within 12 months of initiation of therapy (Barth et al. 2010). Between 53 % and 90 % of these have viruses with clinically important HIV-1 drug-resistance mutations (Gupta et al. 2009; Hamers et al. 2012; Hosseinipour et al. 2009). As such, antiretroviral drug resistance is one of the main threats to the global control of HIV-1.

NVP or EFV in combination with 2 NRTIs forms the foundation of most first-line ART regimens in resource-limited settings. NVP has also been routinely used in regimens for prevention mother-to-child transmission. Due to the extensive use of NNRTIs, there has been a significant increase in NNRTI drug resistance in regions of sub-Saharan Africa (Gupta et al. 2012). The prevalence of NNRTI mutations has increased by 36 % per year in east Africa and by 23 % per year in southern Africa since the inception of ART rollout (Gupta et al. 2012). There has also been a significant increase in transmitted NNRTI resistance in resource-limited settings (Gupta et al. 2012). The spread of NNRTI resistance threatens the success of prevention and first-line and salvage ART therapies.

This threat is of even of greater significance when one considers that the diarylpyrimidine (DAPY) NNRTIs, dapivirine (TMC120), ETV, and RIL, will be increasingly used for the treatment and prevention of HIV-1 infection in resource-limited settings. Many sub-Saharan African countries already have access to ETV, which has been approved for the treatment of HIV infection in ART-experienced individuals. RIL, which has been co-formulated with FTC and TFV, is pending approval as a first-line ART regimen in sub-Saharan Africa. A long-acting RIL formulation is in development as a preexposure prophylaxis agent for use in resource-limited settings (Baert et al. 2009; van't Klooster et al. 2010). Finally, the ASPIRE study is currently assessing whether TMC120 can safely prevent HIV infection when continuously released in the vagina from a silicone ring replaced once a month. Given the escalating frequency of NNRTI-resistant variants present in

ART-naïve and ART-experienced HIV-infected individuals in sub-Saharan Africa, as well as the potential for bidirectional cross-resistance between first-generation NNRTIs (NVP and EFV) and the DAPY analogs, there is a continued need to monitor and understand NNRTI drug resistance in resource-limited settings.

Conclusions

RTIs are routinely used in first-line, second-line, and salvage ART therapies. HIV-1 resistance to all of the FDA-approved RTIs has been documented. In general, there is extensive cross-resistance among the NRTIs, and separately the NNRTIs, although in some instances antagonistic interactions occur. Of concern, there has been a significant increase in circulating and transmitted NNRTI drug resistance in resource-limited settings due to the extensive use of NNRTIs in prevention and treatment strategies for HIV-1 infection. Despite this increase in NNRTI drug resistance, the diarylpyrimidine NNRTIs, dapivirine, etravirine, and rilpivirine, will be increasingly used in resource-limited settings. As such, there is a continued need to monitor and understand NNRTI resistance, particularly in sub-Saharan Africa where non-subtype B HIV-1 predominates.

Acknowledgments Research in the Sluis-Cremer laboratory was supported by grants AI081571, GM068406, and AI071846 from the National Institutes of Health (NIH), United States of America. Grant Schauer was supported by an NIH training grant (T32GM088119).

References

Andries K, Azijn H, Thielemans T et al (2004) TMC125, a novel next-generation nonnucleoside reverse transcriptase inhibitor active against nonnucleoside reverse transcriptase inhibitor-resistant human immunodeficiency virus type 1. Antimicrob Agents Chemother 48:4680–4686

Anta L, Llibre JM, Poveda E et al (2013) Resistance Platform of the Spanish AIDS Research Network. Rilpivirine resistance mutations in HIV patients failing non-nucleoside reverse transcriptase inhibitor-based therapies. AIDS 27:81–85

Arion D, Kaushik N, McCormick S et al (1998) Phenotypic mechanism of HIV-1 resistance to 3′-azido-3′-deoxythymidine (AZT): increased polymerization processivity and enhanced sensitivity to pyrophosphate of the mutant viral reverse transcriptase. Biochemistry 37:15908–15917

Azijn H, Tirry I, Vingerhoets J et al (2010) TMC278, a next-generation nonnucleoside reverse transcriptase inhibitor (NNRTI), active against wild-type and NNRTI-resistant HIV-1. Antimicrob Agents Chemother 54:718–727

Baert L, van't Klooster G, Dries W et al (2009) Development of a long-acting injectable formulation with nanoparticles of rilpivirine (TMC278) for HIV treatment. Eur J Pharm Biopharm 72:502–508

Balotta C, Violin M, Monno L et al (2000) Prevalence of multiple dideoxynucleoside analogue resistance (MddNR) in a multicenter cohort of HIV-1-infected Italian patients with virologic failure. J Acquir Immune Defic Syndr 24:232–240

Barth RE, van der Loeff MF, Schuurman R et al (2010) Virological follow-up of adult patients in antiretroviral treatment programmes in sub-Saharan Africa: a systematic review. Lancet Infect Dis 10:155–166

Biondi MJ, Beilhartz GL, McCormick S, Gotte M (2010) N348I in HIV-1 reverse transcriptase can counteract the nevirapine-mediated bias toward RNase H cleavage during plus-strand initiation. J Biol Chem 285:26966–26975

Boyer PL, Sarafianos SG, Arnold E, Hughes SH (2002) Nucleoside analog resistance caused by insertions in the fingers of human immunodeficiency virus type 1 reverse transcriptase involves ATP-mediated excision. J Virol 76:9143–9151

Brehm JH, Scott Y, Koontz DL et al (2012) Zidovudine (AZT) monotherapy selects for the A360V mutation in the connection domain of HIV-1 reverse transcriptase. PLoS One 7:e31558

Brenner B, Turner D, Oliveira M et al (2003) A V106M mutation in HIV-1 clade C viruses exposed to efavirenz confers cross-resistance to non-nucleoside reverse transcriptase inhibitors. AIDS 17:F1–F5

Chen R, Quinones-Mateu ME, Mansky LM (2004) Drug resistance, virus fitness and HIV-1 mutagenesis. Curr Pharm Des 10:4065–4070

Cherrington JM, Mulato AS, Fuller MD, Chen MS (1996) Novel mutation (K70E) in human immunodeficiency virus type 1 reverse transcriptase confers decreased susceptibility to 9-[2-(phosphonomethoxy)ethyl]adenine in vitro. Antimicrob Agents Chemother 40:2212–2216

Cohen CJ, Molina JM, Cassetti I et al (2013) Week 96 efficacy and safety of rilpivirine in treatment-naive, HIV-1 patients in two Phase III randomized trials. AIDS 27:939–950

Coutsinos D, Invernizzi CF, Xu H et al (2010) Factors affecting template usage in the development of K65R resistance in subtype C variants of HIV type-1. Antivir Chem Chemother 20:117–131

Das K, Bandwar RP, White KL et al (2009) Structural basis for the role of the K65R mutation in HIV-1 reverse transcriptase polymerization, excision antagonism, and tenofovir resistance. J Biol Chem 284:35092–35100

Deval J, Selmi B, Boretto J et al (2002) The molecular mechanism of multidrug resistance by the Q151M human immunodeficiency virus type 1 reverse transcriptase and its suppression using alpha-boranophosphate nucleotide analogues. J Biol Chem 277:42097–42104

Deval J, Courcambeck J, Selmi B et al (2004a) Structural determinants and molecular mechanisms for the resistance of HIV-1 RT to nucleoside analogues. Curr Drug Metab 5:305–316

Deval J, White KL, Miller MD et al (2004b) Mechanistic basis for reduced viral and enzymatic fitness of HIV-1 reverse transcriptase containing both K65R and M184V mutations. J Biol Chem 279:509–516

Deval J, Navarro JM, Selmi B et al (2004c) A loss of viral replicative capacity correlates with altered DNA polymerization kinetics by the human immunodeficiency virus reverse transcriptase bearing the K65R and L74V dideoxynucleoside resistance substitutions. J Biol Chem 279:25489–25496

Ehteshami M, Beilhartz GL, Scarth BJ et al (2008) Connection domain mutations N348I and A360V in HIV-1 reverse transcriptase enhance resistance to 3′-azido-3′-deoxythymidine through both RNase H-dependent and -independent mechanisms. J Biol Chem 283:22222–22232

Faraj A, Agrofoglio LA, Wakefield JK et al (1994) Inhibition of human immunodeficiency virus type 1 reverse transcriptase by the 5′-triphosphate beta enantiomers of cytidine analogs. Antimicrob Agents Chemother 38:2300–2305

Feng JY, Anderson KS (1998) Mechanistic studies examining the efficiency and fidelity of DNA synthesis by the 3TC-resistant mutant (184 V) of HIV-1 reverse transcriptase. Biochemistry 38:9440–9448

Gao HQ, Boyer PL, Sarafianos SG et al (2000) The role of steric hindrance in 3TC resistance of human immunodeficiency virus type-1 reverse transcriptase. J Mol Biol 300:403–418

Girouard M, Diallo K, Marchand B et al (2003) Mutations E44D and V118I in the reverse transcriptase of HIV-1 play distinct mechanistic roles in dual resistance to AZT and 3TC. J Biol Chem 278:34403–34410

Goody RS, Muller B, Restle T (1991) Factors contributing to the inhibition of HIV reverse transcriptase by chain-terminating nucleotides in vitro and in vivo. FEBS Lett 291:1–5

Gotte M, Arion D, Parniak MA, Wainberg MA (2000) The M184V mutation in the reverse transcriptase of human immunodeficiency virus type 1 impairs rescue of chain-terminated DNA synthesis. J Virol 74:3579–3585
Gupta RK, Hill A, Sawyer AW et al (2009) Virological monitoring and resistance to first-line highly active antiretroviral therapy in adults infected with HIV-1 treated under WHO guidelines: a systematic review and meta-analysis. Lancet Infect Dis 9:409–417
Gupta S, Vingerhoets J, Fransen S et al (2011) Connection domain mutations in HIV-1 reverse transcriptase do not impact etravirine susceptibility and virologic responses to etravirine-containing regimens. Antimicrob Agents Chemother 55:2872–2879
Gupta RK, Jordan MR, Sultan BJ et al (2012) Global trends in antiretroviral resistance in treatment-naive individuals with HIV after rollout of antiretroviral treatment in resource-limited settings: a global collaborative study and meta-regression analysis. Lancet 380:1250–1258
Hachiya A, Kodama EN, Sarafianos SG et al (2008) Amino acid mutation N348I in the connection subdomain of human immunodeficiency virus type 1 reverse transcriptase confers multiclass resistance to nucleoside and nonnucleoside reverse transcriptase inhibitors. J Virol 82:3261–3270
Hamers RL, Sigaloff KC, Wensing AM et al (2012) Patterns of HIV-1 drug resistance after first-line antiretroviral therapy (ART) failure in 6 sub-Saharan African countries: implications for second-line ART strategies. Clin Infect Dis 54:1660–1669
Hammond JL, Parikh UM, Koontz DL et al (2005) In vitro selection and analysis of human immunodeficiency virus type 1 resistant to derivatives of beta-2′,3′-didehydro-2′,3′-dideoxy-5-fluorocytidine. Antimicrob Agents Chemother 49:3930–3932
Harrigan PR, Kinghorn I, Bloor S et al (1996) Significance of amino acid variation at human immunodeficiency virus type 1 reverse transcriptase residue 210 for zidovudine susceptibility. J Virol 70:5930–5934
Hooker DJ, Tachedjian G, Solomon AE et al (1996) An in vivo mutation from leucine to tryptophan at position 210 in human immunodeficiency virus type 1 reverse transcriptase contributes to high-level resistance to 3′-azido-3′-deoxythymidine. J Virol 70:8010–8018
Hosseinipour MC, van Oosterhout JJ, Weigel R et al (2009) The public health approach to identify antiretroviral therapy failure: high-level nucleoside reverse transcriptase inhibitor resistance among Malawians failing first-line antiretroviral therapy. AIDS 23:1127–1134
Hu Z, Kuritzkes DR (2011) Interaction of reverse transcriptase (RT) mutations conferring resistance to lamivudine and etravirine: effects on fitness and RT activity of human immunodeficiency virus type 1. J Virol 85:11309–11314
Huang H, Chopra R, Verdine GL, Harrison SC (1998) Structure of a covalently trapped catalytic complex of HIV-1 reverse transcriptase: implications for drug resistance. Science 282:1669–1675
Huang W, Gamarnik A, Limoli K et al (2003) Amino acid substitutions at position 190 of human immunodeficiency virus type 1 reverse transcriptase increase susceptibility to delavirdine and impair virus replication. J Virol 77:1512–1523
Invernizzi CF, Coutsinos D, Oliveira M et al (2009) Signature nucleotide polymorphisms at positions 64 and 65 in reverse transcriptase favor the selection of the K65R resistance mutation in HIV-1 subtype C. J Infect Dis 200:1202–1206
Kagan RM, Lee TS, Ross L et al (2007) Molecular basis of antagonism between K70E and K65R tenofovir-associated mutations in HIV-1 reverse transcriptase. Antiviral Res 75:210–218
Kellam P, Boucher CA, Larder BA (1992) Fifth mutation in human immunodeficiency virus type 1 reverse transcriptase contributes to the development of high-level resistance to zidovudine. Proc Natl Acad Sci 89:1934–1938
Kerr SG, Anderson KS (1997) Pre-steady-state kinetic characterization of wild type and 3′-azido-3′-deoxythymidine (AZT) resistant human immunodeficiency virus type 1 reverse transcriptase: implication of RNA directed DNA polymerization in the mechanism of AZT resistance. Biochemistry 36:14064–14070

Kohlstaedt LA, Wang J, Friedman JM et al (1992) Crystal structure at 3.5 A resolution of HIV-1 reverse transcriptase complexed with an inhibitor. Science 256:1783–1790

Larder BA (1992) 3′-Azido-3′-deoxythymidine resistance suppressed by a mutation conferring human immunodeficiency virus type 1 resistance to nonnucleoside reverse transcriptase inhibitors. Antimicrob Agents Chemother 36:2664–2669

Larder BA, Kemp SD (1998) Multiple mutations in HIV-1 reverse transcriptase confer high-level resistance to zidovudine (AZT). Science 246:1155–1158

Marchand B, Gotte M (2003) Site-specific footprinting reveals differences in the translocation status of HIV-1 reverse transcriptase. Implications for polymerase translocation and drug resistance. J Biol Chem 278:35362–35372

Mas A, Parera M, Briones C et al (2000) Role of a dipeptide insertion between codons 69 and 70 of HIV-1 reverse transcriptase in the mechanism of AZT resistance. EMBO J 19:5752–5761

Matsumi S, Kosalaraksa P, Tsang H et al (2003) Pathways for the emergence of multi-dideoxynucleoside-resistant HIV-1 variants. AIDS 17:1127–1137

Meyer PR, Matsuura SE, Mian AM et al (1998) A mechanism of AZT resistance: an increase in nucleotide-dependent primer unblocking by mutant HIV-1 reverse transcriptase. Mol Cell 4:35–43

Meyer PR, Lennerstrand J, Matsuura SE et al (2003) Effects of dipeptide insertions between codons 69 and 70 of human immunodeficiency virus type 1 reverse transcriptase on primer unblocking, deoxynucleoside triphosphate inhibition, and DNA chain elongation. J Virol 77:3871–3877

Miller V, Ait-Khaled M, Stone C et al (2000) HIV-1 reverse transcriptase (RT) genotype and susceptibility to RT inhibitors during abacavir monotherapy and combination therapy. AIDS 14:163–171

Miranda LR, Gotte M, Liang F, Kuritzkes DR (2005) The L74V mutation in human immunodeficiency virus type 1 reverse transcriptase counteracts enhanced excision of zidovudine monophosphate associated with thymidine analog resistance mutations. Antimicrob Agents Chemother 49:2648–2656

Molina JM, Clumeck N, Redant K et al (2013) Rilpivirine vs. efavirenz in HIV-1 patients with baseline viral load 100,000 copies/ml or less: week 48 phase III analysis. AIDS 27:889–897

Nikolenko GN, Delviks-Frankenberry KA, Pathak VK (2010) A novel molecular mechanism of dual resistance to nucleoside and nonnucleoside reverse transcriptase inhibitors. J Virol 84:5238–5249

Paredes R, Puertas MC, Bannister W et al (2011) A376S in the connection subdomain of HIV-1 reverse transcriptase confers increased risk of virological failure to nevirapine therapy. J Infect Dis 204:741–752

Parikh UM, Koontz DL, Chu CK et al (2005) In vitro activity of structurally diverse nucleoside analogs against human immunodeficiency virus type 1 with the K65R mutation in reverse transcriptase. Antimicrob Agents Chemother 49:1139–1144

Parikh UM, Bacheler L, Koontz D, Mellors JW (2006) The K65R mutation in HIV-1 reverse transcriptase exhibits bi-directional phenotypic antagonism with thymidine analog mutations. J Virol 80:4971–4977

Parikh UM, Zelina S, Sluis-Cremer N, Mellors JW (2007) Molecular mechanisms of bi-directional antagonism between K65R and thymidine analog mutations in HIV-1 reverse transcriptase. AIDS 21:1405–1414

Radzio J, Sluis-Cremer N (2011) Subunit-specific mutational analysis of residue N348 in HIV-1 reverse transcriptase. Retrovirology 8:69

Radzio J, Yap SH, Tachedjian G, Sluis-Cremer N (2010) N348I in reverse transcriptase provides a genetic pathway for HIV-1 to select thymidine analogue mutations and mutations antagonistic to thymidine analogue mutations. AIDS 24:659–667

Ray AS, Murakami E, Basavapathruni A et al (2003) Probing the molecular mechanisms of AZT drug resistance mediated by HIV-1 reverse transcriptase using a transient kinetic analysis. Biochemistry 42:8831–8841

Reardon JE (1992) Human immunodeficiency virus reverse transcriptase: steady-state and pre-steady-state kinetics of nucleotide incorporation. Biochemistry 31:4473–4479

Ren J, Nichols C, Bird L et al (2001) Structural mechanisms of drug resistance for mutations at codons 181 and 188 in HIV-1 reverse transcriptase and the improved resilience of second generation non-nucleoside inhibitors. J Mol Biol 312:795–805

Rimsky L, Van Eygen V, Hoogstoel A et al (2013) 96-week resistance analyses of rilpivirine in treatment-naive, HIV-1-infected adults from the ECHO and THRIVE Phase III trials. Antivir Ther 18(8):967–977

Ross L, Scarsella A, Raffanti S et al (2001) NZT40012 Study Team. Thymidine analog and multinucleoside resistance mutations are associated with decreased phenotypic susceptibility to stavudine in HIV type 1 isolated from zidovudine-naive patients experiencing viremia on stavudine-containing regimens. AIDS Res Hum Retroviruses 17:1107–1115

Schinazi RF, Lloyd RM Jr, Nguyen MH et al (1993) Characterization of human immunodeficiency viruses resistant to oxathiolane-cytosine nucleosides. Antimicrob Agents Chemother 37:875–881

Schuckmann MM, Marchand B, Hachiya A et al (2010) The N348I mutation at the connection subdomain of HIV-1 reverse transcriptase decreases binding to nevirapine. J Biol Chem 285:38700–38709

Selmi B, Boretto J, Sarfati SR et al (2001) Mechanism-based suppression of dideoxynucleotide resistance by K65R human immunodeficiency virus reverse transcriptase using an alpha-boranophosphate nucleoside analogue. J Biol Chem 276:48466–48472

Selmi B, Deval J, Boretto J, Canard B (2003) Nucleotide analogue binding, catalysis and primer unblocking in the mechanisms of HIV-1 reverse transcriptase-mediated resistance to nucleoside analogues. Antivir Ther 8:143–154

Sluis-Cremer N, Arion D, Parniak MA (2000a) Molecular mechanisms of HIV-1 resistance to nucleoside reverse transcriptase inhibitors (NRTIs). Cell Mol Life Sci 57:1408–1422

Sluis-Cremer N, Arion D, Kaushik N et al (2000b) Mutational analysis of Lys65 of HIV-1 reverse transcriptase. Biochem J 348:77–82

Sluis-Cremer N, Temiz NA, Bahar I (2004) Conformational changes in HIV-1 reverse transcriptase induced by nonnucleoside reverse transcriptase inhibitor binding. Curr HIV Res 2:323–332

Sluis-Cremer N, Arion D, Parikh U et al (2005) The 3′-azido group is not the primary determinant of 3′-azido-3′-deoxythymidine (AZT) responsible for the excision phenotype of AZT-resistant HIV-1. J Biol Chem 280:29047–29052

Sluis-Cremer N, Sheen CW, Zelina S et al (2007) Molecular mechanism by which the K70E mutation in human immunodeficiency virus type 1 reverse transcriptase confers resistance to nucleoside reverse transcriptase inhibitors. Antimicrob Agents Chemother 51:48–53

Sluis-Cremer N, Moore K, Radzio J et al (2010) N348I in HIV-1 reverse transcriptase decreases susceptibility to tenofovir and etravirine in combination with other resistance mutations. AIDS 24:317–319

Sluis-Cremer N, Huber K, Brumme C, et al (2013) The E138A mutation in HIV-1 reverse transcriptase is more common in Subtype C than B and decreases susceptibility to NNRTIs. In: 20th conference on retroviruses and opportunistic infections (CROI), Altanta, 3–6 Mar 2013

Sunpath H, Wu B, Gordon M et al (2012) High rate of K65R for antiretroviral therapy-naive patients with subtype C HIV infection failing a tenofovir-containing first-line regimen. AIDS 26:1679–1684

Theys K, Vercauteren J, Snoeck J et al (2013) HIV-1 subtype is an independent predictor of reverse transcriptase mutation K65R in HIV-1 patients treated with combination antiretroviral therapy including tenofovir. Antimicrob Agents Chemother 57:1053–1056

Together we will end AIDS. Joint United Nations Programme on HIV/AIDS. http://www.unaids.org/en/media/unaids/contentassets/documents/epidemiology/2012/20120718_togetherwewillendaids_en.pdf

Ueno T, Shirasaka T, Mitsuya H (1995) Enzymatic characterization of human immunodeficiency virus type 1 reverse transcriptase resistant to multiple 2′,3′-dideoxynucleoside 5′-triphosphates. J Biol Chem 270:23605–23611

van't Klooster G, Hoeben E, Borghys H et al (2010) Pharmacokinetics and disposition of rilpivirine (TMC278) nanosuspension as a long-acting injectable antiretroviral formulation. Antimicrob Agents Chemother 54:2042–2050
Vingerhoets J, Tambuyzer L, Azijn H et al (2010) Resistance profile of etravirine: combined analysis of baseline genotypic and phenotypic data from the randomized, controlled Phase III clinical studies. AIDS 24:503–514
von Wyl V, Ehteshami M, Symons J et al (2010) Epidemiological and biological evidence for a compensatory effect of connection domain mutation N348I on M184V in HIV-1 reverse transcriptase. J Infect Dis 201:1054–1062
Wang J, Smerdon SJ, Jager J et al (1994) Structural basis of asymmetry in the human immunodeficiency virus type 1 reverse transcriptase heterodimer. Proc Natl Acad Sci 91:7242–7246
Whitcomb JM, Parkin NT, Chappey C et al (2003) Broad nucleoside reverse-transcriptase inhibitor cross-resistance in human immunodeficiency virus type 1 clinical isolates. J Infect Dis 188:992–1000
Winters MA, Merigan TC (2005) Insertions in the human immunodeficiency virus type 1 protease and reverse transcriptase genes: clinical impact and molecular mechanisms. Antimicrob Agents Chemother 49:2575–2582
Winters MA, Shafer RW, Jellinger RA et al (1994) Human immunodeficiency virus type 1 reverse transcriptase genotype and drug susceptibility changes in infected individuals receiving dideoxyinosine monotherapy for 1 to 2 years. Antimicrob Agents Chemother 41:757–762
Winters MA, Shafer RW, Jellinger RA et al (1997) Human immunodeficiency virus type 1 reverse transcriptase genotype and drug susceptibility changes in infected individuals receiving dideoxyinosine monotherapy for 1 to 2 years. Antimicrob Agents Chemother 41:757–762
Xu HT, Asahchop EL, Oliveira M et al (2011) Compensation by the E138K mutation in HIV-1 reverse transcriptase for deficits in viral replication capacity and enzyme processivity associated with the M184I/V mutations. J Virol 85:11300–11308
Yap SH, Sheen CW, Fahey J et al (2007) N348I in the connection domain of HIV-1 reverse transcriptase confers zidovudine and nevirapine resistance. PLoS Med 4(12):e335
Zelina S, Sheen CW, Radzio J et al (2008) Mechanisms by which the G333D mutation in human immunodeficiency virus type 1 Reverse transcriptase facilitates dual resistance to zidovudine and lamivudine. Antimicrob Agents Chemother 52:157–163

HIV Drug Resistance in Mothers and Infants Following Use of Antiretrovirals to Prevent Mother-to-Child Transmission

Scott Olson, Quy Ton, and Lisa Frenkel

Contents

S. Olson • Q. Ton
University of Washington, Seattle, WA, USA
e-mail: s.chambers.o@gmail.com; quyton@u.washington.edu

L. Frenkel (✉)
Infectious Diseases/Departments of Pediatrics, Laboratory Medicine and Global Health, University of Washington and Seattle Children's Research Institute, Seattle, WA, USA
e-mail: lfrenkel@u.washington.edu; lfrenkel@uw.edu

M. Gotte et al. (eds.), *Handbook of Antimicrobial Resistance*,
DOI 10.1007/978-1-4939-0694-9_27

Abstract

In the United States and other resource-rich nations, combination antiretroviral therapy (**ART**) that suppresses viral replication below the limits of detection in the plasma is standard of care for prevention of mother-to-child transmission of HIV (**PMTCT**). In many resource-limited communities, financial and infrastructure limitations preclude ART for pregnancy. Instead, abbreviated PMTCT regimens of short-term antiretrovirals (**ARV**) (mono- or dual therapy) that do not suppress viral replication to undetectable levels are recommended. While these less costly approaches achieve significant decreases in the rates of MTCT, selection of HIV drug resistance (**HIV-DR**) has been detected in both mothers and infected infants. This chapter reviews prominent studies that provide insight into HIV-DR related to use of ARV for PMTCT and discusses how recent findings and therapeutic advances have led to policy changes and new directions in this developing field.

Keywords

HIV • Mother-to-child-transmission • Zidovudine • Nevirapine • Drug-resistance

Introduction

Single-dose nevirapine (**sdNVP**) given to the mother at onset of labor and to the infant after birth has been the most common PMTCT regimen used in resource-limited settings and has been part of the World Health Organization (**WHO**) PMTCT recommendations since 2001 (World-Health-Organization 2001). Significant HIV-DR occurs in mothers and in HIV-infected infants treated with sdNVP (Eshleman et al. 2001, 2005a, b, c, 2006; Flys et al. 2005, 2006, 2007a; Palmer et al. 2006; Dross et al. 2010; Micek et al. 2010; Farr et al. 2010) and is associated with an increased risk of virologic failure (defined as non-suppression of HIV replication) when women or infants are treated with non-nucleoside reverse transcriptase (**NNRTI**)-based ART (Jourdain et al. 2004, 2010; Lockman et al. 2007, 2010; Coovadia et al. 2010; Palumbo et al. 2010; Moorthy et al. 2011). However, the effects of drug resistance from sdNVP appears to fade over time (Eshleman et al. 2001; Palmer et al. 2006; Johnson et al. 2005; Loubser et al. 2006; Flys et al. 2007b), with no significant increased risk of virologic failure detected in mothers when NNRTI-based ART is initiated >12–18 months after exposure to sdNVP (Lockman et al. 2010).

NVP resistance is particularly concerning because it confers cross-resistance to efavirenz (**EFV**), another NNRTI, and either NVP or EFV is part of the first-line regimens used globally to treat HIV-infected adults, children, and some infants. The detrimental effect of NVP resistance on the outcome of NNRTI-based ART led the WHO to modify the recommended ARV for PMTCT in 2010 (World-Health-Organization 2010). Currently, sdNVP is only recommended when ART is not prescribed and zidovudine (**ZDV** or **AZT**) is given to the pregnant mother for <4 weeks prior to the onset of labor. The challenges to safe and effective PMTCT include the lack of human capacity, inadequate infrastructure, and insufficient financial backing needed to enact the WHO guidelines. Additionally, under the current WHO guidelines (World-Health-Organization 2010; Moorthy et al. 2009; Fogel et al. 2011a), development of ARV resistance in breastfeeding infants occurs with both recommended regimens: NVP monotherapy prophylaxis of nursing infants (World-Health-Organization 2010; Moorthy et al. 2009; Fogel et al. 2011a) and ART use by breastfeeding mothers (Zeh et al. 2011; Fogel et al. 2011b).

Mechanisms Leading to the Transmission, Selection, and Decay of HIV-DR from sdNVP

Dynamics of HIV-DR

The selection of HIV drug resistance in PMTCT is influenced by the pharmacokinetic properties of the antiretrovirals administered and the genetic barrier posed by a single or a combination of drugs. NVP has a long half-life (~60 h in adults and ~45 h in infants) (Mirochnick et al. 2001; Cressey et al. 2005) and a low "genetic barrier to resistance," with any of several single-base-pair mutations conferring high-level resistance (Richman et al. 1994; Kantor et al. 2001). Lamivudine (**3TC**) and ZDV, nucleoside reverse transcriptase inhibitors (**NRTI**) commonly used in both PMTCT and in first-line ART regimens, have shorter half-lives. 3TC has a low genetic barrier to resistance, with a single-base change conferring high-level resistance, while two or three mutations are required to confer high-level resistance to ZDV (Boucher et al. 1992). Single-base changes conferring resistance to NNRTI and 3TC are estimated to occur on a daily basis due to properties of the viral DNA polymerase (Coffin 1995). However, the likelihood of multiple resistance mutations occurring spontaneously in one virion prior to ARV treatment is exceedingly low (Perelson et al. 1997); therefore, resistance to ZDV and ART occurs by the sequential accumulation of mutations while receiving therapy if there is HIV replication. The selection of ZDV resistance was uncommon when administered for ~10 weeks to mothers for PMTCT (Jourdain et al. 2004; Shapiro et al. 2010), consistent with its moderate genetic barrier to selection of resistance. Based on these findings, ZDV monotherapy is one of two WHO-recommended regimens for pregnant women with CD4 cells counts >350/uL for PMTCT (World-Health-Organization 2010). However, as discussed below, mutants are selected in pregnant women given ZDV for longer periods of time. Because NVP remains detectible in maternal plasma for 1–3 weeks after sdNVP, the administration of a short-course "tail" of ZDV +/− 3TC postpartum decreases viral replication and increases the genetic barrier to resistance, which limits the selection of NVP resistance. Therefore, ARV tails are recommended to reduce resistance when sdNVP is used for PMTCT (World-Health-Organization 2006, 2010).

Individuals administered with mono- or dual-ARV regimens and those who experience virologic failure during ART often experience selection of mutants. These drug-resistant variants infect cells, including populations of long-lived cells that constitute the latent reservoir of viruses. Generally, virions with selected HIV-DR have decreased replication capacity compared to wild-type viruses, and in the absence of selective ARV pressure, the mutants decrease in frequency over time, largely replaced by wild-type virus (Deeks et al. 2001). However, if replication-competent mutants persist in the viral reservoir, these variants rapidly reemerge when an ARV is recycled or an ARV with cross-resistance is administered. The reservoir of mutants selected by sdNVP persist for less time compared to mutants selected by failing ART, presumably because a longer period of selection archives a greater number of viable ARV-resistant viruses in long-lived cells. In mothers and infected infants, NVP-resistant viruses in plasma decay to undetectable levels within several months by consensus sequencing, and generally within 6–12 months using more sensitive assays (Eshleman et al. 2001; Palmer et al. 2006; Johnson et al. 2005; Loubser et al. 2006; Flys et al. 2007b; Wagner et al. 2010). When NVP-based ART is started after a sufficient interval (~12 months), resistant variants generally do not reemerge (Lockman et al. 2007, 2010; Palumbo et al. 2010). However, a threshold concentration of NVP resistance or a time interval between sdNVP and initiation of NVP-based ART that can predict virologic failure of NVP-based ART has not been definitively established.

In contrast to HIV-DR selected by sdNVP, persons directly infected with a drug-resistant virus, commonly called transmitted drug-resistant HIV (**TDR**), have HIV-DR that persists over many years, even without selective drug pressure (Little et al. 1999, 2008). This is likely because acute infection corresponds to the time that viruses infect a large number of susceptible cells, and a proportion of these become quiescent and part of the latent HIV reservoir (Schacker et al. 2000). Also, TDR variants generally have a high replication capacity. In Africa, variable rates of TDR have been observed, ranging from 3 % to 19 %, with significant increases in resistance to NNRTI medications occurring progressively since access to ART has improved (Price et al. 2011; Bennett et al. 2008a, b; Jordan et al. 2008; Maphalala et al. 2008; Myatt and Bennett 2008; Nguyen et al. 2008; Pillay et al. 2008; Shafer et al. 2008; Somi et al. 2008; Gupta et al. 2012). In resource-limited communities, screening tests for drug resistance are not used prior to administering ARV for PMTCT or when initiating ART, as is routine in resource-rich communities. Thus, increasing rates of TDR are of concern for PMTCT as well as general ART programs. The WHO recommends the surveillance of ARV-naïve individuals to monitor rates of TDR and at specific thresholds to strengthen voluntary counseling and testing and adherence programs and address weaknesses in the supply of ARV and other identified programmatic insufficiencies (Bennett et al. 2008a, b).

History of Antiretrovirals Used for PMTCT in Resource-Rich Communities and Associated Resistance

Zidovudine Monotherapy

In 1994, ZDV monotherapy was shown to reduce MTCT by 67.5 % in a randomized placebo-controlled trial conducted in infants given formula in place of breast milk (Pediatric Clinical Trials Group Protocol [PACTG 076]) (Connor and Mofenson 1995). ZDV and other mono- and dual-ARV therapies generally do not suppress viral replication to undetectable levels and therefore can select drug-resistant forms. In spite of a moderate genetic barrier to resistance, ZDV resistance has been detected during pregnancy (Eastman et al. 1998; Frenkel et al. 2006) and has been transmitted to infants (Frenkel et al. 1995).

In an observational study of US pregnant women receiving ZDV for their medical care or PMTCT, ZDV resistance was detected in the blood of 16 of 48 (33 %) women using a sensitive oligonucleotide ligation assay (**OLA**) (Frenkel et al. 2006). ZDV resistance was not associated with low maternal CD4, high HIV-1 RNA levels in the plasma, or with the duration of antiretroviral therapy. The median length of ZDV treatment in women with and without ZDV mutants in the blood was 21.4 and 21.0 weeks, respectively. In contrast, larger studies conducted in mid- or low-resource communities with shorter durations of ZDV, and use of less sensitive assays, have reported lower rates of ZDV resistance (Jourdain et al. 2004; Shapiro et al. 2006).

More recently, among Tanzanian women who received antenatal ZDV (median duration 53 days), sdNVP, and ZDV/3TC postpartum for 1 week, at time of delivery, ZDV resistance was detected in 10 % using a sensitive allele-specific PCR (**AS-PCR**) (Hauser et al. 2012). Over a 16-week follow-up period, however, ZDV resistance was detected in 22 %, suggesting that postpartum ARV tails administered following sdNVP to diminish the emergence of NVP-resistant virus may continue to exert selective pressure for ZDV resistance mutations.

The observations of resistance in a substantial proportion of US (Frenkel et al. 2006) and Tanzanian (Hauser et al. 2012) women with >350 CD4 cells/uL after ZDV argue for studies to evaluate the effect of ZDV monotherapy on subsequent maternal ART, as mutations selected by ZDV monotherapy may be archived in long-lived cells, potentially diminishing the efficacy of subsequent maternal ART containing ZDV or other NRTI.

Combination Antiretroviral Therapy (ART)

In 1996, combination ART revolutionized the treatment of HIV infection (Hammer et al. 1996). Among women taking ART to treat their HIV infection, a lower rate of MTCT was observed compared to those taking ZDV monotherapy (Cooper et al. 2002). Use of ART was associated with diminished rates of transmission to non-breastfeeding infants (1–2 %) in North America and Europe (Lindegren et al. 1999; World-Health-Organization 2009).

ART during gestation became standard of care for PMTCT in resource-rich settings. HIV-infected pregnant women with high CD4 cell counts often elect to stop ART postpartum. When viral replication is suppressed by a ritonavir-boosted protease inhibitor (PI)-based ART regimen, HIV-DR mutations generally are not selected during the elimination of the ARV. However, women treated with less potent regimens, for example, with nelfinavir-based ART, or who have been nonadherent can select HIV-DR during or upon the cessation of ART (Ellis et al. 2011). While studies that use consensus sequencing show overall low rates of resistance following either NNRTI- or PI-based ART for PMTCT (Souda et al. 2013), those using more sensitive assays, such as OLA or AS-PCR, reveal selection of resistant variants below the limit of detection of consensus sequencing (Lehman et al. 2009; Perez et al. 2008; Paredes et al. 2010). The clinical importance of low-frequency variants has not been fully investigated, though there is growing evidence that they may negatively impact the efficacy of later ART (Metzner et al. 2009; Li et al. 2011; Stekler et al. 2011).

Several studies have compared rates of resistance that develop following ART versus mono- or dual-drug combinations for PMTCT. In Kenya ART (ZDV/3TC/NVP) started at 34 weeks' gestation and continued through 6 months of breastfeeding was associated with lower rates of resistance compared to antenatal ZDV plus sdNVP at 3 months post-ARV by AS-PCR (18 % vs. 75 %, $p = 0.007$) (Lehman et al. 2009). In the Kesho Bora study, ART (ZDV/3TC/LVP/rt) started at 34 weeks' gestation and continued through breastfeeding selected less resistance compared to antenatal ZDV plus sdNVP (1.4 % vs. 24 %) (The Kesho Bora Group 2012). Importantly, however, none of the subjects in the ZDV/sdNVP arm who received postpartum ARV tails developed resistance mutations.

History of Antiretrovirals Used for PMTCT in Resource-Limited Communities and Associated Resistance

The Rise of Single-Dose Nevirapine (sdNVP)

In contrast to resource-rich communities, women in resource-limited communities had virtually no PMTCT services in the 1990s. Insufficient infrastructure and a lack of funds and political will resulted in millions of HIV-infected children, including over one million infants in sub-Saharan Africa – the region with the greatest number of HIV-infected women of childbearing age.

In response to these challenges, shortened, simplified, and inexpensive PMTCT regimens were explored. In 1999, the HIVNET 012 trial demonstrated that one oral dose of nevirapine given to mothers during labor and one dose administered to breastfeeding infants shortly after birth reduced MTCT by 50 % at 6 weeks of age and by 38 % at 18 months of age (Jackson et al. 2003). sdNVP does not require refrigeration and thus can be taken by a woman at home when she begins labor.

Given its feasibility and low cost, sdNVP was included in WHO recommendations beginning in 2001 (World-Health-Organization 2001) and quickly became the most common regimen for PMTCT in resource-limited settings. While access to PMTCT programs has improved in recent years, many women receive suboptimal care. A recent random sampling of African sites with PMTCT services found that only 51 % of HIV-exposed infants received NVP (Stringer et al. 2010a).

Unfortunately, sdNVP selects resistant viruses at high rates in both mothers and infected infants: 10–75 % of mothers (Flys et al. 2005; Eshleman et al. 2005a, d; Micek et al. 2010; Johnson et al. 2005; Arrive et al. 2007) and 4–87 % of children (Eshleman et al. 2005b; Micek et al. 2010; Lockman 2008; Lockman and McIntyre 2007; Martinson et al. 2007a). The prevalence of NVP resistance after sdNVP varies across HIV subtypes, with higher rates in subtypes C and D compared to subtype A (Eshleman et al. 2005a; Flys et al. 2006), and detection is increased when evaluated using sensitive assays. A meta-analysis reported a pooled prevalence estimate of 35.7 % among women exposed to sdNVP by consensus sequencing and 62.4 % by sensitive research assays (Arrive et al. 2007).

ARV "Tails" to Prevent Selection of NVP-Resistant HIV

To reduce resistance following sdNVP, a strategy that gives short courses of postpartum ARV, so-called "tails," to suppress viral replication and increase the genetic barrier to resistance has been investigated across many studies. These ARV tails vary in costs and feasibility, but all effectively reduce selection of NVP resistance. Postpartum tails were incorporated into WHO recommendations in 2006 (World-Health-Organization 2006) and continue to be recommended for women receiving sdNVP (World-Health-Organization 2010).

Among women receiving sdNVP, the TOPS study found that 4 or 7 days of postpartum ZDV/3TC significantly diminished NVP resistance compared to untreated controls as detected by consensus sequencing: 11.7 %, 7.3 %, and 59.2 %, respectively ($p < 0.0001$) (McIntyre et al. 2009). Similarly, the BAN trial found that a 7-day tail of ZDV/3TC significantly reduced NVP resistance in mothers assessed by consensus sequencing and AS-PCR (10 % vs. 64 %, $p < 0.0001$) (Farr et al. 2010). More recently, a longer, 21-day ARV tail of either ZDV/3TC, TDF/FTC, or lopinavir/rt (**LPV/rt**) reduced resistance more than a 7-day tail of the same medications by AS-PCR (5 % vs. 18 %, $p = 0.019$), though rates were similar by consensus sequencing (McMahon et al. 2013).

Among mothers receiving antenatal ZDV +/−3TC and sdNVP in labor, the administration of ZDV/3TC for 3-days postpartum decreased NVP resistance compared to historical controls (Chaix et al. 2006). A randomized study administering a single dose of TDF/FTC during labor markedly reduced NVP resistance compared to controls by consensus sequencing (Chi et al. 2007) and by OLA (Chi et al. 2009). A two-dose TDF/FTC tail was similarly effective (Arrive et al. 2009).

In Thailand, where antenatal ZDV was standard of care and hepatitis B is prevalent, tails composed of ZDV/didanosine (**ddI**) +/− lopinavir/rt were investigated because the cessation of 3TC allows HBV to replicate, which can lead to a clinical flare of hepatitis B (Altfeld et al. 1998; Bessesen et al. 1999). One study detected no NVP resistance among women receiving a 1-month tail of ddI/ZDV, which was significantly less compared to historical controls (0 % vs. 10.4 %, respectively, by consensus sequencing and 1.8 % vs. 18.9 % by OLA, $p = <0.001$ for both analyses) (Lallemant and Jourdain 2010). A second study of tails comprised of 1 week of ddI/ZDV/LPV/rt, 1 month of ddI/ZDV, and 1 month of ddI/ZDV/LPV/rt similarly detected no NVP resistance in any group by consensus sequencing and 1.8 %, 7.1 %, and 5.3 % by OLA, respectively, which compared favorably to untreated historical controls with 13.4 % by sequencing and 29.4 % by OLA ($p < 0.001$ for each study arm vs. comparison group) (Van Dyke et al. 2012).

Reuse of sdNVP in Subsequent Pregnancies: HIV Transmission and Maternal/Infant Resistance Risks

Studies of the reuse of sdNVP with subsequent pregnancies have generally shown similar efficacies for PMTCT and similar rates of NVP resistance. Following reuse of sdNVP at median intervals of 21–32 months (Martinson et al. 2007b, 2009; McConnell et al. 2007; Walter et al. 2008), the proportion with NVP resistance mutations after the first compared to subsequent sdNVP did not differ at 6 weeks (Kuhn et al. 2006; Flys et al. 2008), 6 months (Flys et al. 2008), and 12 months (Flys et al. 2008) by consensus sequencing (Kuhn et al. 2006; Flys et al. 2008) or by more sensitive assays (Flys et al. 2008). Similarly, in infected infants the proportion of NVP resistance mutations was similar at 6 weeks (Flys et al. 2008). These data on reuse of sdNVP in subsequent pregnancies indicate that NVP resistance does not reemerge in the mother postpartum at a rate that increases the transmission of drug-resistant HIV via breastfeeding and furthermore suggests that the reservoir of NNRTI mutants following sdNVP is relatively short-lived.

Effects of sdNVP on Efficacy of Subsequent NNRTI-Based ART in Women

Evidence of the negative impact of sdNVP on subsequent NNRTI-based ART began to accumulate when postpartum women in resource-limited settings gained access to ART in the mid-2000s. A subset of Thai women who received antenatal ZDV and were randomized to receive sdNVP or placebo during labor (Lallemant et al. 2004) were first reported to have increased rates of virologic failure when subsequently administered with NVP-based ART to treat their HIV disease (Jourdain et al. 2004). Fewer sdNVP-exposed women had viral suppression (HIV-1 RNA levels <50 copies/mL) compared to placebo-treated women (49 % vs. 68 %, respectively, $p = 0.03$). Consensus sequencing of maternal virus 1–2 months postpartum was not associated with virologic failure; however, detection of NVP resistance in DNA isolated from blood cells collected just prior to the initiation of ART by OLA was linked with failure (Jourdain et al. 2010).

The Mashi trial, among women with or without a history of sdNVP who subsequently took NNRTI-based ART, observed increased rates of virologic failure (18 % vs. 5 %, $p = 0.002$) (Lockman et al. 2007). sdNVP was associated with virologic failure among women who initiated ART within 6 months of sdNVP (42 % vs. 0 %, $p < 0.001$), but not among women who initiated NVP-ART 6 months or more after sdNVP exposure (12 % vs. 7.8 %, $p = 0.39$). These results suggest that drug resistance selected by sdNVP decays over time, which is consistent with multiple studies showing that NVP resistance mutations fade from detection over time (Eshleman et al. 2001; Palmer et al. 2006; Johnson et al. 2005; Loubser et al. 2006; Flys et al. 2007b; Wagner et al. 2010). In pre-ART specimens, NVP resistance mutations K103N and Y181C were detected by AS-PCR in 65 % of subjects at concentrations of 0.1–4.1 % (Rowley et al. 2010). NVP resistance of >0.19 % was associated with virologic failure (86 % of 7 subjects with failure vs. 32 % of 19 without failure; OR = 13, 95 % CI 1.27–133); however, the input of viral templates for PCR amplification was not reported, which likely influenced the nominal concentration determined to be clinically predictive.

The decay of mutants selected by sdNVP to clinically insignificant concentrations has been confirmed in multiple studies. In an observational study in South Africa, an interval of 18–36 months between sdNVP and the initiation of NNRTI-based ART revealed rates of suppression of viral replication comparable to women not exposed to sdNVP (Coovadia et al. 2009). Similarly, long intervals were associated with increased viral suppression in Zambian women (Kuhn et al. 2009). Treatment failure (defined as virologic failure, death, loss to follow-up, or discontinuation of NNRTI-based ART for any reason before 48 weeks) was greater among women who initiated NVP-based ART at an interval of <6 months (41 %, $p = 0.001$) or 7–12 months (37 %, $p = 0.04$), but not if >12 months compared to sdNVP-unexposed women in Zambia, Kenya, and Thailand (Stringer et al. 2010b).

The multi-country OCTANE trial demonstrated the superiority of LPV/rt- compared to NVP-based ART among sdNVP-exposed women but not among NVP-unexposed women (Lockman et al. 2010). Again, the effect of sdNVP appeared to decrease as the interval between sdNVP exposure and ART initiation increased. NVP resistance was detected prior to ART by consensus sequencing in 15 (13 %) women in the NVP group and 18 (15 %) women in the LPV/rt group. Among those with NVP resistance, 73 % in the NVP group compared to only 6 % in the LPV/rt group died or had virologic failure ($p = 0.006$). Analysis of the OCTANE participants revealed that at the time of starting ART with an NNRTI regimen, those women with either K103N or Y181C at a concentration >1 % of the plasma HIV population by AS-PCR testing were at increased risk of virologic failure or death (HR 2.93, 95 % CI 1.27–6.75) (Boltz et al. 2011). This finding supports the assertion that minority variant resistant virus can impact the response to ART and highlights the potential impact of sensitive resistance assays for women who used sdNVP.

Importantly, use of two inexpensive HIV-DR assays, AS-PCR in the OCTANE (Boltz et al. 2011) and OLA in the PHPT-2 trials (Jourdain et al. 2010), detected

NVP resistance associated with virologic failure. These data suggest that testing for HIV-DR prior to ART initiation by point mutation assays may be useful in women after sdNVP to guide the choice of an appropriate ART regimen. While ARV testing is available to a limited degree for clinical care and research studies in Africa and Asia, studies are needed to clarify the clinical relevance of mutations at single versus multiple NVP resistance codons or in virus in plasma versus cells and whether there are specific threshold concentrations of mutants that predict the outcome of NNRTI-based ART.

Effects of sdNVP on HIV-DR in Infants and Subsequent NNRTI-Based ART

In HIV-infected infants exposed to sdNVP, the timing of perinatal HIV acquisition determines the size of the NVP-resistant viral reservoir and whether it persists. A study of Mozambican infants revealed three distinct dynamic patterns of NVP resistance (Micek et al. 2010). Most frequent were infants whose HIV infection had been established in utero prior to administration of sdNVP. Among these infants, mutants were selected to concentrations approaching 100 %, followed by rapid decay by 4–6 months of age. Among a smaller group of infants, who appeared in the midst of acute HIV infection at the time of birth, NVP resistance was selected when their viral population was large enough to contain spontaneously generated mutants prior to administration of sdNVP. These mutants expanded rapidly to high concentrations and apparently entered long-lived cells, as these mutants persisted over time. Among infants infected peri- or postpartum, approximately 30 % acquired pure populations of NVP-resistant virus, which also persisted over time. Given that NVP resistance was not detected in maternal blood or milk at delivery, NVP-resistant variants were most likely transmitted through breastfeeding.

Not surprisingly, following prophylaxis with sdNVP, the treatment of infants with NVP-based ART showed diminished rates of virologic efficacy in the Mashi trial (76.9 % vs. 9.1 %, respectively, $p < 0.001$) (Lockman et al. 2007). NVP resistance was evaluated in specimens collected from 33 infants prior to ART initiation (MacLeod et al. 2010). Consensus sequencing identified NVP resistance in only 11 % infants compared to 39 % infants by AS-PCR. Testing of pre-ART blood plasma and cell samples at a median age of 6.5 months detected NVP resistance in 9 of 16 infants experiencing virologic failure compared to 4 of 17 infants without virologic failure (risk ratio 2.4, CI 0.94–7.8, $p = 0.08$).

A randomized trial (P1060) of NVP- versus LPV/rt-based ART in infants following sdNVP was conducted across multiple African countries (Palumbo et al. 2010). After 24 weeks of ART, treatment failure was greater among infants randomized to NVP- compared to LPV/rt-based ART (39.6 % vs. 21.7 %, respectively, $p = 0.02$). Among those randomized to NVP-ART, the detection of NVP resistance mutations in the pre-ART specimen by consensus sequencing was predictive of treatment failure (83 % with vs. 36 % without detection of NVP resistance failed, $p = 0.02$).

One study of sdNVP-treated infants aimed to capitalize on the decay of NVP resistance by using a novel ART strategy (NEVEREST Study) (Coovadia et al. 2010). All infants initiated LPV/rt-based ART, and those with suppression of viral replication to $\leq$400 copies/mL for $\geq$3 months (median = 10) were then randomized to either continue LPV/rt- or switch to NVP-based ART. The switch occurred at a median of 19 months of age (range 9–43), which in most women given sdNVP is a sufficiently long interval from treatment with sdNVP for NVP resistance to decay to clinically insignificant concentrations (Lockman et al. 2007). However, virologic failure (plasma HIV RNA >1,000 copies/mL) was greater in infants who switched compared to those who continued PI-based ART (20 % vs. 2 %, respectively, $p < 0.001$). Children switched to NVP-ART who had NNRTI mutations detectible by consensus sequencing at switch experienced viral failure at a greater rate compared to those without mutations (10/19 vs. 7/51; $p < 0.02$) (Kuhn et al. 2012).

It is possible that this significant difference in failure rates among NEVEREST infants who switched to NVP-based ART was due to fundamental differences in the reservoir of NVP-resistant virus of infants compared to adult women. While most adult women have rapid decay of NVP resistance, as previously mentioned, a large and persistent reservoir of NVP-resistant viruses is established in a subset of infants following sdNVP, including infants with acute infection at birth (Micek et al. 2010) and who acquired HIV via breastfeeding (Dross et al. 2010). Thus, the NEVEREST infants with virologic failure after the switch to NVP-based ART likely include infants with long-lived reservoirs of ARV-resistant HIV (Little et al. 2008). Indeed, pre-ART consensus (Kuhn et al. 2012) and pyrosequencing (Moorthy et al. 2009) detected high concentrations of NVP mutants in those with virologic failure. The findings that NVP resistance does not predictably decay in infants and that testing of infants for NVP resistance predicts virologic response to NVP-based ART (Palumbo et al. 2010; Moorthy et al. 2011) suggest that in low-resource communities studies are needed to evaluate the feasibility and cost-effectiveness of pre-ART drug resistance testing compared to alternative strategies, such as viral load monitoring during ART.

HIV-DR Associated with Maternal ART or Infant NVP Prophylaxis During Breastfeeding

In resource-limited settings, breastfeeding offers infants protection from disease and death compared to artificial infant formulas, which require mixing with potentially unsanitary water (Nduati et al. 2000; Arvelo et al. 2010; Kunz et al. 2009; Kuhn et al. 2008). Strategies to protect infants from HIV infection while providing them with the beneficial effects of breast milk include two approaches that have been examined in multiple studies: first, administration of ARV prophylaxis directly to infants and, second, maternal ART to reduce HIV load in breast milk. NVP prophylaxis of various durations has been examined in breastfeeding infants (Petra-Study-Team 2002; Moodley et al. 2003; SWEN-Study-Team 2008; Kumwenda et al. 2008;

Coovadia et al. 2011). Across these studies the efficacy of prophylaxis appears to increase with the coverage of the breastfeeding period. Maternal ART was shown to reduce rates of MTCT compared to short-course ZDV plus sdNVP during pregnancy by the Kesho Bora study (de Vincenzi 2011) and during breastfeeding by the Kesho Bora and BAN studies (Chasela et al. 2010).

ARV-resistant virus can be selected by ARV given to the infants as prophylaxis or ARV transferred to the infant in breast milk. In addition, primary infection with drug-resistant virus can occur in the postnatal period by exposure to ARV-resistant virus in breast milk (Dross et al. 2010; Lidstrom et al. 2010). Following sdNVP, rates of NVP resistance in breast milk range from 40 % to 65 %, persist for up to 8 months, and can differ from concurrent plasma viruses (Lee et al. 2005; Kassaye et al. 2007; Hudelson et al. 2010; Gantt et al. 2012).

In the Stopping Infection from Mother-to-child via Breastfeeding in Africa (SIMBA) study, infants were given either daily lamivudine or nevirapine after birth until 1 month after cessation of breastfeeding, while their mothers had received zidovudine and didanosine from 36 weeks' gestation until 1 week postpartum (Giuliano et al. 2006). The HIV-infected infants who received prophylaxis prior to confirmation of diagnosis frequently selected drug-resistant variants, including 12/13 (92.3 %) of those on NVP for a median of 45 days and 9/13 (69.2 %) on 3TC for a median of 14 days.

Multiple studies of daily NVP prophylaxis administered to infants include a randomized controlled trial of 6 weeks of extended-dose nevirapine (SWEN) (SWEN-Study-Team 2008). A higher prevalence of NVP resistance was detected in infants randomized to continue NVP compared to those who only received sdNVP by population sequencing (92 % of 12 % vs. 38 % of 29 infants, $p = 0.002$), which persisted as a majority population through 6 months (Moorthy et al. 2009). In the Post Exposure Prophylaxis of Infants (PEPI) trial in Malawi, infants who had received sdNVP and a week of ZDV after birth were randomized to no additional intervention, daily NVP for 14 weeks, or daily NVP/ZDV for 14 weeks (Kumwenda et al. 2008). While the continuation of NVP and NVP/ZDV conferred similar rates of protection from MTCT, infants with in utero HIV infection had lower rates of NVP resistance if assigned to NVP/ZDV compared to NVP (54.5 % vs. 85.7 %, $p = 0.007$) (Lidstrom et al. 2010). However, the protective effect of ZDV on NVP resistance was lost if infants continued to take ARV beyond 6 weeks of age (83.3 % vs. 87.5 %, $p = 1.0$). In a similar randomized trial (HPTN/IMPAACT 046) of NVP prophylaxis for 6 weeks versus 6 months, NVP was selected for resistant variants in infants infected after 6 weeks of age (75 % in the NVP arm vs. 6 % in the placebo arm at 6 months of age; $p = 0.001$) (Fogel et al. 2013).

ARV concentrations in breast milk of mothers receiving ART appear variable, in part due to sparse sampling. 3TC is concentrated in breast milk with levels 3–5 times higher than in maternal plasma; ZDV concentrations are similar or slightly lower compared to maternal plasma; NVP concentrations are 60–75 % that of plasma; and protease inhibitors penetrate poorly into breast milk (Mirochnick et al. 2009). Studies evaluating ARV levels in the plasma of breastfeeding infants have demonstrated

NVP and 3TC at biologically active levels, while ZDV is typically at lower concentrations (Shapiro et al. 2005), (Mirochnick et al. 2009).

Several studies have evaluated HIV-DR in the HIV-infected infants of mothers receiving ART. HIV-infected PEPI infants whose mothers initiated NVP-based ART during their first year of life had HIV-DR to multiple drugs detected in 30 % ($n = 37$) in association with earlier initiation of postpartum maternal ART and exclusive breastfeeding at initiation of ART (Fogel et al. 2011b). Comparisons of maternal and infant patterns of HIV-DR mutations suggested MTCT of virus resistant to multiple ARV in a subset of infants.

The KiBS study assessed the safety and efficacy of maternal ART (ZDV/3TC plus either NVP or nelfinavir) beginning at 34–36 weeks' gestation and continuing through to 6 months of breastfeeding (Zeh et al. 2011). The cumulative HIV transmission rates assessed at infants' birth, 6 weeks, and 6, 12, and 24 months of age were 2.5 %, 4.2 %, 5.0 %, 5.7 %, and 7.0 %, respectively. A secondary analysis of HIV-DR in 32 HIV-infected infants by consensus sequencing found that the rate of HIV-DR increased over time: 30 % of infants at 6 weeks, 63 % at 14 weeks, and 67 % at 6 months had HIV-DR (Zeh et al. 2011). In contrast to the infants in the PEPI study, only one mother-infant pair had similar patterns of HIV-DR, suggesting that HIV-DR was principally the result of selective pressure from ARV in mothers' breast milk rather than transmitted directly from the mother. Importantly, HIV-infected infants in these studies were not started immediately on LPV/rt-based ART as currently recommended, which would likely preclude the selection of HIV-DR variants (but may incur additional ARV toxicities).

To date, the efficacy of concomitant maternal ART and infant NVP prophylaxis during breastfeeding for PMTCT has not been systematically studied. However, the mothers of a subset of infants participating in HPTN/IMPAACT 046 of NVP prophylaxis initiated ART, thus exposing the infants to both NVP prophylaxis and ARV via maternal milk (Coovadia et al. 2011). All four infants whose mothers started NNRTI-based ART developed NVP resistance, while only 14 % of the infants whose mothers did not start ART developed resistance (Fogel et al. 2011b). Cost and potential NVP toxicity to the infant from the combined prophylactic NVP plus ARV ingested in maternal breast milk may limit this approach.

Modifications of WHO Recommendations for PMTCT to Reduce Use of sdNVP and Increase Maternal ART

The results of the multiple studies described above indicate that the use of sdNVP for PMTCT can negatively impact the outcome of subsequent NNRTI-based ART for mothers and infected infants. As the time interval between sdNVP and the initiation of maternal or infant ART increases, the effect of ARV resistance on treatment outcome diminishes, presumably due to decay of NVP-resistant viruses. However, a threshold time interval, after which NVP resistance is no longer clinically significant, has not been clearly defined, particularly in infected infants. Given that maternal baseline CD4 and viral load (Micek et al. 2012) and HIV-1 subtype affect selection of NVP resistance, this time interval may vary across individuals and geographic regions. Furthermore, in a subset of infected infants, HIV-resistant mutants do not appear to decay but rather persists in the viral reservoir (Micek et al. 2010).

These issues, combined with the growing infrastructure to administer ART to adults, bring into question the balance between providing simplified regimens to reach the greatest number of women and providing more effective therapies that minimize both MTCT and HIV-DR. In response, the WHO PMTCT recommendations changed in two stages. In 2006, ZDV in late gestation was added to sdNVP to further reduce MTCT and postpartum combination ARV tails were recommended to reduce selection of NVP resistance (World-Health-Organization 2006). In 2010, in response to the growing evidence of the negative effect of NVP resistance on the efficacy of maternal and infant ART, the WHO recommended ART or ZDV monotherapy for women with >350 CD4/uL, with sdNVP given only if mothers received fewer than 4 weeks of ART or ZDV (World-Health-Organization 2010). The rationale for continued use of ZDV monotherapy in women with high CD4 cell counts included the high efficacy of ZDV monotherapy in PMTCT (Shapiro et al. 2006), lower cost of ZDV compared to ART, avoidance of the rare but fatal hepatic toxicity associated with NVP-based ART in women with CD4 > 250 cells/uL, and past studies showing that ZDV resistance is rarely selected in women with relatively high CD4 counts who took ~10 weeks of ZDV (Jourdain et al. 2004; Shapiro et al. 2010). As infrastructure has improved, some low-resource communities have adopted ART for PMTCT regardless of a woman's immune (CD4) status (Chimbwandira et al. 2013). However, given the poor access to care in some, especially rural communities (Stringer et al. 2010a), the use of sdNVP may continue for some women.

A WHO update in 2012 discusses the use of ART for PMTCT with continuation of lifelong treatment of the woman, regardless of her CD4 count or clinical status. This strategy, termed "Option B+," was adopted in Malawi and was associated with an increase in PMTCT administration due to the integration of antenatal and HIV care (Chimbwandira et al. 2013). Option B or B+ is gaining support in other resource-poor nations. Some experts express concerns about the higher cost of ART, potential adverse reactions, and lapses in adherence that could select HIV-DR and oppose the blanket recommendation of B+ (Coutsoudis et al. 2013a, b). Few studies evaluate ARV resistance in association with long-term ART in communities without routine testing for HIV-DR.

Conclusions: Future Directions

Since ~1996, ART has nearly eliminated MTCT in North America and Europe. During the past decade, multiple studies have shown that simplified mono- and dual-ARV strategies generally are less effective for PMTCT or have a negative impact on EFV- or NVP-based ART subsequently administered to treat HIV disease in mothers and infants. Given these findings and the increasing access to ART around the world, a number of research and policy experts promote universal ART for pregnant and breastfeeding HIV-infected women to eliminate MTCT (Becquet et al. 2010). Others question the ethics of continuing to conduct research using suboptimal PMTCT regimens given the superiority of ART regimens over suboptimal short-course mono-, dual-, or triple-ARV regimens (Schouten et al. 2013; Goosby 2013; Ammann 2009). While the WHO recommendations have shown a continuing trend away from short-course mono- or dual-ARV, with the 2010 WHO Guidelines avoiding the use of sdNVP when possible (World-Health-Organization 2010), new 2013 Guidelines will likely recommend ART exclusively.

While modeling suggested that HIV-DR prevalence would remain low in Africa (Blower et al. 2001), recent surveillance detected substantial rates of TDR in some communities (Price et al. 2011; Gupta et al. 2012). Continued increases in TDR could undermine PMTCT programs (Geretti 2007; Shet et al. 2006). Expansion of PMTCT could increase the prevalence of HIV-DR viruses and further fuel TDR. Testing for NNRTI resistance before the initiation of ART in communities with high rates of TDR could allow clinicians to select PI-based regimens for affected individuals, which modeling suggests is cost effective in the United States (Sax et al. 2005). Pre-ART testing for HIV-DR should lead to better rates of suppression of viral replication in treated individuals and help prevent the spread of HIV infection by diminishing MTCT and reducing heterosexual transmission from women to their serodiscordant sexual partners (Cohen et al. 2011). Research directed at optimization of operational aspects and cost-effectiveness of testing for HIV-DR prior to ART is needed as ART services expand to allow recognition of virologic failure and better tailoring of post-failure treatment.

The evolution of PMTCT interventions in resource-limited communities during the past decade demonstrates the challenges faced by public health officials who worked to balance the limited infrastructure and resources with effective prevention of MTCT and HIV-DR. As access to ART continues to increase, there is potential to further decrease MTCT. Importantly, both monitoring of HIV-DR and programmatic investments to limit the spread of ARV-resistant variants will be needed to maximize the gains antiretrovirals can deliver to PMTCT.

References

Altfeld M, Rockstroh JK, Addo M, Kupfer B, Pult I, Will H et al (1998) Reactivation of hepatitis B in a long-term anti-HBs-positive patient with AIDS following lamivudine withdrawal. J Hepatol 29(2):306–309 [Case Reports]

Ammann AJ (2009) Optimal versus suboptimal treatment for HIV-infected pregnant women and HIV-exposed infants in clinical research studies. J Acquir Immune Defic Syndr 51(5):509–512

Arrive E, Newell ML, Ekouevi DK, Chaix ML, Thiebaut R, Masquelier B et al (2007) Prevalence of resistance to nevirapine in mothers and children after single-dose exposure to prevent vertical transmission of HIV-1: a meta-analysis. Int J Epidemiol 36(5):1009–1021

Arrive E, Chaix ML, Nerrienet E, Blanche S, Rouzioux C, Coffie PA et al (2009) Tolerance and viral resistance after single-dose nevirapine with tenofovir and emtricitabine to prevent vertical transmission of HIV-1. AIDS 23(7):825–833

Arvelo W, Kim A, Creek T, Legwaila K, Puhr N, Johnston S et al (2010) Case-control study to determine risk factors for diarrhea among children during a large outbreak in a country with a high prevalence of HIV infection. Int J Infect Dis 14(11):e1002–e1007

Becquet R, Bland R, Ekouevi DK, Dabis F, Newell ML (2010) Universal antiretroviral therapy among pregnant and postpartum HIV-infected women would improve maternal health and decrease postnatal HIV transmission. AIDS 24(8):1239–1241

Bennett DE, Bertagnolio S, Sutherland D, Gilks CF (2008a) The World Health Organization's global strategy for prevention and assessment of HIV drug resistance. Antivir Ther 13(Suppl 2):1–13

Bennett DE, Myatt M, Bertagnolio S, Sutherland D, Gilks CF (2008b) Recommendations for surveillance of transmitted HIV drug resistance in countries scaling up antiretroviral treatment. Antivir Ther 13(Suppl 2):25–36

Bessesen M, Ives D, Condreay L, Lawrence S, Sherman KE (1999) Chronic active hepatitis B exacerbations in human immunodeficiency virus-infected patients following development of resistance to or withdrawal of lamivudine. Clin Infect Dis 28(5):1032–1035 [Case Reports]

Blower SM, Aschenbach AN, Gershengorn HB, Kahn JO (2001) Predicting the unpredictable: transmission of drug-resistant HIV. Nat Med 7(9):1016–1020

Boltz VF, Zheng Y, Lockman S, Hong F, Halvas EK, McIntyre J et al (2011) Role of low-frequency HIV-1 variants in failure of nevirapine-containing antiviral therapy in women previously exposed to single-dose nevirapine. Proc Natl Acad Sci U S A 108(22):9202–9207

Boucher CA, O'Sullivan E, Mulder JW, Ramautarsing C, Kellam P, Darby G et al (1992) Ordered appearance of zidovudine resistance mutations during treatment of 18 human immunodeficiency virus-positive subjects. J Infect Dis 165:105–110

Chaix ML, Ekouevi DK, Rouet F, Tonwe-Gold B, Viho I, Bequet L et al (2006) Low risk of nevirapine resistance mutations in the prevention of mother-to-child transmission of HIV-1: agence Nationale de Recherches sur le SIDA Ditrame Plus, Abidjan, Cote d'Ivoire. J Infect Dis 193(4):482–487

Chasela CS, Hudgens MG, Jamieson DJ, Kayira D, Hosseinipour MC, Kourtis AP et al (2010) Maternal or infant antiretroviral drugs to reduce HIV-1 transmission. N Engl J Med 362 (24):2271–2281

Chi BH, Sinkala M, Mbewe F, Cantrell RA, Kruse G, Chintu N et al (2007) Single-dose tenofovir and emtricitabine for reduction of viral resistance to non-nucleoside reverse transcriptase inhibitor drugs in women given intrapartum nevirapine for perinatal HIV prevention: an open-label randomised trial. Lancet 370(9600):1698–1705

Chi BH, Ellis GM, Chintu N, Cantrell RA, Sinkala M, Aldrovandi GM et al (2009) Intrapartum tenofovir and emtricitabine reduces low-concentration drug resistance selected by single-dose nevirapine for perinatal HIV prevention. AIDS Res Hum Retroviruses 25 (11):1099–1106

Chimbwandira F, Mhango E et al (2013) Impact of an innovative approach to prevent mother-to-child transmission of HIV–Malawi, July 2011-September 2012. MMWR Morb Mortal Wkly Rep 62(8):148–151

Coffin J (1995) HIV population dynamics in vivo: implications for genetic variation, pathogenesis, and therapy. Science 267:483–489

Cohen MS, Chen YQ, McCauley M, Gamble T, Hosseinipour MC, Kumarasamy N et al (2011) Prevention of HIV-1 infection with early antiretroviral therapy. N Engl J Med 365(6):493–505 [Multicenter Study Randomized Controlled Trial Research Support, N.I.H., Extramural Research Support, Non-U.S. Gov't]

Connor EM, Mofenson LM (1995) Zidovudine for the reduction of perinatal human immunodeficiency virus transmission: pediatric AIDS Clinical Trials Group Protocol 076 – results and treatment recommendations. Pediatr Infect Dis J 14(6):536–541

Cooper ER, Charurat M, Mofenson L, Hanson IC, Pitt J, Diaz C et al (2002) Combination antiretroviral strategies for the treatment of pregnant HIV-1-infected women and prevention of perinatal HIV-1 transmission. J Acquir Immune Defic Syndr 29(5):484–494

Coovadia A, Hunt G, Abrams EJ, Sherman G, Meyers T, Barry G et al (2009) Persistent minority K103N mutations among women exposed to single-dose nevirapine and virologic response to nonnucleoside reverse-transcriptase inhibitor-based therapy. Clin Infect Dis 48(4):462–472

Coovadia A, Abrams EJ, Stehlau R, Meyers T, Martens L, Sherman G et al (2010) Reuse of nevirapine in exposed HIV-infected children after protease inhibitor-based viral suppression: a randomized controlled trial. JAMA 304(10):1082–1090

Coovadia H, Brown E, Maldonado Y, Mofenson L, Moodley D, Musoke P et al (2011) HPTN 046: efficacy of extended daily infant NVP through age 6 months compared to 6 weeks for postnatal PMTCT of HIV through breastfeeding. In: 18th conference on retroviruses and opportunistic infections. Boston

Coutsoudis A, Goga A, Desmond C, Barron P, Black V, Coovadia H (2013a) Is option B+ the best choice? Lancet 381(9863):269–271

Coutsoudis A, Goga A, Desmond C, Barron P, Black V, Coovadia H (2013b) Is option B+ the best choice? Authors' reply. Lancet 381(9874):1273–1274

Cressey TR, Jourdain G, Lallemant MJ, Kunkeaw S, Jackson JB, Musoke P et al (2005) Persistence of nevirapine exposure during the postpartum period after intrapartum single-dose nevirapine in addition to zidovudine prophylaxis for the prevention of mother-to-child transmission of HIV-1. J Acquir Immune Defic Syndr 38(3):283–288

de Vincenzi I (2011) Triple antiretroviral compared with zidovudine and single-dose nevirapine prophylaxis during pregnancy and breastfeeding for prevention of mother-to-child transmission of HIV-1 (Kesho Bora study): a randomised controlled trial. Lancet Infect Dis 11(3):171–180

Deeks SG, Wrin T, Liegler T, Hoh R, Hayden M, Barbour JD et al (2001) Virologic and immunologic consequences of discontinuing combination antiretroviral-drug therapy in HIV-infected patients with detectable viremia. N Engl J Med 344(7):472–480

Dross S, Beck IA, Micek MA, Blanco AJ, Matunha L, Montoya P et al (2010) Transmission of NVP-resistant HIV-1 to infants by breastfeeding observed after maternal sdNVP. In: 17th conference on retroviruses and opportunistic infections, Montreal

Eastman PS, Shapiro DE, Coombs RW, Frenkel LM, McSherry GD, Britto P et al (1998) Maternal viral genotypic zidovudine resistance and infrequent failure of zidovudine therapy to prevent perinatal transmission of human immunodeficiency virus type 1 in Pediatric AIDS Clinical Trials Group Protocol 076. J Infect Dis 177(3):557–564

Ellis GM, Huang S, Hitti J, Frenkel LM (2011) Selection of HIV resistance associated with antiretroviral therapy initiated due to pregnancy and suspended postpartum. J Acquir Immune Defic Syndr 58(3):241–247 [Research Support, N.I.H., Extramural Research Support, Non-U.S. Gov't]

Eshleman SH, Mracna M, Guay LA, Deseyve M, Cunningham S, Mirochnick M et al (2001) Selection and fading of resistance mutations in women and infants receiving nevirapine to prevent HIV-1 vertical transmission (HIVNET 012). AIDS 15(15):1951–1957

Eshleman SH, Guay LA, Wang J, Mwatha A, Brown ER, Musoke P et al (2005a) Distinct patterns of emergence and fading of K103N and Y181C in women with subtype A vs. D after single-dose nevirapine: HIVNET 012. J Acquir Immune Defic Syndr 40(1):24–29

Eshleman SH, Hoover DR, Chen S, Hudelson SE, Guay LA, Mwatha A et al (2005b) Resistance after single-dose nevirapine prophylaxis emerges in a high proportion of Malawian newborns. AIDS 19(18):2167–2169

Eshleman SH, Hoover DR, Chen S, Hudelson SE, Guay LA, Mwatha A et al (2005c) Nevirapine (NVP) resistance in women with HIV-1 subtype C, compared with subtypes A and D, after the administration of single-dose NVP. J Infect Dis 192(1):30–36

Eshleman SH, Guay LA, Mwatha A, Brown E, Musoke P, Mmiro F et al (2005d) Comparison of mother-to-child transmission rates in Ugandan women with subtype A versus D HIV-1 who received single-dose nevirapine prophylaxis: HIV Network For Prevention Trials 012. J Acquir Immune Defic Syndr 39(5):593–597

Eshleman SH, Hoover DR, Hudelson SE, Chen S, Fiscus SA, Piwowar-Manning E et al (2006) Development of nevirapine resistance in infants is reduced by use of infant-only single-dose nevirapine plus zidovudine postexposure prophylaxis for the prevention of mother-to-child transmission of HIV-1. J Infect Dis 193(4):479–481

Farr SL, Nelson JA, Ng'ombe TJ, Kourtis AP, Chasela C, Johnson JA et al (2010) Addition of 7 days of zidovudine plus lamivudine to peripartum single-dose nevirapine effectively reduces nevirapine resistance postpartum in HIV-infected mothers in Malawi. J Acquir Immune Defic Syndr 54(5):515–523

Flys T, Nissley DV, Claasen CW, Jones D, Shi C, Guay LA et al (2005) Sensitive drug-resistance assays reveal long-term persistence of HIV-1 variants with the K103N nevirapine (NVP) resistance mutation in some women and infants after the administration of single-dose NVP: HIVNET 012. J Infect Dis 192(1):24–29

Flys TS, Chen S, Jones DC, Hoover DR, Church JD, Fiscus SA et al (2006) Quantitative analysis of HIV-1 variants with the K103N resistance mutation after single-dose nevirapine in women with HIV-1 subtypes A, C, and D. J Acquir Immune Defic Syndr 42(5):610–613

Flys TS, Donnell D, Mwatha A, Nakabiito C, Musoke P, Mmiro F et al (2007a) Persistence of K103N-containing HIV-1 variants after single-dose nevirapine for prevention of HIV-1 mother-to-child transmission. J Infect Dis 195(5):711–715

Flys TS, Mwatha A, Guay LA, Nakabiito C, Donnell D, Musoke P et al (2007b) Detection of K103N in Ugandan women after repeated exposure to single dose nevirapine. AIDS 21 (15):2077–2082

Flys TS, McConnell MS, Matovu F, Church JD, Bagenda D, Khaki L et al (2008) Nevirapine resistance in women and infants after first versus repeated use of single-dose nevirapine for prevention of HIV-1 vertical transmission. J Infect Dis 198(4):465–469

Fogel J, Hoover DR, Sun J, Mofenson LM, Fowler MG, Taylor AW et al (2011a) Analysis of nevirapine resistance in HIV-infected infants who received extended nevirapine or nevirapine/zidovudine prophylaxis. AIDS 25(7):911–917

Fogel J, Li Q, Taha TE, Hoover DR, Kumwenda NI, Mofenson LM et al (2011b) Initiation of antiretroviral treatment in women after delivery can induce multiclass drug resistance in breastfeeding HIV-infected infants. Clin Infect Dis 52(8):1069–1076

Fogel JM, Mwatha A, Richardson P, Brown ER, Chipato T, Alexandre M et al (2013) Impact of maternal and infant antiretroviral drug regimens on drug resistance in HIV-infected breastfeeding infants. Pediatr Infect Dis J 32(4):e164–e169

Frenkel LM, Wagner LE 2nd, Demeter LM, Dewhurst S, Coombs RW, Murante BL et al (1995) Effects of zidovudine use during pregnancy on resistance and vertical transmission of human immunodeficiency virus type 1. Clin Infect Dis 20(5):1321–1326

Frenkel LM, McKernan J, Dinh PV, Goldman D, Hitti J, Watts DH et al (2006) HIV type 1 zidovudine (ZDV) resistance in blood and uterine cervical secretions of pregnant women. AIDS Res Hum Retroviruses 22(9):870–873

Gantt S, Payant R, Carlsson J, Micek MA, Blanco AJ, Beck IA et al (2012) Nevirapine-resistant HIV-1 DNA in breast milk after single-dose nevirapine with or without zidovudine for prevention of mother-to-child transmission. J Pediatr Infect Dis Soc 1(3):244–249

Geretti AM (2007) Epidemiology of antiretroviral drug resistance in drug-naive persons. Curr Opin Infect Dis 20(1):22–32

Giuliano M, Galluzzo CM, Germinario EA, Amici R, Bassani L, Deho L et al (2006) Selection of resistance mutations in children receiving prophylaxis with lamivudine or nevirapine for the prevention of postnatal transmission of HIV. J Acquir Immune Defic Syndr 42 (1):131–133

Goosby EP (2013) Is option B+ the best choice? Lancet 381(9874):1272

Gupta RK, Jordan MR, Sultan BJ, Hill A, Davis DH, Gregson J et al (2012) Global trends in antiretroviral resistance in treatment-naive individuals with HIV after rollout of antiretroviral treatment in resource-limited settings: a global collaborative study and meta-regression analysis. Lancet 380(9849):1250–1258

Hammer SM, Katzenstein DA, Hughes MD, Gundacker H, Schooley RT, Haubrich RH et al (1996) A trial comparing nucleoside monotherapy with combination therapy in HIV-infected adults with CD4 cell counts from 200 to 500 per cubic millimeter. AIDS Clinical Trials Group Study 175 Study Team. N Engl J Med 335(15):1081–1090

Hauser A, Sewangi J, Mbezi P, Dugange F, Lau I, Ziske J et al (2012) Emergence of minor drug-resistant HIV-1 variants after triple antiretroviral prophylaxis for prevention of vertical HIV-1 transmission. PLoS One 7(2):e32055

Hudelson SE, McConnell MS, Bagenda D, Piwowar-Manning E, Parsons TL, Nolan ML et al (2010) Emergence and persistence of nevirapine resistance in breast milk after single-dose nevirapine administration. AIDS 24(4):557–561

Jackson JB, Musoke P, Fleming T, Guay LA, Bagenda D, Allen M et al (2003) Intrapartum and neonatal single-dose nevirapine compared with zidovudine for prevention of mother-to-child transmission of HIV-1 in Kampala, Uganda: 18-month follow-up of the HIVNET 012 randomised trial. Lancet 362(9387):859–868

Johnson JA, Li JF, Morris L, Martinson N, Gray G, McIntyre J et al (2005) Emergence of drug-resistant HIV-1 after intrapartum administration of single-dose nevirapine is substantially underestimated. J Infect Dis 192(1):16–23

Jordan MR, Bennett DE, Bertagnolio S, Gilks CF, Sutherland D (2008) World Health Organization surveys to monitor HIV drug resistance prevention and associated factors in sentinel antiretroviral treatment sites. Antivir Ther 13(Suppl 2):15–23

Jourdain G, Ngo-Giang-Huong N, Le Coeur S, Bowonwatanuwong C, Kantipong P, Leechanachai P et al (2004) Intrapartum exposure to nevirapine and subsequent maternal responses to nevirapine-based antiretroviral therapy. N Engl J Med 351(3):229–240

Jourdain G, Wagner TA, Ngo-Giang-Huong N, Sirirungsi W, Klinbuayaem V, Fregones F et al (2010) Association between detection of HIV-1 DNA resistance mutations by a sensitive assay at initiation of antiretroviral therapy and virologic failure. Clin Infect Dis 50 (10):1397–1404

Kantor R, Machekano R, Gonzales MJ, Dupnik K, Schapiro JM, Shafer RW (2001) Human immunodeficiency Virus reverse transcriptase and protease sequence database: an expanded data model integrating natural language text and sequence analysis programs. Nucleic Acids Res 29(1):296–299

Kassaye S, Lee E, Kantor R, Johnston E, Winters M, Zijenah L et al (2007) Drug resistance in plasma and breast milk after single-dose nevirapine in subtype C HIV type 1: population and clonal sequence analysis. AIDS Res Hum Retroviruses 23(8):1055–1061

Kuhn L, Sinkala M, Kankasa MP, Kasonde P, Thea DM, Aldrovandi GM (2006) Nevirapine resistance viral mutations after repeat use of nevirapine for prevention of perinatal HIV transmission. J Acquir Immune Defic Syndr 42(2):260–262

Kuhn L, Aldrovandi GM, Sinkala M, Kankasa C, Semrau K, Mwiya M et al (2008) Effects of early, abrupt weaning on HIV-free survival of children in Zambia. N Engl J Med 359(2):130–141

Kuhn L, Semrau K, Ramachandran S, Sinkala M, Scott N, Kasonde P et al (2009) Mortality and virologic outcomes after access to antiretroviral therapy among a cohort of HIV-infected women who received single-dose nevirapine in Lusaka, Zambia. J Acquir Immune Defic Syndr 52 (1):132–136

Kuhn L, Coovadia A, Strehlau R, Martens L, Hu CC, Meyers T et al (2012) Switching children previously exposed to nevirapine to nevirapine-based treatment after initial suppression with a protease-inhibitor-based regimen: long-term follow-up of a randomised, open-label trial. Lancet Infect Dis 12(7):521–530

Kumwenda NI, Hoover DR, Mofenson LM, Thigpen MC, Kafulafula G, Li Q et al (2008) Extended antiretroviral prophylaxis to reduce breast-milk HIV-1 transmission. N Engl J Med 359 (2):119–129

Kunz A, Frank M, Mugenyi K, Kabasinguzi R, Weidenhammer A, Kurowski M et al (2009) Persistence of nevirapine in breast milk and plasma of mothers and their children after single-dose administration. J Antimicrob Chemother 63(1):170–177

Lallemant M, Jourdain G (2010) Preventing mother-to-child transmission of HIV-protecting this generation and the next. N Engl J Med 363(16):1570–1572

Lallemant M, Jourdain G, Le Coeur S, Mary JY, Ngo-Giang-Huong N, Koetsawang S et al (2004) Single-dose perinatal nevirapine plus standard zidovudine to prevent mother-to-child transmission of HIV-1 in Thailand. N Engl J Med 351(3):217–228
Lee EJ, Kantor R, Zijenah L, Sheldon W, Emel L, Mateta P et al (2005) Breast-milk shedding of drug-resistant HIV-1 subtype C in women exposed to single-dose nevirapine. J Infect Dis 192 (7):1260–1264
Lehman DA, Chung MH, Mabuka JM, John-Stewart GC, Kiarie J, Kinuthia J et al (2009) Lower risk of resistance after short-course HAART compared with zidovudine/single-dose nevirapine used for prevention of HIV-1 mother-to-child transmission. J Acquir Immune Defic Syndr 51 (5):522–529
Li JZ, Paredes R, Ribaudo HJ, Svarovskaia ES, Metzner KJ, Kozal MJ et al (2011) Low-frequency HIV-1 drug resistance mutations and risk of NNRTI-based antiretroviral treatment failure: a systematic review and pooled analysis. JAMA 305(13):1327–1335
Lidstrom J, Li Q, Hoover DR, Kafulafula G, Mofenson LM, Fowler MG et al (2010) Addition of extended zidovudine to extended nevirapine prophylaxis reduces nevirapine resistance in infants who were HIV-infected in utero. AIDS 24(3):381–386
Lindegren ML, Byers RH Jr, Thomas P, Davis SF, Caldwell B, Rogers M et al (1999) Trends in perinatal transmission of HIV/AIDS in the United States. JAMA 282(6):531–538
Little SJ, Daar ES, D'Aquila RT, Keiser PH, Connick E, Whitcomb JM et al (1999) Reduced antiretroviral drug susceptibility among patients with primary HIV infection. JAMA 282 (12):1142–1149 [see comments]
Little SJ, Frost SD, Wong JK, Smith DM, Pond SL, Ignacio CC et al (2008) Persistence of transmitted drug resistance among subjects with primary human immunodeficiency virus infection. J Virol 82(11):5510–5518
Lockman S (2008) Prevention of mother-to-child transmission, drug resistance, and implications for response to therapy. Curr Opin HIV AIDS 3(2):166–172
Lockman S, McIntyre JA (2007) Reduction of HIV-1 drug resistance after intrapartum single-dose nevirapine. Lancet 370(9600):1668–1670
Lockman S, Shapiro RL, Smeaton LM, Wester C, Thior I, Stevens L et al (2007) Response to antiretroviral therapy after a single, peripartum dose of nevirapine. N Engl J Med 356 (2):135–147
Lockman S, Hughes MD, McIntyre J, Zheng Y, Chipato T, Conradie F et al (2010) Antiretroviral therapies in women after single-dose nevirapine exposure. N Engl J Med 363 (16):1499–1509
Loubser S, Balfe P, Sherman G, Hammer S, Kuhn L, Morris L (2006) Decay of K103N mutants in cellular DNA and plasma RNA after single-dose nevirapine to reduce mother-to-child HIV transmission. AIDS 20(7):995–1002
MacLeod IJ, Rowley CF, Thior I, Wester C, Makhema J, Essex M et al (2010) Minor resistant variants in nevirapine-exposed infants may predict virologic failure on nevirapine-containing ART. J Clin Virol 48(3):162–167
Maphalala G, Okello V, Mndzebele S, Gwebu P, Mulima N, Dlamini S et al (2008) Surveillance of transmitted HIV drug resistance in the Manzini-Mbabane corridor, Swaziland, in 2006. Antivir Ther 13(Suppl 2):95–100
Martinson NA, Ekouevi DK, Dabis F, Morris L, Lupodwana P, Tonwe-Gold B et al (2007a) Transmission rates in consecutive pregnancies exposed to single-dose nevirapine in Soweto, South Africa and Abidjan, Cote d'Ivoire. J Acquir Immune Defic Syndr 45(2):206–209
Martinson NA, Morris L, Gray G, Moodley D, Pillay V, Cohen S et al (2007b) Selection and persistence of viral resistance in HIV-infected children after exposure to single-dose nevirapine. J Acquir Immune Defic Syndr 44(2):148–153
Martinson NA, Morris L, Johnson J, Gray GE, Pillay V, Ledwaba J et al (2009) Women exposed to single-dose nevirapine in successive pregnancies: effectiveness and nonnucleoside reverse transcriptase inhibitor resistance. AIDS 23(7):809–816

McConnell M, Bakaki P, Eure C, Mubiru M, Bagenda D, Downing R et al (2007) Effectiveness of repeat single-dose nevirapine for prevention of mother-to-child transmission of HIV-1 in repeat pregnancies in Uganda. J Acquir Immune Defic Syndr 46(3):291–296

McIntyre JA, Hopley M, Moodley D, Eklund M, Gray GE, Hall DB et al (2009) Efficacy of short-course AZT plus 3TC to reduce nevirapine resistance in the prevention of mother-to-child HIV transmission: a randomized clinical trial. PLoS Med 6(10):e1000172

McMahon DK, Zheng L, Hitti J, Chan ES, Halvas EK, Hong F et al (2013) Greater suppression of nevirapine resistance with 21- vs 7-day antiretroviral regimens after intrapartum single-dose nevirapine for prevention of mother-to-child transmission of HIV. Clin Infect Dis 56 (7):1044–1051

Metzner KJ, Giulieri SG, Knoepfel SA, Rauch P, Burgisser P, Yerly S et al (2009) Minority quasispecies of drug-resistant HIV-1 that lead to early therapy failure in treatment-naive and -adherent patients. Clin Infect Dis 48(2):239–247

Micek MA, Blanco AJ, Beck IA, Dross S, Matunha L, Montoya P et al (2010) Nevirapine resistance by timing of HIV type 1 infection in infants treated with single-dose nevirapine. Clin Infect Dis 50(10):1405–1414

Micek MA, Blanco AJ, Carlsson J, Beck IA, Dross S, Matunha L et al (2012) Effects of short-course zidovudine on the selection of nevirapine-resistant HIV-1 in women taking single-dose nevirapine. J Infect Dis 205(12):1811–1815

Mirochnick M, Siminski S, Fenton T, Lugo M, Sullivan JL (2001) Nevirapine pharmacokinetics in pregnant women and in their infants after in utero exposure. Pediatr Infect Dis J 20(8):803–805

Mirochnick M, Thomas T, Capparelli E, Zeh C, Holland D, Masaba R et al (2009) Antiretroviral concentrations in breast-feeding infants of mothers receiving highly active antiretroviral therapy. Antimicrob Agents Chemother 53(3):1170–1176

Moodley D, Moodley J, Coovadia H, Gray G, McIntyre J, Hofmyer J et al (2003) A multicenter randomized controlled trial of nevirapine versus a combination of zidovudine and lamivudine to reduce intrapartum and early postpartum mother-to-child transmission of human immunodeficiency virus type 1. J Infect Dis 187:725–735

Moorthy A, Gupta A, Bhosale R, Tripathy S, Sastry J, Kulkarni S et al (2009) Nevirapine resistance and breast-milk HIV transmission: effects of single and extended-dose nevirapine prophylaxis in subtype C HIV-infected infants. PLoS One 4(1):e4096

Moorthy A, Kuhn L, Coovadia A, Meyers T, Strehlau R, Sherman G et al (2011) Induction therapy with protease-inhibitors modifies the effect of nevirapine resistance on virologic response to nevirapine-based HAART in children. Clin Infect Dis 52(4):514–521

Myatt M, Bennett DE (2008) A novel sequential sampling technique for the surveillance of transmitted HIV drug resistance by cross-sectional survey for use in low resource settings. Antivir Ther 13(Suppl 2):37–48

Nduati R, John G, Mbori-Ngacha D, Richardson B, Overbaugh J, Mwatha A et al (2000) Effect of breastfeeding and formula feeding on transmission of HIV-1: a randomized clinical trial. JAMA 283(9):1167–1174

Nguyen HT, Duc NB, Shrivastava R, Tran TH, Nguyen TA, Thang PH et al (2008) HIV drug resistance threshold survey using specimens from voluntary counselling and testing sites in Hanoi, Vietnam. Antivir Ther 13(Suppl 2):115–121

Palmer S, Boltz V, Martinson N, Maldarelli F, Gray G, McIntyre J et al (2006) Persistence of nevirapine-resistant HIV-1 in women after single-dose nevirapine therapy for prevention of maternal-to-fetal HIV-1 transmission. Proc Natl Acad Sci U S A 103(18):7094–7099

Palumbo P, Lindsey JC, Hughes MD, Cotton MF, Bobat R, Meyers T et al (2010) Antiretroviral treatment for children with peripartum nevirapine exposure. N Engl J Med 363(16):1510–1520

Paredes R, Cheng I, Kuritzkes DR, Tuomala RE (2010) Postpartum antiretroviral drug resistance in HIV-1-infected women receiving pregnancy-limited antiretroviral therapy. AIDS 24(1):45–53

Perelson AS, Essunger P, Ho DD (1997) Dynamics of HIV-1 and CD4+ lymphocytes in vivo. AIDS 11(Suppl A):S17–S24

Perez H, Vignoles M, Laufer N, Gomez A, Coll P, Lottner J et al (2008) Low rate of emergence of nevirapine and lamivudine resistance after post-partum interruption of a triple-drug regimen. Antivir Ther 13(1):135–139

Petra-Study-Team (2002) Efficacy of three short-course regimens of zidovudine and lamivudine in preventing early and late transmission of HIV-1 from mother to child in Tanzania, South Africa, and Uganda (Petra study): a randomised, double-blind, placebo-controlled trial. Lancet 359:1178–1186

Pillay V, Ledwaba J, Hunt G, Rakgotho M, Singh B, Makubalo L et al (2008) Antiretroviral drug resistance surveillance among drug-naive HIV-1-infected individuals in Gauteng Province, South Africa in 2002 and 2004. Antivir Ther 13(Suppl 2):101–107

Price MA, Wallis CL, Lakhi S, Karita E, Kamali A, Anzala O et al (2011) Transmitted HIV type 1 drug resistance among individuals with recent HIV infection in East and Southern Africa. AIDS Res Hum Retroviruses 27(1):5–12

Richman DD, Havlir D, Corbeil J, Looney D, Ignacio C, Spector SA et al (1994) Nevirapine resistance mutations of human immunodeficiency virus type 1 selected during therapy. J Virol 68(3):1660–1666

Rowley CF, Boutwell CL, Lee EJ, MacLeod IJ, Ribaudo HJ, Essex M et al (2010) Ultrasensitive detection of minor drug-resistant variants for HIV after nevirapine exposure using allele-specific PCR: clinical significance. AIDS Res Hum Retroviruses 26(3):293–300

Sax PE, Islam R, Walensky RP, Losina E, Weinstein MC, Goldie SJ et al (2005) Should resistance testing be performed for treatment-naive HIV-infected patients? A cost-effectiveness analysis. Clin Infect Dis 41(9):1316–1323

Schacker T, Little S, Connick E, Gebhard-Mitchell K, Zhang ZQ, Krieger J et al (2000) Rapid accumulation of human immunodeficiency virus (HIV) in lymphatic tissue reservoirs during acute and early HIV infection: implications for timing of antiretroviral therapy. J Infect Dis 181 (1):354–357

Schouten EJ, Jahn A, Chimbwandira F, Harries AD, Van Damme W (2013) Is option B+ the best choice? Lancet 381(9874):1272–1273

Shafer RW, Rhee SY, Bennett DE (2008) Consensus drug resistance mutations for epidemiological surveillance: basic principles and potential controversies. Antivir Ther 13(Suppl 2):59–68

Shapiro RL, Ndung'u T, Lockman S, Smeaton LM, Thior I, Wester C et al (2005) Highly active antiretroviral therapy started during pregnancy or postpartum suppresses HIV-1 RNA, but not DNA, in breast milk. J Infect Dis 192(5):713–719

Shapiro RL, Thior I, Gilbert PB, Lockman S, Wester C, Smeaton LM et al (2006) Maternal single-dose nevirapine versus placebo as part of an antiretroviral strategy to prevent mother-to-child HIV transmission in Botswana. AIDS 20(9):1281–1288

Shapiro RL, Hughes MD, Ogwu A, Kitch D, Lockman S, Moffat C et al (2010) Antiretroviral regimens in pregnancy and breast-feeding in Botswana. N Engl J Med 362(24):2282–2294

Shet A, Berry L, Mohri H, Mehandru S, Chung C, Kim A et al (2006) Tracking the prevalence of transmitted antiretroviral drug-resistant HIV-1: a decade of experience. J Acquir Immune Defic Syndr 41(4):439–446

Somi GR, Kibuka T, Diallo K, Tuhuma T, Bennett DE, Yang C et al (2008) Surveillance of transmitted HIV drug resistance among women attending antenatal clinics in Dar es Salaam, Tanzania. Antivir Ther 13(Suppl 2):77–82

Souda S, Gaseitsiwe S, Georgette N, Powis K, Moremedi D, Iketleng T et al (2013) No clinically significant drug resistance mutations in HIV-1 subtype C infected women after discontinuation of NRTI-based or PI-based HAART for PMTCT in Botswana. J Acquir Immune Defic Syndr 63 (5):572–577

Stekler JD, Ellis GM, Carlsson J, Eilers B, Holte S, Maenza J et al (2011) Prevalence and impact of minority variant drug resistance mutations in primary HIV-1 infection. PLoS One 6(12):e28952

Stringer EM, Ekouevi DK, Coetzee D, Tih PM, Creek TL, Stinson K et al (2010a) Coverage of nevirapine-based services to prevent mother-to-child HIV transmission in 4 African countries. JAMA 304(3):293–302

Stringer JS, McConnell MS, Kiarie J, Bolu O, Anekthananon T, Jariyasethpong T et al (2010b) Effectiveness of non-nucleoside reverse-transcriptase inhibitor-based antiretroviral therapy in women previously exposed to a single intrapartum dose of nevirapine: a multi-country, prospective cohort study. PLoS Med 7(2):e1000233

SWEN-Study-Team (2008) Extended-dose nevirapine to 6 weeks of age for infants to prevent HIV transmission via breastfeeding in Ethiopia, India, and Uganda: an analysis of three randomised controlled trials. Lancet 372:300–313

The Kesho Bora Group (2012) Maternal HIV-1 disease progression 18–24 months postdelivery according to antiretroviral prophylaxis regimen (triple-antiretroviral prophylaxis during pregnancy and breastfeeding vs zidovudine/single-dose nevirapine prophylaxis): The Kesho Bora Group randomized controlled trial. Clin Infect Dis 55(3):449–460

Van Dyke RB, Ngo-Giang-Huong N, Shapiro DE, Frenkel L, Britto P, Roongpisuthipong A et al (2012) A comparison of 3 regimens to prevent nevirapine resistance mutations in HIV-infected pregnant women receiving a single intrapartum dose of nevirapine. Clin Infect Dis 54(2):285–293

Wagner TA, Kress CM, Beck I, Techapornroong M, Wittayapraparat P, Tansuphasawasdikul S et al (2010) Detection of HIV-1 drug resistance in women following administration of a single dose of nevirapine: comparison of plasma RNA to cellular DNA by consensus sequencing and by oligonucleotide ligation assay. J Clin Microbiol 48(5):1555–1561

Walter J, Kuhn L, Kankasa C, Semrau K, Sinkala M, Thea DM et al (2008) Reuse of single-dose nevirapine in subsequent pregnancies for the prevention of mother-to-child HIV transmission in Lusaka, Zambia: a cohort study. BMC Infect Dis 8:172 [Research Support, N.I.H., Extramural Research Support, Non-U.S. Gov't]

World-Health-Organization (2001) Prevention of mother-to-child transmission of HIV: selection and use of nevirapine. Technical notes. World-Health-Organization, Geneva

World-Health-Organization (2006) Antiretroviral drugs for treating pregnant women and preventing HIV infection in infants: towards universal access. World Health Organization, Geneva

World-Health-Organization (2009) Towards universal access: scaling up priority HIV/AIDS interventions in the health sector: progress report 2009. World Health Organization, Geneva

World-Health-Organization (2010) Antiretroviral drugs for treating pregnant women and preventing HIV infection in infants. World Health Organization, Geneva

Zeh C, Weidle PJ, Nafisa L, Lwamba HM, Okonji J, Anyango E et al (2011) HIV-1 drug resistance emergence among breastfeeding infants born to HIV-infected mothers during a single-arm trial of triple-antiretroviral prophylaxis for prevention of mother-to-child transmission: a secondary analysis. PLoS Med 8(3):e1000430

HIV Protease Inhibitor Resistance

Annemarie M. J. Wensing, Axel Fun, and Monique Nijhuis

Contents

Abstract

HIV protease is pivotal in the viral replication cycle and directs the formation of mature infectious virus particles. The development of highly specific HIV protease inhibitors (PIs), based on thorough understanding of the structure of HIV protease and its substrate, serves as a prime example of structure-based drug design. The introduction of first-generation PIs marked the start of combination

A.M.J. Wensing • M. Nijhuis (✉)
Department of Medical Microbiology, University Medical Center Utrecht, Utrecht, The Netherlands
e-mail: a.m.j.wensing@umcutrecht.nl; m.nijhuis@umcutrecht.nl

A. Fun
University of Cambridge, Cambridge, UK
e-mail: af497@cam.ac.uk

M. Gotte et al. (eds.), *Handbook of Antimicrobial Resistance*,
DOI 10.1007/978-1-4939-0694-9_28

antiretroviral therapy. However, low bioavailability, high pill burden, and toxicity ultimately reduced adherence and limited long-term viral inhibition. Therapy failure was often associated with multiple protease inhibitor resistance mutations, both in the viral protease and its substrate (HIV gag protein), displaying a broad spectrum of resistance mechanisms. Unfortunately, selection of protease inhibitor resistance mutations often resulted in cross-resistance to other PIs.

Therefore, second-generation approaches were imperative. Coadministration of a cytochrome P-450 3A4 inhibitor greatly improved the plasma concentration of PIs in the patient. A second advance was the development of PIs that were efficacious against first-generation PI-resistant HIV. Both approaches increased the number of protease mutations required by the virus to develop clinically relevant resistance, thereby raising the genetic barrier towards PI resistance. These improvements greatly contributed to the success of PI-based therapy.

Keywords
Antiretroviral therapy protease inhibitors • Evolution • HIV • Mechanisms of resistance • Protease • Resistance

Introduction into HIV Evolution and Selection of Resistance

HIV has an intrinsic high mutation rate, which is a feature that is common to all RNA viruses. The underlying biochemical mechanism explaining the high mutation rate is the low fidelity of viral RNA polymerase and reverse transcriptase both lacking 3′–5′exonuclease activity, which is a proofreading mechanism that normally amends incorrect base pairs. The estimated mutation rate of HIV-1 is 3.4×10^{-5} per base pair per replication cycle (Mansky and Temin 1995), which, when multiplied with the size of the HIV-1 genome of about 10 kb, translates to approximately one third of all newly generated virus particles containing a nucleotide change in their genome. The high mutation frequency and recombination capacity of the viral reverse transcriptase enzyme in combination with the high turnover rate of HIV in an untreated, infected individual results in the generation of large numbers of genetically distinct viruses, also referred to as a viral quasispecies (Domingo et al. 1996). Within this quasispecies, the most frequent individual variant (wild type) is surrounded by diverse but closely related mutant genomes. The number of mutants is orders of magnitude higher than the number of wild-type viruses. It is therefore predicted that any single genome selected at random from the population is likely to have a mutation relative to wild type, rendering it less fit. Fitness is defined as the replicative adaptability of an organism in its environment. Upon environmental changes (e.g., antiretroviral therapy), the viral population is subject to evolutionary pressure, and its genetic flexibility may allow selection of a mutant virus that has an increased fitness in the new environment (drug-resistant variant). Within an HIV-infected individual, viral fitness is largely reflected by the size of the viral population.

Early estimates suggested that the viral population within an infected individual was virtually infinite and therefore evolution deterministic and antiretroviral resistance inevitable (Coffin 1995). Later it was recognized that the number of HIV variants that produce infectious progeny (i.e., the effective population size) is finite and can be relatively small (Brown 1997; Brown and Richman 1997; Nijhuis et al. 1998; Balagam et al. 2011). This would allow more stochastic viral evolution, although it was also argued that the effective population size is currently underestimated (Kouyos et al. 2006). The majority of mutations in newly produced viral particles result in noninfectious virus. In addition, limited target cell availability, clearance of potentially infectious particles by the host immune system, and epigenetic silencing of infected cells further reduce the effective population size. This relatively small effective population size suggests a population in which only single or double mutants as compared to wild type are present. This model is supported by the observation that current cART (combination antiretroviral therapy) is capable of (fully) inhibiting viral replication, which is unlikely if more genetically diverse variants are present at baseline.

The genetic barrier of an antiretroviral compound is usually defined by the number of resistance mutations conferring virological failure. However, other factors have to be taken into consideration, such as impact of the mutations on viral replication, drug resistance, and recognition by the host immune system. As such the "genetic" barrier towards resistance can also be viewed as the kinetic obstacle for the generation of genetic changes required to overcome selective pressure (Götte 2012).

HIV Protease: Function and Structure

HIV is released from the cell membrane as a noninfectious particle also called the immature virus. During or shortly after the assembled virus particles are released from the infected cells, it undergoes a dramatic structural rearrangement. The transition of the amorphous, noninfectious particle into the mature, infectious virus that is characterized by its election-dense conical core is called maturation (Fig. 1). This transition is triggered by the proteolytic cleavage of the Gag and GagPol precursor polyproteins by the viral enzyme protease (Fig. 1).

HIV protease is a homodimeric aspartic protease that cleaves the Gag polyprotein into six structural viral proteins: matrix (p17, MA), capsid (p24, CA), and nucleocapsid (p7, NC); the p6 protein; and the two spacer peptides p2 (SP1) and p1 (SP2) (Fig. 1a). The GagPol polyprotein is generated through a −1 ribosomal frameshift event that occurs at a 5–10 % frequency (Jacks et al. 1988). This GagPol polyprotein encodes MA, CA, p2, NC, the transframe protein (TFP) and the virally encoded enzymes protease (PR), reverse transcriptase (p66, RT-RH), including its two subunits RT (p51, RT) and RNaseH (p15, RH), and integrase. HIV protease cleaves the unfolded linker regions between the individual folded domains of the encoded Gag and GagPol proteins. The substrate specificity of HIV protease is rather complex; the enzyme recognizes the asymmetric shape of the substrates rather than a specific amino

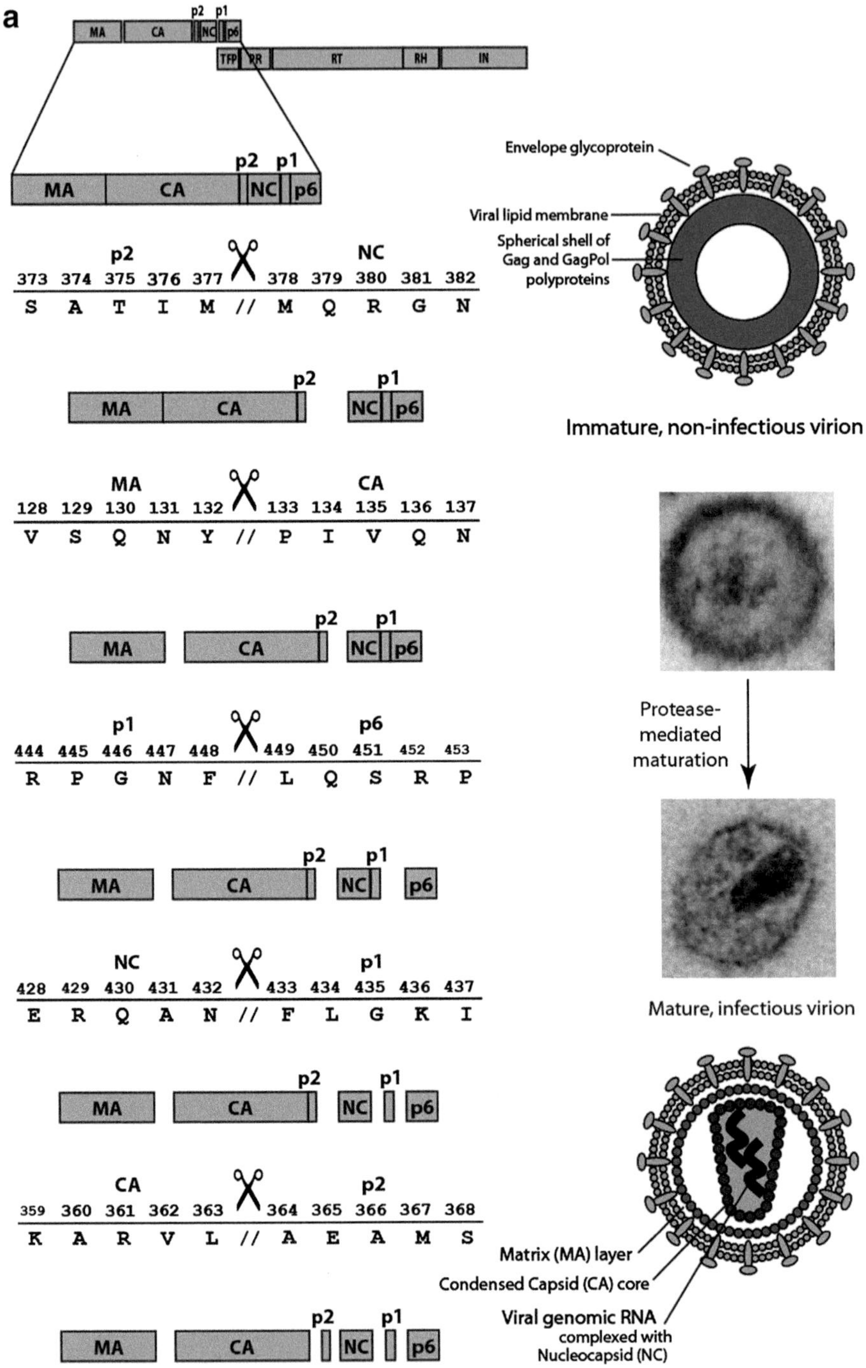

Fig. 1 (continued)

b

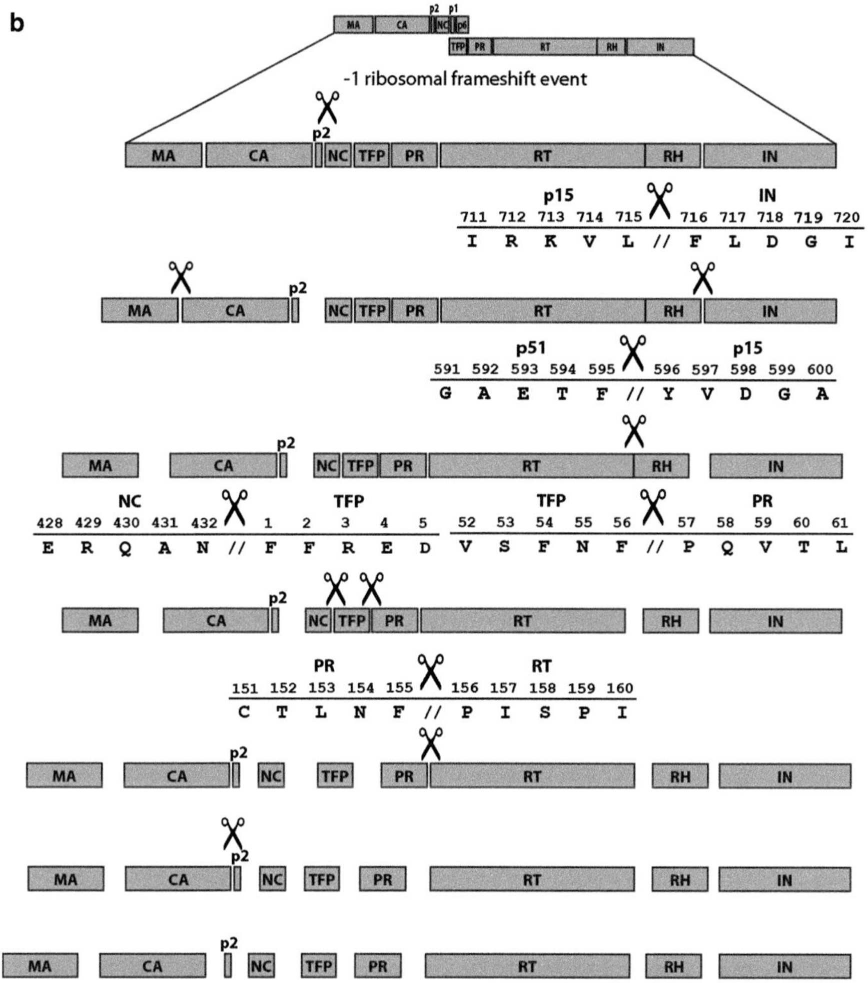

Fig. 1 HIV particle maturation. (**a**) Proteolytic processing of the Gag precursor protein. On the left the five individual cleavage steps are shown with their corresponding amino acid sequences. On the right the transition from the immature noninfectious particle (*top panels*) to infectious virion with its characteristic electron-dense conical is depicted. (**b**) Processing of the GagPol polyprotein that occurs after a −1 frameshift event in the 3′ end of Gag. The amino acid sequences of the cleavage sites are given. The scissors indicate where the viral protease cleaves the precursor GagPol polyprotein

acid sequence (Prabu-Jeyabalan et al. 2002). There is a slight preference for aromatic amino acids and proline at the P1, P1′ positions and large and hydrophobic amino acids at the P2–P2′ position (Fig. 1). There is a discrepancy between the relaxed sequence specificity of the protease enzyme regarding cleavage of peptide substrates in vitro and the very strict requirements for the orderly, precise processing of the Gag and GagPol precursor proteins during virus maturation. The peptides forming the cleavage sites (CS) have a superimposable secondary structure, yielding the so-called substrate "envelope" which fits within the substrate-binding pocket of the viral protease. However, there are a few subtle differences in the way the amino acid side chains protrude from the "envelope." It is thought that these differences in structure play a central role in the highly ordered stepwise process of viral maturation in which all the individual cleavages occur at different rates (Fig. 1a, b; Lee et al. 2012a; Pettit et al. 1994, 2005; Kräusslich et al. 1989; Wiegers et al. 1998; Erickson-Viitanen et al. 1989). First, the scissile bond between p2 and NC (MA-CA-p2↓NC-p1-p6) is cleaved, followed by separation of MA from CA-p2 (MA↓CA-p2) and NC-p1 from p6 (NC-p1↓p6). Finally, the two small spacer peptides p2 (CA↓p2) and p1 (NC↓p1) are removed in the rate-limiting cleavage steps. In case the −1 ribosomal frameshift occurs and the GagPol protein is synthesized, the viral protease also cleaves the Pol-encoded enzymes into its functional units. Similar to cleavage of Gag, the processing cascade starts by cleaving p2/NC(MA-CA-p2↓NC-TFP-PR-RT-RH-IN), followed by MA/CA (MA↓-CA-p2), and releasing the integrase protein at RH/IN (NC-TFP-PR-RT-RH↓IN). Subsequently, the RNaseH domain is removed from RT (NC-TFP-PR-RT↓RH). The following step is excision of the transframe protein from the GagPol junction: NC/TFP(NC↓-TFP-PR-RT) and TFP/PR(TFP↓PR-RT). Finally the mature PR and RT enzymes are released (PR↓RT). Exactly when p2 is removed from capsid, (CA↓p2) in these final stages of processing is not clear but is likely to be one of the last cleavages (Pettit et al. 2005). As indicated above, the exact factors determining the ordered processing of these substrates are not identified, although cleavage appears to be predominantly regulated by the amino acids that are in close proximity to the actual protease cleavage site (positions p4–p3′). However, it is demonstrated that also the context surrounding the processing sites (Lee et al. 2012b) including the p4′and p5′ positions (Nijhuis et al. 2007; Dam et al. 2009) plays a role in determining the cleavage rate of a subset of processing sites.

HIV protease is an aspartic protease and is a symmetrically assembled homodimer consisting of two identical subunits of 99 amino acids (Navia et al. 1989; Wlodawer et al. 1989). Both subunits contribute catalytic residues to the active site (aspartic acid at codon 25). The substrate-binding pocket is at the center of the homodimer and interacts with the substrate sequences in the Gag and GagPol proteins. HIV protease is itself embedded in the GagPol protein, and the mechanism by which the viral protease becomes activated is not yet fully understood. It is known, however, that the viral protease is responsible for its own release from the precursor polyprotein (autoprocessing). Since protease is only active as a dimer, it is thought that autoprocessing is initiated when two protease domains which are still embedded in the GagPol precursor dimerize. Recently, it was shown that autoprocessing at the N-terminus of protease mediates stable dimer formation essential for catalytic activity, leading to the formation of infectious virus. An antiparallel β-sheet interface formed by the four N- and C-terminal residues of each subunit is important for the dimer stability (Agniswamy et al. 2012). The initial cleavage is a transient, intramolecular event, and the low occupancy of the embedded dimer configuration can explain its low enzymatic activity compared to the fully matured protease enzyme (Tang et al. 2008).

HIV Protease Inhibitors and Their Mechanism of Action

The development of HIV protease inhibitors (PIs) is often regarded as a textbook example of structure-based rational drug design. Currently, there are nine PIs approved for clinical use: saquinavir, ritonavir, indinavir, nelfinavir, (fos) amprenavir, lopinavir, atazanavir, tipranavir, and darunavir (Fig. 2). Of these, atazanavir, lopinavir, and darunavir are most frequently used in current clinical practice. Most PIs are prescribed with a concomitant low dose of ritonavir, which is also a cytochrome P450-3A4 inhibitor and thereby improves bioavailability and half-life of the PIs (Kempf et al. 1997). Except for tipranavir, all PIs are competitive peptidomimetic inhibitors, mimicking the natural substrate of the viral protease. These inhibitors contain a hydroxyethylene core, which prohibits cleavage of the inhibitor by the HIV-1 protease (Fig. 2; Kempf et al. 1995; Sham et al. 1998; Craig et al. 1991; Koh et al. 2003; Partaledis et al. 1995; Patick et al. 1996; Robinson et al. 2000; Vacca et al. 1994). Tipranavir contains dihydropyrone ring as a central scaffold instead of a peptidomimetichydroxyethylene core (Fig. 2; Turner et al. 1998).

Inhibition of the initial GagPol processing steps which involves self-cleavage of the embedded HIV protease from the GagPolpolyprotein (autoprocessing) would prevent viral maturation at the earliest stage and therefore be an ideal drug target. However, all PIs have been developed to bind the active site of the mature protease dimer instead of the precursor protein. It was shown that the embedded HIV protease dimer is 10,000 fold less susceptible to a protease inhibitor (ritonavir) than the mature protease dimer (Pettit et al. 2004). Recently, two groups demonstrated independently and using different assays that of all approved PIs, darunavir and tipranavir are the most potent inhibitors of autoprocessing (Davis et al. 2012; Louis et al. 2011). However, both inhibitors are still three orders of magnitude less active against the embedded dimer as compared to the mature viral protease.

As stated above, the HIV protease inhibitors have been designed as competitive inhibitors with a high affinity for the substrate-binding region of the active viral protease dimer. Analysis of inhibitor-protease complexes revealed that tightly binding inhibitors "lock" into the protease active site (Nalam et al. 2010). Furthermore, it was demonstrated that PIs that fit within the substrate envelope, regardless of their affinity, are more active against drug-resistant protease variants than inhibitors that protrude beyond the substrate envelope (Nalam et al. 2010). Tipranavir and darunavir exert an additional mechanism of action by impeding dimerization of the viral protease (Koh et al. 2007). This dual mechanism of action may explain their high genetic barrier towards resistance, although this has not yet been fully elucidated.

Despite its critical role in HIV infectivity, it was until recently unclear where in the virus life cycle inhibition of virus maturation becomes most manifest. It was known that virus maturation was important for early post-entry steps including reverse transcription (Kawamura et al. 1997). Recently, it was shown that inhibition of viral maturation by PIs not only blocks reverse transcription but also post-reverse transcription steps and viral entry (Rabi et al. 2013). This observation is in line with

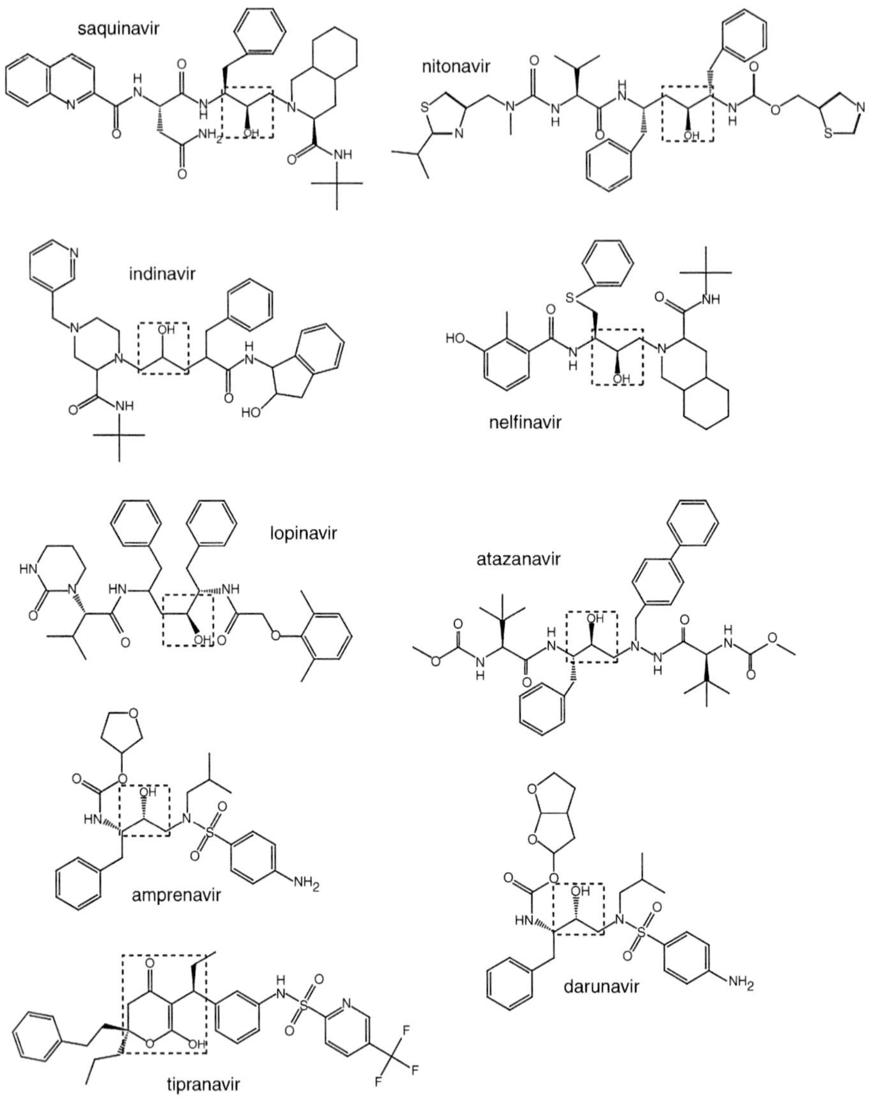

Fig. 2 Chemical structures of the nine PIs currently approved for clinical use. All protease inhibitors are peptidomimetic inhibitors and have a hydroxyethylene core (*dashed boxes*), except tripanavir which contains a dihydropyrone ring (*dashed box*) as a central scaffold

earlier findings that HIV-1 Gag mutants impairing processing are defective in viral entry (Wyma et al. 2004; Murakami et al. 2004; Davis et al. 2006). It was shown that approximately half of the inhibitory effect of PIs becomes manifest at the entry step, most likely reflecting interactions between the unprocessed Gag and the cytoplasmic tail of the viral envelope protein (Rabi et al. 2013). Understanding the mechanisms responsible for the high antiviral potency of PIs and the different steps in the viral life cycle affected by these PIs is essential and also provides insight in the different mechanisms of protease inhibitor resistance.

Mechanisms of HIV Protease Resistance

The International AIDS Society-USA group yearly reviews data on HIV-1 drug resistance to maintain an updated list of mutations associated with PI resistance (Table 1). Currently, major PI resistance mutations have been identified at 15 different protease codons, and an additional 21 protease codons have been included in the update to contain minor mutations (Fig. 3; Johnson et al. 2013). In addition to protease-based PI resistance, also several alternative protease resistance mechanisms have been suggested of which some may provide an explanation for PI therapy failure in the absence of HIV protease mutations.

Protease-Based PI Resistance

Development of PI resistance usually has a biphasic signature reflecting the initial selection of amino acid changes in or near the substrate-binding cleft of the viral protease, e.g., at codons 30, 50, 82, or 84 (Fig. 3). It has been shown that these resistance mutations are mainly selected at those positions where the PIs protrude beyond the substrate-binding envelope, are in direct contact with inhibitor, and result in an overall enlargement of the catalytic region (Nalam et al. 2010; Kolli et al. 2006; Prabu-Jeyabalan et al. 2006). The affinity for the natural substrates (Gag, GagPol) is also slightly altered, often reducing viral replication (Croteau et al. 1997; Gulnik et al. 1995; Nijhuis et al. 1999; Mammano et al. 2000; Mahalingam et al. 1999). These resistance mutations, which are initially selected and reduce the susceptibility to PIs, are called primary or "major" resistance mutations (Tables 1 and 2; Fig. 3; Johnson et al. 2013). In a second step, compensatory or "minor" mutations emerge, e.g., at codons 20, 36, and 71 which by themselves do not have a substantial effect on drug resistance but improve resistance and/or replication of viruses containing major mutations (Table 1; Fig. 3; Johnson et al. 2013; Nijhuis et al. 1999; Mammano et al. 1998, 2000). These amino acid changes can be observed in the viral protease as well as in the substrate (Dam et al. 2009; Nijhuis et al. 1999; Mammano et al. 1998, 2000; Maguire et al. 2002; Borman et al. 1996; Doyon et al. 1996; Zhang et al. 1997; Prado et al. 2002; Kozísek et al. 2012; Kolli et al. 2009; Shibata et al. 2011). The gag substrate changes are mainly observed in the NC/p1 and p1/p6 CS and are thought to increase the affinity of the drug-resistant viral protease, which has an altered substrate-binding pocket, for its substrate.

Occasionally during PI therapy, amino acid insertions ranging from 1 to 6 amino acids are selected at various sites in the viral protease sequence (Kim et al. 2001; Grantz Sasková et al. 2013; Amiel et al. 2011; Winters and Merigan 2005; Winters et al. 2005; Kozísek et al. 2008; Jordan et al. 2009). The insertions may also appear as polymorphism and can be considered as minor mutations since they modestly

Table 1 Mutations in the HIV protease gene associated with resistance to protease inhibitors atazanavir, darunavir, fosamprenavir, indinavir and lopinavir

Drug	Position	Wild type	Mutations
Atazanavir +/- ritonavir	10	L	I, F, V, C
	16	G	E
	20	K	R, M, I, T, V
	24	L	I
	32	V	I
	33	L	I, F, V
	34	E	Q
	36	M	I, L, V
	46	M	I, L
	48	G	V
	50	I	L
	53	F	L, Y
	54	I	L, V, M, T, A
	60	D	E
	62	I	V
	64	I	L, M, V
	71	A	V, I, T, L
	73	G	C, S, T, A
	82	V	A, T, F, I
	84	I	V
	85	I	V
	88	N	S
	90	L	M
	93	I	L, M
Darunavir/ ritonavir	11	V	I
	32	V	I
	33	L	F
	47	I	V
	50	I	V
	54	I	M, L
	74	T	P
	76	L	V
	84	I	V
	89	L	V
Fosamprenavir/ ritonavir	10	L	F, I, R, V
	32	V	I
	46	M	I, L
	47	I	V
	50	I	V
	54	I	L, V, M
	73	G	S
	76	L	V
	82	V	A, F, S, T
	84	I	V
	90	L	M
Indinavir/ ritonavir	10	L	I, R, V
	20	K	M, R
	24	L	I
	32	V	I
	36	M	I
	46	M	I, L
	54	I	V
	71	A	V, T
	73	G	S, A
	76	L	V
	77	V	I
	82	V	A, F, T
	84	I	V
	90	L	M
Lopinavir/ ritonavir	10	L	F, I, R, V
	20	K	M, R
	24	L	I
	32	V	I
	33	L	F
	46	M	I, L
	47	I	V, A
	50	I	V
	53	F	L
	54	I	V, L, A, M, T, S
	63	L	P
	71	A	V, T
	73	G	S
	76	L	V
	82	V	A, F, T, S
	84	I	V
	90	L	M

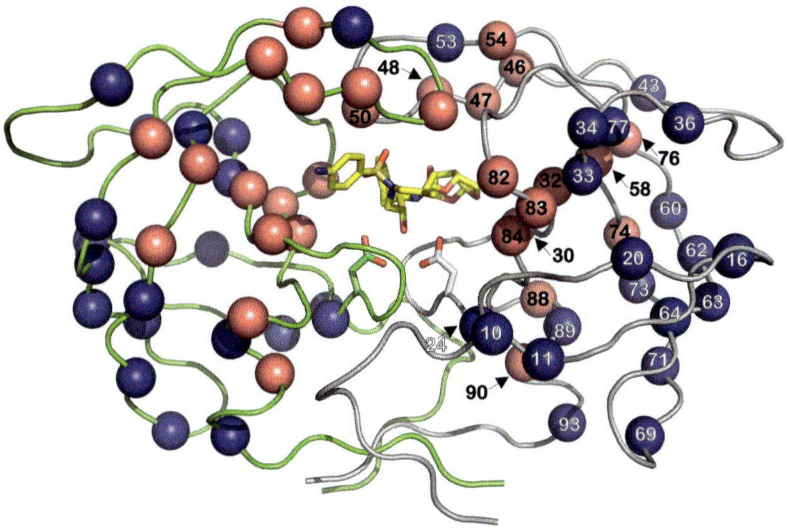

Fig. 3 Three-dimensional structure of the HIV protease dimer. The numbers indicate the amino acids that are associated with PI resistance. In *red* are major (primary) resistance mutations and in *blue* the minor (secondary) resistance mutations. Only one side of the dimer is numbered (*grey* backbone), the corresponding amino acids on the other chain (*green* backbone) are colored but not numbered. The active site aspartates and darunavir bound to the substrate envelope are represented in sticks

improve viral replication (Kim et al. 2001; Kozísek et al. 2008) and only contribute to PI resistance in combination with other mutations either in the PR or in Gag (Kim et al. 2001). Presence of these insertions is positively correlated with protease resistance mutations conferring reduced susceptibility to the contemporary PIs atazanavir, lopinavir, amprenavir, and tipranavir (Kozísek et al. 2008).

Alternative PI-Resistance Mechanisms

Several alternative mechanisms of protease inhibitor resistance have been postulated (Fig. 4).

1. *Improved packaging of viral enzymes*. Duplications of the PTAP motif (Pro-Thre-Ala-Pro) in p6 Gag were identified in patients treated with antiretroviral compounds, and it was proposed that these duplications mediate PI resistance by improved packaging of the viral enzymes (Peters et al. 2001). However, different results were obtained in cross-sectional analyses demonstrating either increased rates (Martins et al. 2011) or comparable rates (Gallego et al. 2003) of PTAP duplications in isolates from antiretroviral therapy-experienced patients versus drug-naïve patients. Furthermore, no effect of p6 Gag insertions was observed on time to virological failure or immunological failure (Brumme et al. 2003),

Table 2 Mutations in the HIV protease gene associated with resistance to protease inhibitors nelfinavir, saquinavir and tipranavir

Nelfinavir

L	D	M	M	A	V	V	I	N	L
10	**30**	36	46	71	77	82	84	88	**90**
F I	N	I	I L	V T	I	A F T S	V	D S	M

Saquinavir/ritonavir

L	L	G	I	I	A	G	V	V	I	L
10	24	**48**	54	62	71	73	77	82	84	**90**
I R V	I	V	V L	V	V T	S	I	A F T S	V	M

Tipranavir/ritonavir

L	L	M	K	M	I	I	Q	H	T	V	N	I	L
10	33	36	43	46	**47**	54	**58**	69	**74**	**82**	**83**	**84**	89
V	F	I L V	T	L	V	A M V	E	K R	P	L T	D	V	I M V

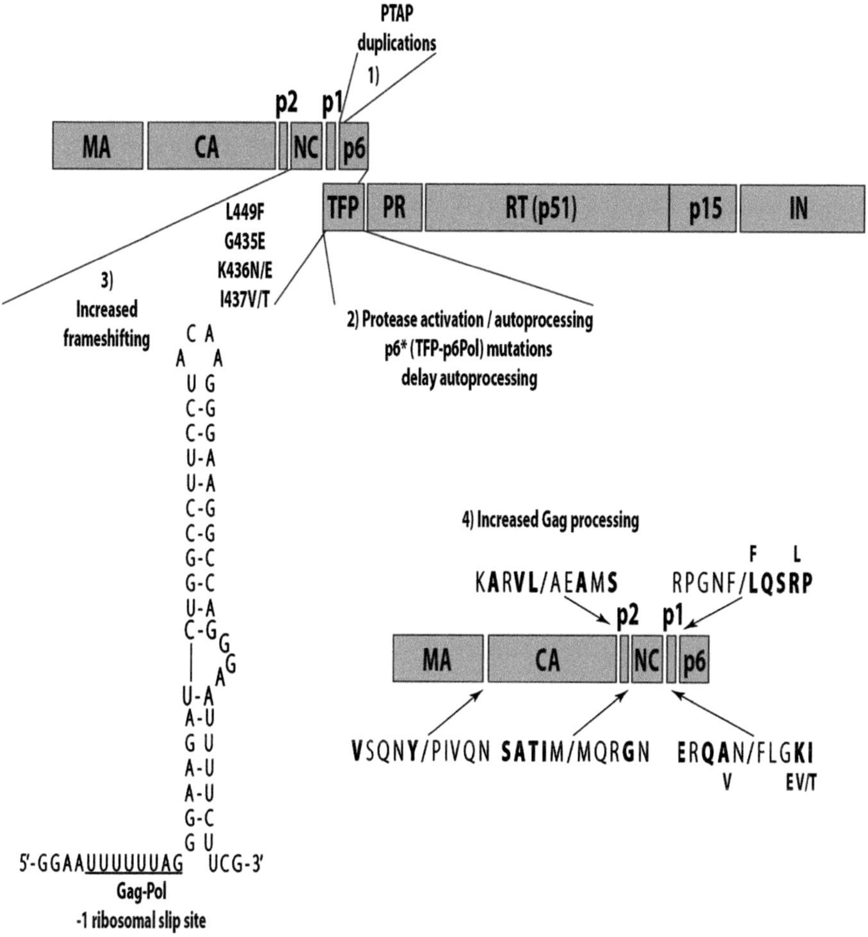

Fig. 4 Proposed alternative mechanisms for protease inhibitor resistance. (*1*) Duplications of the PTAP motif in p6 of Gag. (*2*) Modification of protease activation/autoprocessing. (*3*) Increased GagPol frameshifting. (*4*) Enhanced processing of the Gag substrate. Amino acids associated with protease inhibitor resistance are marked in *bold* and known resistance mutations are indicated

suggesting that these insertions may not be exclusively related to drug resistance but rather reflect (natural) polymorphisms.

2. *Altering protease activation/autoprocessing.* This alternative protease resistance mechanism was proposed based on the observation that mutations in p6* (TFP + p6pol; Figs. 1b and 4) in patient-derived viral isolates can delay Gag autoprocessing and as such decrease PI susceptibility (Whitehurst et al. 2003). The p6* region and especially p6* cleavage is essential for complete activation of the protease and subsequent processing of the viral precursor polyproteins (Ludwig et al. 2008; Paulus et al. 1999, 2004; Tessmer and Kräusslich 1998).

Further research is warranted to investigate the role of mutations in p6* in delayed protease activation and decreased PI susceptibility.

3. *Increased GagPol frameshifting.* Over 15 years ago, an L449F amino acid change in the Gag p1/p6 cleavage site was observed in protease-resistant isolates, and it was suggested that the reduced susceptibility was related to an increased frequency of Gag-Pol ribosomal frameshifting, thereby increasing the levels of the viral enzymes (Doyon et al. 1998). More recent analyses demonstrated that this particular substitution along with other changes in the NC-p1-p6 region of Gag (G435E, K436N, K436N/E, I437V/T) has no effect or only a very modest effect on RNA structure and frameshift efficiency and is therefore unlikely to affect protease susceptibility through this mechanism (Nijhuis et al. 2007; Knops et al. 2012; Girnary et al. 2007).
4. *Enhanced Gag substrate cleavage.* A clear association has been identified between the use of PIs, selection of mutations in protease, and the concurrent substitutions in the viral Gag protein and especially in the protease cleavage sites (Mammano et al. 1998; Zhang et al. 1997; Kolli et al. 2009). Over a decade ago, it was shown that substitutions L449F and P453L in the p1/p6 cleavage site, which do not affect drug susceptibility on their own, reduce PI susceptibility in combination with primary protease mutation I50V (Maguire et al. 2002; Prado et al. 2002). Since then, many Gag cleavage site substitutions have been identified that increase PI resistance in the background of protease mutations, indicating the interactions between the viral protease and its substrate to overcome drug pressure (Fun et al. 2012; Clavel and Mammano 2010).

Interestingly, several mutations in the NC/p1 cleavage site have been identified (A431V, K436E, and/or I437V/T) that confer PI resistance without any mutations in protease (Nijhuis et al. 2007). The Gag-mediated PI resistance was found to be the result of an increased Gag processing (Nijhuis et al. 2007; van Maarseveen et al. 2012). Also emergence of resistance to GS-8374, a potent HIV PI with a unique diethyl-phosphonate moiety, involved a combination of substrate mutations without typical resistance mutations in the viral protease (Stray et al. 2013). Analysis of viral particles indicated that these substrate mutations rendered Gag more susceptible to protease-mediated cleavage in the presence of GS-8374. These data demonstrate that substrate substitutions not only function as compensatory mutations or reduce PI susceptibility in the background of resistance mutations in the viral protease but also represent and alternative PI-resistance mechanism.

Besides mutations in the cleavages sites, mutations outside the Gag cleavage sites have been identified in in vitro selection experiments with different PIs (Stray et al. 2013; Gatanaga et al. 2002) and in patient-derived virus isolates (Parry et al. 2011). These non-cleavage site mutations decrease the potency of the protease inhibitors several fold. The mechanism for the Gag non-cleavage site-mediated resistance is currently not understood.

Several studies evaluated the natural variation within Gag and its cleavage sites (Kolli et al. 2009; Côté et al. 2001; de Oliveira et al. 2003; Verheyen et al. 2009, 2010; Larrouy et al. 2010; Bally et al. 2000; Lambert-Niclot et al. 2012) and suggest that the variation in HIV-1 non-B subtypes is greater than in subtype B (de Oliveira et al. 2003; Verheyen et al. 2009; Larrouy et al. 2011a). The level of conservation differs dramatically between the different CS as within CS (Fig. 1). The p2/NC CS is the most variable of the 5 Gag CS, followed by p1/p6, NC/p1, CA/p2, and finally MA/CA, which is the most conserved CS in subtype B isolates.

Virological failure during boosted-protease inhibitor first-line protease triple combination is usually not associated with the detection of resistance mutations in the viral protease. Thus, alternative protease resistance pathways/mechanisms are being investigated. Substitutions in all gag CS have been described during PI exposure, and amino acid changes in MA/CA (codon 128), NC/p1 (codons 431, 436, and 437), and p1/p6 (codons 449, 452, and 453) are observed most frequently and have been shown to reduce PI susceptibility (Fun et al. 2012).

Further research is needed to investigate if these alternative gag-based PI drug resistance mechanisms play a significant role during boosted-PI therapy failure. In individual cases, gag mutations were shown to be relevant, e. g., that first-line LPV/r failure was associated with the initial selection of the A431V mutation in Gag followed by the 46I and 76V substitution in the viral protease (Nijhuis et al. 2009). Furthermore, it was shown that pre-therapy mutations in the gag CS sequences were significantly associated with virological outcome of a first-line LPV/r single drug regimen in the Monark Trial (Ghosn et al. 2011) and may impact virological response in naïve patients receiving a combination of two protease inhibitors (Larrouy et al. 2010, 2011b). However, other studies have indicated that Gag CS mutations did not significantly contribute to PI-resistance development and virological failure in patients on a (simplified) boosted-PI regimen (McKinnon et al. 2011; Lillemark et al. 2011).

Recently, it was shown that inhibition of viral maturation by PIs also blocks viral entry (Rabi et al. 2013). Approximately half of the inhibitory potential of the inhibitors becomes manifest at this particular step in the viral life cycle, most likely reflecting the interaction between HIV gag and the cytoplasmic tail of the viral envelope protein. The authors studied patients on a PI-based regimen who had detectable viremia and no major PI-resistance mutations in the viral protease and showed that env sequences may contribute to PI failure in a subset of these patients (Rabi et al. 2013). This may provide an explanation for PI therapy failure without the detection of mutations in the viral protease, the target gene of the drugs.

Twenty Years of Protease Inhibitor-Based Therapy

The introduction of cART greatly reduced HIV-associated morbidity and mortality (Palella et al. 1998). Despite this huge achievement, first-generation PI-based cART was characterized by low bioavailability, high pill burden, toxicity, a low genetic barrier to resistance development, and extensive cross-resistance impairing long-term efficacy.

The first protease inhibitor to be licensed was saquinavir in 1995 (Fig. 2). As monotherapy, the drug had failed to establish sustained antiviral efficacy, and selection of resistance characterized by mutations 48V and/or 90M in the protease-coding gene was frequently detected (Jacobsen et al. 1996; Noble and Faulds 1996; Kitchen et al. 1995; Table 1; Fig. 3). Combination of saquinavir with two NRTIs in the ACTG-229 trial resulted in a greater reduction in plasma viral RNA level compared to dual NRTI regimens at 24 weeks. However, efficacy markers tended to return to pretreatment values at 48 weeks (Collier et al. 1996; zidovudine, and zalcitabine. AIDS Clinical Trials Group). Resistance to saquinavir was observed less frequently compared to monotherapy but still occurred in about a quarter of patients using a saquinavir-based triple combination regimen (Jacobsen et al. 1996).

As a result of limited absorption and extensive first-pass metabolism by the hepatic cytochrome P450 3A system, very low oral bioavailability of saquinavir was observed with the initial hard gel formulation (HGC). In order to achieve more adequate absorption, saquinavir had to be taken three times daily with a high-fat meal. To address this problem, saquinavir was later reformulated as a soft-gel capsule (SGC) which provided better systemic exposure.

Ritonavir, approved by the FDA in 1996, was the first protease inhibitor licensed for treatment of HIV infection in the European Union (Fig. 2). Its prolonged absorption phase and half-life permitted the use of a twice-daily dosing schedule (Danner et al. 1995). When used as monotherapy, partial loss of antiviral efficacy was seen 3–4 months following initial impressive decrease in HIV-RNA plasma levels (Danner et al. 1995; Markowitz et al. 1995). Monotherapy of ritonavir was associated with accumulation of resistance characterized by signature mutations at amino acid positions 46, 54, 82, and 84 in the viral protease (Fig. 3; Schmit et al. 1996; Molla et al. 1996). Combination therapy consisting of ritonavir and two NRTIs resulted in significant increase in CD4 cell counts and >2log declines in plasma HIV-RNA levels in observational studies (Mathez et al. 1997; Notermans et al. 1998). In patients with advanced disease, addition of ritonavir to double nucleoside therapy prolonged survival compared to placebo. Unfortunately, the PI was poorly tolerated and use of full dose ritonavir in clinical practice was gradually abandoned.

The other protease inhibitor that became licensed in 1996 was indinavir (Fig. 2). Indinavir, when used as monotherapy, also caused extensive declines in HIV-RNA plasma levels. But over time antiviral efficacy diminished and HIV-RNA almost returned to baseline values at 24 weeks (Stein et al. 1996). Multiple drug resistance-related mutations in the protease-coding region were commonly detected at positions 46, 82, and 84, inducing cross resistance to other PIs (Table 1; Fig. 3; Drusano et al. 1998; Condra et al. 1996). A historical breakthrough was observed when indinavir was combined with zidovudine and lamivudine in patients with prior zidovudine exposure. This triple combination not only dramatically reduced HIV-RNA plasma levels, to below the limit of quantification (at that time <400 copies HIV-RNA/mL) in the majority of patients (Condra et al. 1996; Gulick et al. 1997), but also significantly slowed the progression of HIV disease and mortality (ACTG-320 trial) (Hammer et al. 1997). As a result, triple PI-based combination therapy was implemented as standard of care for treatment of HIV infection in resource-rich areas all over the world. In the long-term, success of indinavir was hampered due to strict intake recommendations and renal toxicity. The drug had to be dosed three times daily preferably on an empty stomach, and a high intake of fluid was needed to prevent indinavir-associated renal toxicity (Plosker and Noble 1999).

Nelfinavir was the fourth protease inhibitor that was registered (Fig. 2). In patients previously exposed to antiretroviral therapy, nelfinavir-based triple combination therapy suppressed HIV-RNA at 28 weeks to below 400 copies/mL in 72 % of patients compared with only 17 % in the control arm of NRTIs and placebo (Gartland and Group 2001). Subsequently, comparable levels of HIV-RNA suppression were observed with a twice-daily dosing regimen which was formally approved in 1999 (Marzolini et al. 2001). Resistance to nelfinavir appeared to be initially driven by the specific protease resistance mutation 30 N, which does not lead to PI cross resistance, followed by changes at amino acid position 88, which also mildly affects susceptibility to several other PIs (Table 1; Fig. 3). In addition, nelfinavir resistance could be observed in the presence of extensive mutational patterns in the viral protease selected by earlier used PIs (Atkinson et al. 2000; Pellegrin et al. 2002; Martinez-Picado et al. 1999). Diarrhea and loose stool frequently limited nelfinavir tolerability.

Second-Generation Protease Inhibitor Therapy; Boosting of Protease Inhibitors

A major advance in the use of protease inhibitors came when it was recognized that ritonavir reduces the metabolism of concomitantly administered PIs through hepatic and intestinal cytochrome P-450 3A4 inhibition, leading to dramatic improvement of bioavailability and half-life of PIs. The first combination used in clinical trials was saquinavir and ritonavir both in therapeutic doses. This combination rapidly pushed HIV-RNA below 200 copies/mL in 80 % of treated individuals (Cameron et al. 1999). Tolerability of a considerable dose of ritonavir remained, however, a concern. The approach really took off when it was found that lower, nontherapeutic doses of ritonavir (100 mg) were sufficient to enhance the pharmacokinetics of coadministrated PIs allowing twice-daily dosing (van Heeswijk et al. 2001).

Boosting of the HGC formulation of saquinavir achieved similar improvement of systemic exposure compared with boosting saquinavir SGC, resulting in reintroduction of the HGC formulation (Kurowski et al. 2003; Cardiello et al. 2003). Boosting of indinavir was not broadly implemented because of high plasma peak levels of the PI leading to enhanced renal toxicity (Voigt et al. 2002; Boyd et al. 2006). Boosting did not greatly enhance the bioavailability of nelfinavir. This limited the efficacy of nelfinavir compared to newly approved PIs and reduced its role for use in pregnancy only until other drugs were found to be a safe and more efficient alternative for this indication as well.

Amprenavir was approved for twice-daily dosing in 1999 (Fig. 2). The combination of amprenavir with two NRTIs was compared to the two NRTIs plus placebo. Although high efficacy of amprenavir versus placebo (89 % vs. 60 % HIV-RNA

<400 copies/mL) was observed at 48 weeks, the intention to treat analysis showed disappointing results with less than 30 % suppressed HIV-RNA in the amprenavir arm (Haubrich et al. 1999). It appeared that many patients prematurely discontinued amprenavir, most likely because of the exceptional pill burden. Furthermore, suboptimal drug concentrations regularly resulting in weak activity of the PI and frequent selection of resistance (Arvieux and Tribut 2005; Sadler et al. 2001). Resistance in the protease-coding region appeared to be somewhat different from the earlier registered PIs and involving key mutations at positions I50V, I54L/M, and V32I + I47V and less commonly I84V (Table 1; Fig. 3; Paulsen et al. 2003).

Introduction of the prodrug fosamprenavir led to improved plasma concentrations and lower pill burden. This formulation showed higher efficacy when combined with two NRTIs compared to nelfinavir-based cART in antiretroviral-naïve individuals in the NEAT trial (Rodriguez-French et al. 2004). Subsequent boosting with ritonavir further improved the efficacy of fosamprenavir-based cART, resulting in suppression of HIV-RNA (<400 copies/mL) in 73 % of naïve individuals at 48 weeks in the KLEAN-trial (Eron et al. 2006). Diarrhea and elevation of fasting cholesterol and triglyceride levels were the most frequent observed adverse events (Eron et al. 2006). There are only limited data available on the efficacy of boosted amprenavir in PI-experienced individuals, but in the CONTEXT trial, viral suppression (<50 copies/mL) in about 50 % of individuals was observed (Arvieux and Tribut 2005; Quercia et al. 2005). Later on, once-daily use of a high dose of boosted fosamprenavir (1,400/100 mg) for combination therapy in therapy-naïve individuals was approved.

Lopinavir (Fig. 2) was the first and thus far only PI co-formulated with a low-dose ritonavir as Kaletra. Lopinavir capsules received approval in 2000 as a twice-daily regimen. Subsequently, the capsules were replaced by pills that were better tolerated and did not require dietary restrictions or refrigeration (Schrader et al. 2008). Efficacy of lopinavir/ritonavir as initial therapy was compared in a randomized placebo controlled study with nelfinavir (three times a day) as comparator with an NRTI backbone in both arms. At 48 weeks, 75 % of individuals on the lopinavir-based regimen had suppressed plasma HIV-RNA (<400 copies/mL) compared to only 63 % in the control arm (Walmsley et al. 2002). Remarkably, no genotypic or phenotypic resistance to lopinavir was observed over 96 weeks in the small group of patients that experienced virological failure (Kempf et al. 2004). Development of resistance during first-line lopinavir-based cART has remained extremely rare but may occur by selection of protease mutations 32I, 47A, and 46I or L33F, I54V, and V82A or combinations of L76V, M46I, and V82A in protease and A431V in gag (Table 1; Figs. 3 and 4) (Nijhuis et al. 2009; Conradie et al. 2004; Friend et al. 2004).

In 2005, once-daily lopinavir was approved based on comparable efficacy with twice-daily lopinavir-based cART. However, the lower Ctrough concentrations observed with once-daily dosing limited registration to antiretroviral-naïve individuals (Johnson et al. 2006a). Lopinavir was the first boosted PI compared head-to-head with an NNRTI as initial therapy. In ACTG study 5142, 48 % of lopinavir-ritonavir recipients versus 61 % of efavirenz recipients (both combined with two NRTIS) maintained plasma HIV-1 RNA at <50 copies/mL through week 96.

Although superior viral suppression was observed in the efavirenz arm, double-class resistance was more frequently detected in this arm. In addition, a significantly better CD4 response was obtained with lopinavir/ritonavir compared with efavirenz (Riddler et al. 2008). Investigations in previously PI-exposed patients demonstrated that the high genetic barrier of lopinavir can be compromised by accumulation of mutations during prior PI-based regimens (Mo et al. 2005). Acquisition of mutations at codons 82, 54, and 46 and less commonly L33F, I50V, and V32I + I47V/A was observed (Table 1; Fig. 3). In PI-experienced patients, lopinavir-/ritonavir-based combination therapy showed superior virological efficacy compared to other at that time available boosted and non-boosted PI-based regimens (Oldfield and Plosker 2006).

The approval of atazanavir in 2003, the first PI that was immediately approved for once-daily dosing, further simplified boosted PI-based combination therapy (Fig. 2). Atazanavir raises plasma bilirubin levels in almost all treated individuals by inhibiting UDP glucuronyltransferase. The bilirubin elevation does generally not result in clinically relevant symptoms. When used unboosted, the drug has only limited effect on fasting cholesterol and triglyceride levels. Unboosted once-daily atazanavir showed equal immunological and superior virological efficacy when compared with nelfinavir twice daily with two NRTIs in antiretroviral-naïve patients (64 % vs. 53 % HIV-RNA suppression <400 copies/mL) (Murphy et al. 2003). Disappointing virological results were obtained in a head-to-head comparison of efavirenz and atazanavir both combined with two NRTIs as first-line regimens. Although plasma HIV-RNA was suppressed below 400 copies/mL in 70 % and 64 % of the atazanavir and efavirenz arms respectively, much lower rates of suppression (32 % and 37 %) were observed in both arms using the more stringent <50 copies/mL criterion (Squires et al. 2004). Soon after the trial, it became apparent that nonstandard collection tubes were possibly responsible for the unexpected low efficacy in both arms (Giordano et al. 2006). Better results were obtained in the Castle study in which once-daily boosted atazanavir was demonstrated as being not inferior to twice-daily lopinavir-ritonavir for the treatment of antiretroviral-naïve patients in the background of a fixed-dose NRTI combination. In both arms, high levels of suppression were observed (78 % vs. 76 % <50 copies/mL) and an increase in CD4 cell counts of more than 200 cells/mm^3 (Molina et al. 2008).

Subsequently, it was recognized that a high genetic barrier to resistance was not limited to lopinavir-ritonavir but could be reached through boosting other PIs. Comparable efficacy and only rarely selection of resistance were demonstrated in several trials comparing lopinavir-ritonavir with either twice-daily boosted fosamprenavir or twice-daily saquinavir in antiretroviral-naive patients (Eron et al. 2006; Molina et al. 2008; Johnson et al. 2006b). Moreover, the use of boosted saquinavir or atazanavir also resulted in better tolerability with lower lipid profiles and less diarrhea compared with lopinavir-ritonavir (Molina et al. 2008; Johnson et al. 2006b; Walmsley et al. 2009).

In PI-experienced individuals, boosted atazanavir with two NRTI proved to be virologically and immunologically non-inferior to twice-daily lopinavir-ritonavir regimens; however, this did not hold up for unboosted atazanavir. Unboosted atazanavir was therefore not approved for use in this patient group (Johnson et al. 2005; Cohen et al. 2005). Selection of resistance in treatment-naive patients experiencing therapy failure during unboosted atazanavir-based regimens was characterized by the I50L mutation in protease which reduced susceptibility to atazanavir, but increased susceptibility to other PIs (Table 1; Fig. 3; Colonno et al. 2004). In contrast, in treatment-experienced patients and patients on boosted therapy, other mutations conferring PI cross-resistance are generally observed including I84V, L90M, A71V/T, N88S/D, and M46I (Table 1; Fig. 3; Pellegrin et al. 2006).

Tipranavir was approved in 2005 (Fig. 2) for the treatment of highly experienced patients with resistance to multiple PIs. Tipranavir is a non-peptidomimetic protease inhibitor and as such less potent than the peptidomimetic PI as described above. Instead of a peptidomimetichydroxyethylene core, tipranavir contains a dihydropyrone ring as a central scaffold (Fig. 2; Turner et al. 1998). Tipranavir is a potent inducer of its own metabolism through induction of the cytochrome P450 expression, which results in a need for double-dose ritonavir boosting. Tipranavir showed superior efficacy in salvage relative to the comparator protease inhibitor (CPI), both with optimized background in heavily pretreated patients with extensive PI resistance in the RESIST trials. At 48 weeks, significantly more patients achieved and maintained treatment response in the boosted tipranavir arm than in the CPI-ritonavir arm (plasma HIV-RNA <400 copies/mL: 33.6 % vs. 15.3 % and <50 copies/mL: 22.8 % vs. 10.2 %). However, tipranavir appeared not to be superior to lopinavir in lopinavir-naïve individuals. Moreover, gastrointestinal system disorders, liver-related toxicity, and elevated lipid profiles were more frequently reported in the boosted tipranavir arm (Gathe et al. 2006; Cahn et al. 2006; Hicks et al. 2006).

During tipranavir in vitro selection experiments, major PI-resistance mutations were observed: V32I, I54V, V82L, and I84V (Table 1; Fig. 3; Doyon et al. 2005). After failure of tipranavir-based cART, mutations at positions 82 and 84 have been reported most frequently (Table 1; Fig. 3; Naeger and Struble 2007). Based on the results in the RESIST study, a weighted genotypic susceptibility list has been reported including a larger number of mutations, T74P, I47V, V82L/T, Q58E, N83D as the strongest predictors of reduced efficacy and I54A/M/V, I84V, M36I, K43T, L10V, and M46L as weaker predictors, whereas L24I, I50L/V, I54L, and L76V were predictors of virological response (Fig. 3; Schapiro et al. 2010). Even though the virological benefits of tipranavir were evident, significant risk of hepatotoxicity, high pill burden, and availability of new treatment options restricted wide uptake.

One such new treatment option was darunavir, a ninth protease inhibitor approved in 2006 (Fig. 2). Although this PI was especially designed to inhibit drug-resistant strains, its powerful antiviral potency and limited adverse events profile rapidly expanded use of the drug into earlier lines of therapy. In the Artemis trial, once-daily darunavir/ritonavir was compared to once- or twice-daily lopinavir-ritonavir with a fixed-dose NRTI backbone in antiretroviral-naïve patients. At week 96, significantly more patients in the darunavir (79 %) than the lopinavir arm (71 %) had a plasma HIV-RNA less than 50 copies/ml. Median CD4 cell count increase from baseline was circa 180 cells/mm^3. Darunavir had a more favorable gastrointestinal and lipid profile compared to lopinavir (Mills et al. 2009). In treatment-experienced patients, the dose-finding Power 1 and 2 studies evaluated the efficacy and safety of boosted darunavir with that of currently approved PIs combined with an optimized background therapy. 96-week efficacy and safety data of both trials confirmed the recommended the 600/100 mg twice-daily dose as the preferred option for pretreated individuals (Arastéh et al. 2009). In a combined analysis of both trials, 39 % of patients receiving boosted darunavir regimens achieved plasma HIV-RNA <50 copies/mL compared to 9 % with comparator PI-based regimens (Arastéh et al. 2009). In the Titan study, twice-daily boosted darunavir was compared to twice-daily lopinavir-ritonavir both with optimized backbone. At 48 weeks, significantly more patients receiving darunavir achieved a plasma HIV-RNA load of <50 copies/mL. CD4 cell count increases were similar in both treatment groups (Madruga et al. 2007). Fewer patients with virologic failure in the darunavir arm than in the lopinavir arm developed resistance (De Meyer et al. 2009).

In vitro selection of darunavir-resistant HIV-1 appears to be slower and less frequent than with other PIs, probably reflecting the particularly strong binding of darunavir to the HIV protease, resulting in a higher intrinsic genetic barrier than observed with the other boosted PIs (De Meyer et al. 2005; King et al. 2004). This makes it very difficult for the PI-naïve virus to escape via the traditional protease-based route and alternative gag substrate-based resistance may be selected (Fig. 4).

Pooled resistance data from the Power trials who initiated boosted darunavir 600/100 mg in PI-experienced patients was used to establish a list of resistance mutations associated with a diminished response to darunavir (de Meyer et al. 2008). The list was updated using data from more trials with therapy-experienced patients, including the following mutations in the protease-coding region: V11I, V32I, L33F, I47V, I50V, I54L/M, T74P, L76V, I84V, and L89V (Table 1; Fig. 3). The presence of more than three darunavir-listed mutations was associated with a median darunavir FC >10 and a diminished virological response (De Meyer et al. 2009). Of interest, some of the darunavir mutations are associated with improved response to tipranavir, which might give additional options for future salvage therapy, if needed at all.

Double Boosting Protease Inhibitor-Based Therapy

Preceding the recent approval of several new antiretroviral compounds, physicians experienced difficulties building an effective regimen for a group of heavily therapy-experienced patients with extensive drug resistance. In this setting of limited therapeutic options, the use of double-boosted PI was explored to gain possible synergistic or added antiviral activity of both drugs and to increase the genetic barrier to PI resistance. Although no large randomized trials assessing the clinical efficacy of double-boosted-PI regimens were reported, several comparative and cohort studies suggested potential utility of combinations such as lopinavir/ritonavir with either saquinavir or atazanavir, or atazanavir plus low-dose ritonavir with saquinavir all in combination with two NRTIs as a backbone (Smith et al. 2005; Gilliam et al. 2006;

Ribera et al. 2006; Manosuthi et al. 2008; von Hentig et al. 2007; Petersen et al. 2007; Stebbing et al. 2009).

A high pill burden, increased risk for toxicity, and lower efficacy compared to standard of care regimens did not make double-boosted PIs an appealing option beyond salvage therapy (Ulbricht et al. 2011). The combination of darunavir with drugs from new classes has resulted in impressive efficacy in heavily pretreated patients discarding the use of double-boosted PIs as salvage therapy in resource-rich settings.

Protease Inhibitor: Mono or Dual Therapy

Although NRTIs had been the cornerstone of cART, the finding that originally to PIs attributed lipoatrophy was mainly induced by these NRTIs fuelled a search for alternative regimens. Moreover, the profound efficacy of boosted PI-based cART and the high genetic barrier to resistance questioned the paradigm of a three-drug regimen. Combined with the challenge of lifelong adherence, high costs of triple therapy, and the risk for selection of multidrug resistance, these considerations led to reevaluation of the concept of mono or dual therapy in several trials.

A dual NRTI-sparing PI-NNRTI combination of lopinavir/r and efavirenz demonstrated comparable efficacy to efavirenz and lopinavir-based cART but extensive elevation of triglyceride levels and a trend towards more NNRTI resistance upon therapy failure (Riddler et al. 2008). More elaborated selection of resistance was also reported with the use of NRTI-sparing regimens of either lopinavir or boosted indinavir with an NNRTI in the ANRS-121 trial (Soulié et al. 2009). The results from these two important trials clearly limited the role for future initiatives using NNRTI/PI combinations as NRTI-sparing regimens. Several trials addressed efficacy of NRTI-sparing regimens using boosted PIs and the integrase inhibitor raltegravir. In the randomized Spartan trial, which was not powered for statistical comparison of efficacy, twice-daily unboosted atazanavir plus raltegravir was compared to once-daily atazanavir plus two NRTIs in therapy naive patients (Kozal et al. 2012). At 24 weeks of treatment, 74.6 % of patients in the dual arm had confirmed virological response, compared with 63.3 % in the standard of care arm. However, patients in the dual arm frequently suffered from grade 4 hyperbilirubinemia and occasionally selected resistance to raltegravir. As a result, this strategy has not been broadly implemented. In an uncontrolled trial, first-line therapy of boosted darunavir plus raltegravir was well tolerated, but virologic failure and selection of integrase resistance mutations were common, particularly in patients with baseline viral load more than 100,000 copies/mL (Taiwo et al. 2011). The same dual combination appeared to be non-inferior to a standard three-drug combination of boosted darunavir with two NRTIs in the randomized controlled NEAT001/ANRS143 trial. A very high percentage of patients received virological control in both arms (93 % in the three-drug arm vs. 89 % in the dual arm). Of note selection of resistance to raltegravir was occasionally observed in the dual arm, while no resistance was detected in the comparator arm (Raffi et al. 84LB, CROI 2014).

Recently a multicenter, randomized, double-blind comparative trial of boosted darunavir plus the CCR5-blocker maraviroc versus the standard of boosted darunavir with two NRTIs in antiretroviral-naïve HIV-infected patients with CCR5 tropic HIV was terminated after preliminary review of week 48 data. Reason of termination was significant inferior efficacy of the dual arm as compared to the comparator arm (http://clinicaltrials.gov/ct2/show/NCT01345630).

A systematic review of monotherapy on the available clinical trials with lopinavir and non-comparative atazanavir monotherapy studies found an absolute risk difference of 10.3 % of failure compared to standard PI-based cART (Bierman et al. 2009). In antiretroviral-naïve patients initiating PI-monotherapy, low-level viremia and development of resistance was also more frequently observed compared to standard of care 3-drug-based regimens (Bierman et al. 2009). However, no significant difference in short-term efficacy was observed in individuals starting monotherapy after induction with full suppressive cART (Bierman et al. 2009). Furthermore, among individuals who successfully controlled HIV after restarting nucleosides, failure rates did not significantly differ between monotherapy groups and standard-regimen groups (Bierman et al. 2009).

A potential explanation for the increased risk of failure with lopinavir monotherapy without induction phase may be insufficient viral suppression by boosted PIs in all body compartments. A lower genetic barrier to resistance for monotherapy than originally foreseen may provide an alternative explanation for increased failure as just two mutations can be sufficient for viral breakthrough during (mono)therapy with lopinavir-ritonavir (Nijhuis et al. 2009; Delaugerre et al. 2009). However, the reported combination of protease mutations M46I plus L76V is not frequently observed in cases of lopinavir-based therapy failure. This indicates that the genetic barrier to resistance is not simply a calculated sum of the two mutations but also includes the selective advantage of these particular mutations in the viral quasispecies.

Maintenance monotherapy with once-daily boosted darunavir, a PI for which it is generally accepted that it has a very high genetic barrier, was performed in two relatively large clinical trials. In the Monet trial, HIV RNA during monotherapy was non-inferior to a three-drug regimen at 48 weeks (84.3 % vs. 85.3 % HIV-RNA <50 copies/mL) (Arribas et al. 2012). At 96 and 144 weeks, non-inferiority was still observed in an ITT analysis considering switches not as failure. However, non-inferiority was not maintained in a TLOVR (time to loss of virological response) switch equals failure analysis (Arribas et al. 2012). Also in the MONOI-ANRS trial, non-inferiority was observed at 48 weeks; however, in the ITT analysis, the rate of success was 87.5 % in the monotherapy arm and 92 % in the three-drug arm. Longer-term data at 96 weeks showed high efficacy rate of darunavir (85 %); nevertheless, there was a consistent small difference favoring the three-drug combination (Katlama et al. 2010). In both studies, patients failing on darunavir/r monotherapy had virtually no emergence of darunavir resistance mutations (Arribas et al. 2012; Katlama et al. 2010).

The Influence of Genetic Diversity on Protease Inhibitor Efficacy and Selection of Resistance

Initial drug design and data on efficacy and selection of drug resistance have focused on subtype B infections. Among subtypes the difference in nucleotide sequence in the protease-coding *pol* gene is approximately 10–15 %, leading to distinct variation at amino acid level. The genetic differences may influence baseline susceptibility of PIs, the genetic barrier for selection of PI drug resistance and mutational pathways (Martinez-Cajas et al. 2009).

In vitro decreased susceptibility to PIs was reported in a limited number of CRF02_AG isolates from therapy-naïve individuals (Fleury et al. 2006; Kinomoto et al. 2005). Caution is warranted by interpretation of these results since deletion clones and phenotypic resistance cutoffs applied are based on subtype B virus backbones. Additional reports on small numbers of non-B HIV-1 isolates with decreased baseline susceptibility or hypersusceptibility for PIs in vitro have been published. Slight differences in protease inhibitor efficiency based on conformational differences with subtype B leading to a more flexible enzyme in several non-B subtypes may explain at least partially these results (Huang et al. 2014). In the absence of clinical trials specifically addressing differences in susceptibility, no obvious differences in susceptibility of non-B isolates compared to subtype B isolates have been observed in clinical practice (Martinez-Cajas et al. 2009; Frater 2002).

Wild-type sequences at several resistance-related codons differ between non-B subtypes and subtype B (van de Vijver et al. 2006). These differences may influence viral replication capacity, the genetic barrier, or specific pathways to resistance (Lisovsky et al. 2010). Examples are the minor mutations 10 V and 36I, which are generally present in non-B viruses and which are included in the tipranavir resistance score (Table 1; Fig. 3; Schapiro et al. 2010; van de Vijver et al. 2006). Diversity in nucleotide sequence may also lead to differential selection of PI-resistant variants on position 82 (van de Vijver et al. 2006; Abecasis et al. 2006).

In addition, the frequency of selection of specific mutational patterns may differ among subtypes. For instance, in subtype C and other non-B subtypes, selection of resistance to nelfinavir preferably occurs via PI cross-resistance pathways including mutation L90M, and to a lesser extent via the, in subtype B most frequently observed, nelfinavir-specific pathway with mutation D30N (Cane et al. 2001; Grossman et al. 2004).

Finally, alternative resistance pathways may be selected among non-B subtypes. This is most extensively described for a PI-resistance pathway that includes positions 89 and 90 in non-B subtypes. In non-B subtypes such as subtype C, F, G, and CRF01_AE, M89 is the consensus amino acid, compared to L89 in subtype B. The M89 polymorphism present in non-B subtypes may lead to the selection of the M89T mutational pathway conferring reduced susceptibility to atazanavir, lopinavir, and nelfinavir (Martinez-Cajas et al. 2012). Acquisition of the mutations M89I and L90M results in decreased susceptibility to nelfinavir in these subtypes (Abecasis et al. 2005). Additional presence of mutation 71T or 74S has been correlated with high levels of resistance to nelfinavir in subtype G viruses (Gonzalez et al. 2008).

The Use of Boosted PIs in Resource-Limited Settings

cART became available in resource-limited settings all over the world after adoption of the Doha-declaration in 2001, enabling countries to circumvent patent rights for essential medicines. Two years later, the World Health Organization (WHO) launched their "3 by 5" initiative as a global target for provision of antiretroviral therapy to three million people by the end of 2005 in resource-limited settings. Even though this goal was not met, the initiative led to massive programmatic rollout of NNRTI-based first-line therapy. By the end of 2013, nearly ten million people were on cART worldwide. For second-line therapy in resource-limited settings, WHO advises a PI-based regimen with lopinavir-ritonavir plus two NRTIs. The important advantage of this choice is that no refrigeration of ritonavir capsules is required as ritonavir is co-formulated with lopinavir tablets. Furthermore, a PI-based regimen is likely to demonstrate still viral efficacy even if the NRTI backbone is compromised by first-line therapy. At present there are only anecdotal data available regarding the efficacy of second-line lopinavir-ritonavir-based regimens in resource-limited settings. One small study showed accumulation of protease mutations among patients with long-term failure on second-line PI-based cART in Nigeria, but more extensive results are needed before firm conclusion on the extent of selection of PI-related resistance can be drawn (Rawizza et al. 2013).

Conclusion

HIV protease plays a crucial role in the viral life cycle, and the introduction of protease inhibitors marked the start of combination antiretroviral therapy. Initially, therapy failure was often associated with the selection of multiple drug resistance mutations, a broad range of resistance mechanisms, and cross-resistance to other PIs. Fortunately, the genetic barrier towards PI resistance could be raised which greatly contributed to the current success of PI-based therapy. Still there are concerns regarding use of PIs that require compelling attention, with respect to toxicity and the potential for development of resistance especially if used as maintenance therapy or if used in resource-limited setting with less frequent monitoring.

Acknowledgements We thank Dr. Pavlina Rezacova from the Institute of Organic Chemistry and Biochemistry Institute of Molecular Genetics in Prague, Czech Republic, for preparing Fig. 3. Funding resource: the Netherlands Organization for Scientific Research (NWO) VIDI Grant (91796349).

References

Abecasis AB, Deforche K, Snoeck J et al (2005) Protease mutation M89I/V is linked to therapy failure in patients infected with the HIV-1 non-B subtypes C, F or G. AIDS 19(16):1799–1806

Abecasis AB, Deforche K, Bacheler LT et al (2006) Investigation of baseline susceptibility to protease inhibitors in HIV-1 subtypes C, F, G and CRF02_AG. Antivir Ther 11(5):581–589

Agniswamy J, Sayer JM, Weber IT, Louis JM (2012) Terminal interface conformations modulate dimer stability prior to amino terminal autoprocessing of HIV-1 protease. Biochemistry 51 (5):1041–1050

Amiel C, Charpentier C, Désiré N et al (2011) Long-term follow-up of 11 protease inhibitor (PI)-naïve and PI-treated HIV-infected patients harbouring virus with insertions in the HIV-1 protease gene. HIV Med 12(3):138–144

Arastéh K, Yeni P, Pozniak A et al (2009) Efficacy and safety of darunavir/ritonavir in treatment-experienced HIV type-1 patients in the POWER 1, 2 and 3 trials at week 96. Antivir Ther 14 (6):859–864

Arribas JR, Clumeck N, Nelson M, Hill A, van Delft Y, Moecklinghoff C (2012) The MONET trial: week 144 analysis of the efficacy of darunavir/ritonavir (DRV/r) monotherapy versus DRV/r plus two nucleoside reverse transcriptase inhibitors, for patients with viral load <50 HIV-1 RNA copies/mL at baseline. HIV Med 13(7):398–405

Arvieux C, Tribut O (2005) Amprenavir or fosamprenavir plus ritonavir in HIV infection: pharmacology, efficacy and tolerability profile. Drugs 65(5):633–659

Atkinson B, Isaacson J, Knowles M, Mazabel E, Patick AK (2000) Correlation between human immunodeficiency virus genotypic resistance and virologic response in patients receiving nelfinavir monotherapy or nelfinavir with lamivudine and zidovudine. J Infect Dis 182 (2):420–427

Balagam R, Singh V, Sagi AR, Dixit NM (2011) Taking multiple infections of cells and recombination into account leads to small within-host effective-population-size estimates of HIV-1. PLoS One 6(1):e14531

Bally F, Martinez R, Peters S, Sudre P, Telenti A (2000) Polymorphism of HIV type 1 gag p7/p1 and p1/p6 cleavage sites: clinical significance and implications for resistance to protease inhibitors. AIDS Res Hum Retroviruses 16(13):1209–1213

Bierman WFW, van Agtmael MA, Nijhuis M, Danner SA, Boucher CAB (2009) HIV monotherapy with ritonavir-boosted protease inhibitors: a systematic review. AIDS 23(3):279–291

Borman AM, Paulous S, Clavel F (1996) Resistance of human immunodeficiency virus type 1 to protease inhibitors: selection of resistance mutations in the presence and absence of the drug. J Gen Virol 77(Pt 3):419–426

Boyd MA, Srasuebkul P, Khongphattanayothin M et al (2006) Boosted versus unboosted indinavir with zidovudine and lamivudine in nucleoside pre-treated patients: a randomized, open-label trial with 112 weeks of follow-up (HIV-NAT 005). Antivir Ther 11(2):223–232

Brown AJ (1997) Analysis of HIV-1 env gene sequences reveals evidence for a low effective number in the viral population. Proc Natl Acad Sci U S A 94(5):1862–1865

Brown AJ, Richman DD (1997) HIV-1: gambling on the evolution of drug resistance? Nat Med 3 (3):268–271

Brumme ZL, Chan KJ, Dong WW et al (2003) Prevalence and clinical implications of insertions in the HIV-1 p6Gag N-terminal region in drug-naive individuals initiating antiretroviral therapy. Antivir Ther 8(2):91–96

Cahn P, Villacian J, Lazzarin A et al (2006) Ritonavir-boosted tipranavir demonstrates superior efficacy to ritonavir-boosted protease inhibitors in treatment-experienced HIV-infected patients: 24-week results of the RESIST-2 trial. Clin Infect Dis 43(10):1347–1356

Cameron DW, Japour AJ, Xu Y et al (1999) Ritonavir and saquinavir combination therapy for the treatment of HIV infection. AIDS 13(2):213–224

Cane PA, de Ruiter A, Rice P, Wiselka M, Fox R, Pillay D (2001) Resistance-associated mutations in the human immunodeficiency virus type 1 subtype c protease gene from treated and untreated patients in the United Kingdom. J Clin Microbiol 39(7):2652–2654

Cardiello PG, Monhaphol T, Mahanontharit A et al (2003) Pharmacokinetics of once-daily saquinavir hard-gelatin capsules and saquinavir soft-gelatin capsules boosted with ritonavir in HIV-1-infected subjects. J Acquir Immune Defic Syndr 32(4):375–379

Clavel F, Mammano F (2010) Role of Gag in HIV resistance to protease inhibitors. Viruses 2 (7):1411–1426
Coffin JM (1995) HIV population dynamics in vivo: implications for genetic variation, pathogenesis, and therapy. Science 267(5197):483–489
Cohen C, Nieto-Cisneros L, Zala C et al (2005) Comparison of atazanavir with lopinavir/ritonavir in patients with prior protease inhibitor failure: a randomized multinational trial. Curr Med Res Opin 21(10):1683–1692
Collier AC, Coombs RW, Schoenfeld DA et al (1996) Treatment of human immunodeficiency virus infection with saquinavir, zidovudine, and zalcitabine. AIDS Clinical Trials Group. N Engl J Med 334(16):1011–1017
Colonno R, Rose R, McLaren C, Thiry A, Parkin N, Friborg J (2004) Identification of I50L as the signature atazanavir (ATV)-resistance mutation in treatment-naive HIV-1-infected patients receiving ATV-containing regimens. J Infect Dis 189(10):1802–1810
Condra JH, Holder DJ, Schleif WA et al (1996) Genetic correlates of in vivo viral resistance to indinavir, a human immunodeficiency virus type 1 protease inhibitor. J Virol 70(12):8270–8276
Conradie F, Sanne I, Venter W, Eron J (2004) Failure of lopinavir-ritonavir (Kaletra)-containing regimen in an antiretroviral-naive patient. AIDS 18(7):1084–1085
Côté HC, Brumme ZL, Harrigan PR (2001) Human immunodeficiency virus type 1 protease cleavage site mutations associated with protease inhibitor cross-resistance selected by indinavir, ritonavir, and/or saquinavir. J Virol 75(2):589–594
Craig JC, Duncan IB, Hockley D, Grief C, Roberts NA, Mills JS (1991) Antiviral properties of Ro 31–8959, an inhibitor of human immunodeficiency virus (HIV) proteinase. Antiviral Res 16 (4):295–305
Croteau G, Doyon L, Thibeault D, McKercher G, Pilote L, Lamarre D (1997) Impaired fitness of human immunodeficiency virus type 1 variants with high-level resistance to protease inhibitors. J Virol 71(2):1089–1096
Dam E, Quercia R, Glass B et al (2009) Gag mutations strongly contribute to HIV-1 resistance to protease inhibitors in highly drug-experienced patients besides compensating for fitness loss. PLoS Pathog 5(3):e1000345
Danner SA, Carr A, Leonard JM et al (1995) A short-term study of the safety, pharmacokinetics, and efficacy of ritonavir, an inhibitor of HIV-1 protease. European-Australian Collaborative Ritonavir Study Group. N Engl J Med 333(23):1528–1533
Davis MR, Jiang J, Zhou J, Freed EO, Aiken C (2006) A mutation in the human immunodeficiency virus type 1 Gag protein destabilizes the interaction of the envelope protein subunits gp120 and gp41. J Virol 80(5):2405–2417
Davis DA, Soule EE, Davidoff KS, Daniels SI, Naiman NE, Yarchoan R (2012) Activity of human immunodeficiency virus type 1 protease inhibitors against the initial autocleavage in Gag-Pol polyprotein processing. Antimicrob Agents Chemother 56(7):3620–3628
De Meyer S, Azijn H, Surleraux D et al (2005) TMC114, a novel human immunodeficiency virus type 1 protease inhibitor active against protease inhibitor-resistant viruses, including a broad range of clinical isolates. Antimicrob Agents Chemother 49(6):2314–2321
de Meyer S, Vangeneugden T, van Baelen B et al (2008) Resistance profile of darunavir: combined 24-week results from the POWER trials. AIDS Res Hum Retroviruses 24(3):379–388
De Meyer S, Lathouwers E, Dierynck I et al (2009) Characterization of virologic failure patients on darunavir/ritonavir in treatment-experienced patients. AIDS 23(14):1829–1840
de Oliveira T, Engelbrecht S, Janse van Rensburg E et al (2003) Variability at human immunodeficiency virus type 1 subtype C protease cleavage sites: an indication of viral fitness? J Virol 77 (17):9422–9430
Delaugerre C, Flandre P, Chaix ML et al (2009) Protease inhibitor resistance analysis in the MONARK trial comparing first-line lopinavir-ritonavir monotherapy to lopinavir-ritonavir plus zidovudine and lamivudine triple therapy. Antimicrob Agents Chemother 53(7):2934–2939

Domingo E, Escarmís C, Sevilla N et al (1996) Basic concepts in RNA virus evolution. FASEB J 10 (8):859–864
Doyon L, Croteau G, Thibeault D, Poulin F, Pilote L, Lamarre D (1996) Second locus involved in human immunodeficiency virus type 1 resistance to protease inhibitors. J Virol 70 (6):3763–3769
Doyon L, Payant C, Brakier-Gingras L, Lamarre D (1998) Novel Gag-Pol frameshift site in human immunodeficiency virus type 1 variants resistant to protease inhibitors. J Virol 72(7):6146–6150
Doyon L, Tremblay S, Bourgon L, Wardrop E, Cordingley MG (2005) Selection and characterization of HIV-1 showing reduced susceptibility to the non-peptidic protease inhibitor tipranavir. Antiviral Res 68(1):27–35
Drusano GL, Bilello JA, Stein DS et al (1998) Factors influencing the emergence of resistance to indinavir: role of virologic, immunologic, and pharmacologic variables. J Infect Dis 178 (2):360–367
Erickson-Viitanen S, Manfredi J, Viitanen P et al (1989) Cleavage of HIV-1 gag polyprotein synthesized in vitro: sequential cleavage by the viral protease. AIDS Res Hum Retroviruses 5 (6):577–591
Eron J, Yeni P, Gathe J et al (2006) The KLEAN study of fosamprenavir-ritonavir versus lopinavir-ritonavir, each in combination with abacavir-lamivudine, for initial treatment of HIV infection over 48 weeks: a randomised non-inferiority trial. Lancet 368(9534):476–482
Fleury HJ, Toni T, Lan NT et al (2006) Susceptibility to antiretroviral drugs of CRF01_AE, CRF02_AG, and subtype C viruses from untreated patients of Africa and Asia: comparative genotypic and phenotypic data. AIDS Res Hum Retroviruses 22(4):357–366
Frater J (2002) The impact of HIV-1 subtype on the clinical response on HAART. J HIV Ther 7 (4):92–96
Friend J, Parkin N, Liegler T, Martin JN, Deeks SG (2004) Isolated lopinavir resistance after virological rebound of a ritonavir/lopinavir-based regimen. AIDS 18(14):1965–1966
Fun A, Wensing AMJ, Verheyen J, Nijhuis M (2012) Human immunodeficiency virus gag and protease: partners in resistance. Retrovirology 9
Gallego O, de Mendoza C, Corral A, Soriano V (2003) Changes in the human immunodeficiency virus p7-p1-p6 gag gene in drug-naive and pretreated patients. J Clin Microbiol 41(3):1245–1247
Gartland M, Group AS (2001) AVANTI 3: a randomized, double-blind trial to compare the efficacy and safety of lamivudine plus zidovudine versus lamivudine plus zidovudine plus nelfinavir in HIV-1-infected antiretroviral-naive patients. Antivir Ther 6(2):127–134
Gatanaga H, Suzuki Y, Tsang H et al (2002) Amino acid substitutions in Gag protein at non-cleavage sites are indispensable for the development of a high multitude of HIV-1 resistance against protease inhibitors. J Biol Chem 277(8):5952–5961
Gathe J, Cooper DA, Farthing C et al (2006) Efficacy of the protease inhibitors tipranavir plus ritonavir in treatment-experienced patients: 24-week analysis from the RESIST-1 trial. Clin Infect Dis 43(10):1337–1346
Ghosn J, Delaugerre C, Flandre P et al (2011) Polymorphism in Gag gene cleavage sites of HIV-1 non-B subtype and virological outcome of a first-line lopinavir/ritonavir single drug regimen. PLoS One 6(9):e24798
Gilliam BL, Chan-Tack KM, Qaqish RB, Rode RA, Fantry LE, Redfield RR (2006) Successful treatment with atazanavir and lopinavir/ritonavir combination therapy in protease inhibitor-susceptible and protease inhibitor-resistant HIV-infected patients. AIDS Patient Care STDS 20 (11):745–759
Giordano M, Kelleher T, Colonno RJ, Lazzarin A, Squires K (2006) The effects of the Roche AMPLICOR HIV-1 MONITOR UltraSensitive Test versions 1.0 and 1.5 viral load assays and plasma collection tube type on determination of response to antiretroviral therapy and the inappropriateness of cross-study comparisons. J Clin Virol 35(4):420–425
Girnary R, King L, Robinson L, Elston R, Brierley I (2007) Structure-function analysis of the ribosomal frameshifting signal of two human immunodeficiency virus type 1 isolates with increased resistance to viral protease inhibitors. J Gen Virol 88(Pt 1):226–235

Gonzalez LM, Santos AF, Abecasis AB et al (2008) Impact of HIV-1 protease mutations A71V/T and T74S on M89I/V-mediated protease inhibitor resistance in subtype G isolates. J Antimicrob Chemother 61(6):1201–1204
Götte M (2012) The distinct contributions of fitness and genetic barrier to the development of antiviral drug resistance. Curr Opin Virol 2(5):644–650
Grantz Sasková K, Kozísek M, Stray K et al (2013) GS-8374, a prototype phosphonate-containing inhibitor of HIV-1 protease, effectively inhibits protease mutants with amino acid insertions. J Virol 88:3586–3590
Grossman Z, Paxinos EE, Averbuch D et al (2004) Mutation D30N is not preferentially selected by human immunodeficiency virus type 1 subtype C in the development of resistance to nelfinavir. Antimicrob Agents Chemother 48(6):2159–2165
Gulick RM, Mellors JW, Havlir D et al (1997) Treatment with indinavir, zidovudine, and lamivudine in adults with human immunodeficiency virus infection and prior antiretroviral therapy. N Engl J Med 337(11):734–739
Gulnik SV, Suvorov LI, Liu B et al (1995) Kinetic characterization and cross-resistance patterns of HIV-1 protease mutants selected under drug pressure. Biochemistry 34(29):9282–9287
Hammer SM, Squires KE, Hughes MD et al (1997) A controlled trial of two nucleoside analogues plus indinavir in persons with human immunodeficiency virus infection and CD4 cell counts of 200 per cubic millimeter or less. AIDS Clinical Trials Group 320 Study Team. N Engl J Med 337(11):725–733
Haubrich R, Thompson M, Schooley R et al (1999) A phase II safety and efficacy study of amprenavir in combination with zidovudine and lamivudine in HIV-infected patients with limited antiretroviral experience. Amprenavir PROAB2002 Study Team. AIDS 13 (17):2411–2420
Hicks CB, Cahn P, Cooper DA et al (2006) Durable efficacy of tipranavir-ritonavir in combination with an optimised background regimen of antiretroviral drugs for treatment-experienced HIV-1-infected patients at 48 weeks in the Randomized Evaluation of Strategic Intervention in multi-drug resistant patients with tipranavir (RESIST) studies: an analysis of combined data from two randomised open-label trials. Lancet 368(9534):466–475
Huang X, Britto MD, Kear JL et al (2014) The role of select subtype polymorphisms on HIV-1 protease conformational sampling and dynamics. J Biol Chem 289:17203–17214
Jacks T, Power MD, Masiarz FR, Luciw PA, Barr PJ, Varmus HE (1988) Characterization of ribosomal frameshifting in HIV-1 gag-pol expression. Nature 331(6153):280–283
Jacobsen H, Haenggi M, Ott M et al (1996) Reduced sensitivity to saquinavir: an update on genotyping from phase I/II trials. Antiviral Res 29(1):95–97
Johnson M, Grinsztejn B, Rodriguez C et al (2005) Atazanavir plus ritonavir or saquinavir, and lopinavir/ritonavir in patients experiencing multiple virological failures. AIDS 19(7): 685–694
Johnson MA, Gathe JC, Podzamczer D et al (2006a) A once-daily lopinavir/ritonavir-based regimen provides noninferior antiviral activity compared with a twice-daily regimen. J Acquir Immune Defic Syndr 43(2):153–160
Johnson M, Grinsztejn B, Rodriguez C et al (2006b) 96-week comparison of once-daily atazanavir/ritonavir and twice-daily lopinavir/ritonavir in patients with multiple virologic failures. AIDS 20 (5):711–718
Johnson VA, Calvez V, Gunthard HF et al (2013) Update of the drug resistance mutations in HIV-1: March 2013. Top Antivir Med 21(1):6–14
Jordan PS, Poon A, Eron J et al (2009) A novel codon insert in protease of clade B HIV type 1. AIDS Res Hum Retroviruses 25(5):547–550
Katlama C, Valantin MA, Algarte-Genin M et al (2010) Efficacy of darunavir/ritonavir maintenance monotherapy in patients with HIV-1 viral suppression: a randomized open-label, noninferiority trial, MONOI-ANRS 136. AIDS 24(15):2365–2374
Kawamura M, Shimano R, Inubushi R et al (1997) Cleavage of Gag precursor is required for early replication phase of HIV-1. FEBS Lett 415(2):227–230

Kempf DJ, Marsh KC, Denissen JF et al (1995) ABT-538 is a potent inhibitor of human immunodeficiency virus protease and has high oral bioavailability in humans. Proc Natl Acad Sci U S A 92(7):2484–2488

Kempf DJ, Marsh KC, Kumar G et al (1997) Pharmacokinetic enhancement of inhibitors of the human immunodeficiency virus protease by coadministration with ritonavir. Antimicrob Agents Chemother 41(3):654–660

Kempf DJ, King MS, Bernstein B et al (2004) Incidence of resistance in a double-blind study comparing lopinavir/ritonavir plus stavudine and lamivudine to nelfinavir plus stavudine and lamivudine. J Infect Dis 189(1):51–60

Kim EY, Winters MA, Kagan RM, Merigan TC (2001) Functional correlates of insertion mutations in the protease gene of human immunodeficiency virus type 1 isolates from patients. J Virol 75 (22):11227–11233

King NM, Prabu-Jeyabalan M, Nalivaika EA, Wigerinck P, de Béthune MP, Schiffer CA (2004) Structural and thermodynamic basis for the binding of TMC114, a next-generation human immunodeficiency virus type 1 protease inhibitor. J Virol 78(21):12012–12021

Kinomoto M, Appiah-Opong R, Brandful JA et al (2005) HIV-1 proteases from drug-naive West African patients are differentially less susceptible to protease inhibitors. Clin Infect Dis 41 (2):243–251

Kitchen VS, Skinner C, Ariyoshi K et al (1995) Safety and activity of saquinavir in HIV infection. Lancet 345(8955):952–955

Knops E, Brakier-Gingras L, Schülter E, Pfister H, Kaiser R, Verheyen J (2012) Mutational patterns in the frameshift-regulating site of HIV-1 selected by protease inhibitors. Med Microbiol Immunol 201(2):213–218

Koh Y, Nakata H, Maeda K et al (2003) Novel bis-tetrahydrofuranylurethane-containing nonpeptidic protease inhibitor (PI) UIC-94017 (TMC114) with potent activity against multi-PI-resistant human immunodeficiency virus in vitro. Antimicrob Agents Chemother 47 (10):3123–3129

Koh Y, Matsumi S, Das D et al (2007) Potent inhibition of HIV-1 replication by novel non-peptidyl small molecule inhibitors of protease dimerization. J Biol Chem 282(39):28709–28720

Kolli M, Lastere S, Schiffer CA (2006) Co-evolution of nelfinavir-resistant HIV-1 protease and the p1-p6 substrate. Virology 347(2):405–409

Kolli M, Stawiski E, Chappey C, Schiffer CA (2009) Human immunodeficiency virus type 1 protease-correlated cleavage site mutations enhance inhibitor resistance. J Virol 83 (21):11027–11042

Kouyos RD, Althaus CL, Bonhoeffer S (2006) Stochastic or deterministic: what is the effective population size of HIV-1? Trends Microbiol 14(12):507–511

Kozal MJ, Lupo S, DeJesus E et al (2012) A nucleoside- and ritonavir-sparing regimen containing atazanavir plus raltegravir in antiretroviral treatment-naïve HIV-infected patients: SPARTAN study results. HIV Clin Trials 13(3):119–130

Kozísek M, Sasková KG, Rezácová P et al (2008) Ninety-nine is not enough: molecular characterization of inhibitor-resistant human immunodeficiency virus type 1 protease mutants with insertions in the flap region. J Virol 82(12):5869–5878

Kozísek M, Henke S, Sasková KG et al (2012) Mutations in HIV-1 gag and pol compensate for the loss of viral fitness caused by a highly mutated protease. Antimicrob Agents Chemother 56 (8):4320–4330

Kräusslich HG, Ingraham RH, Skoog MT, Wimmer E, Pallai PV, Carter CA (1989) Activity of purified biosynthetic proteinase of human immunodeficiency virus on natural substrates and synthetic peptides. Proc Natl Acad Sci U S A 86(3):807–811

Kurowski M, Sternfeld T, Sawyer A, Hill A, Möcklinghoff C (2003) Pharmacokinetic and tolerability profile of twice-daily saquinavir hard gelatin capsules and saquinavir soft gelatin capsules boosted with ritonavir in healthy volunteers. HIV Med 4(2):94–100

Lambert-Niclot S, Flandre P, Valantin MA et al (2012) Resistant minority species are rarely observed in patients on darunavir/ritonavir monotherapy. J Antimicrob Chemother 67(6):1470–1474

Larrouy L, Chazallon C, Landman R et al (2010) Gag mutations can impact virological response to dual-boosted protease inhibitor combinations in antiretroviral-naïve HIV-infected patients. Antimicrob Agents Chemother 54(7):2910–2919

Larrouy L, Lambert-Niclot S, Charpentier C et al (2011a) Positive impact of HIV-1 gag cleavage site mutations on the virological response to darunavir boosted with ritonavir. Antimicrob Agents Chemother 55(4):1754–1757

Larrouy L, Charpentier C, Landman R et al (2011b) Dynamics of gag-pol minority viral populations in naive HIV-1-infected patients failing protease inhibitor regimen. AIDS 25(17): 2143–2148

Lee SK, Potempa M, Swanstrom R (2012a) The choreography of HIV-1 proteolytic processing and virion assembly. J Biol Chem 287(49):40867–40874

Lee SK, Potempa M, Kolli M, Özen A, Schiffer CA, Swanstrom R (2012b) Context surrounding processing sites is crucial in determining cleavage rate of a subset of processing sites in HIV-1 Gag and Gag-Pro-Pol polyprotein precursors by viral protease. J Biol Chem 287 (16):13279–13290

Lillemark MR, Gerstoft J, Obel N et al (2011) Characterization of HIV-1 from patients with virological failure to a boosted protease inhibitor regimen. J Med Virol 83(3):377–383

Lisovsky I, Schader SM, Martinez-Cajas JL, Oliveira M, Moisi D, Wainberg MA (2010) HIV-1 protease codon 36 polymorphisms and differential development of resistance to nelfinavir, lopinavir, and atazanavir in different HIV-1 subtypes. Antimicrob Agents Chemother 54 (7):2878–2885

Louis JM, Aniana A, Weber IT, Sayer JM (2011) Inhibition of autoprocessing of natural variants and multidrug resistant mutant precursors of HIV-1 protease by clinical inhibitors. Proc Natl Acad Sci U S A 108(22):9072–9077

Ludwig C, Leiherer A, Wagner R (2008) Importance of protease cleavage sites within and flanking human immunodeficiency virus type 1 transframe protein p6* for spatiotemporal regulation of protease activation. J Virol 82(9):4573–4584

Madruga JV, Berger D, McMurchie M et al (2007) Efficacy and safety of darunavir-ritonavir compared with that of lopinavir-ritonavir at 48 weeks in treatment-experienced, HIV-infected patients in TITAN: a randomised controlled phase III trial. Lancet 370(9581):49–58

Maguire M, Shortino D, Klein A et al (2002) Emergence of resistance to protease inhibitor amprenavir in human immunodeficiency virus type 1-infected patients: selection of four alternative viral protease genotypes and influence of viral susceptibility to coadministered reverse transcriptase nucleoside inhibitors. Antimicrob Agents Chemother 46(3):731–738

Mahalingam B, Louis JM, Reed CC et al (1999) Structural and kinetic analysis of drug resistant mutants of HIV-1 protease. Eur J Biochem 263(1):238–245

Mammano F, Petit C, Clavel F (1998) Resistance-associated loss of viral fitness in human immunodeficiency virus type 1: phenotypic analysis of protease and gag coevolution in protease inhibitor-treated patients. J Virol 72(9):7632–7637

Mammano F, Trouplin V, Zennou V, Clavel F (2000) Retracing the evolutionary pathways of human immunodeficiency virus type 1 resistance to protease inhibitors: virus fitness in the absence and in the presence of drug. J Virol 74(18):8524–8531

Manosuthi W, Sungkanuparph S, Ruxrungtham K et al (2008) Plasma levels, safety, and 60-week efficacy of a once-daily double-boosted protease inhibitor regimen of atazanavir, saquinavir, and ritonavir. J Acquir Immune Defic Syndr 47(1):127–129

Mansky LM, Temin HM (1995) Lower in vivo mutation rate of human immunodeficiency virus type 1 than that predicted from the fidelity of purified reverse transcriptase. J Virol 69 (8):5087–5094

Markowitz M, Saag M, Powderly WG et al (1995) A preliminary study of ritonavir, an inhibitor of HIV-1 protease, to treat HIV-1 infection. N Engl J Med 333(23):1534–1539

Martinez-Cajas JL, Pai NP, Klein MB, Wainberg MA (2009) Differences in resistance mutations among HIV-1 non-subtype B infections: a systematic review of evidence (1996–2008). J Int AIDS Soc 12:11

Martinez-Cajas JL, Wainberg MA, Oliveira M et al (2012) The role of polymorphisms at position 89 in the HIV-1 protease gene in the development of drug resistance to HIV-1 protease inhibitors. J Antimicrob Chemother 67(4):988–994
Martinez-Picado J, Savara AV, Sutton L, D'Aquila RT (1999) Replicative fitness of protease inhibitor-resistant mutants of human immunodeficiency virus type 1. J Virol 73(5):3744–3752
Martins AN, Arruda MB, Pires AF, Tanuri A, Brindeiro RM (2011) Accumulation of P(T/S)AP late domain duplications in HIV type 1 subtypes B, C, and F derived from individuals failing ARV therapy and ARV drug-naive patients. AIDS Res Hum Retroviruses 27(6):687–692
Marzolini C, Buclin T, Decosterd LA, Biollaz J, Telenti A (2001) Nelfinavir plasma levels under twice-daily and three-times-daily regimens: high interpatient and low intrapatient variability. Ther Drug Monit 23(4):394–398
Mathez D, Bagnarelli P, Gorin I et al (1997) Reductions in viral load and increases in T lymphocyte numbers in treatment-naive patients with advanced HIV-1 infection treated with ritonavir, zidovudine and zalcitabine triple therapy. Antivir Ther 2(3):175–183
McKinnon JE, Delgado R, Pulido F, Shao W, Arribas JR, Mellors JW (2011) Single genome sequencing of HIV-1 gag and protease resistance mutations at virologic failure during the OK04 trial of simplified versus standard maintenance therapy. Antivir Ther 16(5):725–732
Mills AM, Nelson M, Jayaweera D et al (2009) Once-daily darunavir/ritonavir vs. lopinavir/ritonavir in treatment-naive, HIV-1-infected patients: 96-week analysis. AIDS 23 (13):1679–1688
Mo H, King MS, King K, Molla A, Brun S, Kempf DJ (2005) Selection of resistance in protease inhibitor-experienced, human immunodeficiency virus type 1-infected subjects failing lopinavir- and ritonavir-based therapy: mutation patterns and baseline correlates. J Virol 79 (6):3329–3338
Molina JM, Andrade-Villanueva J, Echevarria J et al (2008) Once-daily atazanavir/ritonavir versus twice-daily lopinavir/ritonavir, each in combination with tenofovir and emtricitabine, for management of antiretroviral-naive HIV-1-infected patients: 48 week efficacy and safety results of the CASTLE study. Lancet 372(9639):646–655
Molla A, Korneyeva M, Gao Q et al (1996) Ordered accumulation of mutations in HIV protease confers resistance to ritonavir. Nat Med 2(7):760–766
Murakami T, Ablan S, Freed EO, Tanaka Y (2004) Regulation of human immunodeficiency virus type 1 Env-mediated membrane fusion by viral protease activity. J Virol 78(2):1026–1031
Murphy RL, Sanne I, Cahn P et al (2003) Dose-ranging, randomized, clinical trial of atazanavir with lamivudine and stavudine in antiretroviral-naive subjects: 48-week results. AIDS 17 (18):2603–2614
Naeger LK, Struble KA (2007) Food and Drug Administration analysis of tipranavir clinical resistance in HIV-1-infected treatment-experienced patients. AIDS 21(2):179–185
Nalam MN, Ali A, Altman MD et al (2010) Evaluating the substrate-envelope hypothesis: structural analysis of novel HIV-1 protease inhibitors designed to be robust against drug resistance. J Virol 84(10):5368–5378
Navia MA, Fitzgerald PM, McKeever BM et al (1989) Three-dimensional structure of aspartyl protease from human immunodeficiency virus HIV-1. Nature 337(6208):615–620
Nijhuis M, Boucher CAB, Schipper P, Leitner T, Schuurman R, Albert J (1998) Stochastic processes strongly influence HIV-1 evolution during suboptimal protease-inhibitor therapy. Proc Natl Acad Sci U S A 95(24):14441–14446
Nijhuis M, Schuurman R, de Jong D et al (1999) Increased fitness of drug resistant HIV-1 protease as a result of acquisition of compensatory mutations during suboptimal therapy. AIDS 13 (17):2349–2359
Nijhuis M, van Maarseveen NM, Lastere S et al (2007) A novel substrate-based HIV-1 protease inhibitor drug resistance mechanism. PLoS Med 4(1):152–163
Nijhuis M, Wensing AMJ, Bierman WFW et al (2009) Failure of treatment with first-line Lopinavir boosted with ritonavir can be explained by novel resistance pathways with protease mutation 76V. J Infect Dis 200(5):698–709

Noble S, Faulds D (1996) Saquinavir. A review of its pharmacology and clinical potential in the management of HIV infection. Drugs 52(1):93–112
Notermans DW, Jurriaans S, de Wolf F et al (1998) Decrease of HIV-1 RNA levels in lymphoid tissue and peripheral blood during treatment with ritonavir, lamivudine and zidovudine. Ritonavir/3TC/ZDV Study Group. AIDS 12(2):167–173
Oldfield V, Plosker GL (2006) Lopinavir/ritonavir: a review of its use in the management of HIV infection. Drugs 66(9):1275–1299
Palella FJ, Delaney KM, Moorman AC et al (1998) Declining morbidity and mortality among patients with advanced human immunodeficiency virus infection. HIV Outpatient Study Investigators. N Engl J Med 338(13):853–860
Parry CM, Kolli M, Myers RE, Cane PA, Schiffer C, Pillay D (2011) Three residues in HIV-1 matrix contribute to protease inhibitor susceptibility and replication capacity. Antimicrob Agents Chemother 55(3):1106–1113
Partaledis JA, Yamaguchi K, Tisdale M et al (1995) In vitro selection and characterization of human immunodeficiency virus type 1 (HIV-1) isolates with reduced sensitivity to hydroxyethylamino sulfonamide inhibitors of HIV-1 aspartyl protease. J Virol 69(9):5228–5235
Patick AK, Mo H, Markowitz M et al (1996) Antiviral and resistance studies of AG1343, an orally bioavailable inhibitor of human immunodeficiency virus protease. Antimicrob Agents Chemother 40(2):292–297
Paulsen D, Elston R, Snowden W, Tisdale M, Ross L (2003) Differentiation of genotypic resistance profiles for amprenavir and lopinavir, a valuable aid for choice of therapy in protease inhibitor-experienced HIV-1-infected subjects. J Antimicrob Chemother 52(3):319–323
Paulus C, Hellebrand S, Tessmer U, Wolf H, Kräusslich HG, Wagner R (1999) Competitive inhibition of human immunodeficiency virus type-1 protease by the Gag-Pol transframe protein. J Biol Chem 274(31):21539–21543
Paulus C, Ludwig C, Wagner R (2004) Contribution of the Gag-Pol transframe domain p6* and its coding sequence to morphogenesis and replication of human immunodeficiency virus type 1. Virology 330(1):271–283
Pellegrin I, Breilh D, Montestruc F et al (2002) Virologic response to nelfinavir-based regimens: pharmacokinetics and drug resistance mutations (VIRAPHAR study). AIDS 16 (10):1331–1340
Pellegrin I, Breilh D, Ragnaud JM et al (2006) Virological responses to atazanavir-ritonavir-based regimens: resistance-substitutions score and pharmacokinetic parameters (Reyaphar study). Antivir Ther 11(4):421–429
Peters S, Muñoz M, Yerly S et al (2001) Resistance to nucleoside analog reverse transcriptase inhibitors mediated by human immunodeficiency virus type 1 p6 protein. J Virol 75 (20):9644–9653
Petersen ML, Wang Y, van der Laan MJ, Rhee SY, Shafer RW, Fessel WJ (2007) Virologic efficacy of boosted double versus boosted single protease inhibitor therapy. AIDS 21(12):1547–1554
Pettit SC, Moody MD, Wehbie RS et al (1994) The p2 domain of human immunodeficiency virus type 1 Gag regulates sequential proteolytic processing and is required to produce fully infectious virions. J Virol 68(12):8017–8027
Pettit SC, Everitt LE, Choudhury S, Dunn BM, Kaplan AH (2004) Initial cleavage of the human immunodeficiency virus type 1 GagPol precursor by its activated protease occurs by an intramolecular mechanism. J Virol 78(16):8477–8485
Pettit SC, Lindquist JN, Kaplan AH, Swanstrom R (2005) Processing sites in the human immunodeficiency virus type 1 (HIV-1) Gag-Pro-Pol precursor are cleaved by the viral protease at different rates. Retrovirology 2:66
Plosker GL, Noble S (1999) Indinavir: a review of its use in the management of HIV infection. Drugs 58(6):1165–1203
Prabu-Jeyabalan M, Nalivaika E, Schiffer CA (2002) Substrate shape determines specificity of recognition for HIV-1 protease: analysis of crystal structures of six substrate complexes. Structure 10(3):369–381

Prabu-Jeyabalan M, Nalivaika EA, Romano K, Schiffer CA (2006) Mechanism of substrate recognition by drug-resistant human immunodeficiency virus type 1 protease variants revealed by a novel structural intermediate. J Virol 80(7):3607–3616

Prado JG, Wrin T, Beauchaine J et al (2002) Amprenavir-resistant HIV-1 exhibits lopinavir cross-resistance and reduced replication capacity. AIDS 16(7):1009–1017

Quercia R, Garnier E, Ferré V et al (2005) Salvage therapy with ritonavir-boosted amprenavir/fosamprenavir: virological and immunological response in two years follow-up. HIV Clin Trials 6(2):73–80

Rabi SA, Laird GM, Durand CM et al (2013) Multi-step inhibition explains HIV-1 protease inhibitor pharmacodynamics and resistance. J Clin Invest 123(9):3848–3860

Rawizza HE, Chaplin B, Meloni ST et al (2013) Accumulation of protease mutations among patients failing second-line antiretroviral therapy and response to salvage therapy in Nigeria. PLoS One 8(9):e73582

Ribera E, Azuaje C, Lopez RM et al (2006) Atazanavir and lopinavir/ritonavir: pharmacokinetics, safety and efficacy of a promising double-boosted protease inhibitor regimen. AIDS 20 (8):1131–1139

Riddler SA, Haubrich R, DiRienzo AG et al (2008) Class-sparing regimens for initial treatment of HIV-1 infection. N Engl J Med 358(20):2095–2106

Robinson BS, Riccardi KA, Gong YF et al (2000) BMS-232632, a highly potent human immunodeficiency virus protease inhibitor that can be used in combination with other available antiretroviral agents. Antimicrob Agents Chemother 44(8):2093–2099

Rodriguez-French A, Boghossian J, Gray GE et al (2004) The NEAT study: a 48-week open-label study to compare the antiviral efficacy and safety of GW433908 versus nelfinavir in antiretroviral therapy-naive HIV-1-infected patients. J Acquir Immune Defic Syndr 35(1):22–32

Sadler BM, Piliero PJ, Preston SL, Lloyd PP, Lou Y, Stein DS (2001) Pharmacokinetics and safety of amprenavir and ritonavir following multiple-dose, co-administration to healthy volunteers. AIDS 15(8):1009–1018

Schapiro JM, Scherer J, Boucher CA et al (2010) Improving the prediction of virological response to tipranavir: the development and validation of a tipranavir-weighted mutation score. Antivir Ther 15(7):1011–1019

Schmit JC, Ruiz L, Clotet B et al (1996) Resistance-related mutations in the HIV-1 protease gene of patients treated for 1 year with the protease inhibitor ritonavir (ABT-538). AIDS 10(9):995–999

Schrader S, Chuck SK, Rahn LW, Parekh P, Emrich KG (2008) Significant improvements in self-reported gastrointestinal tolerability, quality of life, patient satisfaction, and adherence with lopinavir/ritonavir tablet formulation compared with soft gel capsules. AIDS Res Ther 5:21

Sham HL, Kempf DJ, Molla A et al (1998) ABT-378, a highly potent inhibitor of the human immunodeficiency virus protease. Antimicrob Agents Chemother 42(12):3218–3224

Shibata J, Sugiura W, Ode H et al (2011) Within-host co-evolution of Gag P453L and protease D30N/N88D demonstrates virological advantage in a highly protease inhibitor-exposed HIV-1 case. Antiviral Res 90(1):33–41

Smith GH, Boulassel MR, Klien M et al (2005) Virologic and immunologic response to a boosted double-protease inhibitor-based therapy in highly pretreated HIV-1-infected patients. HIV Clin Trials 6(2):63–72

Soulié C, Assoumou L, Ghosn J et al (2009) Nucleoside reverse transcriptase inhibitor-sparing regimen (nonnucleoside reverse transcriptase inhibitor + protease inhibitor) was more likely associated with resistance comparing to nonnucleoside reverse transcriptase inhibitor or protease inhibitor + nucleoside reverse transcriptase inhibitor in the randomized ANRS 121 trial. AIDS 23(12):1605–1608

Squires K, Lazzarin A, Gatell JM et al (2004) Comparison of once-daily atazanavir with efavirenz, each in combination with fixed-dose zidovudine and lamivudine, as initial therapy for patients infected with HIV. J Acquir Immune Defic Syndr 36(5):1011–1019

Stebbing J, Scourfield A, Koh G et al (2009) A multicentre cohort experience with double-boosted protease inhibitors. J Antimicrob Chemother 64(2):434–435

Stein DS, Fish DG, Bilello JA, Preston SL, Martineau GL, Drusano GL (1996) A 24-week open-label phase I/II evaluation of the HIV protease inhibitor MK-639 (indinavir). AIDS 10 (5):485–492

Stray KM, Callebaut C, Glass B et al (2013) Mutations in multiple domains of Gag drive the emergence of in vitro resistance to the phosphonate-containing HIV-1 protease inhibitor GS-8374. J Virol 87(1):454–463

Taiwo B, Zheng L, Gallien S et al (2011) Efficacy of a nucleoside-sparing regimen of darunavir/ritonavir plus raltegravir in treatment-naive HIV-1-infected patients (ACTG A5262). AIDS 25 (17):2113–2122

Tang C, Louis JM, Aniana A, Suh JY, Clore GM (2008) Visualizing transient events in amino-terminal autoprocessing of HIV-1 protease. Nature 455(7213):693–696

Tessmer U, Kräusslich HG (1998) Cleavage of human immunodeficiency virus type 1 proteinase from the N-terminally adjacent p6* protein is essential for efficient Gag polyprotein processing and viral infectivity. J Virol 72(4):3459–3463

Turner SR, Strohbach JW, Tommasi RA et al (1998) Tipranavir (PNU-140690): a potent, orally bioavailable nonpeptidic HIV protease inhibitor of the 5,6-dihydro-4-hydroxy-2-pyrone sulfonamide class. J Med Chem 41(18):3467–3476

Ulbricht KU, Behrens GM, Stoll M et al (2011) A multicenter, open labeled, randomized, phase III study comparing lopinavir/ritonavir plus atazanavir to lopinavir/ritonavir plus zidovudine and lamivudine in naive HIV-1-infected patients: 48-week analysis of the LORAN trial. Open AIDS J 5:44–50

Vacca JP, Dorsey BD, Schleif WA et al (1994) L-735,524: an orally bioavailable human immunodeficiency virus type 1 protease inhibitor. Proc Natl Acad Sci U S A 91(9):4096–4100

van de Vijver DA, Wensing AM, Angarano G et al (2006) The calculated genetic barrier for antiretroviral drug resistance substitutions is largely similar for different HIV-1 subtypes. J Acquir Immune Defic Syndr 41(3):352–360

van Heeswijk RP, Veldkamp A, Mulder JW et al (2001) Combination of protease inhibitors for the treatment of HIV-1-infected patients: a review of pharmacokinetics and clinical experience. Antivir Ther 6(4):201–229

van Maarseveen NM, Andersson D, Lepsik M et al (2012) Modulation of HIV-1 Gag NC/p1 cleavage efficiency affects protease inhibitor resistance and viral replicative capacity. Retrovirology 9

Verheyen J, Knops E, Kupfer B et al (2009) Prevalence of C-terminal gag cleavage site mutations in HIV from therapy-naïve patients. J Infect 58(1):61–67

Verheyen J, Verhofstede C, Knops E et al (2010) High prevalence of bevirimat resistance mutations in protease inhibitor-resistant HIV isolates. AIDS 24(5):669–673

Voigt E, Wickesberg A, Wasmuth JC et al (2002) First-line ritonavir/indinavir 100/800 mg twice daily plus nucleoside reverse transcriptase inhibitors in a German multicentre study: 48-week results. HIV Med 3(4):277–282

von Hentig N, Babacan E, Staszewski S, Stürmer M, Doerr HW, Lötsch J (2007) Predictive factors for response to a boosted dual HIV-protease inhibitor therapy with saquinavir and lopinavir in extensively pre-treated patients. Antivir Ther 12(8):1237–1246

Walmsley S, Bernstein B, King M et al (2002) Lopinavir-ritonavir versus nelfinavir for the initial treatment of HIV infection. N Engl J Med 346(26):2039–2046

Walmsley S, Avihingsanon A, Slim J et al (2009) Gemini: a noninferiority study of saquinavir/ritonavir versus lopinavir/ritonavir as initial HIV-1 therapy in adults. J Acquir Immune Defic Syndr 50(4):367–374

Whitehurst N, Chappey C, Petropoulos C, Parkin N, Gamarnik A (2003) Polymorphisms in p1-p6/p6* of HIV type 1 can delay protease autoprocessing and increase drug susceptibility. AIDS Res Hum Retroviruses 19(9):779–784

Wiegers K, Rutter G, Kottler H, Tessmer U, Hohenberg H, Kräusslich HG (1998) Sequential steps in human immunodeficiency virus particle maturation revealed by alterations of individual Gag polyprotein cleavage sites. J Virol 72(4):2846–2854

Winters MA, Merigan TC (2005) Insertions in the human immunodeficiency virus type 1 protease and reverse transcriptase genes: clinical impact and molecular mechanisms. Antimicrob Agents Chemother 49(7):2575–2582

Winters MA, Kagan RM, Heseltine PN, Merigan TC (2005) New two-amino acid insertion near codon 70 of the HIV type 1 protease gene. AIDS Res Hum Retroviruses 21(4):311–313

Wlodawer A, Miller M, Jaskólski M et al (1989) Conserved folding in retroviral proteases: crystal structure of a synthetic HIV-1 protease. Science 245(4918):616–621

Wyma DJ, Jiang J, Shi J et al (2004) Coupling of human immunodeficiency virus type 1 fusion to virion maturation: a novel role of the gp41 cytoplasmic tail. J Virol 78(7):3429–3435

Zhang YM, Imamichi H, Imamichi T et al (1997) Drug resistance during indinavir therapy is caused by mutations in the protease gene and in its Gag substrate cleavage sites. J Virol 71 (9):6662–6670

Index

M. Gotte et al. (eds.), *Handbook of Antimicrobial Resistance*,
DOI 10.1007/978-1-4939-0694-9